THE
MONT REID
SURGICAL HANDBOOK

Second Edition

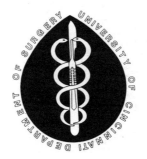

THE
MONT REID
SURGICAL HANDBOOK

Second Edition

Editor-in-Chief
Darryl T. Hiyama, M.D.

Editors

Thomas C. Appleby, M.D.   Joel P. Garmon, M.D.
George W. Daneker, M.D.   John P. Sutyak, M.D.
Mark D. Epstein, M.D.   Steven D. Tennenberg, M.D.

with a Foreword by Josef E. Fischer, M.D.

From the Department of Surgery, University of Cincinnati,
College of Medicine, Cincinnati, Ohio

Illustrations by Jean A. Loos, A.M.I.
Photography by Roger C. West

Mosby
Year Book

St. Louis   Baltimore   Boston   Chicago   London   Philadelphia   Sydney   Toronto

Mosby Year Book
Dedicated to Publishing Excellence

Sponsoring Editor: Nancy E. Chorpenning
Assistant Managing Editor, Text and Reference: Jan Gardner
Production Coordinator: Nancy C. Baker
Proofroom Supervisor: Barbara M. Kelly

2   3   4   5   6   7   8   9   0   Y   R   94   93   92   91

NOTICE

Every effort has been made to ensure that the drug dosage schedules herein are accurate and in accord with the standards accepted at the time of publication. However, as new research and experience broaden our knowledge, changes in treatment and drug therapy occur. Therefore the reader is advised to check the product information sheet included in the package of each drug he or she plans to administer to be certain that changes have not been made in the recommended dose or in the contraindications. This is of particular importance in regard to new or infrequently used drugs.

Library of Congress Cataloging-in-Publication Data

Hiyama, Darryl.
    The Mont Reid surgical handbook.—2nd ed. / Darryl Hiyama:
residents of the University of Cincinnati, Department of Surgery.
        p.   cm.
    Rev. ed of: The Mont Reid handbook / Michael S. Nussbaum, editor
-in-chief.   c1987.
    Includes bibliographical references.
    Includes index.
    ISBN 0-8151-4310-9
    1. Therapeutics, Surgical—Handbooks, manuals, etc.   I. Reid,
Mont.   II. University of Cincinnati, Dept. of Surgery.   III. Mont
Reid handbook.   IV. Title.   V. Title: Surgical handbook.
    [DNLM: 1. Surgery, Operative—handbooks.   WO 39 H676m]
RD49.H59   1990
617.9—dc20   90-12761
DNLM/DLC   CIP
for Library of Congress

CONTRIBUTORS

Steven Albertson, M.D.
Daniel W. Benson, M.D.
Robert J. Brodish, M.D.
Phillip Buffington, M.D.
  (Urology)
Curtis A. Crimmins, M.D.
Christopher B. Davies, M.D.
Steven M. Clark, M.D.
Barry R. Cofer, M.D.
Barry L. Dick, M.D.
Edward J. Diekhoff, M.D.
Joshua D. I. Ellenhorn, M.D.
Elliott J. Fegelman, M.D.
Robert H. Fleming, M.D.
Janice A. Frederick, M.D.
Paul B. Friedman, M.D.
J. Michael Guenther, M.D.
Robert P. Hummel III, M.D.
John Kitzmiller, M.D.
  (Plastic Surgery)
Theodore C. Koutlas, M.D.

Lawrence Kurtzman, M.D.
  (Plastic Surgery)
Boris W. Kuvshinoff II, M.D.
John C. Lucke, M.D.
Pamela A. Martin, M.D.
Ronna G. Miller, M.D.
Richard M. Nedelman, M.D.
Gregory A. Nelcamp, M.D.
Joseph J. Pavlik, M.D.
Troy Payner, M.D.
  (Neurosurgery)
Peter N. Purcell, M.D.
Gary J. Rosenthal, M.D.
Reed Shank, M.D. (Urology)
Anthony Stallion, M.D.
Michael Stanley, M.D.
  (Neurosurgery)
Daniel von Allmen, M.D.
Stuart Weil, M.D.
  (Neurosurgery)
Cathy White-Owen, M.D.

DEDICATION

On occasion we are fortunate enough to meet an individual who personifies our vision of the ideal surgeon. It is to the memory of such an individual, Dr. Ronald Fegelman, that we dedicate this edition of *The Mont Reid Surgical Handbook*. His death in 1988 was a sudden and devastating loss for his family, the surgical residency, and the community.

A graduate of the surgical residency of the University of Cincinnati, Dr. Fegelman devoted his time and energies as a clinical instructor and was a "favorite" among the residents. To many of us, Dr. Fegelman embodied those qualities we strive to develop throughout our training and in our daily lives. He was a knowledgeable and decisive physician, a superb technician, an excellent teacher, and a generous humanitarian.

Dr. Fegelman is sorely missed, and will always be remembered as a surgeon's surgeon.

FOREWORD

Dr. Mont Reid was the second Christian R. Holmes Professor of Surgery at the University of Cincinnati College of Medicine. Trained at Johns Hopkins, he came to Cincinnati in 1922 as the associate of Dr. George J. Heuer, the initial Christian R. Holmes Professor. He became responsible for the surgical residency program, and assumed the Chair in 1931. His death in 1943 was a great tragedy for both the city and the University of Cincinnati College of Medicine. Dr. Reid was beloved by the residents and townspeople. A learned, patient man, he was serious about surgery, surgical education, and surgical research. His papers on wound healing are still classic and can, to this day, be read with profit.

It was under Mont Reid that the surgical residency first matured. In his memory the new surgical suite built in 1948 was named the Mont Reid Pavilion. Part of the surgical suite is still operational in that building, as are the residents' living quarters. *The Mont Reid Surgical Handbook* is written by the surgical residents at the University of Cincinnati hospitals for residents and medical students, and is thus appropriately named. It represents a compilation of the approach taken in our residency program, of which we are justifiably proud. The residency program as well as the Department reflect a basic science physiological approach to the science of surgery. Metabolism, infection, nutrition, and physiological responses to the above as well as the physiological basis for surgical and presurgical interventions form the basis of our residency program, and presumably will form the basis of surgical practice into the 21st century. We hope that you will read it with profit and that you will use it as a basis for further study in the science of surgery.

Josef E. Fischer, M.D.
Christian R. Holmes Professor of Surgery
and Chairman of the Department of Surgery
University of Cincinnati Medical Center
Cincinnati, Ohio

PREFACE TO THE SECOND EDITION

The first edition of *The Mont Reid Handbook* is a remarkable and unique accomplishment. While many "handbooks" are available, few are written by surgery residents for residents and medical students. The notoriety and popularity of the first edition is evidence that a book of this type is in demand.

The success of the first edition is a tribute to the efforts of the residents involved in its production. Many of these same individuals, members of the surgical housestaff of the University of Cincinnati, are involved in the production of the second edition of *The Mont Reid Surgical Handbook*. As before, the chief residents served as the editorial board. The residents in general surgery, as well as representative members from the divisions of urology, plastic surgery, and neurosurgery are the authors.

In creating the second edition, much of the information has been updated to reflect the rapid changes occurring in surgery today. In addition, several chapters have been added covering gastrointestinal endoscopy, surgical infections, urologic problems, and preoperative care. The information included in this edition reflects the education and experience of the authors and the practices adopted at the University of Cincinnati. We have updated the information, but it is by no means exhaustive. It was our intent to create a portable guide and resource for residents and medical students alike. We hope it serves this purpose.

Darryl T. Hiyama, M.D.
Editor-in-Chief
Cincinnati, 1990

PREFACE TO THE FIRST EDITION

We can only instil principles, put the student in the right path, give him methods, teach him how to study, and early to discern between essentials and non-essentials. **Sir William Osler**

The surgical residency training program at the University of Cincinnati Medical Center dates back to 1922 when it was organized by Drs. George J. Heuer and Mont R. Reid, both students of Dr. William Halsted and graduates of the Johns Hopkins surgical training program. The training program was thus established in a strong Hopkins mode. When Dr. Heuer left to assume the chair at Cornell University, Mont Reid succeeded him as chairman. During Reid's tenure (1931–1943) the training program at what was then the Cincinnati General Hospital was brought to maturity. Since then the training program has continued to grow and has maintained the tradition of excellence in academic and clinical surgery which was so strongly advocated by Dr. Reid and his successors.

The principal goal of the surgical residency training program at the University of Cincinnati today remains the development of exemplary academic and clinical surgeons. There also is a strong tradition of teaching by the senior residents of their junior colleagues as well as the medical students at the College of Medicine. Thus the surgical house staff became very enthused when Year Book Medical Publishers asked us to consider writing a surgical handbook which would be analogous to the very successful pediatrics handbook, *The Harriet Lane Handbook* (now in its 11th edition). We readily accepted the challenge of writing a pocket "pearl book" which would provide pertinent, practical information to students and residents in surgery. The six chief residents for 1985–1986 served as editors of this handbook and the contributors included the majority of the surgical house staff in consultation with other specialists who are involved in the direct care of surgical patients and the education of residents and medical students.

The information collected in this handbook is by no means exhaustive.

We have attempted simply to provide a guide for the more efficient management of prevalent surgical problems, especially by those with limited experience. Therefore, this is not a substitute for a comprehensive textbook of surgery, but is rather a supplement which concentrates on those things that are important to medical students and junior residents on the wards, namely the initial management of common surgical conditions. Much of the information is influenced by the philosophies advocated by the residents and faculty at the University of Cincinnati and thus reflects a certain bias. In areas of controversy, however, we have also provided other views and useful references. The index has been liberally cross-referenced in order to provide a rapid and efficient means of locating information.

This handbook would not have been possible without the enthusiastic support and advice of our chairman, Dr. Josef E. Fischer, whose commitment to excellence in surgical training serves as an inspiration to all of his residents. We also would like to acknowledge the invaluable advice provided by several of the faculty members of the Department of Surgery: Dr. Robert H. Bower, Dr. James M. Hurst, and Dr. Richard F. Kempczinski. The authors gratefully acknowledge the helpful input of Dr. Donald G. McQuarrie, Professor of Surgery at the University of Minnesota, for his review of each chapter in the handbook. Also we would like to thank Mr. Daniel J. Doody, Vice President, Editorial, Year Book Medical Publishers, for his patience and guidance in the conception and writing of this first edition of *The Mont Reid Handbook*.

None of this would have been possible were it not for the wordprocessing expertise and herculean efforts of Mr. Steven E. Wiesner. His assistance in the typing and editing of the manuscript was invaluable.

Finally, this handbook is the result of the cumulative efforts of the surgical house staff at the University of Cincinnati as well as those residents who preceded us and taught us many of the principles that are advocated in this book. We wish to thank all of those who worked so diligently on this manuscript in order to make the first edition of *The Mont Reid Handbook* a reality.

Michael S. Nussbaum, M.D.
Editor-in-Chief
Cincinnati, 1987

ACKNOWLEDGMENTS

An undertaking of this magnitude is not accomplished without the efforts of several individuals, who we, the editors, would like to acknowledge.

Only within an environment wholly committed to surgical education can a project such as this have been completed. Our chairman, Dr. Josef Fischer, has maintained an unwavering commitment to the surgical residency. He has directed his relentless energy toward supporting the endeavors of the housestaff in whatever manner possible. We are indebted to him for his guidance, encouragement, and support.

Nancy Chorpenning, the sponsoring editor for this edition, is the force behind this book. She has gently steered, encouraged, and prodded a group of fledgling editors into achieving their goal. We thank her for her patience, enthusiasm, and advice.

Steve Wiesner, our editorial assistant, alone completed the herculean task of word processing the entire manuscript. Production of this edition would have been physically impossible without his determination, energy, and patience. We are extremely grateful to him for his invaluable effort.

Jean Loos, provided the diagrams and illustrations used throughout the book. We thank her for providing her talent, ideas, and efforts to this project.

We would especially like to thank the members of the faculty of the Department of Surgery who enthusiastically reviewed the manuscript. We appreciate the time they spent in applying their experience and knowledge and for providing much needed advice and assistance.

Finally, we thank our families for the love and unwavering support they show for all of our endeavors.

CONTENTS

PART III: PROCEDURES

PART I

PERIOPERATIVE CARE

DOCUMENTATION

Proper documentation is a critical aspect of the care of patients because of the litigation which increasingly accompanies the practice of medicine. The basis for the proper care of each patient is an early assessment of past history and all possible influences on the current illness, including previous hospitalizations, illnesses and operations. A thorough review of systems need not be overly time-consuming, as the medical student and house officer can train themselves to ask questions about related organ systems during the physical examination. Obviously, careful documentation will facilitate the care of the patient during his/her current and subsequent hospitalizations, and should be done with due thoroughness and thought.

A. History and physical on admission (see "Medical Record" section I).
B. Daily progress note in chart stating current status, problems, plans.
C. Procedure notes.
   1. Written note for bedside procedures.
   2. Written and dictated notes for any procedure performed in O.R.
   3. Include basic **findings** and complications.
D. Preoperative, operative, and postoperative notes (see "Medical Record" section III) are mandatory for procedures done in O.R.
E. Dictate operative notes immediately after procedure for optimal accuracy, as important details fade quickly (see "Medical Record" section IV).
F. Dictated discharge summary (see "Medical Record" section V).
   1. Discharge diagnosis.
   2. Operations.
   3. Complications.
   4. Medications and follow-up.
   5. Summary.
G. Accurate documentation serves several roles:
   1. Communication during hospitalization (consultants, nursing).
   2. Provides information for discharge summary.
   3. Medico-legal concerns (see "Medico-Legal Aspects").
H. In the event of litigation, **nothing can be supported without written documentation** in the chart.
I. Document patient's and family's wishes in progress notes, and especially discussions with family and patient.
J. Consultation notes to include history, physical, relevant lab tests, recommendations and plans (operative and/or follow-up).

MEDICAL RECORD

I. THE SURGICAL HISTORY AND PHYSICAL EXAMINATION
A. Meeting the patient.
1. It is important in this initial contact with the patient to gain his/her confidence and convey the assurance that help is available.
2. **Put the patient at ease**, be gentle and considerate, creating an atmosphere of sympathy, personal interest, and understanding.
3. Be certain that the patient is as comfortable as possible for the interview.
4. Make yourself comfortable; sit down and assume a pose suggesting that you are **interested** and concerned about the patient as a person who needs help, and that you have time to listen.
5. **Listen to your patient.** He/she is trying to tell you the diagnosis. Much can be learned by letting the patient "ramble" a little. Discrepancies and omissions in the history are often due as much to overstructuring and leading questions as to an unreliable patient.
6. **Ensure the patient's privacy.**

B. The history.
1. The diagnosis must be established by inductive reasoning and good "detective work".
2. **Pain** — A careful analysis of the nature of pain is one of the most important features of a surgical history. How did the pain begin? Was the nature of onset rapid or gradual? What is the precise character of the pain? Does anything make it better? Worse? Is it constant or intermittent? Is anything else associated with the pain (eating, urination, bowel movement, exercise, etc.)?
3. Assess the patient's reaction to the pain. For example, a patient who is thrashing about and cannot seem to get comfortable may be suffering from renal or biliary colic. Very severe pain due to infection, inflammation or vascular disease usually forces the patient to restrict all movement as much as possible.
4. **Vomiting** — Personally inspect all vomitus when possible. What did the patient vomit? What did it look like? How much? How often? Was the vomiting projectile? Was it associated with pain? The relationship between onset of abdominal pain and onset of vomiting will suggest level of obstruction.
5. **Change in bowel habits** — Common complaint which is often of no significance. Any distinct change, however, toward intermittent constipation and diarrhea must lead one to suspect colon cancer or, more likely, diverticular disease.

6. **Bleeding.**
   a. The clinical history is the best method of screening patients with potential bleeding tendencies.
   b. Any abnormal bleeding from any orifice must be carefully evaluated and should never be dismissed as due to some immediately obvious cause (e.g., hemorrhoids causing rectal bleeding).
   c. Hematemesis or passage of blood per rectum — Character of blood -- does it clot? Is it bright or dark red blood? Is it changed in any way? Coffee-ground vomitus of slow gastric bleeding or dark, tarry stool of upper GI bleeding.
7. **Trauma** — When a patient is subjected to trauma, the details surrounding the injury must be established as precisely as possible (see "Trauma" chapter, part 1, section V).
8. **Family history** — A number of significant surgical disorders are either inherited or are familial in nature (colonic polyposis, MEN syndrome, certain carcinomas, etc.).
9. **Past medical history** is particularly important in assessing patients for potential anesthetic and perioperative risk and complications.
   a. Allergies — specific drug reactions characterize the response (i.e., rash, edema, stridor, anaphylaxis).
   b. Medications — particularly diuretics, corticosteroids, and cardiac drugs. Indicate dose, route, frequency, and duration of usage.
   c. Alcohol, tobacco, or other substance abuse — how much and how long?
   d. Nutritional deficiencies, particularly acute fluid and electrolyte losses, recent weight loss, anorexia.
   e. Major medical illnesses — chronic diseases and hospitalizations (*always* obtain old records or reports from previous hospitalizations).
   f. Previous operations and serious injuries — date, procedure, hospital (again, always obtain previous records or reports of previous operations).
10. **Review of systems** — to make certain that important details of the history are not overlooked, this system review must be formalized and thorough. Record all pertinent positives and negatives.
C. **Physical examination.**
   1. It is again helpful to put the patient at ease. All patients are sensitive and somewhat embarrassed at being examined. Examining room and table should be comfortable, and drapes should be used if the patient is required to undress.
   2. The physical examination should be performed in an orderly and detailed fashion, performing a complete examination in

exactly the same sequence each time so that no step is omitted.

3. Observe the patient's general physique, habitus, and affect. Carefully inspect the hands (many systemic diseases may involve the hands, e.g., cirrhosis, hyperthyroidism, Raynaud's disease, pulmonary insufficiency, heart disease, nutritional disorders).

4. Inspection, auscultation, palpation, and percussion are the essential steps in evaluating both the normal and abnormal ("*Look, listen, feel*").

   a. Compare both sides of the body.
   b. Palpation and percussion should be performed gently, carefully, and precisely.
   c. Auscultation, particularly of the abdomen and peripheal vessels, is essential in evaluating surgical disorders (a Littman type stethoscope is best).

5. Examination of the body orifices — complete examination of the ears, mouth, eyes, rectum, and pelvis is an essential part of *every* complete examination.

D. **The emergency history and physical examination** — In cases of emergency, the routine of history and physical examination must often be truncated with initial efforts directed toward resuscitating the patient. The history may be limited to a single sentence or obtained from family or friends, rescue or ambulance personnel. **Primary considerations** (*ABC's*) — Is the *airway* open, is the patient *breathing*, is *circulation* being maintained, is there massive hemorrhage? Life-saving maneuvers take precedence over performing even a limited physical examination.

E. **Laboratory/radiologic studies.**

1. Objectives of laboratory examination are to: (a) confirm suspected diagnosis; (b) screen for asymptomatic disease that may affect the surgical result; (c) screen for diseases that may contraindicate elective surgery or require treatment before surgery; (d) diagnose disorders that require surgery; and (e) evaluate the nature and extent of metabolic or septic complications.

2. Routine laboratory studies for all patients undergoing major surgery — CBC, electrolyte profile, BUN, creatinine, coagulation studies, urinalysis, hepatic profile, electrocardiogram (over age 40 or history of cardiac disease).

3. Radiologic evaluation — a chest x-ray is indicated in most patients undergoing major surgery. Special x-rays and studies are required in certain specific clinical situations. It is essential when sending a patient for a particular x-ray study that the radiologist be provided with an adequate account of the patient's history and physical and your specific reason for ordering the study.

F. **Assessment and plan.**

1. Following a thorough history and physical exam, one should be able to make a reasonable assessment of the patient's problem, construct a problem list, and develop a diagnostic and therapeutic plan.
2. Discussion — this is a concise and precise summary of the important data relevant to the patient's problem and which supports the tentative conclusions and diagnosis.
3. Problem list — list in order of importance the particular problems identified in the history and physical examination.
4. Plan — list specific plans for further diagnostic evaluation and therapeutic measures.

II. ORDERS — ADMISSION, PREOPERATIVE & POSTOPERATIVE

A. Admit to ward, ICU or recovery room.
B. Diagnosis, operation.
C. Condition.
   1. I = excellent.
   2. II = good.
   3. III = fair.
   4. IV = serious.
   5. V = critical.
D. Vital signs and frequency; record inputs and outputs as indicated; specify neurologic or vascular checks.
E. Parameters to notify physician — BP < 90/60, > 180/110; P > 110; P < 60; T > 101.5; urine output < 30 cc/hr x 2 hr; change in neurologic/vascular status; respiratory distress; respiratory rate > 30/min.
F. Specific orders about EKG and/or invasive monitoring.
G. Activity or position; type of bed; elevation of head or foot of bed as needed; foot-board; measures for prevention of decubiti and thromboembolism (e.g., turn side-to-side q 2 h, OOB to chair tid, ambulate with assistance in the halls bid, TED® hose, calf compression boots).
H. Diet — when in doubt, keep patient N.P.O. until decisions about patient disposition are finalized.
I. IV orders (e.g., D5 1/2 NS + 20 mEq KCl/liter @ 125 cc/hr).
J. Encourage cough and deep breaths; incentive spirometry (atelectasis prophylaxis).
K. Supplemental O_2 and further respiratory care as indicated; humidification as needed.
L. Foley catheter to gravity drainage (if present).
M. NG tube instructions (if present), e.g., Salem Sump to low continuous suction, irrigate q 4 h with 20 cc NS and "pop" blue port q 4 h with 20 cc air; Levin tube to low intermittent suction; irrigate q 4 h with 20 cc NS.
N. Other drains, tubes, dressing care.

O. Medications — dose, route, frequency: sedatives, hypnotics, analgesics, laxatives, antiemetics, antipyretics, antibiotics, patient's regular medications, thromboembolism prophylaxis.
P. Labs and special tests.
Q. X-rays.
R. EKG, EMG, EEG, etc.

III. NOTES — PREOPERATIVE, POSTOPERATIVE & PROGRESS
A. **Date** and **time** all medical record entries.
B. **Preoperative notes.**
    1. Preoperative diagnosis.
    2. Procedure planned.
    3. Anesthesia anticipated.
    4. Laboratory data.
        a. Minor operations — CBC and UA required.
        b. Major operations — CBC, renal profile, UA, PT, PTT, EKG if patient > 40 years old; CXR if patient has not had a normal CXR in past 6 months; type and screen or crossmatch if needed for specific procedure; ABG, hepatic profile, bone profile, and other specific x-rays and labs as indicated by the patient's disease processes.
    5. Identify any specific risk factors related to cardiac, renal, pulmonary, hepatic, coagulation, and nutritional status. Document that potential risks and benefits of intended operation have been explained to the patient (and family or guardian), questions answered, and patient (or guardian) consent to procedure (see "Documentation" chapter).
    6. Allergies.
    7. Current medications and major medical illnesses.
C. **Postoperative note.**
    1. Mental status — neurologic exam, adequacy of pain control.
    2. Vital signs.
    3. Physical exam — including inspection of surgical dressings, wounds, drains.
    4. Laboratory data.
    5. Impression of condition.
    6. Plan.
D. **Progress notes.**
    1. Daily notes written to document status of current problems, and identifying new problems.
    2. Narrative — problem-oriented style. Identify postoperative day number, hospital day number, antibiotic or hyperalimentation day number, etc.
        a. Subjective data (patient's complaints, nurses' observations).
        b. Objective data (vital signs, physical findings, lab data).
        c. Assessment.
        d. Plans — diagnostic, therapeutic, patient education.

3. Flow sheets — for complex data and time relationships, e.g., hyperalimentation data, diabetes control, hemodynamic parameters, etc.

IV. OPERATIVE REPORT

A. Identifying data — patient name, hospital number, dictator's name, date of dictation.
B. Service and Attending Surgeon.
C. Date of procedure.
D. Preoperative diagnosis.
E. Postoperative diagnosis.
F. Procedure performed.
G. Surgeon, assistants.
H. Type of anesthesia used — note the **specific** agents used.
I. Estimated blood loss.
J. Intraoperative fluid administered and blood products given.
K. Specimens — pathology, microbiology, etc.
L. Drains and tubes placed.
M. Complications.
N. Indications for surgery — brief history (reason for surgery).
O. Details of operation — patient position, skin prep and draping, type and location of incision and technique, **specific details of procedure** (including an itemized description of findings, both normal and abnormal, found at the time of surgery), hemostatic technique, closure technique, dressings, disposition of patient, condition of patient, and sponge and needle counts as reported by nursing staff in attendance; send copies to surgeons and referring physicians.

Note: The above description is a formal, dictated note. A written note consisting of "C" through "M" above, plus a brief description of the operative findings, should be recorded in the chart immediately after the procedure. This "Brief Operative Note" will suffice until the formal transcribed operative note is placed on the chart.

V. DISCHARGE SUMMARY

A. Identifying data — patient name, chart number, service, attending surgeon.
B. Dates of admission and discharge.
C. Primary and secondary diagnoses.
D. Operation and procedures performed and dates.
E. Consultations.
F. Discharge medications.
G. Discharge diet.
H. Activity limitations.
I. Disposition and follow-up appointments.
J. Pertinent findings on physical exam, appropriate lab data, and brief narrative description of hospital course.
K. Copies to be sent to attending and referring physicians.

MEDICO—LEGAL ASPECTS

I. CONSENT

A. Formal consent: Every human being of adult years and sound mind has a right to determine what shall be done with his/her own body, and a surgeon who performs an operation without the patient's consent commits an assault for which he/she is liable in damages. Courts held for *Schloendoff v. Society of New York Hospital*, 211 N.Y. 125, 105 N.E. 92, 93 (1914).

1. **Express consent** — consent given by direct words that may be spoken or written. Difficult to prove effective oral consent; always try to obtain written consent.

2. **Implied consent** — no explicit oral or written expression of consent. Consent is **implied** by reasonable inference from the conduct of the patient (e.g., *O'Brien v. Cunard Steamship Co.*: Passenger on a ship who joined a line of people receiving injections was held to have given implied consent to vaccination).

3. **Extension of consent** — consent is limited to those procedures contemplated when consent is given. Subject to two major exceptions:

   a. Context indicates consent generally to treatment for the purpose of remedying a condition rather than a particular procedure. Consents to use of all reasonable steps to remedy the condition, although the method employed may differ from that anticipated.

   b. Modification of consent when the procedure differs from that originally authorized is not necessary when it is not feasible to consult either the patient or someone who can give consent on the patient's behalf, at the time when a treatment decision must be made (i.e., general anesthesia).

4. In the context of having a condition remedied, a patient who submits to a procedure under an express consent, not limited by an expressed prohibition of extension, impliedly consents to such further procedures as are medically justified by facts discovered in the course of the authorized operation, provided the extension procedure does not materially increase the risk to the patient, involve the removal of an organ or limb, and/or terminate the patient's reproductive capacity.

5. Express limitations of consent by patients: If a patient expressly prohibits a specific medical or surgical procedure, consent to that procedure cannot be implied unless circumstances change significantly from those anticipated at the time of the prohibition. Where medical judgment dictates certain procedures, special efforts should be made to convince the patient to withdraw any such obstacles prior to commencement of treatment.

6. Consent limited to specific practitioner: Under special circumstances, such as an emergency that makes substitution
   necessary, a substitution not anticipated by the patient may
   vitiate the patient's consent to the procedure. Where an
   educational program or other special factor makes substitution
   of practitioners desirable, the patient's knowledgeable agreement to the substitution should be carefully documented.

B. **Informed consent** – *different than formal consent*. The physician
   must disclose sufficient information to allow the patient to make
   an informed decision about the surgery.
   1. **Standard of disclosure.**
      a. Reasonable physician standard – information communicated
         to the patient is similar to that given by other physicians
         in similar circumstances. This standard is recognized by a
         minority of states.
      b. Reasonable patient standard – information communicated
         which a reasonable patient in similar circumstances would
         need to make an informed decision. This view is held by
         the *majority* of states.
      c. Physician is liable for negligent nondisclosure if he/she fails
         to disclose the risks or alternatives to proposed course of
         treatment when a reasonable person, in what the physician
         knows or should have known to be the patient's position,
         would likely attach significance to that risk or alternative
         in formulating his/her decision to consent to treatment.
      d. Optimally, the physician performing the procedure obtains
         consent *personally*. It is always wise to have a third party
         present during the discussion of the procedure to serve as
         a witness.
      e. A note should be written in the chart documenting the
         informed consent discussion and all potential risks and
         alternatives.
   2. **Elements of informed consent.**
      a. Patient is competent (over age 18 and of unimpaired mental
         capacity). Consent for minors must be obtained from parent
         or legal guardian.
      b. Consent is voluntary.
      c. Sufficient information is given:
         1) Nature of the procedure.
         2) Probable consequences (desirable and undesirable results
            that will probably occur).
        `*` 3) Possible material risks that may occur.
         4) Alternatives with their probable consequences.
         5) Problems in recuperation.
      d. The information is understood by the patient.

3. **Situations not requiring informed consent.**
    a. **Risks generally known** — when a relatively minor risk is also inherent in a procedure and is common knowledge to a reasonable patient, the risk need not be disclosed (e.g., the 0.013% risk of hepatitis with blood transfusion).
    b. **Patients asks not to be told** — the patient has the right to waive the right to know the procedure's nature, risks, and alternatives.
    c. **Emergency** — any condition which constitutes an immediate danger to the life or health of the patient and which precludes taking the time to obtain consent from the patient or next of kin. The patient record should indicate that a reasonable effort was made to obtain consent.
    d. **Therapeutic privilege** — when it is the physician's opinion disclosure would complicate or hinder treatment, cause psychological harm, or upset the patient so much as to be unable to make a decision, then consent need not be obtained from the patient. The fact that disclosure might create anxiety in a patient is *not* sufficient to warrant application of this exception. Before opting to treat a patient under therapeutic privilege, a physician should obtain consultation with another physician to make an independent determination that there is a real basis to rely on this exception. The physician should document exactly what risks are being withheld from the patient's knowledge and why. The physician is then best advised to disclose those risks to the appropriate next of kin and to document that fact also.

II. COMPETENCY
A. The issue of patient competency ultimately rests with the responsible physician — may require a psychiatric evaluation.
B. Definitions and criteria for competency vary based on local laws, but basically the patient must be:
    1. Communicative in some manner.
    2. Oriented.
    3. Able to manage his/her own affairs.
    4. Able to understand the procedure, risks, benefits and possible complications.
C. In the event of questions regarding competency and consent, legal advice must be sought, especially in non-emergent cases where it may be necessary to make the patient a ward of the court.

III. DNR ("DO NOT RESUSCITATE"):
   SUPPORTIVE CARE OF THE CRITICALLY ILL
A. DNR orders are guided by institutional regulations.

B. If the responsible physician feels a DNR status is appropriate, then discussion with next-of-kin is essential. Considerations:
   1. Lack of significant benefit from further therapy in a given case.
   2. Prolongation of life in terminal illness or end-stage chronic disease is not productive.
   3. Extending or increasing patient's pain, discomfort, mental/emotional suffering by prolonged care in ICU setting.
   4. An accurate progress note describing such discussion and even witnessed by next-of-kin mandatory.
C. Various methods of writing such orders — should address specific issues involved.
   1. "Do not resuscitate in event of cardiac or respiratory arrest."
   2. "No pressors, mechanical ventilatory support, or CPR in event of cardiac or respiratory arrest."
   3. "In the event of cardiac or respiratory arrest, 'Stat-page' the responsible physician."
D. "Graded" DNR (e.g., pressors only, no tube/no ICU, ICU but no tube) may result in complicated situation because of lack of therapeutic endpoint.
E. A DNR status usually implies maintenance of minimal support, but no therapy is to be added to existing regimen.
   1. No labwork.
   2. No antibiotics.
   3. No addition of nutritional support if not already started and consideration of discontinuance.
   4. Mechanical ventilatory support usually continued if already in effect, but no changes in settings.
   5. No increase in pressor support, and consideration of discontinuance.
   6. Continue IV fluids, O_2, analgesics, sedatives, and *especially* nurse and physician care.

FLUIDS AND ELECTROLYTES

I. BASIC PHYSIOLOGY
A. **Body composition** — water content proportional to lean muscle mass.
  1. **Total body water (TBW)** — 50–70% of body weight. Higher in males, decreases with age.
  2. **Intracellular water** — 40% of body weight. Predominantly in muscle.
  3. **Extracellular water** — composed of interstitial (15%) and intravascular (5%) spaces.
  4. **Plasma volume** — 50 cc/kg body weight.
  5. **Blood volume** — 70 cc/kg body weight.
B. **Fluid balance.**
  1. **Basal requirements** — 35 cc/kg/24 hrs or 1500 cc/m^2/24 hrs.
  2. *Increased* in patients with abnormal losses.
    a. Fever — 15% for each 1°C above 37°C.
    b. Tachypnea — 50% for each doubling of rate.
    c. Diarrhea, fistulas, tube drainage, "third–space" losses — best quantified by direct measurement and serial body weights.
  3. **Antidiuretic hormone (ADH)** frequently elevated in surgical and trauma patients; responsible for hyponatremia, hypotonicity, oliguria. ADH preserves **euvolemia** over tonicity.
  4. **Osmolality** — defines "tonicity" of body fluids.
    a. Represents solute concentration per unit solvent.
    b. Important in maintaining fluid equilibrium between compartments.
    c. Chiefly defined by sodium.
    d. Measured in laboratory by freezing–point depression (colligative property).
    e. Calculated by:

$$\text{Osmolality (mOsm/liter)} = (2 \times Na) + \frac{\text{glucose}}{18} + \frac{\text{BUN}}{2.8}$$

C. **Electrolyte metabolism.**
  1. **Sodium** — normal requirements about 100–150 mEq per day. Major importance in determining body tonicity. Serum concentration does *not* reflect total body sodium content.
  2. **Potassium** — normal requirements about 50–100 mEq per day. Major importance in physiology of muscle contraction and depolarization. Greatly affected by acid–base balance, nutritional state, sodium metabolism, and renal function.
  3. **Bicarbonate** — see VI: "Acid–Base Disorders".
  4. **Chloride** — intimately related to sodium metabolism.

5. **Calcium** — major importance in neuromuscular and enzyme physiology. Normal requirements about 1-3 g/24 hrs. Metabolism controlled by vitamin D and parathormone. Physiologically active form exists in ionized state; measurement of ionized fraction more useful clinically. Total serum level must be corrected for albumin:

$$\text{Corrected Ca}^{++} = \left(\begin{array}{cc}\text{normal} & \text{patient's} \\ \text{albumin} & - & \text{albumin}\end{array}\right) \times 0.8 + \begin{array}{c}\text{patient's} \\ \text{calcium}\end{array}$$

6. **Magnesium** — metabolism similar to calcium. Normal requirements about 20 mEq/24 hrs.
7. **Phosphorus** — metabolism related to calcium. An important mediator of chemical energy.

II. ASSESSMENT

A. History.

1. Determine medical conditions which predispose to derangements and which sensitize patient to effects of derangement (congestive heart failure, renal failure, etc.).
2. Usual and present weight, renal function.
3. Significant medications (e.g., steroids, diuretics, cardiac medications).

B. Physical exam — probably *best* method of determining fluid status.

1. Tissue turgor — decreased in contraction of interstitial fluid due to loss of sodium–containing fluids.
2. Body weight.
3. Jugular venous distention and central venous pressure as indicators of volume if cardiac function is stable.
4. Orthostatic symptoms indicative of at least 10% loss of extracellular volume; may be masked by negative chronotropic medications.
5. Edema and rales — due to increased body water and sodium content. Appears in dependent areas (over sacrum, in basilar lung fields) in supine patient.

C. Laboratory.

1. Sodium.
   a. Serum concentration is *not* indicative of total body content.
   b. In acute hypotonic losses, each 3 mEq/liter rise in serum sodium represents about 1 liter deficit of free water.
2. Hematocrit — may change inversely proportional to degree of hydration.
3. Potassium — increased in acidosis, decreased in alkalosis.
4. Urine.
   a. Volume should be ≥ 0.5 cc/kg/hr if adequate intravascular volume, cardiac function, and renal function.

  b. Specific gravity and osmolality — vary inversely with volume status.

  c. **Urinary indices** — obtained from "spot" urine sample and simultaneous serum samples:

	"Prerenal"	"Renal"
BUN	Increased	Increased
Creatinine	Normal	Increased
BUN/creatinine	Increased	Normal
Urine Na$^+$	< 10	> 20
Urine Osmolality	> 500	< 350
*F$_E$Na$^+$	< 1%	> 1%
Response to fluid	Increased output	No response

$$*F_ENa^+ = \frac{\text{urine sodium x serum creatinine}}{\text{serum sodium x urine creatinine}} \text{ x } 100$$

(Note: Urinary indices not valid if diuretics recently administered.)

III. VOLUME DISORDERS

A. Hypovolemia — usually secondary to losses of isotonic fluids (blood, plasma, most GI fluids).

  1. Clinical setting — trauma, prolonged GI losses (vomiting, tube suctioning, diarrhea), "third–spacing" (ascites, pleural effusions, bowel obstruction, crush injury, burns), increased insensible loss.

  2. **Clinical findings** — mental status changes, orthostatic hypotension and/or tachycardia, poor tissue turgor, oliguria, decreased pulse pressure, decreased CVP or PCWP pressures, hypothermia, acute weight loss.

  3. **Laboratory findings.**

    a. Increased BUN out of proportion to creatinine (> 20:1).

    b. Increased hematocrit (3% rise for each liter deficit).

    c. Fractional excretion of sodium (F$_E$Na) < 1%.

    d. Increased urine specific gravity and osmolality.

  4. **Treatment.**

    a. Acute, life–threatening hypovolemia — usually secondary to trauma or major vascular catastrophe. Requires *rapid* isotonic fluid replacement, plasma, and blood; use **peripheral catheters** instead of central lines (unless pre–existing) to lessen complications.

    b. Non–acute hypovolemia — determine volume deficit and associated electrolyte disorders. Usually treated with balanced crystalloids.

1) Bolus therapy — rapid infusion of 250–1000 cc of fluid (depending on cardiac status), frequent monitoring of BP, urine output, HR.
2) Rapidity and volume of replacement tailored to cardiac status; "stiff" ventricles are poorly compliant and do not tolerate fluid overload.
3) Adjust rate and composition of maintenance fluids to replace deficits and ongoing losses.

B. **Hypervolemia** — usually secondary to overenthusiastic parenteral hydration, fluid–retaining state, or mobilization of previously sequestered fluids.

1. **Clinical findings** — weight gain over baseline (**Note:** Fasting patient in ideal fluid balance should lose 0.25–0.5 kg body weight/day from catabolism), pedal or sacral edema, pulmonary rales or wheezing ("cardiac asthma"), jugular venous distention, elevated CVP or PCWP.

2. **Laboratory findings.**
   a. Decrease in hematocrit, albumin.
   b. Chest x-ray — "cephalization" of pulmonary vessels, alveolar infiltrates, pulmonary effusion, cardiomegaly.
   c. Serum sodium may be low, normal or elevated, but total body sodium is usually elevated.

3. **Treatment.**
   a. Water restriction to 1500 cc/day.
   b. Judicious use of diuretics.
   c. Sodium restriction — 1–2 g/day.
   d. Anasarca responds to combined colloid (albumin) infusion followed by parenteral loop diuretics.

IV. COMPOSITION DISORDERS

A. **Hyponatremia** — secondary to increase in body water relative to sodium content. Three forms:

1. **Isotonic ("pseudohyponatremia")** — occurs in presence of hypertriglyceridemia, hyperproteinemia.

2. **Hypertonic** — due to presence of non–sodium osmotic substances (glucose, mannitol) with intracellular water osmotic redistribution.

3. **Hypotonic** — three forms:
   a. **Hypovolemic** — loss of isotonic fluids, replacement with inadequate volume of excessively hypotonic fluid.
   b. **Hypervolemic** — fluid–retaining states (congestive heart failure, nephrosis, hepatic failure, malnutrition).
   c. **Isovolemic** — clinically undetectable increase in total body water. Due to iatrogenic free–water overloading, SIADH, hypokalemia (sensitizes kidney to ADH), renal insufficiency, and "reset–osmostat".

4. **Symptoms** — predominantly neurologic, dependent upon absolute value and rapidity of change. Usually asymptomatic until below 120 mEq/L. Neurosurgical patients are particularly prone to develop symptoms due to presence of cerebral edema.
5. **Treatment.**
   a. Correction of underlying disorder.
   b. Water restriction to < 1500 cc/day.
   c. Potent loop diuretics (furosemide) followed by hourly replacement of sodium and potassium useful in hypervolemic forms.
   d. Hypertonic saline (3%, 5%) is reserved for symptomatic patients. Calculate deficit; rate of infusion should increase sodium by 2–3 mEq/hr, up to 125–130 mEq/L.
   e. Sodium deficit = (140 − measured sodium) (0.6 x kg wt).
B. **Hypernatremia** — always associated with hyperosmolar state.
   1. **Hypovolemic** — loss of hypotonic fluids with inadequate volumes or hypertonic fluids.
   2. **Hypervolemic** — usually iatrogenic (large amounts of parenteral sodium bicarbonate, certain antibiotics). Also seen in disorders of adrenal axis (Cushing's syndrome, Conn's syndrome, congenital adrenal hyperplasia, steroid use).
   3. **Isovolemic** — actually subclinically hypovolemic. Frequently seen in diabetes insipidus.
   4. Rarely develops in patients with access to water due to powerful thirst mechanism.
   5. Major symptoms — thirst, mental status changes, seizures, coma.
   6. **Treatment.**
      a. Reversal of underlying disorder.
      b. Provision of free–water (D_5W):
         Water deficit = (0.6 x kg wt) (serum sodium/140 − 1).
      c. Fluids should be hypotonic; D_5W good choice, as dextrose is metabolized leaving electrolyte–free water.
      d. Replacement should be *slow*; half of calculated deficit over 24 hours, with remaining half over following 24–48 hours (to avoid cerebral edema).
C. **Hypokalemia.**
   1. Redistribution — intracellular uptake of potassium. Significant in acute alkalosis, insulin therapy, anabolism.
   2. Depletion — external losses (GI tract, biliary tree, tube suctioning, fistulas, diarrhea, Zollinger–Ellison syndrome, villous adenoma, Werner–Morrison syndrome); renal losses commonly high in diuretic use, steroid use, renal tubular acidosis.
   3. **Symptoms** — related to muscle weakness, fatigue, decreased deep tendon reflexes (DTR's), prolonged ileus. See hepatic encephalopathy in cirrhotic, insulin resistance in diabetic.

4. **EKG findings** — low voltage, flattened T waves, ST segment depression, prominent V waves.
5. Commonly seen with concomitant metabolic alkalosis.
6. May precipitate digoxin toxicity — A–V block, atrial or junctional dysrhythmias.
7. **Treatment** — assure adequate renal function prior to repletion.
   a. Deficit usually much greater than apparent from serum level.
   b. Treat alkalosis, decrease sodium intake.
   c. Use enteral route preferentially — 20-40 mEq doses (caution in using jejunostomy tubes, as concentrated potassium implicated in jejunal ulcers and strictures).
   d. Peripheral parenteral — 7.5 mEq KCl in 50 cc D5W; central parenteral — 20 mEq in 50 cc D5W.
   e. Parenteral replacement should not exceed 20 mEq/hr in unmonitored setting, 40 mEq/hr in ICU setting.

D. **Hyperkalemia** — normal or elevated body potassium.
   1. **Pseudohyperkalemia** — leukocytosis, hemolysis, thrombocytosis (late phenomenon; avoided by slow drawing of blood, plasma instead of serum samples).
   2. Redistribution — acidosis, hypoinsulinism, tissue necrosis (crush injury, burns, electrocution), re–perfusion syndrome, digoxin poisoning.
   3. Elevated total body potassium — renal insufficiency, excessive intake, mineralocorticoid deficiency, diabetes mellitus, spironolactone use.
   4. Symptoms — weakness, loss of DTR's, diarrhea.
   5. **EKG** — peaked T waves, decreased ST segments, prolonged QRS progressing to sine wave development and ventricular fibrillation.
   6. **Treatment.**
      a. Look for and remove exogenous sources (medications, IV fluids, diet).
      b. Hydration and forced diuresis to promote renal excretion.
      c. Kayexalate® — 20–50 g in 100–200 cc 20% sorbitol orally every 4 hours or 50 g in 200 cc water with 50 g sorbitol as retention enema, repeat every hour as needed.
      d. Emergent measures — if > 7.5 mEq/L or EKG changes present.
         1) Calcium gluconate — 10 cc 10% solution over 2 min.
         2) NaHCO₃ — 1 ampule, repeat in 15 min.
         3) DW50 (1 ampule = 50 g) and regular insulin 10 units IVP.
         4) Hemodialysis or peritoneal dialysis.
      e. **Note:** Only Kayexalate® and dialysis deplete total body potassium. Other measures only temporize by producing extracellular to intracellular shift of potassium.

E. **Hypocalcemia.**
   1. Most frequently seen in hypoalbuminemic patients, with normal ionized fraction.
   2. Ionized calcium may be subnormal with *normal* serum calcium in acute alkalotic states.
   3. If albumin is normal, check parathormone (PTH) level.
      a. Low PTH — hypoparathyroidism, magnesium deficiency.
      b. High PTH — pancreatitis, hyperphosphatemia, hypovitaminosis D, pseudohypoparathyroidism, massive citrated blood transfusions, certain drugs (gentamicin), renal insufficiency, massive soft tissue infection.
      c. Occurs transiently after removal of hyperfunctioning parathyroid adenomas, especially if pre–op alkaline phosphatase elevated.
   4. **Symptoms** — numbness and tingling in extremities, circumoral paresthesias, muscle cramps, tetany.
      a. **Chvostek's sign** — twitching of facial muscles after percussion over masseter muscle (facial nerve).
      b. **Trousseau's sign** — carpopedal spasm induced by inflated BP cuff above systolic pressure for 3 min.
   5. **EKG** — prolonged Q–T interval.
   6. **Treatment.**
      a. **Acute management** — intravenous therapy.
         1) Calcium chloride — 10 cc 10% solution (potential for tissue necrosis if infiltrated).
         2) Calcium gluconate — 10 cc 10% solution.
      b. **Chronic management** — oral therapy.
         1) Calcium carbonate (see V.D.7: "Oral supplements").
         2) Phosphate-binding antacids — improve GI absorption of calcium.
         3) Vitamin D (calciferol) — begin once serum phosphate is normal. Start at 50,000 units/day, up to 200,000 units/day as needed.

F. **Hypercalcemia.**
   1. Usually occurs secondary to malignancy or hyperparathyroidism. Other causes: thiazide diuretics, milk–alkali syndrome, granulomatous diseases, acute adrenal insufficiency, hyperthyroidism, prolonged immobilization (in young patients), Paget's disease of bone.
   2. **Symptoms** — anorexia, nausea and vomiting, abdominal pains, constipation, polyuria, mental status changes.
   3. **Acute hypercalcemic crisis** — serum calcium > 12. Life–threatening, requires immediate treatment.
   4. **Treatment.**
      a. Hydration with normal saline and induced diuresis — promotes renal excretion. Initial treatment of choice.

    b. Steroids — used in lymphomas, multiple myeloma, non–PTH secreting tumors metastatic to bone, vitamin D intoxication. May take several days to become effective.

    c. Mithramycin — used in malignancy. Associated hypercalcemia refractory to other treatments. Use 15–25 μg/kg IVP over 4–6 hrs. Onset of action 12 hrs, peak action at 36 hrs. Duration of effect 3–7 days. Main adverse reaction is marrow suppression.

    d. Calcitonin — malignancy associated with increased PTH. Skin test 1 unit subcutaneously; usual dosage 4 units/kg subcutaneously or IM every 12–24 hrs.

    e. Phosphates — alters calcium–phosphate ion product towards bone deposition. Use only when phosphate levels are normal to avoid metastatic calcification.

G. Hypomagnesemia.

    1. Causes — malnutrition of any type (alcoholism, prolonged fasting, TPN without adequate replacement, short gut syndrome, malabsorption, fistulas), burns, pancreatitis, SIADH, vigorous diuresis, post–parathyroidectomy, primary hyperaldosteronism.

    2. Clinical findings — weakness, fasciculations, mental status changes, seizures, hyperreflexia, cardiac dysrhythmias.

    3. Treatment.

        a. Symptoms require parenteral replacement — $MgSO_4$ 1–2 g (8–16 mEq) IV as 10% solution over 15 min; continue with 1 g IM or IVP every 4–6 hrs.

        b. Oral — magnesium oxide 35–70 mg each day.

        c. Follow replacement with decreasing patellar reflexes, serial measurements, resolution of symptoms.

H. Hypermagnesemia.

    1. Causes — renal insufficiency, adrenal insufficiency, hypothyroidism, excessive intake (e.g., treatment of eclampsia).

    2. Clinical findings — nausea and vomiting, weakness, mental status changes, hyporeflexia, hyperventilation; A–V block, prolonged Q–T interval.

    3. Treatment.

        a. Delete external sources (large amounts found in cathartics, antacids).

        b. IV calcium gluconate for emergent symptoms.

        c. Dialysis in renal failure.

I. Hypophosphatemia.

    1. Causes — hyperalimentation, nutritional recovery after starvation, DKA, malabsorption, phosphate–binding antacids, alcoholism, ATN, prolonged alkalosis.

    2. Clinical findings — weakness, rhabdomyolysis, CNS changes, hemolysis, platelet and granulocyte dysfunction, cardiac arrest.

    3. Treatment.

    a. Oral — Neutraphos® 2 capsules bid–tid (250 mg phosphorus per tab) or Phosphosoda® 5 cc bid–tid (129 mg phosphorus per 1 cc).

    b. Parenteral — if unable to take PO or if severe hypophosphatemia (< 1 mg/dl).

        1) Recent onset — 0.08–0.20 mM/kg over 6 hrs.

        2) Prolonged — 0.16–0.24 mM/kg over 6 hrs.

    c. Follow serum levels closely.

J. Hyperphosphatemia.

    1. Causes — renal insufficiency, hypoparathyroidism, catabolism, vitamin D metabolites.

    2. May produce metastatic calcifications.

    3. Treatment.

        a. Restrict external sources.

        b. Phosphate–binding antacids (Amphogel®, Alternagel®).

V. THERAPY

A. General considerations.

    1. Unless life–threatening, disorders should be corrected *slowly.*

    2. Plan therapy systematically:

	H_2O	Na^+	K^+	Other
Maintenance				
Deficit				
Ongoing losses				
TOTAL				

B. Maintenance (basal fluid and electrolyte requirements).

    1. Adults.

        a. H_2O — 35 cc/kg/day or 1500 cc/m2/day.

        b. Na^+ — 100–150 mEq/day.

        c. K^+ — 50–100 mEq/day.

    2. Pediatric.

        a. H_2O.

            1) 0–10 kg — 100 cc/kg/day.

            2) 11–20 kg — 1000 cc + 50 cc/kg over 10 kg.

            3) > 20 kg — 1500 cc + 20 cc/kg over 20 kg.

        b. Na^+ — 3–4 mEq/kg/day.

        c. K^+ — 2–3 mEq/kg/day.

        d. Ca^{++} — 2 mEq/kg/day.

C. Deficits and ongoing losses.

    1. Frequent measurements of external losses and weight. Usually only used to quantify composition if volume great or losses prolonged.

    2. Replace losses on regular basis if voluminous or prolonged.

3. **Gastrointestinal fluid composition and average daily volumes:**

Type of secretion	Volume (ml/24 h)	Na (mEq/L)	K (mEq/L)	Cl (mEq/L)	HCO₃ (mEq/L)
Salivary	1,500 (500–2,000)	10 (2–10)	26 (20–30)	10 (8–18)	30
Stomach	1,500 (100–4,000)	60 (9–116)	10 (0–32)	130	
Duodenum	..... (100–2,000)	140	5	80	
Ileum	3,000 (100–9,000)	140 (80–150)	5 (2–8)	104 (43–137)	30
Colon	.....	60	30	40	
Pancreas	..... (100–800)	140 (113–185)	5 (3–7)	75 (54–95)	115
Bile	..... (50–800)	145 (131–164)	5 (3–12)	100 (89–180)	35

Ref: Shires GT, Canizaro PC. In: *Principles of Surgery* (Schwartz SI, et al, Eds.), 2nd Ed. New York: McGraw-Hill, 1974, p. 76, with permission.

D. **Replacement therapy.**
   1. Patients with CHF, renal insufficiency, hepatic disorders require more careful monitoring and careful re–evaluation.
   2. Half of calculated deficits should be given over 24 hours, remaining half over 24–48 hours.
   3. Use oral enteric route when possible.
   4. Tube feeds should be diluted or supplemented as needed.
   5. **Parenteral fluids:**

Solution	Na⁺	K⁺	Cl⁻	Base	mOsm/L	Dextrose	Kcal/L
D₅W	–	–	–	–	278	50	170
D₁₀W	–	–	–	–	556	100	340
D₅₀W	–	–	–	–	2780	500	1700
.9% NaCl	154	–	154	–	286	–	–
.45% NaCl	77	–	77	–	143	–	–
3% NaCl	513	–	513	–	1026	–	–
D₅W .9% NaCl	154	–	154	–	564	50	170
D₅W .45% NaCl	77	–	77	–	421	50	170
D₅W .2% NaCl	39	–	39	–	350	50	170
LR	130	4	109	28	272	–	9
D₅W LR	130	4	109	28	524	50	180

   6. **Parenteral additives:**

Solution	Concentration/Ampule	Volume/Ampule
7.5% Sodium bicarbonate	44 mEq Na⁺, HCO₃⁻	50 cc
42% Sodium phosphate	45 mM PO₄, 60 mEq Na⁺	15 cc
46% Potassium phosphate	45 mM PO₄, 66 mEq K⁺	15 cc
7.5% Potassium chloride	20 mEq K⁺, Cl⁻	20 cc
10% Calcium chloride	14 mEq Ca⁺⁺	10 cc
10% Calcium gluconate	4 mEq Ca⁺⁺	10 cc
25% Magnesium sulfate	4 mEq Mg⁺⁺	2 cc
25% Mannitol	12.5 grams	50 cc

7. **Oral supplements.**
   a. **Potassium.**
      1) Kayciel® elixir — 15 cc = 20 mEq KCl.
      2) KCl solution, 5% — 15 cc = 10 mEq KCl.
      3) Slow K® — 1 tab = 8 mEq KCl.
      4) Klyte® powder — package = 25 mEq K citrate, bicarbonate.
   b. **Calcium.**
      1) Titralac® — 1 cc = 1 g $CaCO_3$ = 400 mg Ca^{++}.
      2) OsCal® 500 — 1 tab = 1.25 g $CaCO_3$ = 500 mg Ca^{++}.
      3) Tums® — 1 tab = 500 mg $CaCO_3$ = 200 mg Ca^{++}.

VI. ACID–BASE DISORDERS

A. Physiology.

1. Most enzymatic processes occur over a narrow pH range.
2. Metabolism accounts for large proton load.
3. Three mechanisms responsible for maintaining pH.
   a. **Buffer systems** — bicarbonate–carbonic acid pair most important and rapid buffer system, with proteins, phosphates, hemoglobin, and bone mineral having secondary roles.
   b. **Respiratory system** — eliminates carbon dioxide ("volatile acid") generated during reduction of bicarbonate and by metabolism. Provides rapid and inexhaustible source of acid elimination as long as ventilation not compromised.
   c. **Renal system** — responsible for excretion of "titratable acids," as well as reclamation of filtered bicarbonate and generation of *de novo* bicarbonate; importance demonstrated by acidosis of renal failure.

B. Disorders.

1. **Metabolic acidosis** — due to overproduction or underexcretion of acids or depletion of buffer stores. Characterized by anion gap (normal 8–12): Anion gap = $Na^+ - (Cl^- + HCO_3^-)$.
   a. **Elevated gap** — renal failure, ketoacidosis, lactic acidosis, various toxins (methanol, ethanol, ethylene glycol, salicylates, paraldehyde).
   b. **Normal gap (hyperchloremic)** — renal tubular acidosis, diarrhea, biliary or pancreatic fluid losses, sulfamylon, acetazolamide, ureteral diversions.
   c. **Diagnosis** — characteristically decreased pH, decreased HCO_3, compensatory hypocapnea.
   d. **Treatment.**
      1) Correct underlying disorder.
      2) Mild to moderate acidosis requires no treatment unless complications ensue.
      3) For pH < 7.3 or HCO_3 < 15, treatment may be required.
      4) Base deficit = .3 x wt (kg) x (25 – measured HCO_3).

     5) Overcorrection can result in significant hypokalemia, hypo-calcemia, and decreased O_2 delivery.

2. **Metabolic alkalosis** — due to loss of acid or gain of base; aggravated by hypokalemia, volume contraction.

    a. **"Saline responsive"** — contraction alkalosis, diuretic–induced, protracted vomiting or NG suctioning with closed pylorus, exogenous bicarbonate loading, villous adenoma.

    b. **"Saline unresponsive"** — severe potassium depletion, mineralocorticoid excess.

    c. Diagnosis — elevated bicarbonate and pH, compensatory hypercapnea; frequently associated hypokalemia.

    d. **Treatment.**

       1) Correction of underlying disorder.

       2) Correction of hypovolemia with chloride–containing solutions (0.9% NaCl).

       3) Correction of hypokalemia (assure adequate renal function first).

       4) Provision of acid solutions in refractory cases.

         a) Chloride deficit = wt (kg) x 0.4 x (100 − measured chloride).

         b) Calculate amount of 0.1 N HCl acid solution required to replace deficit.

       5) **Acetazolamide** (Diamox®) — inhibits carbonic anhydrase, preventing renal reclamation and synthesis of bicarbonate. Dosage averages 250-500 mg q 6 h. Loses effect as serum bicarbonate decreases.

       6) For prolonged gastric suctioning, H_2 antagonists may help decrease gastric acid production and minimize acid loss.

3. **Respiratory acidosis** — results from acute or chronic hypercapnea secondary to inadequate ventilation.

    a. Characterized by increased pCO_2, decreased pH.

    b. Acutely, HCO_3 may be normal, while chronic state produces compensatory increase in HCO_3.

    c. **Treatment.**

       1) Any measure designed to improve alveolar ventilation — aggressive pulmonary toilet, treatment of pneumonia, bronchodilators, and avoidance of respiratory depressants.

       2) Mechanical ventilation if conservative measures fail.

       3) If on ventilator, measures to maximize minute volume. Tidal volume of 12–15 cc/kg, then increase rate.

4. **Respiratory alkalosis** — secondary to acute or chronic hyperventilation.

    a. Characterized by hypocapnea and elevated pH.

    b. May produce symptomatic hypokalemia and hypocalcemia.

    c. Causes — anxiety, metabolic encephalopathy, CNS infections, cerebrovascular accidents, early sepsis, pulmonary embolus, hypoxia, early asthma, pneumonia, CHF, cirrhosis; may be seen in severe head injury ("central hyperventilation").

   d. Treatment.
      1) Treat underlying disorder.
      2) If symptomatic, use re-breathing device; 5% CO_2 used in past, but is hazardous and *not* recommended.
 5. Evaluation of acid–base disorders.
   a. Obtain simultaneous blood gas and electrolyte panel.
   b. Calculate anion gap.
   c. Calculate expected compensation from chart and locate on acid–base nomogram (Fig. 1).
   d. If compensation not within predicted values, suspect "mixed" disorder.
   e. Correlate suspected diagnosis with clinical picture:

Disorder	Primary Change	Secondary Change	Effect
Metabolic acidosis	$\downarrow HCO_3$	$\downarrow pCO_2$	Last 2 digits pH = pCO_2
			$HCO_3 + 15$ = last 2 digits pH
Metabolic alkalosis	$\uparrow HCO_3$	$\uparrow pCO_2$	$HCO_3 + 15$ = last 2 digits pH
Respiratory acidosis:			
Acute	$\uparrow pCO_2$	$\uparrow HCO_3$	ΔpH = .08 per 10 Δ in pCO_2
Chronic	$\uparrow pCO_2$	$\uparrow\uparrow HCO_3$	ΔpH = .03 per 10 Δ in pCO_2
Respiratory alkalosis:			
Acute	$\downarrow pCO_2$	$\downarrow HCO_3$	ΔHCO_3 = .2 x Δ in pCO_2
Chronic	$\downarrow pCO_2$	$\downarrow\downarrow HCO_3$	ΔHCO_3 = .3 x Δ in pCO_2

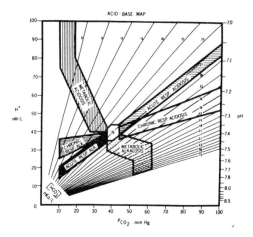

FIGURE 1
Acid–Base Nomogram

N = normal values; A = metabolic acidosis; B = metabolic alkalosis;
D = acute respiratory alkalosis; E = respiratory acidosis; C = compensated respiratory alkalosis; F = compensated respiratory acidosis.

Ref: Goldberg M, et al. *JAMA* 223:269, 1973, with permission.

BLOOD COMPONENT THERAPY AND COAGULATION

The judicious use of blood and blood products is an important aspect of surgical practice. Increasing concerns about transfusion-related infection and limited supplies have led to a critical re-evaluation of the indications and usage of these products. The recommendations made here are derived from guidelines established by the Hoxworth Blood Center and National Institutes of Health.

I. GENERAL CONSIDERATIONS

A. **Estimation of blood volume.**
  1. Total blood volume (TBV) — approximately 7% of body weight (liters).
     a. Male — 77 x body weight = TBV (ml).
     b. Female — 67 x weight = TBV (ml).
     c. Newborn — 80 x body weight = TBV.
  2. Plasma volume = TBV – (TBV x Hct).
B. General indications for use of blood and blood components.
  1. Blood replacement — maintain blood volume; treat shock.
  2. Improve oxygen-carrying capacity — correct anemia.
  3. Maintain hemostasis — correct coagulopathy.
C. **Colloid solutions** — may be used for plasma volume expansion.
  1. **Albumin** (5%, 25%) — commercial product derived from human serum; 5% albumin has oncotic pressure similar to plasma. Indicated in patients with hypovolemia and hypoproteinemia; to induce diuresis (with furosemide) in hypervolemic hypoproteinemic patients; and to reduce gut mucosal edema and feeding intolerance in hypoproteinemic patients (controversial). Rapidly metabolized in catabolic patients. Hepatitis risk low.
  2. **Purified protein fraction** (Plasmanate®) — consists of 83% albumin and 17% globulin. Similar indications as albumin.
  3. **Hetastarch** (Hespan®) — artificial colloid; consists of 6% hetastarch in saline. Plasma volume expansion similar to 5% albumin, but effect decreases over ensuing 24–36 hrs. Contraindicated in bleeding disorders and congestive heart failure.
D. Acellular oxygen-carrying compounds — two currently available: perfluorocarbon emulsions and stroma-free hemoglobin. Not in widespread use, primarily experimental. Inferior to red cell transfusions.
E. Crystalloid solutions — use for acute volume replacement until blood components available. Note: 3 cc crystalloid = 1 cc whole blood.

II. INDICATIONS FOR RED CELL TRANSFUSION

A. **Emergency transfusion** — immediate life–saving need for blood (> 30% loss of blood volume).

1. **Priority** — control hemorrhage, replace loss with crystalloid, then restore oxygen–carrying capacity with blood. Red cell transfusion should begin if > 2 liters of crystalloid fails to produce hemo-dynamic stability.
2. If hemostasis and volume replacement stabilizes patient, trans-fusion can await completion of formal typing and cross-matching.
3. If patient remains unstable, transfusion immediately required in the form of:
   a. O-negative, low-titer ("universal donor") — should be available in critical care areas for immediate use.
   b. Type–specific (ABO, Rh compatible) — no cross–match per-formed; usually safe; available within 10 minutes.
B. **Acute anemia** — studies suggest that oxygen–carrying capacity is adequate at Hgb = 7.0 if intravascular volume is adequate. Current recommendations for transfusion are: Hgb < 8.0; Hct < 24%, unless anemia is symptomatic.
C. **Chronic anemia** — studies suggest wound healing is unimpaired if Hct > 15%; also no evidence that red cell replacement decreased risk of post–op infections. No clear–cut "threshold" for transfusion. In general, use same indications as for acute anemia. Focus of treatment should be on etiology of anemia.

III. **MASSIVE TRANSFUSION**
A. Defined as a single transfusion of > 2 x TBV; > 2.5 liters; or total of 5 liters over 24 hours. Significance arises from the high potential for complications.
B. **Complications** — likely due to tissue damage and hypoperfusion as well as the "storage lesion" of banked blood.
   1. **Hypothermia** — most common. Has severe effect on coagula-tion, platelet function, cardiac function, and acid–base balance. Best treatment is prevention. Recommended maneuvers include use of blood–warming devices, or rapid infusion systems spe-cifically designed for warming and delivering large volumes of blood; raising ambient temperature; and warming IV and irri-gating solutions.
   2. **Citrate toxicity** — results in hypocalcemia; may lead to myo-cardial dysfunction in patients with pre–existing cardiac disease. Treat with calcium supplementation.
   3. **Hyperkalemia** — probably due to elevated extracellular potas-sium content of banked blood; may potentiate cardiac arrythmias, especially in patients with renal insufficiency.
   4. **Acidosis** — due to hypoperfusion and low pH of banked blood.
   5. **Hyperammonemia** — due to accumulation of ammonia in banked blood; may precipitate hepatic encephalopathy in patients with hepatic insufficiency.
   6. **Coagulopathy** — due to consumption as well as dilution of coagulation factors and platelets, as well as the effects of hypo-thermia.

IV. BLOOD COMPONENTS (see Table 1)

A. Whole blood — infrequently used (or available); packed red blood cells reconstituted with crystalloids are safer and as effective. Whole blood has essentially no viable platelets, and decreased levels of Factors V and VIII.

B. **Packed red blood cells (PRBC)** — indicated for treatment of symptomatic anemia in euvolemic patients. One unit has approximately 250 cc of volume; hematocrit of about 65%; each unit should raise the hemoglobin 1 gm/dl and the hematocrit by 3%. Has minimal WBC's and plasma.
   1. **Sedimented PRBC** — Hct approximately 70%. Used for replacement of RBC's in newborns.
   2. **Washed PRBC** — lower risk of disease and antigen transmission. Use in patients with 2 or more documented episodes of febrile or allergic transfusion reactions.

C. **Platelets** — indicated for bleeding due to thrombocytopenia or thrombocytopathy. One unit of platelet concentrate should raise the platelet count by 5,000–10,000 (Foley pt.) in the absence of continued platelet consumption; 8–10 units are usually transfused at one time. Previously allosensitized patients may require **single-donor, HLA–matched platelets** to prevent accelerated immune destruction.

D. **Fresh frozen plasma (FFP)** — indicated for treatment of bleeding in hepatic disease, DIC, dilutional coagulopathy, and specific coagulation factor deficiency; each unit of FFP will increase the level of any clotting factor by 2–3%. Volume is approximately 250 cc/unit. Good source of all clotting factors (including the "labile" Factors X and VIII) although cryoprecipitate is a better source of fibrinogen. Adverse effects include disease transmission and allergic reactions. Requires ABO typing, but not cross–matching.

E. **Cryoprecipitate** — good source of Factor VIII:C, Factor VIII:VWF (von Willebrand factor), fibrinogen and fibronectin. Used to treat acquired hypofibrinogenemia, Factor VIII deficiency.

F. **Specific coagulation factors** — **Factor VIII concentrate** (Hemophilia A), **Factor IX concentrate** (Hemophilia B).

G. **Autologous blood.**
   1. **Preoperative** — patient donates blood prior to proposed operation to be used for himself. Particularly useful when patient has numerous antibodies making cross–match difficult. Blood stored in CPDA–1 has shelf–life of 35 days; frozen cells can be stored up to 2 years.
   2. **Intraoperative/trauma** — useful in major vascular and cardiac surgery, massive hemothorax, or abdominal hemorrhage. Blood is retrieved and either filtered and reinfused or processed and replaced as packed cells. Essentially devoid of clotting factors; *contraindicated* when blood contaminated with feces, bacteria, or malignant cells.

3. Intraoperative hemodilution — removal of 1-3 units immediately prior to cardiopulmonary bypass or other surgery with crystalloid or colloid replacement; whole blood is then stored and reinfused perioperatively. Platelet and coagulation factors remain essentially normal.
4. Post–op — mediastinal or pleural thoracostomy tube drainage may be processed and reinfused as PRBC. Blood should not remain in collecting system more than 4 hrs prior to collection.

TABLE 1
Blood Components

COMPONENT	INDICATIONS	EFFECTS	RISKS	VOLUME	NOTES
Blood Products					
Packed red blood cells (PRBC)	Reduced RBC mass in symptomatic anemia (Hgb ≤ .8)	↑ O_2 carrying capacity, 1 unit yields ↑ Hgb by 1 gm, ↑ Hct by 3-4%	Infectious Allergic Febrile	≈ 250 ml (Hct 70%)	Administer with 0.9 NS or with FFP, 5% albumin or Plasmanate; not D5W, not LR
Leukocyte-depleted RBC's	Repeated (> 3) febrile transfusion reactions	Reduces leukocyte antigens (responsible for febrile reaction)	Infectious ↓ Febrile Allergic	≈ 250 ml	Administer as above; may lose up to 30% of RBC's, so effective; red cell mass is reduced
Leukocyte-poor, saline-washed RBC's	Repeated allergic (urticarial) reactions	↓ WBC's and plasm proteins (responsible for allergic reaction)	Infectious ↓ Febrile ↓ Allergic	≈ 250 ml	
Whole blood	Reduced red cell mass and plasma volume (hemorrhagic shock, burn excision)	Replaces red cell mass, volume, platelets and clotting factors	Infectious Febrile Allergic Circulatory overload	≈ 500 ml	If > 24 hrs old, then ↓ platelet function; ↓ factor V, VIII
Platelets					
Random donor platelets	a) Bleeding secondary to thrombocytopenia b) Prophylactic if < 20,000, clinically stable and intact vascular system c) Prophylactic if < 50,000, during massive transfusion or in perioperative period (48-72 hrs)	1 unit yields ↑ platelet count 5000-10,000, 10 units platelets contains ≈ 500 ml plasma (= 2 units FFP)	Infectious Allergic Febrile	≈ 50 ml	1) Usually pooled 6-8 units 2) Not indicated in consumptive process, e.g., ITP or untreated DIC 3) Use type specific for Rh(·) pre-menopausal women; if not possible, consider Rhogam®
Single donor platelets	Use as above for patients with HLA sensitization to platelets	Equivalent to 6-8 units, therefore ↑ platelet count by 30,000-60,000	Infectious Allergic Febrile	≈ 300 ml	Typed to ABO and HLA, not used prophylactically to prevent HLA sensitization
Granulocytes	To increase circulating granulocytes in septic, neutropenic patients (< 500 PMN/mm³)	Varies	Infectious ↑ Allergic ↑ Febrile	≈ 500 ml	Controversial
Plasma Products					
Fresh frozen plasma (FFP)	Correction of multiple coagulation factor deficiencies	Source of labile and stable clotting factors, ↑ 2-3% per unit, ↑ II, VII, IX, X, XI	Infectious Allergic Febrile	≈ 220 ml	1) ABO compatible 2) Rarely indicated if PT/PTT are less than 1.5 x normal
Single donor plasma	Treatment of stable clotting factor deficiencies		Infectious Allergic Febrile	≈ 220 ml	1) ABO compatible 2) Is supernatant of cryoprecipitate, no V or VIII, not used in DIC
Cryoprecipitate	Hemophilia A, von Willebrands, hypofibrinogenemia, XIII deficiency	↑ VIII (80-120 units) ↑ Fibrinogen ≈ 250 mg ↑ XIII ↑ Fibronectin	Infectious (high)	15 ml	Pooled product, therefore ↑ infectious risk

V. COMPLICATIONS
A. Infectious.
1. Hepatitis:
   a. Non–A, non–B (hepatitis C) — 1:100 transfusions, 30-50% of these develop chronic active hepatitis, 10% of these develop cirrhosis.
   b. Hepatitis B — 1:200 – 1:300.
2. HIV — 1:40,000 – 1:250,000.
3. Others — CMV, HTLV I and II, EBV, papovavirus.

B. Transfusion reactions — overall incidence of 5%.
1. **Acute intravascular hemolytic reaction** — occurs in 0.06:1000 transfusions; 1:100,000 are fatal. Due to ABO incompatibility after red cell transfusion (not with plasma components or platelets). Usual cause is clerical error.
   a. Presentation — fever, chills, tachycardia, tachypnea, flank pain, chest pain; progresses to shock, hemoglobinuria, oliguria, and DIC. Symptoms usually begin with infusion of first 100 cc. In the anesthetized patient, only signs may be fever, tachycardia, and excessive intraoperative bleeding.
   b. **Treatment** — immediately stop transfusion and start IV hydration to restore blood pressure and induce diuresis. Administer mannitol 25–50 mg IV. Alkalinize urine with $NaHCO_3$ 1 ampule in liter of Ringer's lactate. Draw blood from patient for cross–match, CBC, bilirubin, BUN, and creatinine, as well as urine specimen. Return unused blood product and patient's cross–match specimen to blood bank for analysis.
2. **Delayed extravascular hemolytic reaction** — incompatibility of minor blood groups (Kell, Kidd, Duffy, etc.).
   a. Presentation — may include fever, anemia, indirect hyperbilirubinemia, jaundice, and hemoglobinuria. Symptoms develop several days post–transfusion.
   b. **Treatment** — ensure adequate hydration and diuresis; follow renal function closely; avoid nephrotoxic agents.
3. **Allergic reaction** — due to passive transfer of donor antigen to sensitized recipient. Incidence 1.6:1000.
   a. Presentation — fever, chills, flushing, urticaria, pruritis; severe reactions may present with anaphylaxis. Symptoms appear after more than half of unit is infused.
   b. **Treatment** — mild reaction treated with diphenhydramine 50 mg IV or PO. If effective, transfusion may be resumed. Severe reactions may require epinephrine and steroids, and should be treated as a hemolytic transfusion reaction (see above). Future transfusions should use washed PRBC's.
4. **Febrile reaction** — due to antibodies to donor leukocyte antigens. Incidence 3:1000.

    a. Presentation — fever, chills, headache, and flushing usually appear after more than half of unit is infused.

    b. Treatment — antipyretics (acetaminophen). Patients with a history of > 3 episodes of febrile reaction should receive washed or frozen PRBC's.

  5. Circulatory overload — seen in patients with pre-existing cardiac or renal disease. Transfusion should be performed over 3–4 hours and IV diuretics administered between transfusions.

VI. COAGULATION SYSTEM

A. Blood vessels — most common factor in surgical bleeding is inadequate mechanical hemostasis.

B. Platelets — normal value 150,000 – 350,000. Most invasive procedures safe with platelet count > 50,000; spontaneous bleeding not seen until count < 10,000 – 20,000.

C. Coagulation factors:

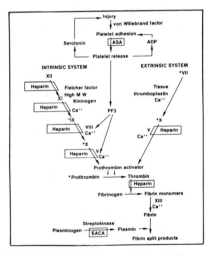

Ref: Condon RE, Nyhus LM: *Manual of Surgical Therapeutics*, 5th Ed. Boston: Little, Brown & Co., 1981, p. 284, with permission.

VII. DIAGNOSIS OF COAGULOPATHY

A. **History** — best screening "test".
1. Family history of coagulopathy (hemophilia A or B, von Willebrand's disease).
2. Abnormal bleeding during previous procedures (oral surgery, biopsies, lacerations).
3. Illnesses — liver disease, biliary obstruction, renal disorders, blood dyscrasias, carcinoma; massive transfusion, trauma, obstetric emergency.
4. Medications — warfarin compounds, aspirin, dipyridamole, nonsteroidal anti–inflammatory agents, antibiotics (especially cephalosporins).

B. **Examination.**
1. Physical findings of diseases mentioned above.
2. Petechiae, purpura, epistaxis, hemarthroses, deep muscle hematomas.
3. Hematuria, menorrhagia, heme–positive stool.

C. **Laboratory** (actual times vary between labs).
1. Quantitative platelet count.
2. Prothrombin time (10–12.5 sec) — evaluates production of thrombin and fibrin polymers by extrinsic pathway; used to monitor coumadin therapy.
3. Activated partial thromboplastin time (23–37 sec) — evaluates production of thrombin and fibrin polymers by intrinsic pathway; used to monitor heparin therapy.
4. Thrombin time — measures polymerization of fibrinogen. Abnormal in presence of heparin, dysfibrinogenemia or DIC.
5. Fibrinogen concentration — 150–350 mg/dl.
6. Fibrin split products — measure of fibrinolysis. Elevated in trauma patients, but greatest elevation seen in primary fibrinolytic states and DIC.
7. Bleeding time — useful measure of platelet function and vessel integrity. Normal IVY bleeding time is 2–6 minutes.

VIII. COAGULOPATHY STATES

A. **Congenital.**
1. **Hemophilia A** (classical) — Factor VIII deficiency; most common congenital coagulopathy. Major surgery or trauma requires factor levels greater than 50–100% of normal to achieve adequate hemostasis.
2. **Hemophilia B** ("Christmas disease") — decreased Factor IX activity. Clinically similar to hemophilia A. Treated with Factor IX concentrates.
3. **Von Willebrand's disease** — due to deficient levels of Factor VIII:VWF. Characterized by prolonged bleeding time and reduced Factor VIII activity. Treated with plasma infusions and intravenous DDAVP.

B. **Acquired.**

1. **Vitamin K deficiency** — due to inadequate intake, malabsorption, lack of bile salts, biliary obstruction, TPN, antibiotics; etiology of hemorrhagic disease of newborns. Treated with parenteral vitamin K (5–10 mg IV slowly; 10–20 mg IM daily for 3 days); produces results in 6–12 hours. Fresh frozen plasma improves coagulopathy sooner.
2. **Hypothermia** — deleterious effect on coagulation system and platelet function (see "Massive Transfusion").
3. **Coumadin** — blocks synthesis of vitamin K–dependent factors. Treated by vitamin K and/or plasma infusions.
4. **Heparin** — augments activity of antithrombin III. Half-life is approximately 4–6 hours. Protamine given IV reverses activity (1 mg for each 100 units of heparin; dosage decreased appropriately for half-life and last dose given).
5. **Hepatic disease** — major site of synthesis of all coagulation factors except VIII. Also has central role in clearing blood of fibrin degradation products. Treated by addressing underlying disease. Administration of large amounts of fresh frozen plasma; vitamin K has minimal effect.
6. **Renal failure** — produces *reversible* platelet dysfunction; improves with reduction of azotemia.
7. **Thrombocytopenia** — spontaneous bleeding is not seen until platelet count less than 10,000–20,000. Below 100,000 bleeding may occur after major trauma or surgery. Causes include: marrow failure or replacement, sequestration in splenomegaly, destruction by autoantibody, sepsis, prosthetic valves, DIC. Treatment by transfusion of platelets; one unit should raise platelet count approximately 10,000 if no ongoing losses.
8. **Thrombocytopathy** — drugs are most common cause of qualitative platelet disorder; includes chemotherapeutic agents, thiazides, alcohol, aspirin, nonsteroidal anti-inflammatory agents, high molecular weight dextran.
9. **Disseminated intravascular coagulation (DIC)** — secondary to intravascular release of thromboplastic substances with subsequent activation of coagulation followed by clot lysis. Caused by trauma, sepsis, malignancy, burns, obstetricial accidents (retained dead fetus, abruptio placentae, amniotic fluid embolus), envenomation, prolonged shock, intravascular hemolysis, and anaphylaxis. Large amounts of fibrin degradation products (FDP) worsen coagulopathy by inhibiting fibrin polymerization. Diagnosis made by appropriate clinical setting; diffuse bleeding from wounds, incisions, and venipuncture sites; prolonged PT and PTT, decreased platelet count and fibrinogen level; elevated FDP; and "microangiopathic" blood smear. **Treatment** directed at reversing primary disorder, replacement of blood components (red cells, platelets, fresh frozen plasma, cryoprecipitate) and vitamin K. Use of heparin is advocated by some, but not widely accepted. Mortality due to sepsis or organ failure.

NUTRITION

A large proportion of hospitalized patients are malnourished to some degree. This may be due to several causes, either singly or in combination: (a) decreased oral intake, (b) impaired absorption, and/or (c) increased requirements due to hypermetabolism.

I. **NUTRITIONAL ASSESSMENT**
A. **Subjective global assessment** [Detsky AS, et al. *JPEN* 8:153, 1984].
   1. A clinical impression performed on the basis of history (attention to recent reduction in oral intake, recent weight loss, underlying disease, and functional status).
   2. No single laboratory test is more accurate than subjective global assessment of nutritional status on admission.
   3. Physical examination — wasting of muscle mass and fat, presence of edema or ascites, glossitis, skin lesions (vitamin deficiencies).
B. **Static nutritional assessment** ("anthropomorphics") including height, weight, skinfold thickness, and muscle circumference.
   1. Useful in assessing **population at risk,** but little predictive value in assessment of *individual* patient.
   2. Weight change or unintentional weight loss is important.
      a. Weight loss of $\geq$ 10% of ideal body weight (IBW) from usual suggests mild to moderate malnutrition.
      b. Weight loss of $\geq$ 20% suggests severe malnutrition.
      c. Weight loss of $\geq$ 30% is premorbid.
C. **Biochemical indicators of malnutrition.**
   1. Visceral proteins — **Albumin:** adequate indicator of malnutrition in absence of other causes of hypoalbuminemia (check for urinary albumin loss). Synthesis decreases with malnutrition.
      a. Long half–life (21 days) and extravascular space distribution make it unreliable as a short–term index of nutrition to be followed during acute illness.
      b. Albumin > 3.5 g/dl suggests adequate nutritional status; < 3.0 g/dl suggests malnutrition.
   2. Rapid–turnover proteins — shorter half–life; earlier indicator of nutritional depletion. Absolute levels less important than falling levels which suggest ongoing malnutrition.
      a. **Transferrin:** half–life of 8 days; a more sensitive indicator of malnutrition, although anemia may stimulate transferrin synthesis. Level < 220 mg/dl suggests malnutrition.
      b. **Thyroxin–binding prealbumin (TBPA):** half–life of 2 days.
      c. **Retinol–binding protein (RBP):** half–life of 12 hours.
D. **Immunologic function** — malnutrition is associated with decreased cellular and humoral immunity.
   1. Complement levels, measurements of neutrophil function, and opsonic index may be useful measurements of response to infection, but are not widely available for clinical use.

    2. Delayed cutaneous hypersensitivity — reflects cellular immunity. Anergy to antigens suggests malnutrition. Anergy may also occur with cancer, severe infection, renal or hepatic failure, post chemo- or radiation therapy.

    3. Total lymphocyte count — calculated as WBC x % lymphocytes. Count < 1500 cells/mm^3 suggests severe malnutrition.

E. Nitrogen balance.

    1. Calculate from intake and excretion of nitrogen.

        a. $Nitrogen_{Balance} = N_{Intake} - N_{Excretion}$.

        b. Total nitrogen loss (g/day) = 24–hour urinary urea nitrogen (UUN) (g/day) + [.20 x 24–hour UUN (g/day)] + 2 g/day.

    2. Useful in unusual cases and as a research tool.

    3. Requires accurate 24–hour urine collection.

II. NUTRITIONAL REQUIREMENTS IN SIMPLE STARVATION AND STRESS

A. Basic needs.

    1. In basal state, caloric requirements are 25 kcal/kg/day, and protein needs are 1 g protein/kg/day.

    2. In stressed multiple–trauma patient, needs may increase up to 35 kcal/kg/day and 1.5 g protein/kg/day.

B. Determination of caloric needs on individual basis.

    1. Calculate basal energy expenditure (BEE) using the **Harris-Benedict equation:**

        BEE (Men) = 66.47 + 13.75 W + 5.0 H − 6.76 A

        BEE (Women) = 65.10 + 9.56 W + 1.85 H − 4.68 A

        BEE (Infants) = 22.10 + 31.05 W + 1.16 H

        W = weight in kg; H = height in cm; A = age.

    2. Calculate increase in energy needs imposed by **activity** (i.e., BEE x activity) using **Calvin–Long activity factor:**

        Confined to bed: 1.2

        Out of bed: 1.3

    3. Calculate increase in energy needs imposed by **injury** (i.e., BEE x activity factor x injury factor) using **Calvin–Long injury factor:**

        Minor operation: 1.2

        Skeletal trauma: 1.35

        Major sepsis: 1.60

        Severe thermal injury: 2.10

    4. Indirect calorimetry — measurements of the patient's oxygen consumption and carbon dioxide production.

        a. Determines resting energy expenditure by measuring respira- tory gas exchange (i.e., O_2 consumption, CO_2 production).

        b. Useful for more precise assessment in critically ill patients. Needs specialized resources in an intensive care unit.

        c. Gives index of fuel utilization — respiratory quotient (RQ) = VCO_2/VO_2. RQ carbohydrate = 1.0; mixed substrate =

0.80; lipid = 0.70; lipogenesis > 1.0 (also induced spuriously by hyperventilation); ketogenesis < 0.70. In our institution, RQ of 0.8–1.0 is desirable; < 0.70 suggests "underfeeding" and > 1.0 "overfeeding".

   d. Despite sophistication, must be treated as part of total clinical assessment without relying on results as sole determinant.

III. INDICATIONS FOR NUTRITIONAL SUPPORT

The application of nutritional support is guided by an assessment of the patient's clinical and nutritional status.

A. Factors.
   1. Age — in a previously healthy adult, adequately hydrated and mildly catabolic.
      a. Up to age 60 will tolerate up to 14 days of starvation.
      b. 60–70 years will tolerate up to 10 days of starvation.
      c. > 70 years will tolerate 5 days of starvation.
   2. Previous state of health — the pre–existing health status, including prior nutritional status. Patients with chronic medical problems (i.e., diabetes mellitus; COPD; renal, cardiac, or hepatic insufficiency) are probably at more nutritional risk than those patients described in section A.1 above. Determine nutritional status and "reserves" by biochemical measurements.
   3. Current condition — assess metabolic demands.
      a. Presence of severe trauma, sepsis, or burns.
      b. Recent major operation.
      c. High–dose corticosteroid therapy.

B. Preoperative nutritional supplementation — requires consideration of the above and anticipated duration of dietary deprivation. If evidence of moderate to severe malnutrition exists, 7–10 days of preoperative nutritional support may be beneficial.

C. Postoperative nutritional supplementation — in the malnourished patient, postoperative nutrition is necessary until adequate oral intake is resumed. For the healthy patient, follow guidelines (see "Factors" above).
   1. If the GI tract is functional, enteral nutrition is preferable. Placement of a nasoenteric feeding tube for short–term feeding is recommended. An alternative is placement of needle catheter jejunostomy (NCJ), which can be used for longer periods of time with improved patient comfort.
   2. If prolonged support is anticipated, a feeding gastrostomy or jejunostomy should be considered (see below).

IV. ENTERAL NUTRITION

A. Indications — functional GI tract, inadequate oral intake.

B. Short–term supplementation — for nasogastric or nasointestinal feeds, use small–bore (7–9 Fr) soft tubes to minimize erosion and aspiration complications and improve patient comfort.

1. **Nasogastric (NG).**
   a. Adequate gastric emptying required.
   b. Alert patient with intact gag reflex.
2. **Nasointestinal** — patients with higher risk of aspiration (i.e., loss of gag reflex, neurologic impairment).
3. **Needle catheter jejunostomy (NCJ).**
   a. Placed intraoperatively at time of upper GI surgery, pancreaticobiliary surgery, or multiple–trauma patient undergoing laparotomy.
   b. Catheter should be placed **distal** to any site of operation, although with care, patients with colonic anastomoses safely tolerate NCJ feedings.
   [Note: The position of any of these tubes *must* be confirmed by x-ray *prior* to initiating tube feedings.]
C. **Long–term supplementation** (> 6 weeks).
   1. **Gastrostomy** — placed operatively or percutaneously.
      a. Adequate gastric emptying required.
      b. Evidence of reflux or impaired gag is contraindication.
      c. Can use intermittent gavage feeds, blenderized meals.
   2. **Jejunostomy** — placed operatively.
      a. Anticipate long–term enteral supplementation in patient for whom gastrostomy is contraindicated.
      b. Usually requires continuous infusion.
D. **Products.**
   1. **Oral supplements.**
      a. Indications — supplementation of an oral diet.
      b. Must be palatable (however, flavoring makes these supplements hyperosmolar).
      c. Examples — Ensure®, Ensure Plus®, Sustacal®, Carnation Instant Breakfast®.
   2. **Tube feedings.**
      a. Blenderized (pureed) diet.
         1) Primarily used with gastrostomies (large–bore tubes).
         2) Indicated for patients with inability to masticate or swallow.
         3) Quality control is difficult, but inexpensive and easy to prepare.
      b. Polymeric — Isocal®, Osmolite®.
         1) Complete diet, with intact protein; generally lactose-free.
         2) Iso–osmolar, fairly well tolerated.
      c. High–caloric density — Magnacal®.
         1) Complete diet, with intact protein; generally lactose-free.
         2) Hyperosmolar — needs either gastric administration for osmotic dilution or dilution with water for intestinal infusion.

3) Indicated in those patients with increased caloric needs and decreased volume tolerance.
4) May provoke diarrhea.
d. Monomeric — Vivonex TEN®, Criticare HN®.
1) Amino acids with or without peptides as protein source. May not be as efficiently absorbed as more complete proteins.
2) Requires no digestion.
3) Essentially complete small-bowel absorption (low residue).
4) Hyperosmolar — cautions as above.
e. Disease–specific formulas.
1) Renal failure — Amin–Aid®.
a) Elemental diet, essential L–amino acids, reduced nitrogen.
b) Hyperosmolar.
c) Best when administered by tube (not very palatable).
2) Acute or chronic hepatic failure — HepaticAid II®.
a) Enriched with branched chain amino acids.
b) Low in aromatic and sulfur–containing amino acids.
c) May be used as tube feeding or to supplement a protein–restricted oral diet.
d) If the patient is in hepatic coma, remain vigilant for gastric aspiration if feeding by the gastric route.

E. **Administration.**
1. Generally, all types of tube feedings should be iso-osmolar (i.e., 300 mosm) for initial administration. Hypertonic feeds require dilution.
2. Gastric feeding — due to the greater diluting capacity of the stomach, feedings should first be advanced in **concentration.** Then, once the hyperosmolar feedings are tolerated at full strength, the rate may be increased. Bolus feeds may be used.
3. Intestinal feedings — increase **rate first,** then concentration. Osmolality > 400 mosm/L may not be tolerated. Continuous drip feeds are recommended. Bolus feeds should be avoided.
4. Elevate the head of the bed (at least 30 degrees) and check gastric residuals (less than 100 cc every 4 hrs).
5. Metoclopramide (Reglan®) 10 mg IV or PO q 6 h may aid gastric emptying.
6. Most feeds can be started at 40 cc/hr and advanced by 20 cc/hr increments at 12–hr intervals as tolerated.
7. If the infusion is stopped for any prolonged period of time, the tube must be flushed with water in order to prevent clogging.
8. If there is any question about the position of the tube, it should be confirmed radiographically.

F. **Major complications of enteral feeding.**
1. Aspiration pneumonia — can be minimized by jejunal feeding and by precautions indicated under "Administration" below.

2. Feeding intolerance — evidenced by vomiting, abdominal distention, cramping, diarrhea. Treat by decreasing infusion rate or diluting feedings. In obtunded patients, gastric tube feeding is associated with a high mortality due to aspiration pneumonia *unless* extreme vigilance is exercised.
3. Diarrhea — > 5 stools per day.
    a. Minimized by a continuous, appropriate administration schedule, assuming intact GI function and no pancreatic insufficiency; rule out antibiotic–associated colitis.
    b. May be a symptom of too rapid advancement of hyperosmolar feeding.
    c. Minimized by clean technique in formula preparation and administration (avoid bacterial overgrowth in formulation). Time limits on formula life and duration of administration should be observed.
    d. Treatment — depending upon severity, one may either decrease administration rate or add an antidiarrheal agent:
        1) Diphenoxylate (Lomotil®) elixir 2.5–5 mg per GT q 6 h prn (primarily antiperistaltic; watch for atropine effects).
        2) Loperamide (Imodium®) elixir 2–4 mg q 6 h prn (increases small bowel absorption; may be helpful in short gut).
        3) Psyllium seed (Metamucil®) 1 package in 6 oz water bid (bulking agent).
4. Metabolic — in general, the metabolic complications are the same as for parenteral nutrition. Hyperglycemia is due to a continuous glucose infusion and should be treated with frequent, short–acting insulin, or a peripheral drip.
5. Hyperosmotic non–ketotic coma — caused by too many calories and not enough free water to excrete the obligatory renal osmotic load.

V. PARENTERAL NUTRITION
A. Indications.
1. Enteral feeding contraindicated or not tolerated.
2. Presence of malnutrition.
B. Role in primary therapy.
1. Efficacy demonstrated in the following situations:
    a. Gastrointestinal fistulas — allows for total bowel "rest" while providing adequate nutrition. Rate of spontaneous closure is increased, but doesn't affect overall mortality.
    b. Short bowel syndrome — to maintain nutritional status until remaining bowel can undergo hypertrophy. May be required for long–term survival.
    c. Acute tubular necrosis — mortality rate is decreased, with earlier recovery from renal failure. Hypercatabolism of renal failure is met by TPN.

    d. Major burns — enables provision of massive amounts of calories to meet energy requirements in combination with enteral feeding. Must rotate catheter site every 72 hrs to prevent development of catheter sepsis. In contrast to routine hyperalimentation catheter care, catheter should be multipurpose (i.e., used for crystalloid antibiotics, etc.). Can usually provide all caloric needs via enteral nutrition once ileus resolves.

    e. Acute–on–chronic hepatic insufficiency — normalization of amino acid profiles results in improved recovery from hepatic encephalopathy and possibly decreased mortality.

  2. Efficacy not completely established:

    a. Inflammatory bowel disease — Crohn's disease limited to small bowel responds best. Course of ulcerative colitis not affected, but allows for bowel rest and improved post–op course when given prior to ileoanal pull-through operations.

    b. Anorexia nervosa.

C. Supportive therapy.

  1. Efficacy established:

    a. Radiation enteritis.

    b. Acute GI toxicity due to chemotherapeutic agents.

    c. Hyperemesis gravidarum.

  2. Efficacy not yet established:

    a. Preoperative nutritional support for malnourished patients. Studies have shown improvement in metabolic endpoints, but no statistically significant improvement in mortality or complication rate.

    b. Cardiac cachexia.

    c. Pancreatitis.

    d. Respiratory insufficiency with need for prolonged ventilatory support.

    e. Prolonged ileus (> 5 days).

    f. Nitrogen–losing wounds.

D. Indications currently under investigation:

  1. Cancer — generally, nutritional support indicated in patients undergoing antineoplastic therapy (e.g., surgery, radiation, chemotherapy) during times of ileus, GI mucosal damage, etc; goal of nutritional support is for weight **maintenance**, not gain.

  2. Sepsis — some evidence exists concerning use of 45% branched chain amino acid (BCAA) solution to improve hepatic protein synthesis as well as improve septic encephalopathy.

E. Basic composition of formulations (Tables 1 and 2).

  1. Carbohydrate — dextrose used exclusively in U.S. Concentrations range from 15% to 47%.

  2. Amino acids — either balanced or disease–specific (renal, hepatic, stress formulations).

3. Lipid emulsions.
   a. Available as 10% or 20% solutions (1 kcal/cc or 2 kcal/cc, respectively).
   b. Infusion of 1000 ml of 10% solution per week is adequate to prevent essential fatty acid deficiency (EFAD).
   c. Important to check baseline measurements of serum triglycerides to avoid exacerbation of pre–existing hypertriglyceridemia.
   d. Lipid emulsion substituted for carbohydrate calories in certain situations (carbohydrate overfeeding, TPN hepatotoxicity).
   e. Safe to provide up to 25% of total calories as lipid, but never exceed 60%.
4. Minor components (see Table 2).
   a. Vitamins.
   b. Trace elements.
   c. Insulin and electrolytes.

TABLE 1: TPN Solutions — Composition

Type of TPN	Volume (ml)	Amino acids (g) (%)	Dextrose (g) (%)	Non-protein cal. (kcal)	Total cal. (kcal)
Central standard formula	1000	42.5 (4.25%)	250 (25%)	850	1000
Modified base central formula	1000	42.5 (4.25%)	150 (15%)	510	680
Renal formula	750	12.75 (1.7%)	350 (46.6%)	1190	1250
Hepatic formula	1000	30.6 (3.5%)	350 (25%)	1190	990
Stress formula	1000	52 (5.2%)	175 (17.5%)	595	903
Peripheral formula	1000	30 (3%)	50 (5%)	170	300

TABLE 2: Additional Components to TPN Solution

Trace Elements (add to 1st bottle each day):

Zn — 3.0 mg		Stress formula
Cu — 1.2 mg	Se — 60 mg	Hepatic formula
Cr — 12 µg		Modified base central formula
Mn — 0.3 mg		

Vitamins (add to 1st bottle each day): MVI — 12 (1 amp. 10 cc)
Vitamin K (add to 2nd bottle every Monday):
   5 mg (for patients not requiring anticoagulants)

Electrolytes and Insulin:

	Usual	Range
Na+ (mEq/L)	20–50	0–150
K+ (mEq/L)	13–40	0–80
Cl⁻ (mEq/L)	10–27	0–150
Ca++ (mEq/L)	4.7	0–10
Mg++ (mEq/L)	8	0–15
P (mM)	14	0–21
Acetate (mEq/L)	45–81	45–220
Human regular insulin (units/L)	0–25	0–60

Electrolytes may be adjusted as appropriate. Some patients with ongoing electrolyte losses may require up to 140 mEq/L NaCl, 80 mEq/L K+.

F. **Central formulas** — administered via central line into vena cava.
    1. **Standard central formula.**
        a. The majority of patients requiring parenteral nutrition can use this standard formula.
        b. The same formulation can be administered in a modified substrate form which contains 15% dextrose and is designed to have fat emulsion administered daily to substitute for some of the carbohydrate calories. This modified base formulation is used in patients who cannot tolerate a higher glucose load, show evidence of carbohydrate overfeeding, or patients with C.O.P.D. and marginal pulmonary reserve.
    2. **Renal formulation.**
        a. Amino acid source is Nephramine® (essential L-amino acids).
        b. Indicated in patients with acute tubular necrosis who cannot tolerate modest fluid administration and are not suffering from severe hyperkalemia.
        c. Useful in preventing rise in potassium and BUN, and may delay dialysis.
        d. Higher concentration of glucose than central formula; start at lower rate.
        e. Once the patient has been converted to chronic dialysis, parenteral nutrition should be changed to a more balanced formulation (e.g., standard, central or cardiac).
    3. **Cardiac formulation.**
        a. Contains a balanced amino acid protein source in hypertonic dextrose in order to give reduced volume in patients with fluid intolerance.
        b. The similarity in glucose substrate concentration to renal formula makes this a good transition from renal formulation to a balanced amino acid formulation.
    4. **Hepatic formulation.**
        a. 50% of patients with chronic liver disease who present with grade 0 (no encephalopathy) or grade 1 (fluctuating confusion) hepatic encephalopathy will tolerate standard central formulation at low doses, 50–60 g protein equivalent/24 hrs.
        b. Indicated for patients with grade 2 (impending stupor) or greater (3 — stupor, 4 — coma, unresponsive to pain) hepatic encephalopathy or who fail standard central formula.
        c. Efficacy of hepatic formulation has been demonstrated only with glucose as the source of calories.
        d. Hepatic formulation is enriched with 35% BCAA, alanine, arginine, and reduced amounts of aromatic and sulfur-containing amino acids.
    5. **Stress formulation.**
        a. 5% amino acid formulation with 45% BCAA (high in leucine).

    b. Contains dextrose @ 17.5% in response to the decreased calorie : nitrogen requirements and glucose intolerance seen in the stressed patient.

    c. Indicated in critically ill, hypermetabolic, traumatized, or septic patients.

    d. Lipid emulsions may be added as an additional source of calories.

G. Peripheral parenteral nutrition.

    1. Contains 3% amino acids in 5% dextrose.

    2. To provide adequate calorie : nitrogen ratio, the equivalent of 500 ml of 10% lipid emulsion should be administered with each liter of peripheral formulation to a maximum of 100 g fat/day.

    3. Indicated in patients without central venous access or in whom central venous catheterization is contraindicated (*Candida* sepsis, blood dyscrasias, thrombosis).

    4. Difficulties include increased cost and difficulties with venous access due to phlebitis.

    5. Peripheral parenteral nutrition may be indicated for 3–5 days of nutritional support in patients who may not be able to take an adequate oral intake.

    6. Only major advantage is elimination of risks associated with central venous catheterization.

H. Administration.

    1. Central formulation should always be infused through a new line (subclavian).

    2. The tip of the catheter should reside within the innominate vein, preferably SVC (*not* right atrium or subclavian vein !); this should be documented in the patient's chart.

    3. Insertion of this catheter is never an emergency; patient should be stable, well hydrated, and without serious coagulopathy.

I. Subclavian catheter insertion.

J. Infusion.

    1. Rate.

        a. All formulations begin at 40 ml/hr with exception of renal and cardiac formulations, which generally begin at 30 ml/hr due to higher glucose content, and modified formulations, which begin at 60 ml/hr.

        b. Rate increased in increments of 20 ml/hr per day (if blood sugar well controlled) until caloric needs are matched.

        c. With renal and cardiac formulations, advance in increments of 10 ml/hr each day.

    2. With exception of lipid emulsion, the catheter cannot be used for any other infusion of maintenance fluid, medication, blood products, or CVP readings.

K. Monitoring.

    1. Vital signs every 6 hours.

2. Urine S & A's every 6 hours. Fingerstick glucose determinations are more accurate if the patient is glucose intolerant.
3. 24–hour I & O's.
4. Weigh patient every other day.
5. Twice-weekly blood work — electrolytes, glucose, liver enzymes, calcium, phosphorus, PT, PTT, CBC, short–turnover proteins, if available.

L. **Complications.**
   1. **Technical** (placement).
      a. **Pneumothorax** — should occur < 3% of all insertions in elective, well–prepared patients.
      b. Injury to subclavian artery, brachial plexus — avoid by keeping angle of needle path < 10°.
      c. Tip in internal jugular vein — may try to reposition over a Cordis wire or 2–Fr. Fogarty catheter and re-X-ray.
   2. **Late technical** — thrombosis of subclavian vein or SVC.
      a. Clinically silent in up to 35% of patients.
      b. If clinically apparent, treat with:
         1) Local heat.
         2) Remove catheter.
         3) Heparinization until symptoms resolve.
         4) Long–term anticoagulation is usually unneccessary, but should be considered for continued symptoms.
      c. Prophylactic heparin is of little benefit in prevention of thrombosis.
   3. **Septic complications** (see Fig. 1).
      a. Catheter sepsis — clinical sepsis in a patient receiving parenteral nutrition for which no anatomic septic focus is identified, and which resolves following removal of the catheter.
      b. Major source of catheter sepsis is bacteria from the skin around the insertion site of the catheter and, thus, catheter sepsis is best prevented by *meticulous* adherence to dressing change protocols.
   4. **Metabolic complications** (see Table 3).
      a. Disorders of glucose metabolism.
         1) Hyperglycemia (blood sugar > 200 mg/dl).
            a) From either parenteral or tube feeding may lead to hyperosmolar, hyperglycemic, non–ketotic dehydration with shock and death resulting if untreated.
            b) If blood sugar is > 200 mg/dl, the rate of infusion of the formulation should not be increased; S.Q. regular insulin should be administered acutely and the amount of insulin in each liter of solution should be increased appropriately.
            c) If urine glucose 3+ or greater, obtain STAT blood glucose.

2) Hypoglycemia — rare complication.
   a) If TPN is suddenly discontinued for any reason, intravenous administration of any 5% dextrose solution is sufficient to prevent hypoglycemia.
   b) Rarely occurs with endogenous insulin response to very high rates of infusion. Treat by slowing infusion.
b. Liver dysfunction due to excess carbohydrate stored in liver as fat.
c. Deficiency states.
   1) Requirements for electrolytes, vitamins, and trace elements vary according to age, previous nutritional state, disease, and external losses.
   2) As patients become anabolic, there is an increased requirement for intracellular ions (potassium, magnesium, phosphate).
   3) Deficiencies of trace elements and vitamins are generally avoided by the administration (daily) of recommended amounts.

FIGURE 1
Algorithm for Management of Suspected TPN Catheter Sepsis

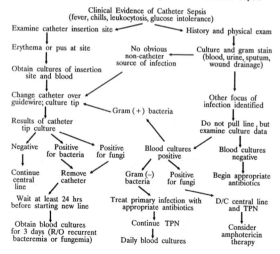

TABLE 3
Metabolic Complications of Intravenous Hyperalimentation

COMPLICATION	ETIOLOGY	TREATMENT
Hyperglycemia (which can progress to hyperosmolar non–ketotic coma)	Excessive rate of glucose administration; inadequate endogenous insulin; increased insulin needs secondary to glucocorticoids or infection	Start subcutaneous insulin based on capillary blood sugars q6h; add insulin to hyperalimentation solution after needs are established
Metabolic acidosis	Excessive chloride content of amino acid solutions or added sodium chloride; excessive base or bicarbonate loss unrelated to solution (e.g., pancreatic fistula)	
Hypophosphatemia	Inadequate administration	Add phosphate as potassium or sodium salt
Hyperphosphatemia	Excessive phosphorus administration or inability to excrete phosphorus, as in renal failure	Reduce or eliminate phosphorus in solutions
Hyperkalemia	Excessive administration or inability to excrete potassium, as in renal failure	Reduce or eliminate potassium
Hypokalemia	Inadequate administration or increased losses due to excretion (stool or urine) or anabolism	Add potassium
Hypercalcemia	Excessive calcium or vitamin D administration	Reduce vitamin D or calcium
Hypocalcemia	Inadequate calcium administration or excessive phosphorus administration, particularly in osteomalacia	Increase calcium administration
Hypermagnesemia	Excessive magnesium administration, especially with renal impairment	Reduce or eliminate magnesium
Hypomagnesemia	Inadequate provision of magnesium, particularly in anabolic situations	Appropriate supplementation
Essential fatty acid deficiency	Continuous feeding of hypertonic dextrose or true deficiency from prolonged severe malnutrition (rare)	IV fat emulsion or cyclic hyperalimentation for first, IV fat emulsion for second
Azotemia	Excessive amino acid administration or reduced renal function	Reduce amino acid load
Elevation in liver enzymes	Continuous infusion of glucose (? essential fatty acid deficiency)	Cyclic hyperalimentation Intralipid® or Liposyn® daily
Anemia	Excessive diagnostic blood tests; inadequate iron, copper, B_{12}, folate, protein replacement	Limit phlebotomies; appropriate supplements
Rare deficiencies (copper, zinc, chromium)	Inadequate administration	Appropriate replacement

Ref: Hardy SP. Hardy's *Textbook of Surgery*. Philadelphia: JB Lippincott, 1983, p. 103, with permission.

ANESTHESIA

While most patients are seen preoperatively by an anesthetist or anesthesiologist, the surgeon should generally be familiar with anesthesia and its influence on surgical patients. Such knowledge is helpful in emergency situations and allows the surgeon to better prepare the patient. Many ancillary local techniques are commonly used by the surgeon.

I. **PREOPERATIVE ASSESSMENT AND PREPARATION**
A. American Society of Anesthesiologists classification (Dripps Classification) (see "Preoperative Preparation" section II. C.).
B. Indications for delaying or postponing surgery (see "Preoperative Preparation").
   1. Uncontrolled medical disease (cardiac, respiratory, hepatic, renal, endocrine).
   2. Upper respiratory infection.
   3. Improper resuscitation prior to emergency surgery.
   4. Recent food ingestion (commonly wait 6 hours after ingestion).
   5. No informed consent.
C. **Preoperative medication** — usually ordered by anesthesiologist.
   1. Goals of preoperative medication.
      a. Anxiety relief.
      b. Sedation.
      c. Analgesia.
      d. Amnesia.
      e. Antisialagogue effect.
      f. Increase gastric fluid pH and decrease fluid volume.
      g. Prophylaxis against allergic reactions.
   2. Principles of preoperative medication.
      a. Use a combination of 2 or more drugs in low doses (e.g., meperidine, diazepam, ranitidine).
      b. Sedative effect of narcotics, tranquilizers, or barbiturates in low doses.
      c. Decrease anesthetic needs.
      d. Anticholinergics reduce secretions and vagal activity.

II. **MUSCLE RELAXANTS**
A. Achieves skeletal muscle relaxation without deep levels of anesthesia. Depolarizing agents mimic the action of acetylcholine, while non–depolarizing agents compete for cholinergic receptors on the post–synaptic membrane. The choice of an agent depends upon the desired duration of effect and the potential side–effects, particularly cardiovascular. The degree of neuromuscular blockade is assessed by electrical stimulation of peripheral motor nerves.
B. **Depolarizing agents.**
   1. **Succinylcholine** [Anectine®] — dose: 1 mg/kg.

    a. Onset of action: 1 min; duration: 5–15 min.
    b. Most commonly used agent.
    c. Side–effects — may cause hyperkalemia in cases of severe muscle damage (i.e., burns, crush injury). Can cause bradycardia and hypotension, post–op muscle pain (secondary to fasciculations). May cause malignant hyperthermia in combination with inhalational agent.
    d. *Contraindicated* in eye injury due to increased intraocular pressure.

C. Non-depolarizing agents.
    1. d–Tubocurarine — dose: 0.5 mg/kg.
       a. Onset of action: 5–8 min; duration: 30–90 min.
       b. Undergoes hepatic degradation, useful in patients with renal failure.
       c. Side–effects — may cause bronchospasm and hypotension due to histamine release and ganglionic blockade.
    2. Pancuronium [Pavulon®] — dose: 0.04–0.1 mg/kg.
       a. Onset of action: 2–3 min; duration: 30–90 min.
       b. Side–effects — interacts with halothane to increase ventricular irritability. May cause **tachycardia** and **hypertension** due to vagolytic effect.
    3. Atracurium [Tracrium®] — dose: 0.4–0.5 mg/kg.
       a. Onset of action: 2–3 min; duration: 20–40 min.
       b. Side–effects — less histamine release than d–tubocurarine and pancuronium. No cumulative effect.
    4. Vecuronium [Norcuron®] — dose: 0.1-0.2 mg/kg.
       a. Onset of action: 2–3 min; duration: 20–40 min.
       b. Very little histamine release, less cardiovascular effects than other neuromuscular blocking agents.

D. Reversal of neuromuscular blockade — non–depolarizing agents can be antagonized by anticholinesterase drugs. Atropine (0.6–1.2 mg) or glycopyrrolate should be added to block muscarinic side–effects (salivation, bronchospasm and bradycardia).
    1. Edrophonium — dose: 10 mg slow IV.
    2. Neostigmine [Prostigmine®] — dose: 0.5–2 mg slow IV.
    3. Pyridostigmine — dose: 10 mg slow IV.

III. INTRAVENOUS ANESTHESIA

A. May be used as induction agents, supplemental anesthesia agents, or as the sole anesthetic agent. Does not have the reversibility of inhalational anesthetics, and has no effect on skeletal muscle relaxation.

B. Ultrashort–acting barbiturates.
    1. Thiopental [Pentothal®] — dose: 4–7 mg/kg over 30–45 sec.
       a. Onset: immediate; duration: awakening may occur in 5–10 min due to redistribution. Often used for induction.

    b. Side–effects — causes myocardial depression and peripheral vasodilatation; use with caution in patients with coronary artery disease and shock. Induces histamine release. Decreases cerebral flow and intracranial pressure.

  2. Methohexital [Brevital®] — dose: 1 mg/kg.

    a. Onset: immediate. Often used for induction and intubation, but respiratory depression may be prolonged.

    b. Side–effects — myocardial depression, significant hypotension. *Contraindicated* in patients with **porphyrias**.

C. Ketamine [Ketalar®] — dose 6–12 mg/kg IM, 1–3 mg/kg IV.

  1. Dissociative anesthetic with good analgesia. Minimal respiratory depression, maintains hypoxic pulmonary vasoconstrictive reflexes. Does not relieve visceral sensation. Useful in burn, pediatric and thoracic surgery.

  2. Side–effects — causes tachycardia, hypertension, increased cardiac output and myocardial oxygen demand. Emergence hallucinations, can be avoided by pretreatment with benzodiazepine.

D. Benzodiazepines — very little analgesic effect; produces good amnesia, and depending upon dose and route of administration, can produce a range of consciousness from sedation to unconsciousness.

  1. Diazepam [Valium®] — dose: 10 mg IM 1–2 hrs pre–op; or 5–10 mg slow IVP (do not exceed 2.5 mg/min) for sedation.

    a. Useful as pre–op medication, or sedation for endoscopic or minor surgical procedures. Use cautiously in elderly or cachectic patients.

    b. Side–effects — respiratory depression, disorientation, unpredictable IM absorption.

  2. Midazolam [Versed®] — dose: 0.07–0.08 mg/kg deep IM 1–2 hrs pre–op; or 0.07–0.1 mg/kg IV for sedation.

    a. Short duration of action. Useful as pre–op medication, or for minor surgical procedures. Use cautiously in elderly patients (reduce dose by 1/2). Water soluble, predictable IM absorption.

  3. Lorazepam [Ativan®] — dose: 0.05 mg/kg deep IM up to 4 mg; 2 hrs pre–op. Recommended in liver disease; more predictable IM absorption than diazepam.

E. Narcotics — useful in high doses as sole anesthetic agent.

  1. Fentanyl [Sublimaze®] — dose: 0.04 mg/kg IV.

    a. Short–acting agent, 50 times more potent than morphine. Minimal myocardial effect. Useful in cardiac surgery.

    b. Side–effects — dose–related respiratory depression, increased muscle tone, occasional truncal rigidity ("wooden chest").

    c. Reversible with **naloxone** [Narcan®] 0.04 mg IVP. **Caution:** short half–life of naloxone can result in return of opioid effect; analgesic effects will also be reversed.

F. **Neuroleptanalgesia.**
1. Combination of tranquilizer and narcotic analgesic.
2. **Droperidol + fentanyl** [Innovar®] (50:1) — preanesthetic used in conjunction with general anesthetic.
3. Amnesia, analgesia and somnolence without complete unconsciousness.

G. **Balanced anesthesia.**
1. Combination of IV drugs to produce amnesia, analgesia, sedation and muscular relaxation.
2. Rapid onset of unconsciousness.
3. Advantageous by giving smaller doses of several drugs; avoid major side–effects of any one drug.
4. Difficult to monitor degree and duration of anesthesia and multiple drug interactions.

IV. **INHALATIONAL ANESTHESIA**

A. Induction is achieved via short–acting barbiturate or inhalation of O_2–anesthetic mixture.
1. Well controlled, closely monitored, easily reversed.
2. **MAC (Minimum Alveolar Concentration)** — the best expression of the potency of inhalation agents. The MAC is the minimum alveolar concentration that prevents 50% of patients from responding by movement to a skin incision.
3. Rapidity of induction of inhalation anesthesia depends upon inspired concentration, volume of pulmonary ventilation, solubility of the agent in blood, and cardiac output clearing the agent from the alveoli.

B. **Nitrous oxide** (MAC > 100%).
1. The most commonly used. Nonflammable, odorless (good patient acceptability). Rapid recovery, quickly reversible, low potency, but a potentiator of other inhalational anesthetics or narcotics (diminished amounts of other agents). Causes increased peripheral resistance and cardiac depression.
2. Complications:
a. **Diffusion anoxia** — O_2 administration post–op to prevent hypoxia.
b. Expansion of air–filled cavities, e.g., bowel (dangerous in bowel obstruction), pneumothorax.

C. **Halothane** [Fluothane®] (MAC = 75%).
1. Potent, rapid onset of action. Bronchial smooth muscle relaxant (excellent for asthmatics).
2. Complications:
a. Myocardial depression, profound hypotension.
b. Sensitized myocardia to catecholamines with increased risk of **ventricular arrhythmias.**
c. Potent vasodilator — increased cerebral perfusion and intracranial pressure (harmful with CNS space occupying lesions).

    d. Halothane hepatitis (accumulative with repeat exposures)
— marked by elevation of LFT's 2 to 5 days post–op and
preceded by fever and eosinophilia. More likely in females.
D. Enflurane [Ethrane®] (MAC = 120%).
1. Rapid induction, quick recovery, has profound muscle relaxation.
2. Complications:
    a. Similar cardiovascular effects as with halothane, yet less
likely to produce arrhythmias.
    b. Potential to elicit grand mal seizures at high MAC with
hyperventilation.
E. Isoflurane [Forane®] (MAC = 130%).
1. Potent muscle relaxant, with minimal hepatic, CNS, or renal
impairment. Less cardiovascular depression than enflurane or
halothane.
2. Complications — increased incidence of coughing and **laryngo-
spasm.**

V. MALIGNANT HYPERTHERMIA

A. 1 : 50,000 adults, 1 : 15,000 children — highest incidence in young,
athletic males. A genetic predisposition exists. **Halothane** and
succinylcholine are most often involved, but may occur with all
anesthetic agents. May occur during induction, anesthesia, or post–
op.
B. Clinical signs — be suspicious of:
1. Masseter rigidity occurs following succinylcholine administration.
2. Unexplained tachycardia.
3. Arrhythmias.
4. Tachypnea.
5. Dark blood in surgical field.
6. Fever is a *late* sign (may reach 107°F).
7. Cyanosis.
8. Development of metabolic or respiratory acidosis.
C. Treatment.
1. Discontinue anesthetic agent and change all tubing.
2. Hyperventilate with 100% O_2.
3. **Dantrolene sodium** (1–10 mg/kg) — treatment of choice, can
also be used prophylactically with suspected family history.
4. $NaHCO_3$ — for severe metabolic and respiratory acidosis.
5. Iced cooling of IV fluids and patient.
6. Procainamide 1 g IV — effective in arresting "runaway" metabolism.
D. Late complications.
1. Consumptive coagulopathy.
2. Acute renal failure.
3. Hypothermia.
4. Pulmonary edema.
5. Skeletal muscle swelling.

6. Neurologic sequelae.
7. Suspected family members should undergo evaluation.

VI. LOCAL ANESTHETICS

A. Local analgesia/anesthesia without risks of general anesthesia. Used in spinal, regional and local anesthesia.
B. **Limit** total anesthetic dose to prevent seizures.
   1. Add vasoconstrictor to slow vascular absorption.
   2. Avoid inadvertent vascular injection by pre–injection aspiration.
   3. Impending toxicity — muscle twitching, restlessness, sleepiness.
   4. Treatment of toxicity — Trendelenburg position, O$_2$, IV Valium® (5–10 mg), Thiopental® (50–100 mg).
C. **Never** inject solutions containing epinephrine into digits, ear, tip of nose, or penis because of ischemic risk.
D. **Commonly used local anesthetics:**

Generic name	Trade name	Maximum dose avg. (mg/kg)	adult (mg)	Duration (hrs)
procaine	Novocaine®, Planocaine®	14	1000	0.5
lidocaine	Xylocaine®, Xylotox®	7	500	1-2
mepivacaine	Carbocaine®	7	500	1-2
tetracaine	Pontocaine®, Pantocaine®	1.5	100	2-3
bupivacaine	Marcaine®	3	225	5-7

E. For most local procedures, 0.5% Xylocaine® or Carbocaine® is usually sufficient.

VII. SPINAL ANESTHESIA

A. Injection of local anesthetic into subarachnoid space.
   1. Order of blockade — preganglionic sympathetic fibers, somatic sensory fibers, somatic motor fibers.
   2. Denervation can extend about 2 spinal segments above the anesthetic areas.
B. **Level of anesthesia** is controlled by specific gravity of injected mixture (hyperbaric solution, e.g., D$_{10}$W) and adjusting Trendelenburg position.
C. Best for procedures below the umbilicus.
   1. L1 dermatome — pubic crest.
   2. T10 dermatome — umbilicus.
   3. T6 dermatome — xiphoid.
   4. T4 dermatome — nipple.
D. **Complications:**
   1. Diminished sympathetic tone, vasodilatation, hypotension, and decreased cardiac output.

2. **Spinal headache** produced by leakage of CSF from puncture site occurring about 36–48 hrs post spinal puncture.
   a. Most frequent after use of large–bore spinal needles. Uncommon when finer needles used.
   b. May last for weeks.
   c. Treatment — bedrest, prone position, IV hydration, "epidural blood patch" (5–10 cc patient's blood injected into epidural space).
3. Intercostal paralysis if agent extends into thoracic area.
4. Total spinal (above C3) block of all intercostal and phrenic nerves, requires ventilatory and hemodynamic support.
5. Urinary retention.
E. **Contraindication** — coagulopathy.

VIII. EPIDURAL ANESTHESIA

A. **Epidural space.**
   1. Bordered by the dura mater internally and the spinal canal periosteum.
   2. Contains fat and blood vessels.
   3. Opioid receptors in spinal cord allow opioid epidural administration for acute/chronic pain states.
B. Anesthetic injection blocks sympathetic/parasympathetic ganglia and motor/sensory impulses.
C. Less dependent on position of patient than spinal anesthesia.
D. Larger amounts of local anesthetic required (*vs.* spinal).
E. **Surgical advantages.**
   1. Blockade of all nerve functions without requirements for endotracheal intubation.
   2. In combination with light general anesthesia, lessens post–op complications.
   3. Better post–op pain control with maintenance of spontaneous breathing and upper airway reflexes.
F. **Surgical disadvantages.**
   1. Profound hypotension if block above T5.
   2. Infection of indwelling catheter (especially immunocompromised patients).
   3. Respiratory depression (especially epidural opioid administration). May last much longer than equivalent IV dose.
   4. More demanding technically.
   5. 5–10 times more drug required.
   6. Urinary retention.
   7. CNS toxicity.
   8. Blood coagulopathies are a *contraindication* due to potential epidural hematoma.

IX. CAUDAL ANESTHESIA

A. Injection at S5 through sacrococcygeal membrane.

B. No spinal headache.
C. Continuous anesthesia for long procedures; useful for rectal surgery.
D. Similar degree of hypotension as with spinal anesthetic, yet lessened amount of motor paralysis.

X. REGIONAL NERVE BLOCKS

A. **Cervical block** (anterior divisions of C1 – C4).
   1. Provides anesthesia in anterior / posterior cervical triangles between jaw and clavicles with relaxation of strap musculature.
   2. Lateral approach – injection at midpoint of posterior border of SCM to anesthetize superficial cervical plexus. Fan out with 10–20 cc 1% lidocaine.
   3. 2nd, 3rd, and 4th nerves individually blocked at anterior tubercles of transverse processes using 5 cc 1% lidocaine at 4th process just above midpoint of posterior border of SCM where external jugular crosses the muscle.
   4. **Note:** Cervical block also blocks phrenic nerve. Bilateral block will produce phrenic paralysis → hypoventilation → **disaster!**
B. **Intercostal block** (12 thoracic nerves) [Figs. 1 & 2].

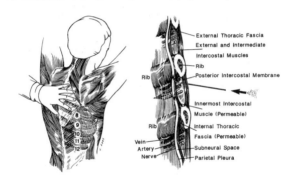

External Thoracic Fascia
External and Intermediate Intercostal Muscles
Rib
Posterior Intercostal Membrane
Innermost Intercostal Muscle (Permeable)
Internal Thoracic Fascia (Permeable)
Subneural Space
Parietal Pleura
Rib
Rib
Vein
Artery
Nerve

FIGURE 1   FIGURE 2

   1. Intercostal nerve courses from intervertebral foramen to rib angle along subcostal groove: nerve–inferior, artery–middle, vein–superior.
   2. May also provide anesthesia of abdominal wall (T5 – T11 must be blocked).

3. Technique.
   a. Prone position for bilateral block; lateral position for unilateral block.
   b. Insert needle over selected rib at 5 cm from posterior midline until needle point touches rib. Walk down rib (2–3 cm); aspirate (no air or blood); inject 3–4 cc 1% lidocaine.
   c. For successful intercostal space block, 3 intercostal nerves (one on each side) must be anesthetized.
C. **Wrist and hand blocks** [Figs. 3–6].
   1. Hand procedures may be performed through blockage of the median, ulnar and radial nerves, or with wrist bracelet infiltration. Minor procedures in digits can be accomplished using a digital block.
   2. General considerations:
      a. Always complete the sensory exam prior to injection.
      b. Do *not* use epinephrine or inject into an infected area.
      c. Always aspirate prior to injection to avoid intra–arterial infection.
   3. **Median nerve** — located between tendons of palmaris longus (PL) and flexor carpi radialis (FCR) with wrist flexed. Enter 2 cm proximal to the distal crease and just radial to the PL tendon or 1 cm ulnad of the FCR tendon. Penetrate to a length of 1 cm and inject 5 cc 1% lidocaine (Figs. 3 & 4).
   4. **Ulnar nerve** — medial to ulnar artery and lateral to flexor carpi ulnaris (FCU). Enter to the ulnar side of the FCU and just proximal to the pisiform bone, aiming about 1.5 cm below tendon. Aspirate, then inject 5 cc 1% lidocaine (Figs. 3 & 4).
   5. **Radial nerve** — superficial branch of radial nerve located in anatomical snuff box; inject 5 cc 1% lidocaine in snuff box (Figs. 3–5).
   6. **Wrist bracelet** —achieved by individual block of median, ulnar and radial nerves and subcutaneous infiltration of wrist circumferentially.
   7. **Digital block** — inject 1–2 cc 1% lidocaine into web space just dorsal to palmar (plantar) and dorsal skin junction. Then redirect needle dorsally and inject additional 1 cc to include dorsal branch. Avoid circumferential injections in the digits (Figs. 3 & 6).
D. **Femoral nerve block.**
   1. Level below inguinal ligament.
   2. NAV (nerve–artery–vein) — lateral to medial.
   3. Lateral to artery with 5–10 cc 1% lidocaine.
   4. Most combine lateral femoral cutaneous nerve block (L2, L3) — beneath inguinal ligament, just medial to anterior superior iliac spine (fanwise) with 5–10 cc 1% lidocaine.

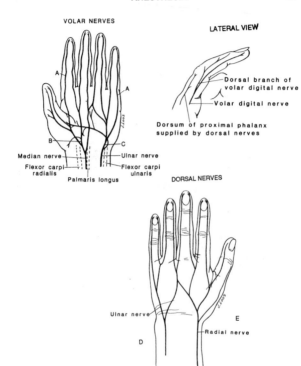

FIGURE 3

Anatomy of sensory nerve blocks and sites for injection:
A, volar digital nerve; B, median nerve; C, ulnar nerve; D,
dorsal branch of ulnar nerve; E, dorsal branch of radial nerve.

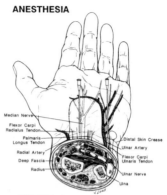

Median Nerve
Flexor Carpi Radialus Tendon
Palmaris Longus Tendon
Radial Artery
Deep Fascia
Radius
Distal Skin Crease
Ulnar Artery
Flexor Carpi Ulnaris Tendon
Ulnar Nerve
Ulna

FIGURE 4

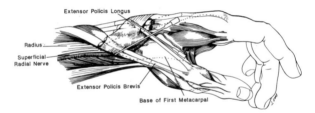

Extensor Policis Longus
Radius
Superficial Radial Nerve
Extensor Policis Brevis
Base of First Metacarpal

FIGURE 5

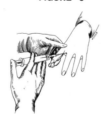

FIGURE 6

E. **Ankle nerve block.**
1. Must block anterior/posterior tibial nerves.
2. Knee flexed with sole of foot on table.
3. Anterior tibial nerve located between tendons of tibialis anticus and extensor hallucis longus, with liberal infiltration of 1% lidocaine.
4. Posterior tibial nerve located medial to calcaneous tendon, lidocaine as above.
5. Add superficial "bracelet" cutaneous block and posterolateral compartment block (deep infiltration) for sural nerve block.

F. **Bier block** (intravenous regional anesthesia).
1. Excellent for forearm, hand or foot procedures.
2. Usually limited to 1 hr.
3. Double pneumatic tourniquet applied above elbow (calf).
4. Initially inflate above venous pressure to distend vein, venipuncture with 22–gauge IV.
5. Release tourniquet, exsanguinate extremity with elevation and wrap with elastic bandage, inflate distal tourniquet then proximal tourniquet, then release distal tourniquet ($>$ 100 mm Hg above arterial).
6. 0.5% lidocaine injection IV 3 mg/kg.
7. With onset of tourniquet pain (at 45 min), inflate distal tourniquet and release proximal tourniquet for slow release of lidocaine into systemic circulation.

References

P. Prithvi Raj: *Handbook of Regional Anesthesia*. New York: Churchill Livingstone, 1985.

J. Adriani: *Labat's Regional Anesthesia – Techniques and Clinical Applications*. St. Louis, MO: W.H. Green, 1985.

XI. **LOCAL ANESTHESIA FOR INGUINAL / FEMORAL HERNIA REPAIR (7 STEPS)**

A. Intraepidermal wheal 2–3 cm above and slightly lateral to anterior superior iliac spine (Fig. 7). At least 5 cc of anesthetic injected superiorly, horizontally and inferiorly (fanwise) deep to the external oblique muscle to anesthetize the ilioinguinal and iliohypogastric nerves which lie deep to the external and internal oblique muscles (Fig. 7).

B. Anesthetic injected subcutaneously and intradermally in a medial direction toward the umbilicus (anesthetize the 11th thoracic nerve), inferiorly toward the anterior superior iliac spine and obliquely in the direction of the proposed line of incision (Fig. 8).

C. Multiple injections of small amounts are placed just under the external oblique fascia (Fig. 9).

D. Injections about the base of the spermatic cord (Fig. 10).

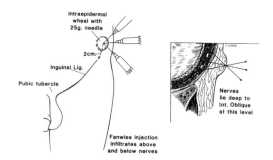

FIGURE 7

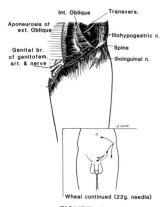

FIGURE 8

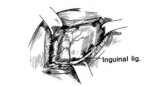

FIGURE 9

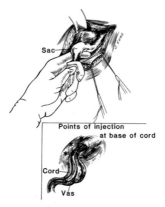

FIGURE 10

E. 3-5 cc of anesthetic injected into the pubic tubercle and in the area in proximity to Cooper's ligament (Fig. 11).

F. Injections of the peritoneal sac under direct vision (Fig. 12).

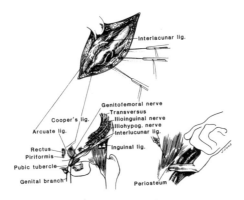

FIGURE 11

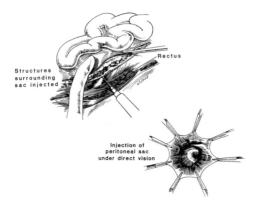

FIGURE 12

XII. ACUTE POSTOPERATIVE PAIN MANAGEMENT

A. **Patient–controlled analgesia (PCA).**
   1. Allows patient to self–administer narcotics with a programmable infusion pump.
   2. Attempts to provide optimal pain relief and safety by avoiding peak and trough levels out of the therapeutic range caused by delays in administration, improper dosage, and pharmacokinetic and pharmacodynamic variability.
   3. Pumps are programmable to be able to deliver on demand intermittent boluses, continuous infusion, or a continuous background infusion with intermittent bolus doses.
   4. The time interval between doses, dose, and/or infusion rate are determined by the physician.
   5. Morphine and meperidine are used often for intermittent dosing because of an intermediate duration of action. Typical morphine bolus doses are 0.5–3.0 mg with a 5–20 minute lockout interval.
   6. A loading dose is administered post–op in the recovery room prior to starting PCA therapy. When fully awake, the patient is given the control button. If the initial dose is inadequate or causes excessive drowsiness, the subsequent doses are increased or decreased accordingly.
   7. Bolus doses and/or infusion rates are often increased at night to provide more sedation and rest.
   8. Potential complications are respiratory depression, tolerance, physical dependence, nausea, vomiting, and pruritis.
B. **Intrathecal analgesia.**
   1. Provides short–term analgesia (24 hours).
   2. Morphine is drug of choice. Dosage is 0.5 mg or less.
   3. Local anesthetics are not used because of a shorter duration of action and dose–dependent side–effects of hypotension and motor block.
   4. Limited to single–dose administration by risk of spinal headache and nerve damage from multiple punctures.
   5. Side–effects are respiratory depression, nausea and vomiting.
C. **Epidural analgesia** — attempts to provide pain relief without high systemic levels and side–effects of analgesics. Narcotics or local anesthetics can be used.
   1. Advantages.
      a. Prevents muscle spasm and splinting, avoiding pulmonary complications.
      b. Less sedation allows earlier ambulation.
      c. Earlier return of GI function postoperatively.
      d. Excellent for patients with rib fractures, especially those with pulmonary contusion.
   2. Catheter tip placed at vertebral level corresponding to targeted dermatome.
   3. Narcotic analgesics.

     a. Effect is most likely by direct action on spinal cord.
     b. Number of nerve roots involved affected by lipid solubility, infusion rate (continuous infusion), and volume of dose (intermittent dosing).
     c. Narcotics with poor lipid solubility (morphine) have greater nerve root spread, slower onset of action and longer duration of action.
     d. Side–effects are respiratory depression, pruritis, nausea, vomiting, and urinary retention.
     e. Relative contraindication in COPD.

4. Local anesthetics.
     a. Blocks conduction and operation of nerve impulses of spinal nerves and of spinal cord.
     b. Number of nerve roots involved affected by infusion rate or volume of intermittent dose.
     c. Bupivacaine used most frequently because of rapid onset of action, good analgesia, long duration, and absence of motor block.
     d. Side–effects are hypotension, motor block, systemic toxicity and urinary retention. Epidural blocks above T5 can cause decreased BP, SV, CO, and TPR.
     e. Contraindications are severe heart disease, shock, and hypovolemia.

5. Dosing.
     a. Intermittent dosing causes peak systemic levels above those required for analgesia, causing more side–effects.
     b. Continuous infusion prevents peaks and troughs of intermittent dosing. Side–effects occur slowly over time.
     c. Combining infusions of local anesthetics and narcotics lowers the total dose of each, reducing the chance of side–effects.
     d. Continuous infusion of local anesthetics should be weaned off slowly over 2–4 hours as increased fluid mobilization secondary to vasoconstriction can occasionally cause pulmonary edema.

PREOPERATIVE PREPARATION

The preparation of the patient for surgery begins with establishing a diagnosis and determining the course of surgical management. This requires thoughtful consideration of both the risks and benefits of a contemplated operation. Much of preoperative care involves optimizing the patient's physiologic status and taking steps to prevent peri– and postoperative complications.

I. NEED FOR OPERATION

A. **Determine relative risks and benefits of surgery.** Requires consideration of:
   1. Natural history of disease if left untreated.
   2. Benefit of surgical therapy *vs.* medical therapy.
   3. Urgency of operation – may limit the amount of time available for preoperative preparation.
   4. Patient's physiologic reserve and overall ability to undergo anesthesia and operation.

II. ASSESSING OPERATIVE RISK

The age, preoperative physiologic status, and urgency and magnitude of the planned operation are major determinants of operative morbidity and mortality.

A. Age.
   1. Elderly patients often have either limited reserve or impaired function of the major organ systems: cardiovascular, pulmonary, renal, hepatic, and immunologic.
   2. True even for "healthy" septuagenarian –"There is nothing like an operation or an injury to bring a patient up to chronological age" (W.R. Howe).

B. Urgency of operation – in one study, emergent nature of surgery **doubled** risk of **operative mortality** in low– and moderate–risk patients.

C. **Organ system dysfunction** – impairment of more than one organ system, disease severity, and adequacy of control profoundly influences risk of operative mortality. American Society of Anesthesiologists classification of physical status (**Dripps–ASA Scale**):
   1. ASA I – healthy individual with no systemic disease, undergoing elective surgery; patient not at extremes of age.
   2. ASA II – individual with one–system, well–controlled disease. Disease does not affect daily activities. Other anesthetic risk factors, including mild obesity, alcoholism and smoking incorporated at this level.
   3. ASA III – individual with multiple system disease or well–controlled major system disease. Disease status limits daily activity.

4. ASA IV — an individual with severe, incapacitating disease. Normally, disease state is poorly controlled or end–stage. Danger of death due to organ failure is always present.
5. ASA V — patient in imminent danger of death. Operation is last resort attempt at preserving life. Patient with little chance for survival. Always an emergency procedure.
6. Each class above may be subclassified with an "E" denoting emergency procedure.

Relation of Physical Status to Anesthetic Mortality
Anesthetic Mortality

Physical status (ASA Classification)	# Patients	# Deaths	Ratio deaths/ patients
I	16,192	0	0/16,000
II	12,154	7	1/1740
III	4,070	11	1/370
IV	720	17	1/40
V	87	4	1/20

Adapted from Dripps RD, Lamont A, and Eckenhoff JE: *J.A.M.A.*, Vol. 178, No. 3, p. 216, with permission. Copyright 1961, American Medical Association.

D. The following conditions identify those patients at risk for increased perioperative and postoperative morbidity and mortality:
   1. Cardiovascular (see Goldman Criteria below) — coronary artery disease; congestive heart failure; presence of arrhythmias; vascular heart disease; or severe hypertension.
   2. Respiratory (see "Respiratory Care" section III) — smoking history > 20 pack–years; morbid obesity; pre–existing pulmonary disease (pO_2 < 60 mmHg; pCO_2 ≥ 50 mmHg; FEV_1/FVC < 70%); thoracic or upper abdominal surgery; pulmonary hypertension.
   3. Renal — renal insufficiency (BUN ≥ 50 mg/dl; creatinine > 3.0 mg/dl); highest risk in **acute** renal failure.
   4. Hepatic — cirrhosis, hepatitis (see "Cirrhosis").
   5. Endocrine — diabetes mellitus; steroid therapy (adrenal insufficiency); hyper– or hypothyroidism.
   6. Hematologic — anemia, leukopenia, thrombocytopenia, coagulopathy.
E. Risk for cardiac complications in non–cardiac surgery (**Goldman criteria**).
   1. Computation of the cardiac risk index.

Computation of Cardiac Risk Index

Item	Points
History	
Age > 70	5
MI within 6 months	10
Physical	
S3 gallop or JVD	11
Important valvular aortic stenosis	3
Electrocardiogram	
Rhythm other than sinus or PACs on preoperative ECG	7
More than 5 PVCs per min at any time prior to surgery	7
Poor general medical status	3
$PO_2 < 60$ or $PCO_2 > 50$	
$K^+ < 3.0$ or $HCO_3^- < 20$ mEq/L	
BUN > 50 or creatinine > 3 mg/dl	
Abnormal SGOT	
Chronic liver disease	
Bedridden due to non–cardiac cause	
Operation	
Intraperitoneal, intrathoracic, aortic surgery	3
Emergency surgery	4
Total Points	**53**

2. Risks of cardiac complications in unselected patients over age 40 years who underwent major non–cardiac surgery:

Class by Cardiac Risk Index	Point Total	No or Only Minor Complication (n=2048)	Life-Threatening Complication (n=60)	Cardiac Deaths (n=33)
I (n=1127)	0 - 5	1118 (99%)	7 (0.6%)	2 (0.2%)
II (n=769)	6 - 12	735 (96%)	25 (3%)	9 (1%)
III (n=204)	13 - 25	175 (86%)	23 (11%)	6 (3%)
IV (n=41)	≥ 26	20 (49%)	5 (12%)	16 (39%)

Ref: Adapted from Goldman L, et al: *N. Engl. J. Med.* 297:845, 1977. Reprinted by permission of *New England Journal of Medicine*.

3. General concepts.
   a. Class III and IV patients warrant routine preoperative consultation.
   b. Class IV — life–saving procedures only.
   c. 28 of the 53 points are potentially correctable preoperatively.
   d. Index correctly classified 81% of the cardiac outcomes.
   e. Criticisms — cardiac risks only and based on mixed patient population (e.g., vascular patients have higher morbidity and mortality).

III. INTERVENTION TO REDUCE OPERATIVE RISK

A. Emergent operations — procedure should not be delayed for most situations. **Note:** Volume–depleted patients (e.g., those with intestinal obstruction, peritonitis, perforated viscus, etc.) should undergo fluid and electrolyte repletion *prior* to operation.

B. Cardiovascular.

1. **Coronary artery disease** (CAD) — history of angina or previous MI increases risk for new MI or sudden death. Risk of MI following recent infarction:

	Steen (1978)	Rao (1983)
0–3 months	27%	5.8%
4–6 months	11%	2.3%
> 6 months	5%	1%

   a. Suspected CAD should be evaluated by EKG, exercise thallium scan or dipyridamole thallium scan and MUGA. Coronary angiography may be indicated.
   b. Coronary artery bypass grafting has been shown to decrease risk of post-op MI.
   c. Patients with severe disease should undergo major operations with perioperative Swan–Ganz monitoring to assess cardiac output and filling pressures (see "Cardiac and Hemodynamic Monitoring").

2. **Congestive heart failure** (CHF) — risk factors for post–op CHF are CAD, elderly patients, and major operations.
   a. Pre–existing CHF should be optimally controlled (e.g., diuretics, digoxin).
   b. Preoperative Swan–Ganz monitoring recommended to guide manipulation of hemodynamic performance (i.e., fluids, inotropes, vasodilators) and guide perioperative fluid management.

3. **Arrhythmias** — optimal medical control required prior to operation (see "Cardiac and Hemodynamic Monitoring"). High grade block and bradyarrhythmias may require temporary or permanent pacing prior to operation.

4. **Valvular heart disease** — management of CHF and arrhythmias same as above (also see section VI below).

5. **Hypertension** (HTN) — no increased risk for non–labile mild HTN and diastolic blood pressure (DBP) < 110 mmHg.
   a. Anti–hypertensive agent should be continued to time of surgery, except monoamine oxidase inhibitors (should discontinue 2 weeks before surgery).
   b. New onset HTN; DBP > 110 mmHg, SBP > 250 mmHg; or suspicion of unusual causes of HTN should lead to further work–up and treatment.

        c. Should check for evidence of end–organ deterioration (e.g., renal insufficiency, CHF).

C. **Respiratory.**
1. Discontinue smoking as long before surgery as possible. May take up to **8 weeks** to decrease risk of pulmonary complications.
2. ABG, pulmonary function tests for suspected or documented pulmonary disease or patients undergoing thoracic surgery.
3. Initiate or continue use of bronchodilators (e.g., inhalants, theophylline) for patients with bronchospastic disease (COPD or asthma).
4. Utilize chest physiotherapy as indicated; initiate incentive spirometry and cough, deep breathing exercises **preoperatively.**
5. Pneumonia, bronchitis – delay elective surgery; treat with pulmonary toilet and antibiotics.
6. Swan–Ganz monitoring – consider use perioperatively for fluid management.

D. **Renal.**
1. Reduce azotemia – peritoneal or hemodialysis, maintenance of nutrition.
2. Correct electrolyte abnormalities – K^+, Na^+, Ca^{++}.
3. Optimize volume status – ultrafiltration, diuretics; consider use of Swan–Ganz monitoring.

E. **Hepatic** (see "Cirrhosis").

F. **Endocrine** (see "Perioperative Care of Diabetic Patient" and section VII below).

H. **Hematologic** (see "Blood Component Therapy and Coagulation").

IV. GENERAL PREOPERATIVE PREPARATION

A. Overall assessment of patient, history, physical examination, and operative risk (see section II above).

B. Documentation of indications for procedure, informed consent (see "Medical Record" and "Medico–Legal Aspects").

C. **Routine preoperative laboratory evaluation.**
1. Labs – CBC, urinalysis, platelet count, electrolytes, BUN, creatinine, PT, PTT.
2. Room–air arterial blood gas (ABG) if predisposed to respiratory insufficiency (> 20 pack–year smoker, can't blow out match, short of breath on 1–2 flights of steps, etc.), or if anticipate prolonged postoperative ventilatory support.
3. X-rays – PA and lateral chest x-ray unless previously normal within the past six months or < 35 years old; x-rays of specific areas of interest in relation to the upcoming procedure.
4. EKG if patient over 35 years old or if otherwise indicated by past cardiac history.

D. Blood Order (number of units; T & S = type & screen):

Abdominal aortic aneurysm repair -- 6
Abdominal perineal resection -- 4
Amputation (lower extremity) -- 2
Aorto-femoral bypass -- 4
Aorto-iliac bypass -- 4
Augmentation mammoplasty -- T & S
Cardiac bypass -- 4
Carotid endarterectomy -- T & S
Cholecystectomy +/- common bile duct exploration -- T & S
Colectomy -- 2
Colostomy, gastrostomy -- T & S
Esophageal resection -- 2
Exploratory laparotomy -- 2
Femoral popliteal bypass -- 4
Gastrectomy -- 2
Hemorrhoidectomy -- T & S
Hepatectomy -- 6
Ileofemoral bypass -- 4
Lobectomy -- 2
Nephrectomy -- 2
Mastectomy -- 2
Pancreatectomy -- 4
Parathyroidectomy -- T & S
Pneumonectomy -- 2
Portacaval shunt -- 6
Renal transplant -- 2
Small bowel resection -- 2
Splenectomy (elective) -- 2
Splenorenal shunt -- 6
Sympathectomy -- T & S
Thyroidectomy -- T & S
Tracheostomy -- 2
Vein stripping -- T & S
Wedge resection -- T & S

E. Skin preparation.

1. Hair removal is best performed the day of surgery with an electric clipper. Shaving the night prior to surgery is associated with an increased risk of infection (Alexander JW, et al. *Arch. Surg.* 118:347, 1983).

2. Preoperative (the night before) scrub or shower of the operative site with a germicidal soap (Hibiclens®, pHisoHex®, etc.).

F. Preoperative antibiotics.

1. When used, should have an **established blood level** at the time of initial skin incision. The best time to administer antibiotics is when the patient first *arrives in the operating room*.

2. **Indications for prophylactic antibiotics.**

   a. Clean, contaminated procedures — GI/GU tract, GYN, respiratory tract.

   b. Contaminated procedures, i.e., trauma.

   c. Insertion of synthetic material (e.g., vascular grafts, artificial valves, prosthetic joints).

   d. High–risk patients.

      e. Patient with prosthetic heart valves or history of valvular heart disease (see VI: Bacterial Endocarditis Prophylaxis).

G. Respiratory care.
1. Preoperative incentive spirometry on the evening *prior* to surgery when indicated (upper abdominal operations, thoracic operations, patient predisposed to respiratory insufficiency).
2. PFT's when indicated (see "Respiratory Care").
3. Nasotracheal suctioning and bronchodilators for moderate to severe COPD.

H. Decompression of GI tract — NPO after midnight.

I. Access and monitoring lines.
1. At least one 18–gauge IV needed for initiation of anesthesia.
2. Arterial catheters and central or Swan–Ganz catheters when indicated (see "Hemodynamic and Cardiac Monitoring").

J. Thromboembolic prophylaxis when indicated (see "Thromboembolic Prophylaxis and Management of DVT").

K. Void on call to the operating room.

L. Pre–op sedation as ordered by anesthesiologist (see "Anesthesia").

M. Special considerations.
1. Maintenance medications (i.e., antihypertensives, cardiac medications, anticonvulsants, etc.) may be given the morning of surgery with a sip of water before routine operations.
2. Preoperative diabetic management (see "Care of the Diabetic Patient").
3. SBE prophylaxis (see VI below).
4. Perioperative steroid coverage (see VII below).

N. Stomas — marking of site by stomal therapist in elective situations (see "Enterostomal Therapy").

V. BOWEL PREP

The purpose of a bowel preparation is to remove all solid and most liquid from the bowel, and to reduce the bacterial population in anticipation of procedures or complications of procedures that may contaminate the wound and the peritoneal cavity.

A. Non–colonic surgery.
1. Stomach decompression prior to induction of anesthesia by remaining NPO after midnight before surgery or by NG suction.
2. Bowel preparation required if any of the upper or lower GI tract is to be opened.
    a. Surgery may involve colon, e.g., extensive surgery for gynecologic malignancy or abdominal masses which impinge upon the colon or where there is a potential for mechanical or ischemic bowel damage (aneurysmectomy).
    b. Achlorhydria, gastric carcinoma, prolonged H_2 blocker usage, and obstructive peptic ulcer disease will allow bacterial growth in the stomach. One should consider using an oral

antibiotic prep (i.e., neomycin) for gastric surgery in these patients (see below).

B. **Colonic surgery** — mechanical or whole gut lavage prep with or without oral antibiotic prep. Many variations exist.
   1. Mechanical prep.
      a. Day 1 — clear liquid diet, laxative of choice (castor oil 60 cc, Milk of Magnesia® (MOM) 30 cc, magnesium citrate 250 cc), tap water or soap–suds enema until clear.
      b. Day 2 — clear liquid diet, NPO, IV fluids, laxative of choice.
      c. Day 3 — operation.
   2. Whole gut lavage — GoLYTELY® (a polyethylene glycol base, electrolyte balanced solution).
      a. Day 1 — GoLYTELY® 5 liters po or per NG tube over 5 hrs.
      b. May include metaclopramide 10 mg po to reduce bloating and nausea.
      c. Clear liquid diet after above.
      d. Day 2 — operation.
   3. Oral antibiotic prep — mechanical prep or whole gut lavage should be completed prior to the administration of the oral antibiotic prep.
      a. Nichols–Condon prep — on day prior to surgery neomycin 1 g and erythromycin base 1 g po at 1 *p.m.*, 2 *p.m.*, 11 *p.m.* for case scheduled at 8 *a.m.* (Nichols RL, et al. *Ann. Surg.* 176:227, 1972).
      b. Metronidazole (500 mg) po may be substituted for erythromycin base in the Nichols–Condon prep (less nausea than with erythromycin base).
   4. Perioperative IV antibiotics may be used in conjunction with or in place of the oral antibiotic prep.
      a. These antibiotics should be administered immediately pre-operatively (see above) and intra–operatively (every 6 hrs) for prolonged operations. Any further doses postoperatively have not been shown to be effective in the prevention of wound infection; however, most surgeons administer at least 1 dose of antibiotic postoperatively, and it is common to continue the antibiotic for 24 hrs postoperatively.
      b. Choice of antibiotic — need broad coverage of enteric organisms (gram negatives, anaerobes), e.g., gentamicin and clindamycin (or metronidazole), cefazolin and metronidazole, cefoxitin, or cefotetan.

VI. BACTERIAL ENDOCARDITIS PROPHYLAXIS

A. **Indications** — patients with the following are particularly vulnerable to bacteriologic seeding during very transient bacteremia.
   1. Prosthetic valve.
   2. Congenital valve disease.

3. Rheumatic valve disease.
4. History of endocarditis.
5. Idiopathic hypertrophic subaortic stenosis.
6. Mitral valve prolapse with murmur (Barlow's syndrome).
B. Antibiotic recommendations:

PREVENTION OF BACTERIAL ENDOCARDITIS[1]

	Dosage for Adults	Dosage for Children
DENTAL AND UPPER RESPIRATORY PROCEDURES[2]		
Oral[3] – Penicillin V	2 g 1 hr before procedure and 1 g 6 hrs later	> 60 lbs: adult dosage; < 60 lbs: 1/2 the adult dose
Penicillin allergy: Erythromycin	1 g 1 hr before procedure and 500 mg 6 hrs later	20 mg/kg 1 hr before procedure and 10 mg/kg 6 hrs later
Parenteral[3,4] – Ampicillin	2 g IM or IV 30 min before procedure	50 mg/kg IM or IV 30 min before procedure
plus Gentamicin	1.5 mg/kg IM or IV 30 min before procedure	2.0 mg/kg IM or IV 30 min before procedure
Penicillin allergy: Vancomycin	1 g IV infused *slowly over 1 hr*, beginning 1 hr before procedure	20 mg/kg IV infused *slowly over 1 hr*, beginning 1 hr before procedure
GASTROINTESTINAL AND GENITOURINARY PROCEDURES[2]		
Parenteral[3,4] – Ampicillin	2 g IM or IV 30 min before procedure	50 mg/kg IM or IV 30 min before procedure
plus Gentamicin	1.5 mg/kg IM or IV 30 min before procedure	2.0 mg/kg IM or IV 30 min before procedure
Penicillin allergy: Vancomycin	1 g IV infused *slowly over 1 hr*, beginning 1 hr before procedure	20 mg/kg IV infused *slowly over 1 hr*, beginning 1 hr before procedure
plus Gentamicin	1.5 mg/kg IM or IV 30 min before procedure	2.0 mg/kg IM or IV 30 min before procedure
Oral[3] – Amoxicillin	3 g 1 hr before procedure and 1.5 g 6 hrs later	50 mg/kg 1 hr before procedure and 25 mg/kg 6 hrs later

Notes:

1. For patients with valvular heart disease, prosthetic heart valves, most forms of congenital heart disease (but not uncomplicated secundum atrial septal defect), idiopathic hypertrophic subaortic stenosis, and mitral valve prolapse with regurgitation.

2. Data are limited on the risk of endocarditis with a particular procedure. For a review of the risk of bacteremia with various procedures, see Everett ED and Hirschmann JV, *Medicine* 56:61, 1977, and Shorvon PJ, et al, *Gut* 24:1078, 1983. For some useful guidelines on which procedures justify prophylaxis, see Shulman ST, et al, *Circulation* 70:1123A, 1984.

3. Oral regimens are more convenient and safer. Parenteral regimens are more likely to be effective; they are recommended especially for patients with prosthetic valves, those who have had endocarditis previously, or those taking continuous oral penicillin for rheumatic fever prophylaxis.

4. A single dose of the parenteral drugs is probably adequate, because bacteremias after most dental and diagnostic procedures are of short duration. However, one or two follow–up doses may be given at 8–12 hr intervals in selected patients, such as hospitalized patients judged to be at higher risk.

Ref: *The Medical Letter*, Vol. 28, #707, p. 22, 1986 with permission.

VII. STEROIDS
A. Indications.
1. *Any* patient currently on steroids, or those who have taken them *within 1 year*.
2. Preoperative for adrenalectomy.
3. Known history of adrenal insufficiency.
4. History of adrenal or pituitary surgery, surgery for renal cell carcinoma, or seminoma therapy.

B. Endogenous cortisol output.
1. Normal unstressed adult − 8–25 mg/day.
2. Adult undergoing major surgery − 75–100 mg/day.

C. Guide to steroid coverage.
1. Correct electrolytes, blood pressure, and hydration if necessary.
2. **Hydrocortisone** phosphate or hemisuccinate, 100 mg IVPB on call to operating room.
3. Hydrocortisone phosphate or hemisuccinate, 100 mg IVPB in recovery room and every 6 hrs for the first 24 hrs.
4. If progress is satisfactory, reduce dosage to 50 mg every 6 hrs for 24 hrs, then taper to maintenance dosage over 3 to 5 days. Resume previous fluorocortisol or oral steroid dose when patient is taking oral medications.
5. Maintain or increase hydrocortisone dosage to 200–400 mg per 24 hrs if fever, hypotension, or other complications occur.

    6. If patient has potassium wasting, may switch to methylprednisolone (Solumedrol®).

Note: High-dose (300-600 mg/day) regimens are potentially deleterious secondary to impaired wound healing, increased catabolism, electrolyte abnormalities, increased infectious complications.

D. Relative potencies of corticosteroids:

DRUG	Equivalent Anti-inflammatory Dose (mg)	Relative Anti-inflammatory Potency	Relative Mineralo-corticoid Activity	Duration of Action
Hydrocortisone (Cortisol®, Cortef®)	20.0	1.0	1.0	8-12 h
Cortisone	25.0	0.8	0.8	8-12 h
Prednisone (Deltasone®)	5.0	4	0.8	12-36 h
Prednisolone (Delta-Cortef®)	5.0	4	0.8	12-36 h
Methylprednisolone (Solu-Medrol®, Medrol®)	4.0	5	0.5	12-36 h
Triamcinolone (Aristocort®, Kenacort®)	4	5	0	12-24 h
Dexamethasone (Decadron®, Hexadrol®)	.75	25	0	36-72 h
Betamethasone (Celestone®)	.60	25	0	36-72 h
9-alpha fluorocortisol (Florinef®) [mineralocorticoid]	0.0	10	125	---

RESPIRATORY CARE

I. RISK FACTORS FOR PULMONARY COMPLICATIONS
A. Site of incision — increased risk with thoracotomy, upper abdominal incision.
B. Prolonged anesthesia (> 3.5 hours).
C.* Smoking history — 20 pack–years, productive cough.
D.* COPD — pCO_2 45–50 mm Hg, FEV_1/FVC < 70%.
E.* Obesity.
F.* Age > 60 years.
G. Use of NG tube.

Preoperative pulmonary function tests (PFT's), with or without bronchodilators, and arterial blood gases are indicated for patients undergoing thoracic or upper abdominal surgery or who have suspected or documented pulmonary disease (*).

II. PULMONARY COMPLICATIONS
A. Atelectasis.
B. Pneumonia.
C. Pulmonary edema.
D. Acute bronchospasm.
E. Pulmonary embolism.
F. Adult respiratory distress syndrome (ARDS).

III. MEASURABLE PULMONARY FUNCTION DERANGEMENTS
A. **Restrictive** — reduction of lung volumes without loss of flow rates. Causes include:
   1. Extrinsic — skeletal deformity, space occupying lesions in chest cavity, obesity, extensive pleural scar, previous thoracotomy.
   2. Intrinsic — deposition of material in alveoli or interstitium which makes the lung stiff (e.g., interstitial fibrosis, interstitial edema, silicosis, or granulomatous disease).
   3. Muscular weakness (e.g., myasthenia gravis, polio).
B. **Obstructive** — reduction of airflow.
   1. Asthma — intermittent reversible obstruction.
   2. Bronchitis — obstruction secondary to thickening of bronchial walls.
   3. Emphysema — airway collapse on expiration secondary to destruction of alveolar walls.
   4. Mixed — chronic obstructive pulmonary disease (COPD) connotes a mixed disorder which may include all three of the above components.

C. **Diffusion defects** — measurement of how much slower gas traverses a membrane divided by the pressure pushing the gas through the membrane (partial pressure gradient of a gas across a membrane).
   1. Loss of alveolar membranes (emphysema).
   2. Thickening of membranes (fibrosis, granuloma, edema, silicosis, etc.).
   3. Decrease in ventilation or perfusion.
   4. Removal of a portion of lung.
D. **Mismatch of ventilation and perfusion** (V/Q mismatch).
   1. An area of lung which is perfused but not ventilated = shunt unit (i.e., pulmonary edema, atelectasis, pneumonia).
   2. Decreased ventilation with persistent blood flow (i.e. obstructive diseases) — may be reversible with O_2 therapy.
   3. Ventilation persists, but without perfusion (i.e., pulmonary embolism) — enlarged dead space where no gas exchange occurs [dead space units].

IV. PREVENTING PULMONARY COMPLICATIONS
A. Preoperative.
   1. Quit smoking — may require 8 weeks to influence risk of complications.
   2. Pre–op education, incentive spirometry — beneficial for patients at risk for complications.
   3. Bronchodilator therapy if indicated by PFT results.
B. Postoperative.
   1. Pain control — judicious use of narcotics; consider use of intercostal block or epidermal analgesia (see "Anesthesia").
   2. Early ambulation.
   3. Remove nasogastric tube ASAP.

V. TREATING PULMONARY COMPLICATIONS
A. Atelectasis — incentive spirometry; early mobilization, adequate analgesics.
B. Pneumonia — pulmonary toilet, appropriate antibiotics. Fiberoptic bronchoscopy may be required for toilet and to obtain diagnostic cultures.
C. Pulmonary edema — correct volume overload, optimize cardiac junction.
D. Acute bronchospasm — bronchodilators.
E. Pulmonary embolism (see "Thromboembolic Prophylaxis & Venous Thromboembolism").
F. **ARDS** — acute respiratory failure characterized by non–cardiogenic pulmonary edema (interstitial and alveolar).
   1. Decreased compliance, increased V/Q mismatch, and pulmonary shunt.

2. Possible causes — sepsis; fat embolism; drug overdosage; aspiration; severe pancreatitis; massive transfusions; allergic reactions; smoke inhalation.
3. Clinical signs — tachypnea; tachycardia; mental confusion; respiratory alkalosis from hypocarbia (early), hypoxia (late); CXR shows bilateral "fluffy" infiltrates.
4. Diagnosis — ABG, CXR, clinical findings.
5. **Treatment** — mechanical ventilation with PEEP.
   a. Increased FRC, decreases shunt.
   b. Treat underlying cause of ARDS.

VI. TYPES OF PULMONARY FUNCTION TESTS

A. **Spirometry** — most frequently performed PFT. Only measures ability of the patient to move air. Marked dependency on technique and patient cooperation.
   1. **Lung volumes** (Fig. 1):

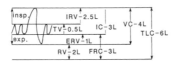

FIGURE 1

   a. TV = Tidal Volume — quiet normal breathing.
   b. IRV = Inspiratory Reserve Volume — from end of tidal inspiration to maximum inspiration.
   c. IC = Inspiratory Capacity — from end of tidal expiration to maximum inspiration.
   d. ERV = Expiratory Reserve Volume — from end of tidal expiration to maximum expiration.
   e. RV = Residual Volume — volume of air remaining in the thorax after maximum expiration; measured by various gas dilution tests, radiographic tests and/or body plethysmography.
   f. FRC = Functional Residual Capacity — from end of tidal expiration to complete thoracic airlessness.
   g. VC = Vital Capacity — from maximum inspiration to maximum expiration.
   h. TLC = Total Lung Capacity — total volume of air in the thorax at maximum inspiration; measured by various gas dilution tests, radiographic tests and/or body plethysmography.

i. FVC = Forced (or Fast) Vital Capacity — vital capacity performed from TLC to RV at maximum effort (Fig. 2).

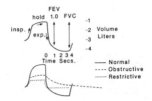

FIGURE 2

j. $FEV_{1.0}$ = Forced Expiratory Volume in One Second — airway obstruction may be inferred from a reduction of the amount of air that can be expelled in one second.

k. MEFR = Maximum Expiratory Flow Rate — expiratory air flow in liters per minute, calculated from FVC.

l. MMEFR = Mid-Maximum Expiratory Flow Rate — measured at midpoint of expiratory effort.

m. MVV = Maximal Voluntary Ventilation — the maximum volume of air the patient can shift per minute, expressed in liters/min. Useful as an indicator of physiologic reserve and the patient's ability to cooperate with maximal effort.

2. Specific disorders.

   a. Restrictive — all lung volumes are reduced.

   b. Obstructive — flow rates are reduced, especially FEV_1 and ratio of FEV_1 to FVC.

      1) Improvement may occur (if there is a reversible component) following bronchodilator administration.

      2) Lung volumes are large, but may not be usable since the majority is RV and trapped gas.

B. **Diffusing capacity** — assessment of ability of oxygen to transfer from the alveolar gas to the pulmonary capillary blood (D_LO_2 = diffusing capacity of the lung for oxygen).

1. Measurement.

   a. D_LO_2 is technically difficult to perform.

   b. Carbon monoxide (CO) diffuses 0.8 times as rapidly as O_2, but binds to hemoglobin 200 times as tenaciously. Therefore, measurement of uptake of a known amount of CO over a known amount of pressure will characterize the diffusing capacity of the lung (D_LCO ml/min/mm Hg).

   2. Characteristics.
      a. Diffusing capacity is grossly proportional to the total effective surface area available for gas exchange.
      b. Dependent on the character of the alveolar capillary membrane and the volume of hemoglobin in the alveolar capillary.
      c. Helpful in assessing the presence of emphysema (decreased D_LCO) in a patient with airway obstruction.
   3. Clinical use.
      a. Intrinsic restrictive diseases — thickened alveolar capillary membrane, decreased D_LCO.
      b. Anemia, lung resection, CO poisoning, pulmonary micro-embolization will all decrease D_LCO.
      c. Early left ventricular failure and polycythemia may elevate D_LCO.

C. Mismatch of ventilation and perfusion.
   1. Arterial blood gases and mixed venous blood gases are used to assess the amount of ventilation/perfusion mismatch.
   2. Radioisotope ventilation–perfusion scan may help in assessing this physiologic problem.

VII. PULMONARY RESECTION CRITERIA

A. The predicted postoperative FEV_1 should exceed 800 cc to provide adequate respiratory reserve for a functional existence. The use of preoperative radionucleotide scanning may aid in the prediction of post–resection FEV_1.

B. Preoperative criteria:

Procedure	MVV	FEV_1	FEV 0.25–0.75	Mortality
Pneumonectomy	> 55%	> 2 L	> 1.6 L	4.4%
Lobectomy	> 40%	> 1 L	> 0.6 L	0%
Wedge Resection	≥ 40%	> 0.6 L	> 0.6 L	0.2%

VENTILATORY SUPPORT

I. DEFINITIONS
A. IMV − Intermittent Mandatory Ventilation.
1. Ventilator delivers a preset tidal volume at a preset rate.
2. Remainder of patient's minute ventilation is self–generated and independent of the ventilator.
3. Theoretical problem − mechanical volume delivered at the peak of spontaneous inspiration or during exhalation; no apparent clinical significance. Synchronized IMV (SIMV) or Intermittent Demand Ventilation (IDV) demonstrate no advantage over IMV.
4. **Criticism** − patient's respiratory drive, and therefore contribution to minute ventilation, may be quite variable.

B. CMV − Controlled Mechanical Ventilation.
1. Ventilator delivers a preset tidal volume at a preset rate.
2. No allowance is made for gas flow upon spontaneous effort by the patient.
3. Usually reserved for intraoperative use with anesthesia or apneic patients.
4. Requires heavy sedation or paralysis.

C. ACMV − Assist Controlled Mechanical Ventilation.
1. Ventilator delivers a preset tidal volume each time the patient makes an inspiratory effort.
2. Entire minute ventilation is ventilator generated.

D. FIO_2 − fractional inspired concentration of oxygen.
E. PaO_2 − partial pressure of O_2 in arterial blood.
F. PAO_2 − alveolar oxygen concentration:

$$PAO_2 = (P_B - P_{H_2O})\ FIO_2 - PECO_2/R$$

P_B = barometric pressure, about 740 torr;
P_{H_2O} = water vapor pressure at body temp. = 47 torr;
$PECO_2 \approx PACO_2$ (measured);
$R = V_{CO_2}/V_{O_2}$ (respiratory quotient, usually 0.8).

G. Q_{sp}/Q_t − "shunt" − the fraction of total cardiac output which passes through the pulmonary circuit without being oxygenated.
H. $A–aDO_2$ − alveolar arterial oxygen gradient.
I. PEEP − positive end expiratory pressure.

II. CRITERIA FOR INITIATION OF VENTILATORY SUPPORT
A. Inadequate ventilation.
1. Apnea.
2. Deteriorating alveolar ventilation.
   a. pH < 7.25.
   b. Rising P_aCO_2 − in appropriate clinical setting, especially with falling pH; $P_aCO_2 > 60$ mmHg.

3. Usually results from increased airway impedence, neuromuscular impairment or decreased drive.

B. Inadequate oxygenation.
   1. Falling P_aO_2.
      a. P_aO_2 < 70 mmHg on 50% O_2 mask.
      b. P_aO_2 < 55 mmHg on room air (in appropriate clinical setting).
   2. Usually results from venous admixture due to pulmonary edema, consolidation or atelectasis.

C. Common clinical entities requiring ventilatory support.
   1. Severe pulmonary edema.
   2. Suspected or impending ARDS (sepsis, shock, prolonged hypotension, massive transfusion, severe pancreatitis, head trauma, multiple trauma).
   3. Massive resuscitation in the face of multiple trauma.
   4. Severe chest trauma (flail chest, pulmonary contusion).
   5. COPD/bronchospasm.
   6. Coma (lack of drive, provides airway protection).

III. VENTILATOR TYPES

A. Time–cycled ventilator.
   1. Timed delivery of gas flow; tidal volume = flow rate x inspiratory time.
   2. Delivers relatively constant tidal volume to ventilator circuit.
   3. Allows precise control and variability in waveform of delivered gas.
   4. Examples: IMV–Bird, Foregger 210, Emerson.

B. Volume–cycled ventilator.
   1. Inspiratory gas flow terminated after pre–selected volume delivered into circuit.
   2. Pressure in circuit determined by tidal volume and lung compliance. Patient–delivered tidal volume varies with changes in pressure (compliance).
   3. Examples: Bennett (MA-1, MA-2, MA-2+2, 7200), Ohio 560, Bourns Bear 1, Monaghan 225, Siemons Servo 900.

C. Pressure–cycled ventilator.
   1. Gas flow continued until preset pressure developed.
   2. Tidal volume = flow rate x time until pressure is reached.
   3. Variable volume if circuit pressure varies (changes in compliance).
   4. Examples: Bird Mark 6, 7, 8, 9, 10, 14, 17; Bennett PR-1, PR-2.

D. High–frequency ventilators.
   1. Five types.
      a. High–frequency positive pressure ventilation.
      b. Jet ventilation.
      c. Flow interruption.

    d. Oscillation.
    e. Percussive ventilation.
  2. Mechanisms of gas transport (theoretical):

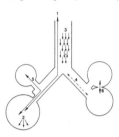

1, Direct alveolar ventilation (bulk gas flow). **2**, Enhanced diffusion across alveolar capillary membrane. **3**, **4**, **5**, Interregional mixing of gases from one time constant to another (pendeluft). **6**, Improved collateral ventilation between alveolar units.

Ref: Hurst JM, Davis K Jr, Branson RD: High frequency ventilation in clinical surgery. In Baker RJ (ed): *Problems in General Surgery.* Philadelphia: JB Lippincott, Oct-Dec 1987, p. 455, with permission.

  3. Physiologic effects.
    a. Lower mean airway pressure. **Note:** The site of pressure measurement is important to avoid unintentional PEEP.
    b. Cardiac output — no clear benefit.
    c. Lung volume — increased.
    d. Mucociliary clearance — decreased.
  4. Clinical indications.
    a. Closed head injury — maintains lower intracranial pressure.
    b. Large pulmonary air leaks/flail chest with contusions — prevents over-PEEPing undamaged lung.
    c. Hemodynamic instability — less depression of cardiac output.
    d. Refractory respiratory failure — promising in investigational setting).

IV. CLINICAL GUIDELINES
A. Inspired oxygen concentration.
  1. FIO_2 ideally maintained < 50% to avoid O_2 toxicity.
  2. Higher levels of FIO_2 may be necessary when initiating therapy; use PEEP to wean FIO_2.

    3. Maintain Hgb saturation > 90% or intra–pulmonary shunt < 15–20%.

B. Tidal volume.

    1. Initially 10–15 cc/kg body weight. Tidal volume may need to be increased in individuals with respiratory acidosis despite adequate frequency of ventilation.

    2. Problem: Ventilator setting and actual delivered volume may be different. Actual tidal volume being delivered is most accurately assessed by measuring flow with a spirometer at the endotracheal tube.

C. Ventilatory rate.

    1. IMV is preferred to ACMV because it allows a lower mean intrathoracic pressure and the patient is allowed to breathe spontaneously, thus preventing disuse and facilitating weaning.

    2. Problem: Tachypnea despite apparently adequate levels of IMV ventilation. Inadequate inspiratory flow rates and increased resistance to air flow through ventilator flow circuit are common problems. If the patient generates negative inspiratory pressures > –5 cm H_2O, this may indicate inadequate flow through the circuit. In this event, it is often helpful to pressurize the inflow circuit with a continuous positive airway pressure (CPAP) system.

D. PEEP.

    1. Positive pressure is maintained at end expiration, thus preventing complete "emptying" of the lung.

    2. Maintains functional residual capacity (FRC) above the critical closing volume (i.e. the volume at which alveolar collapse begins).

    3. Decreases V/Q (ventilation/perfusion) mismatching which results from perfusion of collapsed alveoli (decreases intra–pulmonary shunt).

    4. Re–expands collapsed alveoli, prevents alveolar collapse.

    5. Improves pulmonary compliance and therefore reduces the work of breathing.

    6. May be applied as CPAP via tight–fitting mask in non–intubated patients.

E. Adjusting PEEP.

    1. PEEP is usually begun at 5 cm H_2O and increased in increments of 2–3 cm.

    2. Optimal setting.

        a. Continue to increase PEEP until pulmonary shunt < 15–20% or the P_AO_2/FIO_2 ratio exceeds 250.

        b. Alternatively, adjust PEEP until attaining adequate oxygenation (Hgb saturation > 90%) at non–toxic levels of FIO_2 (< 50%).

        c. Problem: Higher levels of PEEP ("over–PEEPing") may decrease cardiac output. Adjustment at higher levels must consider circulatory volume effects.

F. **Monitoring.**
    1. Swan–Ganz catheters – Indications: PEEP > 15, heart disease, head injury, expected large volume shifts.
    2. Arterial line – frequent blood gas determinations.

V. **WEANING FROM VENTILATORY SUPPORT**
A. Initiated only after the primary process responsible for pulmonary insufficiency has been reversed.
B. **Priorities of weaning.**
    1. Decrease FIO_2 to < 50% (below toxic level).
    2. Decrease mechanical rate.
        a. Reduces mean intrathoracic pressure and frequency of exposure to peak inspiratory pressure (PIP).
        b. Minimizes barotrauma.
        c. Improves V/Q matching.
    3. Decrease PEEP.
        a. Increments of 2–3 cm per step.
        b. Check PO_2 and/or shunt, and if satisfactory, reduce PEEP again.
        c. Allow approximately 6 hrs between successive drops in PEEP.
        d. Decrease PEEP to a base of 5 cm H_2O (approximates end expiratory pressure in extubated patients as a result of epiglottic closure; so–called "physiologic PEEP").

VI. **CRITERIA FOR EXTUBATION**
A. **Traditional extubation criteria.**
    1. Ventilation (mechanical) factors.
        a. Vital capacity > 15 cc/kg.
        b. Negative inspiratory force < –25 cm H_2O.
        c. Respiratory rate < 30.
        d. Spontaneous tidal volume ≥ 5 cc/kg.
        e. 48% false–negative prediction of outcome.
    2. Oxygenation factors – P_aO_2 > 300 mmHg on FIO_2 of 100%.
B. **"Blow by" T–piece trial** should be *avoided*.
    1. Fails to provide physiologic levels of PEEP.
    2. Promotes alveolar collapse.
C. **Gas exchange criteria** – trial of room air CPAP.
    1. IMV rate of zero, FIO_2 of 21% and CPAP of 5 cm H_2O.
    2. After 1/2 hour, extubate if:
        a. P_aO_2 > 55 torr (FIO_2 = .21).
        b. Ventilatory rate < 30 breaths/min.
        c. pH > 7.35.
        d. P_{CO_2} < 45 torr (previously eucapneic patient).
        e. Is 94% predictive of the patient tolerating extubation.
        f. Modify criteria for patients with underlying pulmonary disease, e.g., hypoxemia (chronic), CO_2 retention.

CARDIOPULMONARY MONITORING

I. **MONITORING**
   Basic principle of periodic objective assessment of patient's clinical condition.

A. **"Vital signs"** — evaluation of pulse, blood pressure, temperature, respiratory rate. In its simplest form, these parameters are measured using a watch, thermometer, and sphygmomanometer. While such assessments made at 4 or 8 hour intervals are adequate for the "stable" patient, the seriously ill patient requires closer evaluation on a more frequent schedule. *Continuous* assessment is the ideal situation.

B. **Monitoring techniques** — invasive *vs.* non–invasive.
   1. **Non–invasive.**
      a. Continuous ECG monitoring — heart rate, rhythm.
      b. Apnea monitoring — respiratory drive.
      c. Pulse oximetry — arterial O_2 saturation.
      d. Capnography — end–tidal CO_2.
      e. Ultrasonic blood pressure monitor (Dinamap®) — blood pressure.
   2. **Invasive.**
      a. Arterial catheterization — blood pressure.
      b. Central venous catheterization — central venous pressure (CVP).
      c. Pulmonary artery catheterization — CVP, pulmonary artery systolic (PAS) and diastolic (PAD) pressures, pulmonary artery occlusion pressure (PAO), cardiac output.
   3. In practice, often a combination of non–invasive and invasive techniques are applied. Invasive monitoring (placement of intravascular catheters) provides more direct measurement and provides data from which other measurements can be calculated.

C. **Indications for invasive monitoring.**
   1. Complex surgical procedures associated with large volume shifts.
   2. Circulatory instability.
   3. Fluid management problems.
   4. Deteriorating cardiac function.
   5. Deteriorating pulmonary function.
   6. Inappropriate response to volume challenge.
   7. Unexplained hypoxemia.
   8. Severe head injury.
   9. Need for PEEP in head injury.

II. PULMONARY MONITORING

A. **Apnea monitoring** — sensitive to chest wall motion. Monitors respiratory rate, alarms usually set for bradypnea or apnea.

B. **Pulse oximetry** — non–invasive; transcutaneous measurement of arterial oxygen saturation by light absorption technique. Probe is attached to body areas where capillary beds are accessible (i.e., fingernail bed, earlobes, toes). Does not function under conditions of hypoperfusion or inadequate pulsatile flow.

C. **Capnography** – direct measurement of end–tidal CO_2.

III. HEMODYNAMIC MONITORING TECHNIQUES

A. **Indirect monitoring of blood pressure** — sphygmomanometer (notoriously inaccurate in hypotensive conditions; wide inter-observer variation), ultrasonic blood pressure monitor. Work well in euvolemic patients. Doppler devices give no measure of diastolic pressure.

B. **Arterial catheterization** — provides direct measure of arterial pressure as well as arterial access for sampling. In conjunction with continuous EKG monitor, affords indirect evaluation of electromechanical function of the heart.

    1. The displayed pressure tracing is a synthesis of harmonics of the ejection pressure of the ventricular stroke volume into the elastic arterial tree. Diastolic run–off pressures represent the relationship between systemic vascular resistance, arterial pressure, and intravascular blood volume. An undamped arterial pressure tracing will show a distinct dicrotic notch separating the systolic and diastolic pressures.

        a. In hypovolemia with decreased stroke volume, a smaller pressure wave will be generated.

        b. If rate of myocardial contraction is diminished, there will be prolongation of the upslope of arterial pressure tracing.

    2. **Access for arterial blood samples.**

        a. Sequential analysis of blood gas tensions and acid/base status in the arterial blood are necessary in any acute illness involving cardiovascular or respiratory dysfunction.

        b. Access to other blood samples necessary to chart the progression of multisystemic illness.

        c. Arterial blood cultures.

            1) Fungal organisms may be more reliably cultured from arterial blood.

            2) Risk of catheter–induced sepsis is a danger with any invasive monitoring — sequential arterial cultures are necessary whenever these catheters are maintained for a long period of time. Arterial catheter colonization occurs much less frequently than venous catheters.

    3. Pitfalls.

        a. Arterial BP is not the "*sine qua non*" of shock and should not be used as the sole criterion of effectiveness of therapy.

   b. Blood pressure measurement alone is inadequate to assess
      the relationship between systemic resistance and cardiac
      output. If there is a question about low cardiac output or
      the level of peripheral resistance, then cardiac output
      should be determined.
   4. Method of insertion — see "Vascular Access Techniques".
C. **Central venous pressure (CVP) monitoring** — permits assessment
   of the ability of the right ventricle to accommodate the volume
   being returned to it.
   1. Accurate method of estimating right ventricular filling pressure
      (relevant in interpreting right ventricular function).
   2. CVP is a function of 4 independent forces:
      a. Volume and flow of blood in the central veins.
      b. Compliance and contractility of the right side of the heart
         during filling of the heart.
      c. Venomotor tone of central veins.
      d. Intrathoracic pressure.
   3. **Clinical uses of CVP catheter.**
      a. Infusion of TPN in order to provide adequate nutrition
         during critical illness.
      b. Infusion of vasoactive substances, hypertonic solutions, or
         chemically irritating medications for prolonged period of
         time.
      c. Aspiration of venous samples for chemical analysis (cannot
         be utilized as a substitute for true mixed venous blood).
      d. Head injury — increasing right atrial pressure will result in
         increased intracranial blood volume and may increase intra-
         cranial pressure (ICP).
      e. Sensitive in reflecting increased transmyocardial pressure in
         pericardial tamponade.
   4. Pitfalls of using CVP in critically ill patient.
      a. Water manometer system cannot reliably represent right
         ventricular filling pressure — transducer–monitor system is
         necessary. Transducer systems also need to be accurately
         zeroed: position of transducer is critical.
      b. Misinterpretation of CVP data when extrapolating informa-
         tion relative to left ventricular performance in critically ill
         patients.
         1) In normal situations right ventricular filling pressure
            may correlate with left ventricular filling pressures.
         2) In specific pathophysiologic states (e.g., ARDS, cor
            pulmonale, pulmonary fibrosis, pulmonary hypertension,
            myocardial contusion, septic shock), when invasive moni-
            toring is utilized, right and left atrial pressures differ
            significantly.
         3) CVP cannot be substituted for assessment of left ven-
            tricular performance in thes situations. Since the major

risks encountered in puncturing a central vein are essentially the same for the placement of a CVP catheter or a pulmonary artery catheter, one should consider the latter if your objective is to measure cardiovascular dynamics. In a critically ill patient, the better choice is the placement of a pulmonary artery catheter.

5. Method of insertion — see "Vascular Access Techniques".

D. **Balloon–tipped pulmonary artery catheter (Swan-Ganz® catheter):**
   1. Advantages over CVP measurements.
      a. Allows independent assessment of right and left ventricular function which may be quite dissimilar during critical illness.
      b. Permits measurement of pulmonary arterial diastolic and wedge pressures that approximates left atrial filling pressure (preload).
      c. Continuous monitoring of pulmonary artery systolic and mean pressures reflects the changes in pulmonary vascular resistance (PVR) secondary to hypoxemia, pulmonary edema, pulmonary emboli, and pulmonary insufficiency.
      d. Allows sampling of global mixed venous blood which will help discriminate between effects of pulmonary pathophysiology or changes in cardiac output upon arterial oxygen tension.
         1) Useful in determining adequacy of cardiac output with relation to oxygen delivery and oxygen consumption.
         2) Allows calculation of arteriovenous oxygen content difference ($A-V_{DO_2}$) and physiologic shunt (Qsp/Qt) which is helpful in the management of respiratory failure (see E – Formulas).
      e. Permits accurate, reproducible measurement of cardiac output by thermodilution technique.
      f. Permits monitoring of right ventricular filling pressure through the CVP access port.
      g. With addition of a few calculations, a wealth of cardiovascular data is available (see E – Formulas).
      h. Evaluation of myocardial function — preload, contractility, and afterload (Table 1).
         1) Myocardial perfusion pressure can be estimated from the difference between systemic diastolic pressure and pulmonary capillary wedge pressure.
         2) Heart rate and systolic pressure can be combined to provide a "time tension index".
         3) Systemic vascular resistance (SVR) as an estimation of aortic impedence (afterload) can be calculated.
         4) Effect of therapeutic interventions can be quantitated in terms of physiologic cost of therapeutic interventions.
      i. Specialized pulmonary artery catheter permits atrial, ventricular or sequential A–V pacing simultaneously.

TABLE 1

DETERMINANTS OF CARDIAC OUTPUT

Determinant	Definition	Effect on Cardiac Output	Measurement	Treatment
Preload	Length of myocardial fibers at end-diastole which is the result of ventricular filling pressure	Direct, up to physiologic limit	End-diastolic volume and pressure of the ventricles Pulmonary capillary wedge pressure Pulmonary diastolic pressure Direct left atrial pressure measurements CVP (right atrial)	Volume expansion Pericardiocentesis Reduction of PEEP
Contractility	The inotropic state of the myocardium; Length/tension/velocity relationship of myocardium independent of initial length and afterload	Direct	Ventricular function curves Ejection fraction Vmax Vcf PEP/LVET dP/dt iP	Dopamine Norepinephrine Epinephrine Isoproterenol Dobutamine Digitalis Glucagon GKI
Afterload	Systolic ventricular-wall stress which is produced by the force against which the myocardial fibers must contract	Inverse, as long as coronary flow is maintained	Aortic pressure for left ventricle Pulmonary artery pressure for right ventricle	Diuretics Phentolamine Sodium nitroprusside Nitroglycerine Intra-aortic balloon pumping External counterpulsation
Pulse Rate	The number of cardiac systoles per minute	Direct, above 60 and below 180 per minute	ECG Count pulse	Bradycardia: Atropine Pacemaker Tachycardia: Digitalis Lidocaine Electroversion

Ref: Hardy JD. *Textbook of Surgery.* Philadelphia: JB Lippincott, 1983; p. 54, with permission.

2. Clinical situations where PA catheter is useful — myocardial infarction, acute respiratory failure, sepsis, peritonitis, multiple trauma, noncardiogenic pulmonary edema, near–drowning, over-doses, pulmonary edema in pregnancy, fat emboli, and the elderly or critically ill patient undergoing non–cardiac surgical procedures (see "Preoperative Preparation").

3. **Technical specifications.**
   a. Distal lumen (tip of catheter) — lies in the pulmonary artery. Connected to transducer for continuous pressure monitoring. Blood withdrawn from this lumen (slowly) when the balloon is deflated is global mixed venous blood.
   b. Balloon lumen — when balloon is inflated and catheter correctly positioned, the pressure tracing from the distal lumen will change from an arterial (PA) to a venous (pulmonary capillary wedge) tracing. The balloon should never remain inflated longer than 30–60 seconds.
      1) When air is injected using a syringe and the plunger does not come back on its own, balloon rupture should be suspected.
      2) The balloon should be inflated slowly and gently, stop-ping inflation as soon as the pressure tracing changes, thereby avoiding over-inflation and potential pulmonary artery rupture.
      3) A permanent wedge tracing despite balloon deflation suggests that the catheter tip is too distal (lodged in the wedge position) to the pulmonary tree. This situation may lead to pulmonary infarction or pulmonary artery rupture. The catheter should be re-positioned as soon as this is noted.
   c. Proximal lumen — lies 30 cm proximal to distal lumen. When catheter is in proper position, this lumen lies in the SVC or right atrium. Can be used to monitor CVP and infuse fluids. Also, in utilizing thermodilution cardiac output, this lumen is the "injectate–port" for the iced injectate.
   d. Thermistor — located at the distal end of catheter; when connected to cardiac output computer, allows measurement of "core" temperature and calculation of thermodilution cardiac output when iced saline is injected in the proximal lumen. Integrity of thermistor should be checked prior to catheter placement.

4. Method of insertion — see "Vascular Access Techniques".

E. **Formulas.**
   1. **Mean arterial pressure (MAP):**
      $$MAP = DP + 1/3 (SP–DP) \quad [\text{normal} = 80–90 \text{ Torr}]$$
   2. **Stroke volume (SV):**
      $$SV = CO/HR \quad [\text{normal} = 50–60 \text{ ml}]$$

3. **Cardiac index (CI):**
   CI = CO/BSA   [normal = 3.5–4 ICU population]
4. **Stroke index (SI):**
   SI = SV/BSA   [normal = 35–40 ICU population]
5. **Right ventricular stroke work (RVSW):**
   RVSW = SV x (MPA–CVP) x .0136   [normal = 10–15 gram/meters]
6. **Left ventricular stroke work (LVSW):**
   LVSW = SV x (MAP–PAO) x .0136   [normal = 60–80 gram/meters]
   Ratio = LVSW/PAO
7. **Systemic vascular resistance (SVR)** (also referred to in the literature as total peripheral resistance):
   $$SVR = \frac{(MAP–CVP) \times 80}{CO}$$
   [normal = 800–1200 dynes/sec/cm^{-5}]
8. **Pulmonary vascular resistance (PVR):**
   $$PVR = \frac{(MPA–PAO) \times 80}{CO}$$
   [normal = 100–200 dynes/sec/cm^{-5}]
9. **Myocardial oxygen consumption** (correlate – a fair calculated measure of how much O_2 the heart is requiring):
   $$MVO_2C = \frac{SP \times HR}{100}$$
   [higher values = greater consumption]
10. **Alveolar PO_2:**
    $PAO_2 = (PB–P_{H_2O})\, FiO_2 – PECO_2/R$
    PB = Barometric pressure (760 mmHg at sea level).
    P_{H_2O} (at body temp.) = 47 mmHg.
    $PECO_2 \approx PACO_2$.
    R = 0.8 (assumed).
    Thus: $PAO_2 = (760–47)\, FiO_2 – PaCO_2/0.8$
11. **Capillary O_2 content:**
    $Cc'O_2 = (PAO_2) \times .0031 + Hb \times 1.39 \times 1$
    (assumes 100% Hb sat.)
    [normal = 18.3 ml/100 ml]
12. **Mixed venous O_2 content:**
    $CvO_2 = PvO_2 \times .0031 + Hb \times 1.39 \times$ Ven Sat
    [normal = 13 ml/100 ml]
13. **Arterial O_2 content:**
    $CaO_2 = PaO_2 \times .0031 + Hb \times 1.39 \times$ Art Sat
    [normal = 18 ml/100 ml]
14. **O_2 delivery:**
    O_2 Del = C_A x CO x 10   [normal = 1000 ml/min]

15. **A–V O$_2$ difference (A-V$_{DO_2}$):**
    A-V$_{DO_2}$ = Ca – Cv [normal = 3.5–4.5 ml/100 ml]
16. **O$_2$ consumption:**
    O$_2$ Cons = (Ca – Cv) x CO x 10 [normal = 250 ml/min]
17. **O$_2$ utilization:**
    % Util = Ca – Cv/Ca [normal = 0.2–0.25]
18. **Shunt (intrapulmonary):**
    $$Qsp/Qt = \frac{Cc'O_2 - CaO_2}{Cc'O2 - CvO2}$$ [normal < 0.10]
19. **Body surface area (BSA):**
    Use DuBois' BSA chart (see Reference Data)
20. **Rate pressure product (RPP)** — a reflection of how "hard" the heart is working (correlates poorly with myocardial oxygen consumption): RPP = HR x SP

IV. CARDIAC MONITORING
Surgeons should be versed in basic ECG interpretation and dysrhythmia recognition.

A. **Rate** — at a standard paper speed of 25 mm/sec, each 5-mm block is 0.2 sec in duration. Bradycardia is < 60 BPM (beats per min), whereas tachycardia is > 100 BPM.

B. **Rhythm** — cardiac rhythm is described as *regular* or *irregular*.

C. **Axis** (see Fig. 1) — an estimate of the cardiac axis can be obtained from line leads I and AVF:
   1. Normal axis is between +120° and –30°. The QRS complex will be above the isoelectric line in I and AVF (+I, +AVF).
   2. LAD (left axis deviation) is –30° to –90°; QRS is positive in lead I and negative (below isoelectric line) in AVF (+I, –AVF).
   3. RAD (right axis deviation) is +120° to –90°; QRS is negative in I, and above or below isoelectric line in AVF (–I, +/–AVF).
   4. Alternatively, the mean cardiac axis will be perpendicular to a frontal QRS complex with a net amplitude of ZERO.

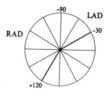

FIGURE 1

D. **Waves, intervals, and segments** — by analyzing the "PQRST" complex in systematic fashion, EKG interpretation is simplified, and pathology can be readily identified.
1. **P waves.**
   a. Reflect electrical activity of the atria. Abnormalities include "P pulmonale" or tall P wave (> 2.5 mm) in lead II, III, AVF. This reflects RA pathology in conditions such as pulmonary hypertension, COPD, pulmonary embolus, and tricuspid stenosis or insufficiency.
   b. "P mitrale" is wide P waves (> .10 sec) in lead II, or a notched P wave in lead VI. Left atrial pathology, secondary to mitral stenosis or regurgitation, may cause P mitrale.
2. **P–R interval** — normally 0.12 to 0.20 sec, but may be as long as 0.14 sec in young individuals. A–V block is reflected in the P–R interval.
   a. **First degree** — delayed A–V conduction, with prolonged P–R.
   b. **Second degree.**
      1) "Type I" (Wenckebach) — P–R interval is progressively prolonged until a QRS is dropped.
      2) "Type II" — P–R intervals are constant, but QRS complexes are unexpectedly dropped.
   c. **Third degree** — atrial and ventricular activity are independent. Conduction is interrupted.
3. **QRS complex** — reflects ventricular activity. Normal QRS width is up to .09 sec.
   a. **LVH** — increased leftward forces result in large R waves in leads I, AVL, V_5 and V_6 ("large" = > 20 mm high in limb leads and > 30 mm in precordial leads). Inverted T waves and depressed ST segments will accompany this finding, and is called a "strain" pattern.
   b. **RVH** — increased rightward forces lead to large S waves in I, AVL, V_5 and V_6, as well as tall R waves in V_1 and/or V_2. Again, an "RV strain" pattern is manifested as inverted T waves and depressed ST segments in leads with dominant R waves.
   c. **LBBB** — a mid–conduction delay causes prolonged ventricular depolarization in left bundle branch block; the QRS interval will be > 0.12 sec. Note that ventricular hypertrophy criteria are invalid if LBBB is present (see above). The following will be seen in LBBB:
      1) Broad R waves in I, AVL, V_5 and V_6.
      2) Broad S waves in V_1 and/or V_2.
      3) Absent septal Q waves in I, AVL, V_5 and V_6.
   d. **RBBB** — a terminal delay in ventricular conduction results in characteristic changes. Again, the QRS will be > 0.12 sec in duration, and will have:

1) Broad R waves in V_1.
2) Broad S waves in I, AVL, V_5 and V_6.

4. **ST segment changes** — may be the only changes seen in infarction or ischemia.
   a. ST depression seen in subendocardial infarction, myocardial ischemia, and in patients on digitalis.
   b. ST elevation seen in transmural infarction, LV aneurysm, and pericarditis.

5. **T waves** — this indicator of depolarization changes the morphology in several clinical settings:
   a. Ventricular hypertrophy (see above).
   b. Transient ischemia.
   c. Late transmural infarction.
   d. CVA's.
   e. High/low serum potassium.

V. DYSRHYTHMIAS: RECOGNITION AND MANAGEMENT

A. **Bradycardia** (rate < 60 beats/min).
   1. **Sinus bradycardia.**
      a. Decreased rate from within the sinus node (disease; increased parasympathetic tone; drugs: digitalis or β–blockers).
      b. Rhythm — regular.
      c. **Therapy** (Fig. 2) — treatment is required only when accompanied by hypotension, angina, dyspnea, altered mental status, myocardial ischemia or ventricular ectopy.
   2. **Second–degree A–V block, Möbitz Type I (Wenckebach)** occurs at level of A–V node and is often due to increased parasympathetic tone or drug effect (digitalis, propranolol). Usually transient. Characterized by a progressive prolongation of the PR interval indicative of decreasing conduction velocity through the A–V node before an impulse is completely blocked. Usually only a single impulse is blocked; then the cycle is repeated. The atrial rhythm is usually regular.
   3. **Second–degree A–V block, Möbitz Type II** occurs below level of A–V node either at the bundle of His (uncommon) or bundle branch level. Associated with an organic lesion in the conduction pathway. Poor prognosis; development of complete heart block should be anticipated. The P–R interval does not lengthen prior to a dropped beat. Atrial rhythm is usually regular. Treatment usually required: placement of transvenous pacemaker.

B. **Sinus tachycardia.**
   1. Increased rate within sinus node from demands for higher cardiac output (exercise, fever, anxiety).
   2. Rate ≥ 100.
   3. P wave — upright in I, II, AVF.
   4. **Therapy** — none specific, but treat underlying cause.

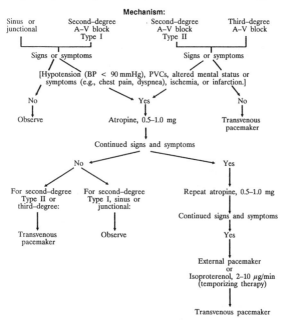

BRADYCARDIA

Slow Heart Rate (< 60 beats/min)
[A solitary chest thump or cough may stimulate cardiac electrical activity.]

FIGURE 2
Treatment for Bradycardia

Ref: Standards and guidelines for cardiopulmonary resuscitation (CPR) and emergency cardiac care (ECC). *JAMA* 255:2949, 1986, with permission. Copyright 1986, American Medical Association.

C. **Paroxysmal supraventricular tachycardia (PSVT) / paroxysmal atrial tachycardia (PAT).**
1. Sudden onset of tachycardia originating in atria, lasting minutes to hours.
2. Rate — atrial rate 160–200.
3. Rhythm — regular.
4. P waves — may not be present, i.e., buried in previous T wave.
5. P–R — normal or prolonged.
6. QRS — normal with rapid rate.
7. RBBB or less often LBBB with PAT/SVT may appear like ventricular tachycardia, but can be discerned by presence of P waves and BBB.
8. **Therapy** (Fig. 3) — dependent upon whether patient is stable or unstable.

UNSTABLE	STABLE
Synchronous cardioversion 75–100 Joules	Vagal maneuvers (carotid sinus massage, Valsalva)
↓	↓
Synchronous cardioversion 200 Joules	Verapamil, 5 mg IV
↓	↓
Synchronous cardioversion 360 Joules	Verapamil, 10 mg IV (in 15–20 min)
↓	↓
Correct underlying abnormalities	↓
↓	Cardioversion, digoxin,
Pharmacological therapy + cardioversion	β–blockers, pacing as indicated

FIGURE 3
Treatment for Paroxysmal Supraventricular Tachycardia

Ref: ibid., *JAMA* 255:2948, with permission. Copyright 1986, American Medical Association.

a. If conversion occurs, but PSVT recurs, repeated electrical cardioversion is *not* indicated. Sedation should be used as time permits.
b. Other therapies may include α–receptor stimulation (phenylephrine 30–60 mg/500 ml D5W to raise systolic BP 30–40 mm Hg in patients who are not significantly hypertensive) or edrophonium 1 mg IV; if no response, use up to 10 mg and watch for bronchospasm.

D. **Premature atrial contraction (PAC).**
1. Originates in atria, not in sinus node. May be caused by stimulants (caffeine, tobacco, ETOH), drugs, hypoxia, digitalis intoxication.
2. Rate — variable.

3. Rhythm — irregular.
4. P wave — abnormal, premature; may be buried in preceding T.
5. P–R — normal or prolonged (PAC with first–degree A–V block).
6. QRS — normal or wide if aberrancy (usually RBBB). QRS absent with complete block.
7. **Therapy** — discontinue stimulating factor (drug), correct hypoxia.

E. **Atrial flutter** (Fig. 4).

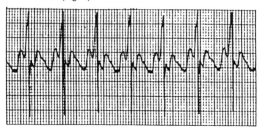

FIGURE 4
Atrial Flutter

Atrial rate is 250 per minute and rhythm is regular. Every other F (flutter) wave is conducted to ventricles (2:1 block), resulting in regular ventricular rhythm at rate of 125 per minute.

Ref: American Heart Association. *Textbook of Advanced Cardiac Life Support*. Dallas, TX: American Heart Association, 1987, p. 71, with permission.

1. "F–wave", "sawtooth" or "picket–fence" waves between QRS complexes with varying conduction ratios, best seen in leads II, III and AVF. Seen in organic heart disease (mitral or tricuspid valve) or coronary disease.
2. Rate — atrial rate about 300/min (220–350); ventricular rate about 150/min, but varies with ratio (2:1, 3:1, etc.).
3. Rhythm — atrial regular.
4. P waves — absent.
5. Flutter waves between QRS complexes. **Hint:** Turn EKG upside down to see waves.
6. QRS — normal, may be aberrant.
7. **Therapy.**
   a. If clinically symptomatic (hemodynamically), low–voltage DC countershock.

  b. Drugs to increase degree of A–V block (digitalis, propranolol).
  c. Overdrive pacemaker – atrial pacing at a rate faster than
   the intrinsic atrial rate may result in the conversion of atrial
   flutter to NSR or to atrial fibrillation.
  d. Watch for development of atrial fibrillation with digitalis
   or pacing.

F. Atrial fibrillation.
 1. Originates from multiple areas within atria, with only a small
  area of depolarization. May occur with digitalis intoxication.
 2. Rate – atrial rate 400–700 (may not be clearly seen); ventricular
  rate 60–180 (variable).
 3. Rhythm – irregularly irregular.
 4. P waves – absent.
 5. QRS – normal.
 6. Therapy.
  a. Digitalis to prolong A–V conduction.
  b. Synchronized DC cardioversion if clinically significant (pulmonary edema, low BP). Precautions include holding digitalis 24–48 hrs if possible, normalizing potassium and renal
   function, and stopping if ventricular arrhythmias occur.
  c. Quinidine, procainamide.
  d. Propranolol.

G. Premature ventricular contraction (PVC) [Fig. 5].

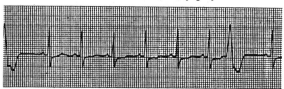

FIGURE 5
Premature Ventricular Contraction

Ref: ibid., p. 75, with permission.

 1. Early depolarization arising within a ventricle from one or more
  sites. Ventricles depolarize sequentially, followed by a compensatory pause (usually twice the regular sinus interval).
 2. Rate – variable.
 3. Rhythm – variable, irregular.
 4. P wave – usually obscured in previous S or T wave, or may
  be present.

5. QRS — prolonged, bizarre ≥ 0.12 sec. Complexes may have different appearances with different ectopic sites.
6. ST segments — slope away from QRS (inverted).
7. T waves — inverted.
8. Variations.
   a. Bigeminy — alternating normal beats and PVCs.
   b. Trigeminy — every third beat is a PVC.
   c. R–on–T — PVC falls on previous T wave; is especially dangerous because it may precipitate ventricular tachycardia or ventricular fibrillation.
9. Therapy (Fig. 6).

Assess for Need for Acute Suppressive Therapy

Rule out treatable cause
Consider serum potassium
Consider digitalis level
Consider bradycardia
Consider drugs

Lidocaine, 1 mg/kg

If not suppressed, repeat lidocaine, 0.5 mg/kg every 2–5 min, until no ectopy, or up to 3 mg/kg given

If not suppressed, procainamide, 20 mg/min, until no ectopy, or up to 1,000 mg given

If not suppressed, and not contraindicated, bretylium, 5–10 mg/kg over 8–10 min

If not suppressed, consider overdrive pacing

Once ectopy resolved, maintain as follows:
After lidocaine, 1 mg/kg ... lidocaine drip, 2 mg/min
After lidocaine, 1–2 mg/kg ... lidocaine drip, 3 mg/min
After lidocaine, 2–3 mg/kg ... lidocaine drip, 4 mg/min
After procainamide ... procainamide drip, 1–4 mg/min (check blood level)
After bretylium ... bretylium drip, 2 mg/min

FIGURE 6
Treatment for Premature Ventricular Contraction

Ref: op. cit., *JAMA* 255:2949, with permission. Copyright 1986, American Medical Association.

H. **Ventricular tachycardia (VT)** [Fig. 7].
1. Three or more PVCs together; may or may not cause clinical symptoms.
2. Rate — ≥ 100; usually ≤ 220.
3. Rhythm — variable, usually regular.
4. P waves — may be present or not.

5. QRS — wide; usually no Q in $V_{5,6}$.

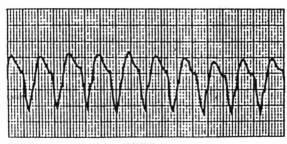

FIGURE 7
Ventricular Tachycardia

Ref: op. cit., American Heart Association, p. 78, with permission.

6. Fusion beats — early sinus–like, later like PVC. These occur prior to and at the end of a run of ventricular tachycardia; thus, are characteristic.
7. Therapy (Fig. 8).
8. Unstable — symptoms (e.g., chest pain, dyspnea), hypotension (systolic BP < 90 mm Hg), CHF, ischemia, or infarction.
9. If patient becomes unstable at any time, move to "unstable" arm of algorithm.
10. Sedation should be considered for all patients, including those defined as unstable, except those who are hemodynamically unstable (e.g., hypotensive, in pulmonary edema or unconscious).
11. If hemodynamically stable, a precordial thump may be employed prior to cardioversion.
12. Once VT has resolved, begin IV nfusion of the anti-arrhythmic agent that has aided resolution of the VT. If hemodynamically unstable, use lidocaine if cardioversion alone is unsuccessful, followed by bretylium. In all other patients, the recommended order of therapy is lidocaine, procainamide, and then bretylium.

I. **Torsade de pointes.**
   1. A form of ventricular tachycardia characterized by gradual alteration in the amplitude and direction of the electrical activity.
   2. Treated differently than other types of VT.
      a. Electrical pacing is treatment of choice.

     b. Magnesium sulfate + isoproterenol and lidocaine have also been reported as effective.

     c. Quinidine–like drugs are *contraindicated*.

  3. Polymorphic VT (PVT) can masquerade as *torsade de pointes* — pay close attention to the length of the QT interval of complexes preceding the tachycardia.

     a. When QT interval is long, pacing is indicated.

     b. If QT interval is normal, the arrhythmia is more likely to be PVT, and may therefore respond to antiarrhythmic drugs.

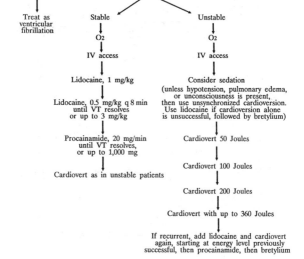

FIGURE 8

Treatment for Sustained Ventricular Tachycardia

Ref: op. cit., *JAMA* 255:2946, with permission. Copyright 1986, American Medical Association.

J. Ventricular fibrillation (Figs. 9 and 10).

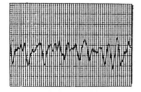
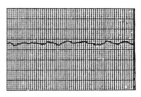

FIGURE 9 (Coarse) Ventricular Fibrillation FIGURE 10 (Fine)

Ref: op. cit., American Heart Association, p. 78, with permission.

1. Multiple areas of ectopic ventricular activity, but no effective pumping of the heart; hence, no cardiac output. It is a common cause of cardiac arrest due to ischemia or infarction. Amplitude of activity determines "coarse" vs. "fine" ventricular fibrillation.
2. Rate – rapid, disorganized.
3. Rhythm – none.
4. P, QRS, ST, T waves all undefinable.
5. **Therapy** (Fig. 11).
6. Pulseless ventricular tachycardia should be treated identically to ventricular fibrillation.
7. Check pulse and rhythm after each shock. If ventricular fibrillation recurs after transiently converting (rather than persists without ever converting), use whatever energy level has previously been successful for defibrillation.
8. The value of sodium bicarbonate is questionable during cardiac arrest, and it is *not* recommended for the routine cardiac arrest sequence. Consideration of its use in a dose of 1 mEq/kg is appropriate at the point noted in the sequence above. One–half of the original dose may be repeated q 10 min if it is used.
K. Ventricular asystole (agonal rhythm).
1. No effective electrical activity, resulting in no contraction.
2. P waves, QRS, ST, T waves may appear in ever–increasing intervals until no impulses or only isolated impulses are seen.
3. Asystole should be confirmed in two leads.
4. **Therapy** (Fig. 12).
5. The value of sodium bicarbonate is questionable during cardiac arrest, and it is *not* recommended for the routine cardiac arrest sequence.

WITNESSED ARREST   **UNWITNESSED ARREST**
Check pulse — if no pulse → precordial thump   Check pulse — if no pulse
Check pulse — if no pulse

CPR until a defibrillator is available
↓
Check monitor for rhythm — if VF or VT
↓
Defibrillate, 200 Joules (check pulse, rhythm after each shock)
↓
Defibrillate, 200–300 Joules
↓
Defibrillate with up to 360 Joules
↓
CPR if no pulse
↓
Establish IV access
↓
Epinephrine, 1:10,000, 0.5–1.0 mg IV push (repeat every 5 min)
↓
Intubate if possible
↓
Defibrillate with up to 360 Joules
↓
Lidocaine, 1 mg/kg IV push (may repeat 0.5–1 mg/kg every 8 min up to 3 mg/kg)
↓
Defibrillate with up to 360 Joules
↓
Bretylium, 5 mg/kg IV push
↓
Consider bicarbonate (1 mEq/kg, then 1/2 dose every 10 min)
↓
Defibrillate with up to 360 Joules
↓
Bretylium, 10 mg/kg IV push
↓
Defibrillate with up to 360 Joules
↓
Repeat lidocaine or bretylium
↓
Defibrillate with up to 360 Joules

FIGURE 11
Treatment for Ventricular Fibrillation

Ref: op. cit., *JAMA* 255:2946, with permission. Copyright 1986, American
Medical Association.

If rhythm is unclear and possibly ventricular fibrillation,
defibrillate as for ventricular fibrillation.
if asystole is present (confirmed in at least two leads):

↓

Continue CPR

↓

Establish IV access

↓

Epinephrine, 1:10,000, 0.5–1.0 mg IV push (repeat every 5 min)

↓

Intubate when possible

↓

Atropine, 1.0 mg IV push (repeated in 5 min)

↓

Consider bicarbonate (1 mEq/kg initially, then 1/2 dose every 10 min)

↓

Consider pacing

FIGURE 12
Treatment for Ventricular Asystole

Ref: ibid., *JAMA* 255:2947, with permission. Copyright 1986, American
Medical Association.

L. **Electromechanical dissociation** (Fig. 13) — electrical activity (usually QRS–type activity) depicted on EKG, but no pulse.

Continue CPR

↓

Establish IV access

↓

Epinephrine, 1:10,000, 0.5–1.0 mg IV push (should be repeated every 5 min)

↓

Intubate when possible
(If intubation can be accomplished simultaneously with other techniques,
then the earlier the better; however, epinephrine is more important
initially if the patient can be ventilated without intubation.)

↓

Consider bicarbonate
(The value of sodium bicarbonate is questionable during cardiac arrest
and is not recommended for the routine cardiac arrest sequence.
Consideration of its use in a dose of 1 mEq/kg is appropriate at this point.
One-half of the original dose may be repeated every 10 min if it is used.)

↓

Consider hypovolemia, cardiac tamponade, tension pneumothorax,
hypoxemia, acidosis, pulmonary embolism

FIGURE 13
Electromechanical Dissociation

Ref: ibid., *JAMA* 255:2947, with permission. Copyright 1986, American
Medical Association.

M. Atrioventricular blocks.
    1. First–degree block (Fig. 14).

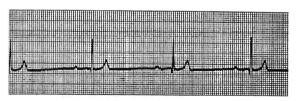

FIGURE 14
First–Degree Atrioventricular Block

Ref: op. cit., American Heart Association, p. 80, with permission.

    a. Delayed impulse transmission from atria to ventricle.
    b. Rhythm — regular.
    c. Rate — variable.
    d. P wave — normal shape; P–R interval is beyond normal
        (> 0.20 sec).
    e. QRS — normal.
    f. Treatment — none usually necessary; watch for second and
        third–degree blocks.
    2. Second–degree block, Type I (Wenckebach) [Fig. 15].

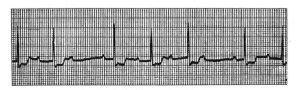

FIGURE 15
Type I (Wenckebach) Second–Degree Atrioventricular Block

Ref: ibid., p. 81, with permission.

    a. Atrial rate is higher than ventricular, since not all impulses are transmitted through to ventricles. Atrial rate is regular despite dropped beats.
    b. Rhythm — atrial regular, ventricular irregular.
    c. Rate — atrial > ventricular.
    d. P wave — normal; progressive lengthening of P–R interval until the impulse is not conducted and the beat is dropped, i.e., R–R is progressively shorter.
    e. QRS — normal.
    f. **Treatment** (see Fig. 2) —Type I occurs with increased parasympathetic tone or drugs (digitalis, propranolol); therapy is usually not required; watch for third–degree block.

3. **Second–degree block, Type II** (Fig. 16).

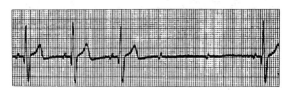

FIGURE 16
Type II Second–Degree Atrioventricular Block

Ref: ibid., p. 82, with permission.

    a. Block occurs at bundle–branch level or bundle of His, and is reflective of organic disease; thus, poorer prognosis.
    b. Rhythm — atrial regular, ventricular irregular.
    c. Rate — atrial > ventricular.
    d. P wave — normal; not all followed by QRS.
    e. QRS — intermittent dropped QRS complexes; following dropped beat, next beat usually has normal P; dropped beats may occur in succession; QRS may be wide in bundle–branch block.
    f. **Therapy** (see Fig. 2) — watch closely for third–degree block to develop; may need pacer.

4. **Third–degree block** (Fig. 17).

    a. Disorganized rhythm, as atrial impulses are not conducted to the ventricles; atrial beats and ventricular beats are therefore independent.
    b. Rhythm — atrial regular, ventricular regular but unrelated.
    c. Rate — atrial rate may be normal; ventricular rate 40–60 if block at A–V node, < 40 if block within ventricle.

    d. P waves — normal, regular interval.
    e. P–R — variable.
    f. QRS — variable intervals unrelated to P wave; may be wide if block in ventricles.
    g. Therapy (see Fig. 2).
        1) May be caused by drugs (digitalis, propranolol) or MI.
        2) Watch for asystole.
        3) If ventricular rate slow, give atropine (bradycardia).
        4) May require pacemaker.
        5) Consider isoproterenol.

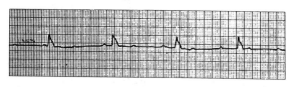

FIGURE 17
Third–Degree Atrioventricular Block

Ref: ibid., p. 83, with permission.

N. Wolff–Parkinson–White syndrome.
    1. Rate — normal.
    2. Rhythm — regular.
    3. P wave — normal.
    4. P–R — short secondary to slurred upstroke of QRS (delta wave).
    5. QRS — prolonged.
        a. (+) QRS in V_1 = Type A.
        b. (–) QRS in V_1 = Type B.
O. Drug reactions.
    1. Digoxin.
        a. Therapeutic reactions.
            1) P–R prolonged.
            2) QT shortened.
            3) ST changes opposite to QRS.
            4) Lower T amplitude.
        b. Toxic reactions.
            1) Bradycardia.
            2) A–V block.
            3) Arrhythmias.

       4) Toxicity increased in hypoxia, low potassium, acidosis.

2. Quinidine.
  a. Therapeutic reactions.
     1) Lower P amplitude.
     2) P–R slightly prolonged.
     3) QRS, QT prolonged (correlates with drug level).
  b. Toxic reactions.
     1) P–R significantly prolonged.
     2) SA node or A–V block.
     3) QRS prolonged > 50% of initial.
     4) Multifocal PVCs.

P. Electrolyte disturbances.
  1. Potassium elevated.
    a. Earliest – tall "tented" T; later wide QRS (like LBBB).
    b. P waves wide, flat (like atrial fibrillation).
    c. Intraventricular block.
    d. Serial EKG correlates with level.
    e. Worse in low sodium or calcium, or acidosis.
  2. Potassium low.
    a. QT prolonged; flat, broad T which may also be inverted.
    b. ST depression.
    c. U wave present.
    d. Supraventricular and ventricular ectopy.
    e. Worse with digitalis intoxication.
  3. Calcium elevated.
    a. QT shortened (smaller ST segment).
    b. PR prolonged; A–V block and/or QRS prolonged if severe.
    c. Ventricular instability (PVCs, ventricular tachycardia).
  4. Calcium low – QT prolonged (long ST).
  5. Magnesium low – QT prolonged.

WOUND HEALING, CARE, AND COMPLICATIONS

The body's capacity to repair tissue damage forms the foundation of all surgical practice. The healing process generally proceeds without complications; however, deficient healing and wound infection continue to be leading causes of morbidity in surgical patients. Current clinical wound care is based on knowledge of the relevant physiology and pathophysiology involved.

I. PHYSIOLOGY OF WOUND HEALING

Orderly repair involves a series of morphologic, chemical, and physical events that result in the production of scar tissue.

A. **Inflammatory phase** — the initial response to injury. Intensity and duration are related to the degree of wound **contamination** and local **tissue damage.** After transient vasoconstriction lasting 5–10 minutes, all local small vessels dilate. Capillaries become abnormally permeable, allowing egress of blood cells and plasma proteins with formation of an inflammatory exudate and edema. **Leukocytes** actively migrate into the wound, and phagocytosis removes cellular debris and injured tissue fragments. Vascular and early inflammatory responses are mediated by **histamines** (released by mast cells), **kinins**, and **prostaglandins.**

B. **Epithelialization** — involves **migration** of cells from the marginal basal layer of the epidermis across the denuded wound area. Begins **24 hours** after wounding. A monolayer is formed, and these cells differentiate and divide. However, normal architecture is never attained and the epidermis is thin and fragile.

C. **Cellular phase** — begins at 48–72 hours. Local perivascular pleuripotential mesenchymal cells in the extravascular tissues migrate into the wound and transform into fibroblasts. The cells migrate along fibrin strands which act as a physical barrier to fibroblast penetration. Factors from platelets and macrophages induce neovascularization. The new capillary buds produce fibrinolysin, which allows them to progress through areas of clot.

D. **Proliferative phase** and collagen synthesis — an active **synthesis of collagen** as well as ground substance (proteoglycans) begins around day 5 and the wound begins to gain strength. Collagen content increases steadily for **3 weeks**, then begins to plateau. After **5 weeks** the fibroblasts decrease in number and the capillary network becomes organized. Wound contraction will occur in open wounds due to the development of contractile **myofibroblasts.** This draws the wound edges together until balanced by equal tension in the surrounding skin.

E. **Scar remodeling** — the predominant phase after 3 weeks; continues for the life of the wound. Collagenases break down old collagen as fast as new collagen is synthesized, forming a dynamic equilibrium. Increase in tensile strength correlates with increased crosslinks between collagen strands and alignment of collagen fibers along lines of tension. Scar tissue *never* reaches the tensile strength of unwounded tissue.

II. TYPES OF WOUND HEALING

A. **Primary intention** — healing occurs when tissue is cleanly incised and reapproximated and repair occurs without complication.

B. **Secondary intention** (spontaneous healing) — an open wound heals by contraction, granulation, and spontaneous epithelialization. Contraction is limited by laxity of surrounding skin, and epithelialization extends only a few millimeters over an open wound.

C. **Tertiary intention** (delayed primary closure) — occurs when a wound is closed after a period of secondary healing. This allows contaminated wounds to be surgically closed after 4–5 days with decreased risk of infection.

III. MANAGEMENT OF SOFT TISSUE WOUNDS

A. **Traumatic wound care.**
   1. Initiate treatment only after more urgent problems have been dealt with. Initial control of arterial and venous bleeding is best done with **direct pressure**.
   2. Obtain x-rays for suspected foreign bodies or underlying fractures.
   3. With adequate light, assistance, instruments, and aseptic technique, begin systematic search for other injuries, including nerves, vascular structures, tendons, joints, ducts (lacrimal/parotid), or bone. Frequently, these injuries are best dealt with under OR conditions.
   4. Cleanse skin around wound, avoiding the wound itself, as antiseptic agents are damaging to exposed tissues. Use povidone-iodine (Betadine®) for extremity and trunk wounds; chlorhexidine (Hibiclens®) or hexachlorophene (pHisoHex®) for facial wounds. Isolate wound with sterile drapes. Cut hair as needed, but avoid shaving eyebrows or hairline.
   5. Anesthetize with local agents as appropriate if there is no history of allergy (see "Anesthesia" — local anesthetics). **Avoid** use of epinephrine.
   6. Gentle saline irrigation can decrease the number of bacteria in a wound. A 60 cc syringe/19 gauge IV catheter can be used. A surfactant such as pluronic F–68 or Poloxamer 188 can be used to remove grease or dirt.
   7. Obtain hemostasis by clamping bleeding vessels under **direct vision**.
   8. Excise devitalized tissue as well as any remaining foreign bodies.

B. **Wound closure.**
   1. Wounds with minimal bacterial contamination, controllable hemorrhage, and little or no necrotic tissue/foreign bodies may be closed primarily.

     a. Close wounds without tension with the least reactive suture, staples or tape. Avoid closure of subcutaneous tissue.

     b. Observe wound periodically for drainage or infection.

  2. Avoid primary closure for:

     a. Inflamed, infected wounds ($> 10^5$ organisms/g tissue).

     b. Dirty, neglected, or old (> 6 hours, except on face/scalp) wounds or wounds contaminated with manure or feces.

     c. Missile, crush or wounds sustained in mass casualty situation.

     d. Wounds in which adequacy of debridement is uncertain.

     e. Human and animal bites, except for selected bites to the face.

  3. Treatment of open wounds should include cleansing and debridement and packing with fine–meshed gauze.

  4. Antibiotics are indicated for cellulitis in the tissues surrounding the wound, infected wounds in immunocompromised individuals, abscesses in the central area of the face, and all human–bite wounds, which must be considered infected from infliction.

  5. Delayed primary closure — may be performed after 4 or more days of dressing changes in the absence of devitalized tissue, significant bacterial contamination, or clinical signs of inflammation. Tape strips or interrupted suture (with nothing buried) is preferable.

C. Dressings.

  1. For **clean surgical wounds**, dressing should be left in place 48–72 hours to allow time for epithelialization. The ideal dressing is sterilely applied, splints the skin around the incision, absorbs excess drainage, and approximates the permeability of the skin (i.e., Tegaderm®/Telfa®). Dressing should be removed earlier if saturated by blood or serum, or there is suspicion of infection.

  2. For **contaminated wounds**, following initial cleansing and debridement, the wound should be packed to keep the wound open, promote hemostasis, and act to debride the wound. The wet–wet or wet–dry dressing should be changed every 6–8 hours or more often as needed.

     a. Normal saline is an isotonic, all–purpose solution that is non–toxic to tissues.

     b. Dakin's solution, 2% boric acid, 0.25% acetic acid, and povidone–iodine have also been used for more heavily contaminated or superficially infected wounds, although their use may inhibit granulation.

D. Tetanus and rabies prophylaxis.

  1. Tetanus is a rare condition caused by the cytotoxin of *Clostridium tetanii*. Symptoms include headache, tetanic contractions, stiffness of jaw muscles, and trismus. May progress to opisthotonus and respiratory arrest.

2. Tetanus–prone wounds are **old** (> 6 hrs), **deep** (> 1 cm), **contaminated** wounds, especially those involving rusty metals, manure, feces, or soil. Missile, crush, stellate or avulsion wounds with devitalized tissue are also at risk.
3. Adequate immunization for adults requires at least **three** injections of toxoid, with a booster every 10 years. In children < 7 years, immunization requires four injections of DPT. A fifth dose may be given at 4–6 years of age. Thereafter, adult type (Td) is recommended for routine or wound boosters.
4. Specific measures for patients with wounds.
   a. Previously immunized individuals.
      1) If the patient is fully immunized and the last dose of toxoid was given within 10 years, for non–tetanus–prone wounds no booster of toxoid is indicated. For tetanus-prone wounds and if **more than five years** has elapsed since the last dose, 0.5 ml of adsorbed toxoid should be given. If excessive prior toxoid injections have been given, this booster may be omitted.
      2) When the patient has had 2 or more prior injections of toxoid and received the last dose more than 10 years previously, 0.5 ml of adsorbed toxoid should be given for both tetanus– and non–tetanus–prone wounds. Passive immunization is not necessary.
   b. Individuals *NOT* adequately immunized (or unknown).
      1) For non–tetanus–prone wounds, 0.5 ml of adsorbed toxoid should be given.
      2) For tetanus–prone wounds, 0.5 ml of adsorbed toxoid and 250 units (or more) of human tetanus immune globulin should be given using different needles, syringes, and sites of injection. Administration of antibiotics should be considered, although their effectiveness in prophylaxis is unproven.
   c. **Note:** Adequate wound care and debridement are important parts of tetanus prophylaxis in all patients.
5. Rabies prophylaxis.
   a. Indicated for bites by carnivorous wild animals (esp. skunks, raccoons, foxes, and coyotes) and bats, but not for bites by domestic animals (unless thought to be rabid) or rodents such as mice, rats, or squirrels.
   b. Previously unimmunized persons should receive five 1–ml doses of human diploid cell vaccine (HDCV) by IM injection on days 0, 3, 7, 14, and 28. Rabies immune globulin (RIG) 20 IU/kg (preferable) or equine anti–rabies serum (ARS) 40 IU/kg should be given only if available prior to day 8, with half the dose infiltrated in the area of the wound and the remainder given IM. RIG or ARS is not indicated after day 8.

IV. WOUND COMPLICATIONS

A. Factors affecting wound healing.

1. Age — probably not important as an independent factor.
2. Anemia — associated hypovolemia with wound hypoperfusion are more important than the absolute level of hemoglobin.
3. Blood supply.
4. Chemotherapy — all are deleterious to healing, with the greatest effects in early stages. Should delay use until 4–7 days after operation.
5. Diabetes — uncontrolled hyperglycemia (> 250) impairs leukocyte function, leading to increased susceptibility to infection. This is largely reversed by good blood glucose control.
6. Immunosuppressants.
   a. Cyclosporine has no effect.
   b. Azathioprine effects are like prednisone.
7. Liver failure (jaundice).
8. Malnutrition.
9. Obesity.
10. Pre–existing disease — particularly neoplasia.
11. Radiation therapy — dose related; both acute and chronic effects are seen. Delaying initiation until POD 4–6 will significantly decrease incidence of wound complications.
12. Sepsis.
13. Steroids — impair healing at every phase.
14. Tension — leads to hypoperfusion and wound hypoxia.
15. Tissue trauma — poor surgical technique.
16. Uremia — healing is improved by careful dialysis and nutritional supplementation.

B. Management of wound complications.

1. One–half of all postoperative complications are wound related, with infection being the most common.
2. **Wound infection** — results from imbalance between number and virulence of bacteria, host defense mechanisms, and wound environment.
   a. Greater incidence with prolonged preoperative stay, shaving the evening prior to operation, breaks in surgical technique, longer duration of operation, abdominal operations, poor surgical technique (mass ligatures, hematomas, necrotic tissue), presence of foreign bodies, presence of drains, wound hypoperfusion, advanced age, pre–existing disease.
   b. Usually noted 3–6 days post–closure with presence of fever and fluctuant, tender, and/or cellulitic wound.
   c. **Treatment** — open wound, culture exudate, debride wound as necessary, then treat as contaminated wound. Antibiotics are useful if significant **cellulitis** or **systemic sepsis** present.

    d. *Staph.* and *Strep.* are the most common pathogens, particularly with implanted prostheses, unless a hollow viscus has been entered, then consider gram–negative bacilli.

    e. Necrotizing fascitis — usually polymicrobial infection. Overlying skin may show only a mild edema. **Aggressive** surgical debridement is essential, with removal of all necrotic tissue. Skin and subcutaneous tissue can often be preserved. Colonic diversion may be indicated if perineum involved. Penicillin/clindamycin/aminoglycoside combinations are appropriate empiric antibiotic treatment with modification according to culture data.

    f. Gas–forming infections — present with early signs of sepsis, progressing to crepitance and shock. Caused by synergistic gram–negative and microaerophilic gram–positive organisms. Often seen in diabetics. **Clostridial myonecrosis** is a rapidly progressive form involving muscle with characteristic "bronze" discoloration of skin over wound.

        1) Treat non–clostridial infections with broad–spectrum antibiotics (including anaerobes), and debridement and drainage. Monitor closely.

        2) Treat clostridial infections with early aggressive debridement and high–dose penicillin. May require early amputation if poor response to treatment. Hyperbaric oxygen adds little to overall survival.

3. Wound collections — hematoma/seroma.

    a. Use closed–suction drains in procedures prone to seroma formation. If seroma forms after removal of drain, treat with intermittent sterile aspirations. May need to re–insert drain if seroma persists. Control regional edema or infection with compression stockings and antibiotics as indicated.

    b. Hematomas must be evacuated and hemostasis obtained if bleeding ongoing. The wound may be resutured if there are no signs of infection.

4. Vascular compromise.

    a. Caused by wound edge necrosis, intrinsic vascular disease, undermined wound edges, excessive tension, sutures fixed with excess tension.

    b. Treat with debridement and local care with antibiotics for cellulitis/sepsis.

5. Wound dehiscence.

    a. Superficial — separation of wound edges at skin or subcutaneous level due to lack of tensile strength or infection. May re–close if not infected, otherwise treat as open contaminated wound.

    b. Fascial — separation of deep fascia (abdomen) with potential evisceration. Evisceration of omentum or bowel is associated with 15% mortality.

1) No one incision or type of closure is most prone to dehiscence. The most common causes are technical error, local ischemia, increased intra–abdominal pressure, sepsis, and obesity. Typically occurs at POD 5–8 with sudden drainage of pink, sero-sanguinous ("salmon-colored") fluid as sentinel sign.

2) If **evisceration** occurs, place a sterile towel moistened with saline over contents and arrange transfer to OR immediately. Repair dehiscence with mass closure of heavy stainless–steel wire or monofilament permanent suture. Minor fascial separations may be dealt with expectantly, with later repair of the resultant hernia. Larger fascial separation should be repaired (see Section IV.-A).

c. **Retention sutures** — used to prevent evisceration in the event of fascial dehiscence in patients at high risk; extraperitoneal placement preferred. These are removed at 14–21 days if healing proceeds without complication.

V. INDICATIONS FOR PROPHYLACTIC ANTIBIOTICS

A. Clean–contaminated wounds — anticipated violation of GI, GU or respiratory tracts.

B. Contaminated wounds — trauma.

C. Insertion of synthetic material — vascular grafts, artificial valves, prosthetic joints.

D. Patients with prosthetic heart valves or history of valvular heart disease.

E. High–risk patients.

VI. PRINCIPLES OF DRAIN MANAGEMENT

A. Rarely indicated for non-infected wounds unless large amount of dead space remains or fluid collection anticipated. Remove after 2 days if used, unless amount of drainage significant.

B. **Closed–suction drains** are preferable, as they have the lowest incidence of infection.

C. Intra–abdominal drains.

1. Clean cases — use only closed–suction drains. Remove with suction off when drainage minimal. Penrose drains (if used) require gravity to be effective.

2. Abscesses — Penrose drains, large axiom sumps, or large closed–suction drains may be used. Purpose is to establish a tract. Leave in 7–10 days or longer if productive. May advance Penrose drains 4 cm/day when patient afebrile.

MANAGEMENT OF THE DIABETIC PATIENT

Diabetes is the most common metabolic disease that surgeons encounter. Poorly–controlled diabetes may result in an increased risk of infection. Neutrophil function may be impaired when blood sugars exceed 250 mg/dl. Complications such as diabetic ketoacidosis, malignant hyperglycemia and hyperosmolar coma are ever–present threats in poorly–controlled diabetes.

I. GENERAL PRINCIPLES AND ASSESSMENT

A. **Diagnosis** — fasting plasma glucose > 140 mg% in the non–stressed patient or > 175 mg% in the stressed patient.
B. Stress produces glucose intolerance (infection, surgery, anesthetic, trauma, steroid treatment, pregnancy).
   1. Altered glucose metabolism in the normal patient.
   2. Aggravates pre–existing diabetes.
C. Predilection for electrolyte/water/acid–base imbalance.
D. **Preoperative management** of the diabetic patient.
   1. Requires preoperative control prior to performing elective procedures.
   2. Pre–op correlation of serum glucose with fingerstick glucose and urine S & A (see IV–A, below).
   3. Correct electrolyte abnormalities, especially hypokalemia.
   4. Maintain adequate hydration.

II. PERIOPERATIVE MANAGEMENT

A. **Preoperative.**
   1. Patients on an oral hypoglycemic agent — discontinue one day preoperatively.
   2. Schedule early *a.m.* operation if possible.
   3. Start IV containing dextrose (i.e., D51/2 normal saline) the night prior to surgery at 50–75 cc/hr (minimum carbohydrate requirement is 100 g/day).
   4. Give 1/3 to 1/2 of usual dose and type (i.e., NPH, Lente, Regular) of insulin subcutaneously (SC) in *a.m.* of surgery.
   5. Some prefer continuous IV infusion of regular insulin for perioperative control of the brittle diabetic.
B. **Postoperative.**
   1. Continue IV dextrose.
   2. Follow glucose q 4-6 h by serum glucose determination, fingerstick glucose, urine S & A. Supplement with regular insulin SC or IV (see Sliding Scale, IV–A, below).
   3. Adjust insulin dose with resumption of oral diet or enteral feeding.
   4. Resume oral hypoglycemic agent when feasible.

III. MANAGEMENT OF HYPERGLYCEMIA

A. Acceptable range of serum glucose 150–200 mg/dl. Hyperglycemia and ketonemia and ketonuria suggests **diabetic ketoacidosis**.

B. **IV fluids.**
   1. When glucose > 250 mg/dl use normal saline plus potassium chloride (no dextrose).
   2. Add dextrose to IV when glucose < 250 mg/dl.
   3. Follow serum glucose, electrolytes, and blood pH every 4 hrs and correct accordingly.

C. **Insulin treatment.**
   1. IV administration — rapid response, accurate dosing. Useful in severe hyperglycemia (glucose > 400 mg/dl).
      a. Bolus injection — rapid response, short half–life. Start with 5–10 units IV bolus. Need to supplement with continuous infusion, IM, or SC administration.
      b. Continuous infusion — more accurate control. Start with 1–2 units/hr. Increase every hour as needed.
   2. Intramuscular (IM) — intermediate absorption, longer half–life than IV bolus.
   3. Subcutaneous (SC) — least reliable absorption in hypoperfused patients; advantageous in well–perfused patient because of longer half–life.

D. **Ultimate control of hyperglycemia** may depend on surgical intervention (i.e., drainage of abscess, amputation, removal of infected line, etc.).

IV. METHODS OF MONITORING GLUCOSE, AND TREATMENT

A. **Serum glucose sliding scale** (if fingerstick glucose is used, must establish correlation with serum glucose).

Glucose	Regular Insulin (SC)
0–200	0
201–250	5 U
251–300	8 U
301–350	10 U
351–400	12 U
> 400	call M.D.

Adjust sliding scale according to response to above parameters.

B. **IV insulin infusion scale:**

Patient

"A"	"B"
Thin	Obese
Minimum illness, minimum surgery	Severe illness, major surgery
Usual insulin requirement < 50 U/day	Usual insulin requirement > 50 U/day
Infusion fluid: 1 L sodium chloride (0.45 mol/L) plus 20 mEq/L potassium chloride plus 500 U heparin* plus 50 U rapid acting insulin	Infusion fluid: 1 L sodium chloride (0.45 mol/L) plus 20 mEq/L potassium chloride plus 500 U heparin* plus 100 U rapid acting insulin.

Blood Glucose Concentration (mg/dl)	Infusion Rate (ml/hr)	"A" Insulin (U/hr)	"B" Insulin (U/hr)
0–50	5	0.25	0.50
5–100	10	0.50	1.00
100–150	15	0.75	1.50
150–200	20	1.00	2.00
200–250	25	1.25	2.50
250–300	30	1.50	3.00
300–350	35	1.75	3.50
350–400	40	2.00	4.00
> 400	50	3.00	6.00

* Does not anticoagulate patient, but does maintain the IV line patent.

Ref: Schade DS. *Med. Clin. N. Am.* 72:1531, 1988, with permission.

C. **Urine sugar and acetone (S & A)** — generally not reliable unless correlation with serum glucose is established and double–voided specimen obtained; may be useful as "screening" for glycosuria or ketonuria.

V. TYPES OF INSULIN

A. **Human insulin (Humulin)** should be used as the standard class of insulin (as opposed to bovine or porcine). Useful in the sensitive diabetic with antibodies to animal–derived insulin.

B. **Insulin characteristics** (see "Formulary"):

Action	Insulin	Onset	Peak	Duration
Short	Regular	1/2–1 hr	2–4 hrs	6 hrs
	Semilente	1/2–1 hr	4–8 hrs	12–16 hrs
Intermediate	NPH	1–2 hrs	8–12 hrs	18–24 hrs
	Lente	1–2 hrs	8–12 hrs	18–24 hrs
Long	Protamine zinc	4–8 hrs	12–24 hrs	36 hrs
	Ultralente	4–8 hrs	12–24 hrs	36 hrs

VI. COMPLICATIONS

A. **Hypoglycemia** (< 50 mg/dl) — dangerous situation, especially under anesthesia when symptoms are masked. Treat with intravenous D50.

B. **Hyperglycemia.**
   1. Leukocyte dysfunction when serum glucose > 250 mg/dl.
   2. Increased infection rate.
   3. Poor wound healing in diabetics (may not be directly related to hyperglycemia).
   4. Osmotic diuresis/dehydration — electrolyte abnormalities.
   5. Extreme:
      a. Diabetic ketoacidosis (DKA).
      b. Hyperglycemic, hyperosmotic non–ketotic coma (HHNK).

Reference:

Diabetic ketoacidosis. In: Campbell JW, Frisse M (eds), *Manual of Medical Therapeutics*, 24th Ed. Boston: Little, Brown and Company, 1983, pp. 345-349.

THROMBOEMBOLIC PROPHYLAXIS AND MANAGEMENT OF VENOUS THROMBOEMBOLISM

I. INTRODUCTION

A. **Deep venous thrombosis (DVT)** is a common problem in surgical patients of all types.

B. **Estimates of DVT** after surgical procedures in unprotected patients:
   1. General surgery (intra-abdominal) — 25%.
   2. Total hip replacement — 40–58%.
   3. Post-partum — 3%.
   4. Prostatectomy — 50%.
   5. Trauma — 20%.

C. **Non–fatal** — DVT results in significant morbidity, prolonged hospitalization, and can lead to post-phlebitis syndrome and chronic venous atresia disease.

D. **Pulmonary embolism (PE)** occurs about 600,000 times annually in the U.S., 50,000 deaths/year and contributes to another 150,000 deaths. About 10% of the deaths occur within the first hour.

E. **Pathogenesis** — there are 3 primary factors, known as **Virchow's Triad,** occurring singly or in combination, which play a role in the pathogenesis of DVT:
   1. Stasis.
   2. Endothelial injury.
   3. Hypercoagulability.

F. **Signs and symptoms** of DVT are nonspecific (leg swelling, pain) and often absent.
   1. In patients suspected of having DVT based on signs and symptoms, less than 50% actually will have DVT.
   2. Signs and symptoms are present in only about 50% of patients documented to have DVT by venography.

G. **Pulmonary thromboembolism** — can occur from iliofemoral and pelvic veins, the IVC, as well as from ovarian, subclavian and internal jugular veins and cavernous sinuses of the skull. Calf vein thrombosis is common, but only rarely gives rise to emboli unless they propagate into the femoral vein.

II. FACTORS THAT INCREASE THE RISK OF DVT

A. Age > 60.

B. Malignancy (especially prostate and pancreatic cancer, and carcinomatosis).

C. Prior history of DVT, PE, or varicose veins.

D. Prolonged immobilization or bed rest.

E. Cardiac disease, especially congestive heart failure.

F. Pregnancy.
G. Oral contraceptives.
H. Hypercoagulability.
I. Obesity.
J. Pelvic surgery.
K. Trauma.

III. PROPHYLAXIS

A. Mechanical methods.

1. **Leg elevation and early ambulation** — reduces thrombosis rate by 25–60%.
2. **Graduated compression stockings** — increases the velocity of femoral venous blood flow and lowers the incidence of DVT by a small amount. However, stockings must be well fitted.
3. **Pneumatic compression boots** — a device that intermittently inflates and deflates, resulting in compression of the limb, usually the calves.
   a. Mechanism of action is both by propulsion of blood flow from calves to heart and by activation of a fibrinolytic mechanism. In one study, boots were found to be effective in preventing DVT even when placed on the arms.
   b. Effective at reducing DVT in surgical patients including orthopedic hip patients. Reduces the incidence of DVT by 2/3 on neurosurgery patients and 50–75% in general surgery patients.
   c. Pneumatic compression boots do not increase the risk of bleeding, which is especially important in neurologic and ophthalmologic patients. Patient compliance can be a problem.

B. Pharmacologic agents.

1. **Coumadin®**.
   a. Effective in surgical patients, including hip patients.
   b. Disadvantages.
      1) Must be started 2–3 days pre-op.
      2) May result in unacceptable intra– and post–op bleeding.
      3) Need to monitor the prothrombin time (PT).
2. **Heparin** — binds to anti–thrombin III and accelerates its action. Can be used at "therapeutic" doses in high–risk patients, but usually given as "low–dose heparin".
   a. Low–dose heparin — 5,000 units SQ beginning 2 hrs before surgery, then every 8–12 hrs thereafter; 12–hr regimens are equally effective as 8 hrs.
   b. Shown to be effective in reducing DVT occurrence by 2/3 and PE by 1/2 in general, urologic and recently orthopedic patients.
   c. For morbidly obese patients, a "micro–heparin drip" at 1 unit/kg/hr is more effective.

    d. There may be a small increase in the incidence of bleeding complications, although low–dose heparin does not increase the partial thromboplastin time (PTT). Thrombocytopenia is a potential side–effect.

  3. Heparin with dihydroergotamine (**Embolex®**) – dihydroergotamine is thought to constrict capacitance vessels and accelerate venous return.

    a. Reduces DVT incidence more than heparin alone.

    b. Contraindicated in patients with angina, a history of stroke or TIA's, or peripheral vascular disease.

  4. **Dextran-40** (low molecular weight dextran) – decreases RBC adhesiveness, platelet aggregation, and causes hemodilution.

    a. Has been shown to be effective DVT prophylaxis, particularly in high–risk patients.

    b. Disadvantages include a small increase in clinical bleeding, volume overload in patients with cardiac compromise, and allergic reaction in 1% of patients.

    c. Recommended dose 15–20 cc/hr continuous IV infusion perioperatively.

  5. **ASA** – only shown to help in hip surgery patients, although there is a high failure rate.

C. **Prophylactic IVC filter placement** – used in extremely high–risk patients who have contraindication to other forms of prophylaxis. Obviously is not effective against DVT, only PE.

D. Regional anesthesia compared to general anesthesia has been shown to be less thrombogenic and to lower the incidence of PE.

IV. AN APPROACH TO PROPHYLAXIS

A. **Determine risk of patient.**

  1. Low risk – age under 40; ambulatory, uncomplicated or minor surgery.

  2. Moderate risk – age over 40; abdominal, pelvic or thoracic surgery.

  3. High risk – age over 40; hip surgery, prior DVT or PE, presence of malignancy, immobility.

B. **Prophylaxis of choice:**

  1. All patients should be out of bed and ambulating as soon as possible after surgery.

  2. Low–risk patients probably do not need prophylaxis.

  3. Moderate–risk patients should have either pneumatic compression boots or low–dose heparin prophylaxis.

  4. High-risk patients should probably have a combination of therapies – pneumatic compression boots plus low–dose heparin or Dextran-40. Full anticoagulation with Coumadin® or caval interruption can be considered. There is no data to support or refute combination therapy as more effective than either therapy alone in high-risk patients.

5. Prophylaxis should be started *prior* to the institution of anesthesia.
6. **Special considerations.**
   a. Ophthalmology and neurosurgery patients with intracranial or spinal lesions are *not* considered candidates for prophylaxis with anticoagulants since even minor bleeding can have disastrous consequences.
   b. Those at high risk should be watched closely for the development of clinical signs and symptoms of DVT and also objectively tested frequently (i.e., every 3–4 days) for DVT. Duplex ultrasound scanning has been shown to be 88% sensitive for clinically significant DVT of the lower extremities. The radioactive fibrinogen uptake test is sensitive for calf vein thrombosis, but insensitive for thigh and iliac vein thrombosis. Contrast venography is the gold standard, but impractical for screening serial evaluation.

V. TREATMENT OF DVT AND PE
A. Most difficult part of treatment is making the diagnosis!
B. **Objectives of treatment.**
   1. Prevent death from PE.
   2. Reduce morbidity from acute event.
   3. Prevent post–phlebitic syndrome (symptoms of chronic edema, induration, pain, pigmentation and ulceration of extremity).
   4. Minimize complications of treatment.
C. **Anticoagulation** — standard treatment for both DVT and PE.
   1. A heparin bolus (100-150 units/kg) is given IV, followed by a constant infusion of heparin (starting at 1,000 U/hr) and titrated to keep the PTT at 60–70 sec. PTT's are checked at least daily and 4–6 hours after the initial bolus and any change in the rate of heparin infusion. Heparin infusion is usually continued for 6–10 days until the patient is "in range" on Coumadin®.
   2. Oral anticoagulants (Coumadin®) are started 3–5 days after initiating heparin and continued for 3 months. PT's are kept 1½ times normal (usually 17–20 seconds).
   3. Contraindications include recent neurosurgical or ophthalmic surgery or hemorrhage, serious active bleeding or malignant hypertension. Relative contraindications include severe hypertension, recent major surgery, recent major trauma, recent stroke, active GI bleed, bacterial endocarditis, severe hepatic or renal failure.
D. **Thrombolytic therapy** (streptokinase, urokinase, TPA).
   1. Promotes rapid clot lysis (heparin for the most part prevents clot propagation only), may preserve venous valve function.
   2. Useful in patients who have massive PE or who are hypertensive or severely hypoxic due to the mechanical effect of

clot producing occlusion of a significant portion of the pulmonary circulation.
E. **Venal caval interruption** (Greenfield filter).
   1. Prevents further embolism of thrombus > 3 mm in size.
   2. Indications.
      a. Recurrent thromboembolism in spite of adequate anticoagulation.
      b. PE in a patient with a contraindication to coagulation.
      c. Complication of coagulation.
      d. Chronic recurrent PE with pulmonary hypertension.
F. **Venous thrombectomy** — not indicated for routine iliofemoral DVT, but may be necessary for venous gangrene (phlegmasia cerulea dolens).
G. **Pulmonary embolectomy** (rarely necessary).
   1. **Transvenous** — suction–cap tipped catheter is passed via the jugular or femoral vein and clot is removed from pulmonary vasculature. Useful with massive PE where there is a contraindication to fibrinolytic therapy.
   2. **Open embolectomy** — usually through a median sternotomy with cardiopulmonary bypass. Mortality is greater than 50%.

SURGICAL INFECTIONS

I. DEFINITIONS

A. **Infection** — invasion of the body by pathogens and the reaction of the host to the organism and its toxins. A **surgical infection** is an infection that requires surgical treatment or has developed as a consequence of surgery.

B. **Virulence** — refers to the tissue–invading powers of a pathogen.

C. **Bacteremia** — the presence of bacteria in the circulation, with or without systemic toxicity.

D. **Septicemia** — the presence of bacteria and their toxins in the circulation, with characteristics of systemic toxicity.

E. **Toxemia** — toxins are present in the circulation, but the micro-organisms producing them need not be. Toxemia may result from infection by a toxin producing bacteria (*Clostridia* of gas gangrene) or result from ingestion of toxins without true infection (botulinum or staphylococcal enterotoxin).

F. **Abscess** — localized collection of pus surrounded by inflamed tissue. Treatment requires incision and drainage, and open wound management.

II. DIAGNOSIS

A. **Signs and symptoms** — 5 signs of inflammation: dolor (pain), rubor (redness), calor (heat), tumor (swelling), and functio laesa (loss of function). In addition:
  1. Local — fluctuance, crepitance, drainage.
  2. Systemic — fever, rigors, tachycardia, tachypnea, leukocytosis.

B. **Culture techniques.**
  1. Aspiration of fluid collection — send for gram stain and culture (aerobic and anaerobic).
  2. Aspiration of *edge* of cellulitic areas (may instill 1–2 cc sterile non–bacteriostatic saline prior to aspiration to increase yield).
  3. Wound or fluid swab.
  4. Tissue biopsy.
  5. Blood cultures — to document bacteremia, take (2) sets each time from peripheral venous and/or via indwelling catheters, at time of fever or at timed intervals.

C. **Imaging techniques.**
  1. Ultrasound — good for defining nature of fluid collections; localizing intra–abdominal abscesses.
  2. CT scan — more accurate than ultrasound, especially useful in obese patients. CT guidance for percutaneous drainage.
  3. Tagged (radiolabelled) WBC scan — uses patient's WBCs labelled with Indium, cells are re–administered to patient and

pool at sites of inflammation. Very non–specific and poor localization.

4. Gallium scan – this technique and above may be useful in localizing **occult** abscesses; both can take 12–72 hours for complete information.

5. MRI – no definite advantage to current techniques.

III. THERAPY FOR SURGICAL INFECTIONS – PRINCIPLES

A. Incision and drainage of purulent material.

B. Debridement of necrotic or devitalized tissue.

C. Removal of foreign bodies.

D. Open wound management – pack wound open, dressing changes.

E. Antibiotics.

1. Empiric choice based on likely pathogens.

2. Adjust according to culture results.

3. Should result in clinical improvement in 24–48 hours.

4. Requires adequate blood supply to infected tissues.

IV. SUPERFICIAL SURGICAL INFECTIONS

A. **Cellulitis** – nonsuppurative inflammation of subcutaneous tissues.

1. Presents with swelling, redness and pain; often fever and chills.

2. *Streptococci* and *Staphylococci* are the most common organisms, although gram–negative bacilli may be responsible, particularly in diabetic patients.

3. Failure to improve on antibiotics by 72 hours suggests abscess formation, requiring incision and drainage.

B. **Lymphangitis** – inflammation of lymphatic channels manifested by red streaking.

1. Often accompanies cellulitis.

2. Swelling of regional lymph nodes is usually seen.

3. Usually responds to appropriate antibiotic therapy.

C. **Erysipelas** – acute spreading *Streptococcus* cellulitis and lymphangitis. Lesions are raised with defined margins.

D. **Furuncle** ("boil") – abscess in a sweat gland or hair follicle.

E. **Carbuncle** – multilocular suppurative extension of a furuncle into the surrounding subcutaneous tissues. Usually caused by *Staphylococci*.

F. **Impetigo** – intraepithelial abscesses, usually caused by *Staphylococci* or *Streptococci*; contagious.

V. DEEP SURGICAL INFECTIONS

A. **Necrotizing fasciitis.**

1. A life–threatening infection, often seen in diabetics, manifesting as extensive necrosis of the subcutaneous tissue and superficial fascia with widespread undermining of the surrounding tissues

and severe systemic toxicity. Often presents in the perineum (Fournier's gangrene).

2. Usual causal organisms are anaerobic *Streptococci*, coagulase–positive *Staphylococcus*, and *Bacteroides*, although gram–negative organisms are found in 10% of the cases.

3. May complicate minor wounds or procedures such as perirectal/anal abscesses, appendectomy and hemorrhoidectomy.

4. Involved skin is pale red without distinct borders, and with blisters or bullae. Red areas progress to purple. Edema and crepitance is prominent.

5. Diagnosis may be confirmed by a serosanguinous exudate, necrotic fascia with undermining, and a gram stain smear of the pus or fluid showing gram-positive organisms and leukocytes.

6. Treatment — aggressive wide debridement and antibiotics (gram–negative and anaerobic coverage recommended). Hyperbaric O_2 may be helpful.

B. **Myonecrosis.**
   1. Muscle invasion caused by anaerobic *Streptococci*, *Staphylococcus* or *Clostridium perfringens*.
   2. Treatment — wide debridement and antibiotics.
   3. Clostridial myonecrosis is rapidly progressive infection in which a 24–hour delay in treatment may be fatal.

C. **Meleney's progressive synergistic gangrene.**
   1. Usually occurs around a thoracic or abdominal incision, ostomy site, or around surgical drains and retention sutures.
   2. Appears as a superficial ulcer with gangrenous skin (eschar) and a purple, erythematous border.
   3. Synergistic infection with *Staphylococcus aureus* and a micro-aerophilic or anerobic *Streptococcus*.
   4. Treatment — wide excision and high–dose penicillin or vancomycin.

D. **Meleney's ulcer.**
   1. A chronic, burrowing ulcer caused by non–hemolytic anaerobic or microaerophilic *Streptococci*.
   2. Begins as a small ulcer following trauma, surgery, or from an infected lymph node.
   3. Treatment — debridement and antibiotics, followed by a skin graft if necessary.

E. **Antibiotic–associated (pseudomembranous) colitis.**
   1. Caused by overgrowth of *Clostridium difficile*.
   2. Diagnosis made upon isolation of organism or its toxin from the stool.
   3. Most frequently follows the use of clindamycin, ampicillin, or cephalosporins, but may be associated with virtually all antibiotics.

4. Presents with watery, non–bloody diarrhea. Fever, abdominal pain and leukocytosis may be present. Sigmoidoscopy reveals yellow–white, exudative plaques or pseudomembranes.
5. Treatment — discontinue offending antibiotic; oral vancomycin (metronidazole is an alternative). Cholestyramine is sometimes used to bind the toxin.

F. **Tetanus.**
   1. Results from toxin produced by *Clostridium tetani* growing at a contaminated site. Incubation period is usually 7–10 days.
   2. Presents with headache, irritability, tremors, spasms, seizures. Death commonly occurs from respiratory failure or aspiration pneumonia. Recovery is usually complete. Diagnosis is made on clinical grounds.
   3. **Treatment.**
      a. Debride wound of necrotic tissue.
      b. Tetanus immune globulin (TIG) 3,000 units IM and 1,000 units into wound. High–dose penicillin 20 million units/day IV.
      c. Sedation, manage airway (may require tracheostomy).
      d. Active immunization required.
   4. **Prophylaxis.**
      a. < 6 years — 3 courses of DPT (diphtheria, pertussis, tetanus).
      b. > 7 years — 3 courses of tetanus toxoid.
      c. Booster dose every 5–10 years.
      d. For previously immunized patients:
         1) Last dose of toxoid within 10 years:
            a) Non–tetanus prone wound — no therapy.
            b) Tetanus prone wound — 0.5 cc toxoid.
         2) Last dose of toxoid more than 10 years — if 2 or more previous injections of toxoid, give 0.5 cc toxoid for both tetanus and non–tetanus prone wounds.
      e. For non–immunized patients:
         1) Non–tetanus prone wound — 0.5 cc toxoid.
         2) Tetanus prone wound — 0.5 cc toxoid and 250 cc TIG given at another site. Follow up with 2 or more doses of toxoid to complete the active immunization series.

G. **Intra–abdominal abscess.**
   1. Localized collection of pus walled off from the rest of the peritoneal cavity by inflammatory adhesions and viscera.
   2. Usually polymicrobial, with both aerobic/anaerobic organisms.
   3. Clinical manifestations — fever (initially intermittent but eventually sustained) and leukocytosis. Paralytic ileus, abdominal distention and anorexia are frequently seen. Abdominal tenderness and pain may be present with a mid–abdominal or pelvic abscess, but are less frequently seen with a subphrenic or retroperitoneal abscess.

4. Diagnosis — usually made by ultrasound or CT scan with confirmatory aspiration for gram stain and culture.
5. Drainage may be effected percutaneously (80% successful) or by open surgical drainage, either transabdominally, by a flank approach (for retroperitoneal abscess), or by a transrectal or transvaginal approach (for pelvic abscess).
6. Lesser sac abscesses usually result from pancreatic abscesses, infected pseudocysts or perforated peptic ulcers. Due to their inaccessibility, they should be drained by open surgical technique.

H. Wound infections.

1. Expected wound infection rates depend on the type of operation performed.
   a. Clean: 1.5–5.1% (skin, vascular).
   b. Clean–contaminated: 7.7–10.8% (GI, GU, GYN, and respiratory tract surgery).
   c. Contaminated: 15.2–16.3% (penetrating trauma, spillage from prepped bowel).
   d. Dirty: 28–40% (bowel perforation, gross pus, gangrene).
2. Conditions associated with increased wound infection rates — malnutrition, cirrhosis, steroid therapy, immunosuppressive drugs, leukopenia.
3. **Wound infection:** definition is based on **clinical criteria** — any wound that drains pus, whether or not bacteria are identified; any wound that is opened by the surgeon for any reason; any wound considered by the surgeon to be infected.
4. **Superficial wound infections** — accounts for 75% of wound infections.
   a. Involves the skin and subcutaneous tissues, and are exterior to the fascia and muscles.
   b. Diagnosis/clinical signs and symptoms — fever, erythema, drainage of pus, identification/culture of micro-organisms, wound erythema with seroma (no pus or bacteria seen), fluctuance, non–healing, tenderness.
   c. **Management — open wound.**
      1) Complicated wounds (extreme obesity, uncooperative patient, necrotizing soft tissue infection, fascial dehiscence, intestinal fistula, deep wound infection) should be explored in the OR.
      2) Prep area widely.
      3) Open wound where signs or symptoms are greatest.
      4) Make generous skin opening, often along entire length of incision.
      5) Palpate/probe wound with finger, inspect fascia digitally or visually.
      6) Obtain culture — send fluid in capped syringe for Gram stain, aerobic and anaerobic cultures; send swab.

7) Pack wound with normal saline wet-to-dry dressing, initiate TID wound care. Showers are helpful to clean wound.

8) Wound may be closed secondarily when all infection is cleared and healthy granulation tissue present throughout.

9) Use systemic antibiotics if significant cellulitis is present, patient is immunocompromised, presence of prosthetic device elsewhere, signs of systemic infection are present.

5. **Deep wound infections.**

a. Involves the muscles and fascia and structures deep to them (intra–abdominal).

b. Signs and symptoms include those of a superficial wound infection, and in addition — fascial dehiscence, drainage between fascial sutures, evisceration, ileus.

c. **Management.**

1) Explore wound in OR.

2) For evisceration — explore intra–abdominal wound to rule out abscess or fistula, debride fascia if necrotic, re-close fascia, consider retention sutures, leave skin and subcutaneous tissues open.

3) For intra–abdominal abscesses — leave wound open, place drains into cavity.

VI. POSTOPERATIVE FEVER

A. To the surgical intern and the rest of the surgical team, fever is a painfully common complication in the postoperative period. A systematic approach is helpful, both in the elucidation of the simple and treatable causes of postoperative fever such as atelectasis, and in the early diagnosis of the more serious complications such as intra–abdominal abscess.

B. Fever that presents within the first 24–48 hrs of surgery is generally related to atelectasis and often amenable to such simple interventions as incentive spirometry and getting the patient out of bed. Important exceptions to this are aspiration and wound infection with *Clostridia* or Group A *Streptococci*.

C. The genitourinary tract is a common source of infection and fever, particularly after instrumentation. Unspun urine can be easily inspected under the microscope. The presence of bacteria in each high-powered field correlates well with the presence of infection.

D. Wound infections typically present with fever 3–7 days after surgery, except as noted above. They are associated with local signs of infection — dolor (pain), rubor (redness), and calor (heat) — as well as grossly purulent discharge at times.

E. Infection of IV sites should always be suspected, since it is often unclear when a particular IV line was placed. Failure to identify an infected IV site can lead to the complication of septic thrombophlebitis, requiring total excision of the vein. Deep venous thromboses typically produce fevers 7–10 days postoperatively. Aggressive prophylaxis has helped to reduce this complication.

F. Intra–abdominal abscesses also present most commonly 7–10 days postoperatively. They often require a high degree of suspicion and a CT scan for diagnosis.
G. Less common sources of fever which must be considered are:
   1. Pulmonary embolus.
   2. Sinuses — particularly after placement of an endotracheal or NG tube.
   3. Salivary glands/parotid gland — check amylase.
   4. Prostate gland.
   5. Peri–rectal abscesses.
   6. Ears and throat.
   7. Drug fevers.
   8. Factitious fever.
H. The presence of new and often unrelated disease should never be overlooked.
   1. Cholecystitis/acalculous cholecystitis.
   2. Appendicitis.
   3. Endocarditis.
   4. Tuberculosis.
   5. Neoplasm.
   6. Connective tissue/autoimmune disease.

VII. PRINCIPLES OF ANTIBIOTIC THERAPY
A. **Types of antibiotics.**
   1. Bacteriostatic — prevents growth and multiplication of bacteria, but does not kill them. The defense mechanisms of the host then clear the infection.
   2. Bactericidal — actually kills the bacteria. Must be employed in patients with an impaired immune system.
B. **Selection of antibiotics.**
   1. **Empiric** choices should be based on *likely* infective organisms, often related to endogenous flora of involved organ.
   2. **Specific** choice is made for activity directed against the *known* infective microorganism (based on culture results).
   3. Other factors.
      a. Minimize potential side–effects.
      b. Assure adequate contact between the drug and the infective organism.
      c. Utilize/maximize host defenses to augment the antibacterial effect of the antibiotic.
C. **Complications of antibiotic therapy.**
   1. Direct toxicity — drug fever, rashes, anaphylaxis, neurologic (seizures), GI symptoms, renal dysfunction, blood/bone marrow dyscrasias, visual and auditory losses.

2. Emergence of resistant strains.
3. Superinfection with microorganisms not covered by the current antibiotic regimen (gram–negative bacteria, *Candida*).

D. **Antibiotic prophylaxis.**
   1. Directed at preventing infection from contaminated or potentially contaminated wounds. Contamination may occur through a break in aseptic technique, patient's skin flora, respiratory, GI or genitourinary tract.
   2. Indications.
      a. Contaminated wounds, prosthetic devices (either the implantation or existence of, such as heart valves or permanent vascular access devices), immunosuppressed state, trauma, obesity, shock, surgery on the respiratory, GI or genitourinary tract.
      b. Unless there is gross contamination during surgery, antibiotics may be discontinued after 24–48 hours.
   3. Intestinal asepsis — involves both antibiotics (systemic and intraluminal) and mechanical cleansing. See "Preoperative Preparation" section V for further details.

VIII. ANTIMICROBIAL AGENTS

Antibiotics should be selected with regard to a particular microorganism and not a specific disease. Base therapy on culture and sensitivity data.

A. **Penicillins** — bactericidal.
   1. Possess beta–lactam ring which blocks cell wall synthesis, resulting in bacteriolysis.
   2. Some semisynthetic penicillins possess activity against beta–lactamase producing organisms (methicillin, nafcillin) or are active against *Pseudomonas* (ticarcillin, piperacillin, carbenicillin).
   3. Ampicillin has slightly less gram–positive activity than penicillin–G, but much broader gram–negative coverage. Bacteriostatic against enterococcus, but when combined with an aminoglycoside it becomes bacteriocidal. When combined with sulbactam, a competitive inhibitor of beta–lactamase, this preparation has excellent gram–positive, gram–negative, and anaerobic coverage.

B. **Cephalosporins** — bactericidal.
   1. Similar mechanism of activity as penicillin. Broad–spectrum coverage and beta–lactamase resistant. Allergic cross–reactivity to penicillin in 5–10% of cases.
   2. Does not possess activity against enterococcus or methicillin–resistant *Staphylococci*.
   3. Cephalosporins currently fall into one of three generations with increased gram–negative and anti–pseudomonal activity, but somewhat decreased gram–positive coverage seen with the higher generations.

    a. 1st generation — examples are cephalothin/cefazolin (IV) and cephradine/caphalexin (PO). Ideal prophylactic agents for clean and clean–contaminated cases. Good gram–positive coverage.

    b. 2nd generation — examples are cefotetan (IV q 12 h) and cefoxitin (IV q 6 h). Ideal prophylactic agents for clean–contaminated cases, particularly involving GI tract. Possess gram–positive and gram–negative coverage.

    c. 3rd generation — examples are cefotaxime, ceftizoxime, ceftriaxone and ceftazidime. Ideal agents for selected infections, including pneumonias and selected intra–abdominal infections, particularly to avoid aminoglycoside toxicity risks. Possess broader coverage, including variable *Pseudomonas* coverage.

C. Aminoglycosides — bactericidal.

    1. Broad range of gram–negative and gram–positive coverage, but used mainly for gram–negative infections.

    2. Toxicity is mainly renal (5–15%) and auditory.

    3. Gentamicin and tobramycin are the most commonly used.

    4. Dosage is usually 4–5 mg/kg/day divided into 2 or 3 doses.

    5. Levels must be checked initially after the first or second dose and then every 3 or 4 days to ensure adequate therapeutic plasma levels and to prevent toxicity.

D. Carbapenems (thienamycins) — example is imipenam/cilastin. Effective as single agent therapy in intra–abdominal infections due to its broad spectrum and minimal toxicity.

E. Quinolones — example is ciprofloxacillin. Excellent broad–spectrum coverage in PO formula.

F. Monobactams — example is aztreonam. Excellent activity toward gram–negatives and beta–lactamases.

G. Specialized drugs.

    1. Clindamycin.

        a. Possesses good gram–positive and anaerobic activity.

        b. Most commonly used in treating intra–abdominal infections and aspiration pneumonia.

        c. Major problem is overgrowth of enteric *Clostridium difficile*, manifesting as pseudomembranous enterocolitis. Treatment is with PO vancomycin or PO/IV metronidazole.

    2. Metronidazole.

        a. Excellent bactericidal activity against most anaerobic organisms, as well as trichomonal, amoebic and giardic activity.

        b. Used frequently as part of prophylaxis in GI surgery.

        c. Has disulfuram–like (Antabuse®) activity; therefore, alcohol should be avoided during and for 1–2 weeks after use.

        d. Other major toxicity is a stocking–glove peripheral neuropathy and convulsions with long–term use.

3. **Vancomycin.**
   a. Bactericidal for gram–positive organisms.
   b. Indications include methicillin–resistant *Staphylococcus aureus,* enterococcal infections in penicillin–resistant patients and *Clostridium difficile* enterocolitis.
   c. Major problems are ototoxicity and phlebitis at IV site. Serum levels should be monitored.
4. **Erythromycin** — bacteriostatic, but may be bactericidal in high doses.
   a. Possess good gram–positive activity with some anaerobic spectrum, good substitute for penicillin when patient allergic.
   b. Bacterial resistance is common during long–term treatment.
   c. Frequently causes GI upset when given orally, venous sclerosis/burning when given IV.
5. **Tetracycline** — bacteriostatic.
   a. Broad spectrum with combined gram–positive and gram–negative activity.
   b. Active against *Treponema pallidum*, mycobacterium, tuberculosis, *Actinomyces, Rickettsiae,* mycoplasma and *Chlamydia*.
   c. Also active against 50% of *Bacteroides*.
   d. Do not use in children or expectant mothers due to permanent discoloration of teeth.
6. **Chloramphenicol** — bacteriostatic.
   a. Broad–spectrum coverage.
   b. Oral form associated with aplastic anemia.
   c. In infants, associated with fetal circulatory collapse (Gray syndrome).
   d. Should only be used when no other suitable choice is available (i.e., rickettsial disease, psittacosis or lymphopathia venereum in a patient unable to tolerate tetracycline).

H. **Antifungal agents.**
1. **Amphotericin B.**
   a. The only parenteral antifungal antibiotic for the treatment of systemic fungal infections.
   b. Test dose of 1 mg is given followed by daily increased (5-10 mg) doses until 30-50 mg/day is reached. Maximum of 15-30 mg/kg total dose is usually adequate. Dose must be given in D_5W. Pretreatment with tylenol, benadryl, and hydrocortisone is recommended.
   c. Major toxicity is renal. Dosage should be adjusted for renal insufficiency (dose every other or every 3rd day). Avoid dehydration and hyponatremia during use.
2. **Nystatin/clotrimazole.**
   a. Nonabsorbed antifungal agent used primarily as prophylactic agent to prevent GI overgrowth of *Candida* in patients on broad–spectrum antibiotics or immunosuppression.

    b. Also used topically for fungal infections of the skin.

    3. Ketoconazole — provides oral alternative to amphotericin B.

I. Antiviral agents — include acyclovir, amantadine and vidarabine.

IX. AIDS (ACQUIRED IMMUNODEFICIENCY SYNDROME)

A. General.

1. Each year, as the number of cases of AIDS has steadily increased, each branch of medicine has had to modify its thinking with respect to this potentially transferable and definitely fatal disease. As of April 1989, the CDC has reported more than 94,000 cases of AIDS and 270,000 cases are predicted by 1991. Seventeen cases of seroconversion in health care workers involved with AIDS patients have been reported, including at least two AIDS–related deaths in surgical residents.

2. Surgeons are at particularly high risk of exposure to the virus. As the prevalence of AIDS increases, we will be asked more frequently to evaluate and treat the spectrum of AIDS associated surgical disease. In addition, we will continue to be called upon to treat every–day surgical problems in an increasing number of incidentally sero–positive patients. In the operating suite alone, glove punctures occur 30–50% of the time and needle sticks occur in 6–20% of all major cases. The acute setting in our emergency rooms is even less controlled.

3. With this onslaught of potential exposures, physicians have struggled with questions such as mandatory preoperative HIV testing, refusal to perform surgery in AIDS patients, and consent for HIV testing after finger sticks. Widespread screening tests, however, have proven disastrously cost–ineffective, in view of the low incidence of the disease. Also, with a known sero-conversion window of 3–6 months between exposure to the HIV virus and a positive ELISA test, the arguments become a moot point. It is imperative that every patient be considered infected.

4. General precautions such as Sharps containers and goggles have already become standard in many medical centers. Just as physicians have treated bubonic plague and tuberculosis, and in doing so have risked their own lives for the good of their patients, now we must face AIDS. At a time when we have no vaccine and no cure for AIDS, common sense and routine precautions, for all patients, are our best defense.

B. The virus and serotesting.

1. A retrovirus (HIV) that attaches to a receptor site on the patient's T4 (helper) lymphocyte and is engulfed. The virus' RNA is encoded into the cell's DNA, resulting in production of large numbers of active virions. These virions are released when the cell is stimulated to divide. Further cell infection leads to destruction of T4 cells and impairment of T4 immune function.

2. Serotesting.
   a. ELISA — good screening test.
   b. Western blot — definitive, confirmatory test.
C. **Clinical stages of HIV infection and AIDS.**
   1. Acute retroviral infection.
      a. Occurs in 10–20% of patients infected by virus.
      b. Clinically a mononucleosis–like illness with a macular red rash, splenomegaly, occasional neurologic symptoms.
      c. Antibodies can be detected 2–6 weeks following this illness; prior to this they are sero–negative, but can transmit the disease.
   2. Asymptomatic, seropositive.
      a. This represents the largest group of patients and poses the greatest threat to health care workers.
      b. Incidence of seropositivity in asymptomatic patients:
         1) Homosexual men: 17–67%.
         2) IV drug abusers in the New York metropolitan area: 50–87%.
         3) Hemophilia A: 72–82%.
         4) Prostitutes: Los Angeles — 4%, San Francisco — 6%, Miami — 19%.
         5) Army recruits: 0.15% (but is high as 1.22% in certain subgroups).
         6) Blood donors: 0.038%.
         7) Study from Baltimore's Johns Hopkins Hospital ER: critically ill — 3%, young trauma patients — 16%.
   3. Generalized lymphodenopathy.
      a. Of these patients, 10% per year progress to AIDS.
      b. Sometimes have systemic illness with fever and weight loss.
   4. AIDS.
      a. Manifested by an opportunistic infection or presence of an epidemic malignancy (Kaposi's sarcoma, B–cell lymphoma, undifferentiated lymphoma).
      b. AIDS–related surgical problems include:
         1) Need for permanent vascular access.
         2) Symptomatic splenomegaly and AIDS–related thrombocytopenia.
         3) GI involvement by Kaposi's or lymphoma — obstruction, perforation, bleeding.
         4) Enterocolitis (CMV) — perforation, bleeding.
         5) Peritonitis — cryptococcus, mycobacterium.
      c. Mortality (3 month) following surgery in these patients is very high.
         1) Elective surgery: 40%.
         2) Emergent surgery: 75–80%.

PART II

SPECIALIZED PROTOCOLS IN SURGERY

TRAUMA

Trauma is the leading cause of death in the first four decades of life in the United States, surpassed only by cancer and atherosclerosis as the cause of death in all age groups. Nearly 70 million injuries occur annually, 10–15 million of which are disabling and about 175,000 are fatal. Trauma occurs at an incidence of 1000 per million population and occupies 12% of all hospital beds. The annual cost of trauma care in the United States is about $100 billion.

Death from trauma has a trimodal distribution:

1. Seconds to minutes of injury — these are due to lacerations of the brain, brain stem, high spinal cord, heart, aorta and other large vessels. These patients can rarely be salvaged.
2. Minutes to few hours of injury ("golden hour") — these are due to subdural and epidural hematomas, hemopneumothorax, ruptured spleens, liver lacerations, femur fractures or multiple injuries with significant blood loss. Rapid assessment and resuscitation during this period can reduce trauma deaths ... and it is toward this period that Advanced Trauma Life Support (ATLS) techniques are aimed.
3. Several days to weeks of injury — these are due to sepsis and organ failure.

The following chapter is based on the ATLS course (from the American College of Surgeons Committee on Trauma) with some adaptations as practiced at the University of Cincinnati Medical Center.

GENERAL CONSIDERATIONS

I. INITIAL ASSESSMENT AND MANAGEMENT — OVERVIEW

A. Primary survey: ABC's — life-threatening conditions are identified and simultaneous management begun.
1. A — Airway maintenance with C–spine control.
2. B — Breathing.
3. C — Circulation with hemorrhage control.
4. D — Disability: neurologic status.
5. E — Exposure: completely undress the patient.

B. Resuscitation phase — Shock management is initiated, oxygenation is reassessed and hemorrhage control is re-evaluated. Tissue aerobic metabolism is assured by perfusion of all tissue with well oxygenated red blood cells. Volume replacement with crystalloid and blood (if needed) is begun. A Foley and nasogastric tube are placed, if not contraindicated.

C. **Secondary survey** — Only begins after primary survey is completed and resuscitation has begun. This is a head–to–toe evaluation of the patient. It utilizes the look, listen and feel techniques in a systematic total body/system evaluation (tubes and fingers in every orifice). A complete neurologic exam completes the secondary survey. Chest, C-spine and pelvic x-rays are obtained. Special assessment procedures (peritoneal lavage, other x-rays, blood/urine tests) are performed.

D. **Definitive care phase** — The patient's less life–threatening injuries are managed. In–depth management, fracture stabilization and splinting, any necessary operative intervention and stabilization in preparation for transfer are undertaken.

II. PRIMARY SURVEY — DETAILS

A. **Airway and C–spine/upper airway management.**
   1. General concepts — the upper airway is assessed to ascertain patency. Maneuvers to establish a patent airway must be cognizant of the possibility of a C–spine injury. A C–spine injury should be assumed in all patients, especially those with injuries above the clavicle.
   2. Airway obstruction — awareness.
      a. Altered level of consciousness — **TIPPS** on the vowels (**AEIOU**):

T — trauma		A — alcohol	
I — infection		E — epilepsy	
P — psych		I — insulin	
P — poison		O — opiates	
S — shock		U — urea/metabolic	

      b. Head, neck and facial trauma — typical injury mechanism is the unbelted passenger/driver thrown into the windshield or dashboard.
   3. Airway obstruction — recognition. The most important question to a trauma patient is "How are you?" No response implies altered level of consciousness. Positive, appropriate verbal response indicates a patent airway, intact ventilation and adequate brain perfusion.
      a. **Look** — agitation (hypoxia), obtundation (hypercarbia), facial trauma.
      b. **Listen** — snoring and gurgling sounds imply partial pharynx occlusion; hoarseness implies laryngeal obstruction/trauma.
      c. **Feel** — air movement.
   4. **Airway obstruction — management.**
      a. Objectives — maintain an intact airway, protect the airway in jeopardy and provide an airway when none is available. These principles must be applied assuming that a C–spine injury is present.

    b. Chin lift.

    c. Jaw thrust.

    d. Suction — remove blood and secretions.

    e. Oropharyngeal airway.

    f. Nasopharyngeal airway — may also be used to facilitate placement of a nasogastric tube when a cribriform plate fracture is suspected.

    g. Esophageal obturator airway (EOA) — its use is controversial, do not remove in the unconscious patient until an endotracheal airway is placed.

    h. Preintubation ventilation — mandatory for the hypoxic or apneic patient, use bag–valve face–mask.

    i. Endotracheal intubation — orally or nasally, neck extension must be avoided, nasal route is preferred for the non–apneic patient with a non–cleared C–spine, apneic patients should be orally intubated with manual cervical immobilization, confirm endotracheal tube placement by auscultation and chest x-ray, intubation is contraindicated in the presence of severe maxillofacial injuries (one attempt with the patient prepped and locally anesthetized for surgical cricothyroidotomy may be acceptable in selected patients).

  5. Surgical airways.

    a. Indications — inability to intubate the trachea (glottic edema, oropharyngeal hemorrhage), contraindication to intubation (severe maxillofacial injuries, larynx fracture).

    b. Needle cricothyroidotomy — preferred for children under age 12, place 12 or 14 gauge plastic cannula into trachea, connect to wall O_2 at 15 L/min (40–50 PSI) with Y–connector or side hole cut in tubing, use intermittent ventilation by placing thumb over opening in system (one second on, four seconds off), effective for only 30–45 min due to poor CO_2 elimination.

    c. Surgical cricothyroidotomy — contraindicated in children under age 12, surgically prep and locally anesthetize the area, stabilize thyroid cartilage and make transverse skin incision over lower half of cricothyroid membrane, incise cricothyroid membrane, insert scalpel handle or tracheal spreader to open airway, insert endotracheal tube or tracheostomy (5–7 mm) and secure.

B. Breathing.

  1. General — expose patient's chest to adequately assess ventilation. Ventilate with a bag–valve device until the patient is stable.

  2. Three traumatic conditions that most often compromise ventilation are:

    a. Tension pneumothorax.

    b. Open pneumothorax.

    c. Flail chest with pulmonary contusion.

C. **Circulation.**

   1. Cardiac output — rapid assessment can be obtained from:

    a. Pulse — assess quality, rate, regularity; site of palpable pulse is related to systolic BP (radial > 80, femoral > 70, carotid > 60).

    b. Skin color.

    c. Capillary refill — test on hypothenar eminence, thumb or toenail bed; color should return within two seconds.

   2. Bleeding.

    a. Identify exsanguinating hemorrhage and control it — direct pressure on wound.

    b. Pneumatic splints and MAST suit often helpful.

    c. Major intrathoracic and intra–abdominal bleeding requires rapid operative repair, usually after brief resuscitative period.

D. **Disability** — brief neurologic evaluation.

   1. AVPU — determine level of consciousness.

    a. A — Alert.

    b. V — responds to Vocal stimuli.

    c. P — responds to Painful stimuli.

    d. U — Unresponsive.

   2. Pupillary size and reaction.

   3. More detailed evaluation is done during secondary survey.

E. **Expose** — completely undress patient.

III. RESUSCITATION PHASE

After the primary survey is completed and especially after an adequate airway has been established, the resuscitation phase begins.

A. **Oxygen.**

   1. Nasal cannula or face–mask delivery for conscious patients with adequate airways.

   2. Ventilatory support for intubated patients.

   3. Monitor ABGs and/or pulse oximetry O_2 saturation (unreliable in shock).

B. **Fluid resuscitation** — Hypovolemia and shock in trauma is almost always due to blood loss. Access to the circulation for crystalloid or blood resuscitation is mandatory (see Table 1).

TABLE 1
Estimated Fluid and Blood Requirements

	Class I	Class II	Class III	Class IV
Blood Loss (ml)	up to 750	750–1500	1500–2000	≥ 2000
Blood Loss (% BV)	up to 15%	15–30%	30–40%	≥ 40%
Pulse Rate	< 100	> 100	> 120	≥ 140
Blood Pressure	Normal	Normal	Decreased	Decreased
Pulse Pressure (mm Hg)	Normal or increased	Decreased	Decreased	Decreased
Capillary Blanch Test	Normal	Positive	Positive	Positive
Respiratory Rate	14–20	20–30	30–40	> 35
Urine Output (ml/hr)	≥ 30	20–30	5–15	Negligible
CNS–Mental Status	Slightly anxious	Mildly anxious	Anxious and confused	Confused-lethargic
Fluid Replacement (3:1 Rule)	Crystalloid	Crystalloid	Crystalloid + blood	Crystalloid + blood

1. IV's.
   a. Location (order of preference).
      1) Antecubital.
      2) Peripheral upper extremity veins.
      3) Saphenous.
      4) Femoral.
      5) Jugular.
      6) Subclavian.
      7) Central lines — rarely used for resuscitation. Use only in extreme situations or when CVP monitoring is needed (suspected pericardial tamponade), place on same side of pneumothorax or subcutaneous emphysema.
   b. Type (order of preference).
      1) Percutaneous 14 or 16 gauge angiocath.
      2) Large bore, single lumen catheter (8 Fr Traumacath, sterile IV tubing, 8 Fr pediatric feeding tube).
      3) Cutdown (antecubital, saphenous, cephalic) — 8 Fr pediatric feeding tube, sterile IV tubing, 8 Fr Traumacath.
   c. Number of lines.
      1) 2 lines for stable patients (systolic BP > 100).
      2) 3 lines for marginally stable patients (systolic BP 80–100).
      3) 4–6 lines for unstable patients (systolic BP < 70–80).
      4) Lines on both sides of the diaphragm when injuries are suspected on both sides of the diaphragm.
2. Laboratory studies.
   a. As soon as the first large–bore IV line is established and before infusion of IV fluid, 30–60 cc of blood is withdrawn and sent for STAT blood studies, including:

      1) Type and cross for 6 units or more, depending upon the injury.
      2) Complete blood count and platelet count.
      3) PT, PTT.
      4) Electrolytes, including calcium, creatinine, BUN, glucose, and measured osmolality.
      5) Ethanol level.
      6) Sickle cell prep as needed.
      7) Pregnancy test as needed.
    b. ABG.
    c. Urinalysis (also dipstick urine).
    d. Osmolality measured (serum and urine).
    e. Urine toxicology screen and serum toxicology screen as indicated.
    f. Liver, bone, and cardiac enzyme profiles as indicated.
    g. Serum amylase.
3. Crystalloid resuscitation.
    a. Initial fluid bolus is 1–2 L of isotonic electrolyte solution, preferably Ringer's lactate (20 cc/kg in pediatric patients).
    b. Response (↑ BP, ↓ pulse, ↑ pulse pressure, ↑ CNS state, ↑ skin circulation, ↑ urinary output) to initial fluid bolus determines degree of shock and dictates decision regarding blood replacement.
      1) Rapid response — patient responds and remains stable as fluids are slowed, indicates class I (or less) hemorrhage without ongoing losses, no further fluid bolus or blood required.
      2) Transient response — initial response but subsequent deterioration, indicates class II–III hemorrhage and ongoing losses, continued fluid administration and initiation of blood transfusion are indicated.
      3) Minimal or no response — indicates class IV hemorrhage with or without ongoing losses, rapid blood administration and surgical intervention are needed, also consider error in diagnosis (tension pneumothorax, pericardial tamponade, cardiogenic shock).
4. Blood replacement.
    a. Type O blood — for class IV exsanguinating hemorrhage, Rh negative preferable for females.
    b. Type–specific, saline crossmatched — for class II–III hemorrhage, usually ready in 10 min.
    c. Crossmatched — usually ready in 30–60 min, have available in all patients and use when needed and ready.
    d. Platelets and fresh frozen plasma should be given for multiple transfusion–induced coagulopathy.
    e. Calcium (2 ml of 10% CaCl₂ solution) — only needed while blood is being transfused at > 100 ml/min.

5. **Military anti–shock trousers (MAST).**
    a. Mechanism of action — translocation of blood from the lower extremities, increased peripheral vascular resistance, increased myocardial afterload; it can raise BP but is not a substitute for and should not delay volume replacement.
    b. Indications.
        1) Pelvic fractures — splinting and hemorrhage control.
        2) Soft tissue hemorrhage — tamponade.
        3) Leg fractures — stabilization.
        4) Stabilize circulation for transport.
        5) Maintaining upper torso perfusion when IV's or volume replacement is inadequate.
    c. Contraindications (first 2 are absolute).
        1) Pulmonary edema.
        2) Circulatory instability due to myocardial dysfunction.
        3) Head injuries.
        4) Intrathoracic bleeding.
        5) Diaphragmatic rupture.
    d. Use.
        1) Remove only after shock state is reversed; deflate gradually with abdominal compartment first, then each leg sequentially; if BP falls $\geq$ 5 mmHg, reinflate and increase volume resuscitation.
        2) Leave in place once deflated, may take to OR if patient unstable.
6. **Assessment of resuscitation.**
    a. Organ perfusion — urine output, CNS status, skin circulation.
    b. Circulatory parameters — BP, pulse, pulse pressure.
C. **ECG monitoring.**
D. **Foley catheterization** — monitor urinary output and decompress bladder in preparation for DPL.
    1. Immediate insertion *contraindicated* in suspected urethral injury, usually associated with pelvic fracture.
        a. Blood at the meatus.
        b. Scrotal or perineal hematoma.
        c. High–riding prostate (or non–palpable prostate) — rectal exam must be performed prior to Foley insertion.
    2. Prior to Foley insertion in suspected urethral injury, obtain:
        a. Urethrogram — use 20 ml of contrast (60% Renografin) diluted with 20 ml saline; inject gently into meatus, obtain AP and oblique x-ray views, look for disruption or extravasation.
        b. Cystogram — after Foley placed, fill bladder with 50 cc of 60% Renografin; if no extravasation, fill bladder to 250–

300 cc by gravity, clamp Foley and obtain AP and oblique x-rays; lastly obtain post–evacuation film.

E. Nasogastric tube placement.
1. Indications — to relieve and prevent gastric dilatation, to remove gastric contents and prevent aspiration (especially prior to intubation), to obtain gastric sample for analysis, to rule out GI bleeding, to decompress stomach prior to DPL.
2. Contraindications (pass NG tube via mouth) — suspected cribriform plate fractures (head trauma with non–clotting [CSF containing] blood coming from ears, nose or mouth) to avoid intracranial placement, maxillofacial trauma.

IV. SECONDARY SURVEY
Involves complete examination of patient in systematic fashion.

A. Head — scalp lacerations, depressed skull fractures, pupillary size and reactivity, fundoscopic and otoscopic exam, visual acuity.

B. Maxillofacial trauma — palpate bones, assess bony stability, palpate mandible and assess bite.

C. Neck — remove front of cervical collar and note swelling, feel and listen to carotids, assess jugulars, palpate trachea, palpate cervical spine posteriorly, crepitance, penetrating injuries, assume C–spine injury, remove helmet with in–line traction after lateral C–spine film obtained.

D. Chest — observe excursion, palpate bony thorax, identify penetrating injuries, sucking chest wounds and flail chest, palpate clavicles, crepitance, auscultate lung fields and heart sounds (pneumothorax, hemothorax, pulmonary contusion, cardiac tamponade).

E. Abdomen — observe and re–examine frequently, distention, bowel sounds, palpate for tenderness.

F. Rectum — digital exam to assess for blood, prostate, sphincter tone.

G. Genitourinary — observe for priapism, perineal hematoma.

H. Fractures — observe for deformities and palpate all long bones, palpate pelvic stability.

I. Pulses — examine throughout.

J. Back/skin — log roll and examine/palpate entire spine and back, lacerations, abrasions.

K. Neurologic — mental status, GCS, cranial nerves, motor and sensory exam, reflexes, Babinski's.

L. X–rays.
1. Initial mandatory films include:
   a. Lateral C–spine.
   b. AP chest x-ray (usually supine until spine cleared).
   c. AP pelvis.

2. Secondary films include:
    a. C–spine series — additional lateral films if not all vertebra seen, AP, odontoid view.
    b. T–spine series — AP and lateral.
    c. L–spine series — AP and lateral.
    d. Specific bony films to evaluate suspected areas of injury — facial, skull, extremities.
    e. Upright chest x-ray — obtained after spine is cleared in blunt trauma, to fully evaluate mediastinum.
M. **Diagnostic peritoneal lavage (DPL)** — see Specific Injuries and Protocols, II. D. below and Trauma Appendix.

V.   HISTORY/MECHANISM OF INJURY

A. **Pertinent past medical history (AMPLE):**
    1. A — Allergies.
    2. M — Medications.
    3. P — Past illnesses.
    4. L — Last meal.
    5. E — Events preceding injury.
B. **Nature of injury.**
    1. Motor vehicle accident (MVA).
        a. Type of collision.
        b. Speed of accident.
        c. Use of seat belts.
        d. Condition of windshield -- head trauma.
        e. Condition of steering wheel — blunt chest trauma.
        f. Location of patient in car at time of impact.
        g. Need for extrication.
    2. Stab wound.
        a. Type of weapon.
        b. Length of knife.
        c. Sex of attacker.
            1) Male — upward thrust.
            2) Female — downward thrust.
    3. Gunshot wound.
        a. Caliber of gun.
        b. Distance from patient that gun was fired.
        c. Patient's position when shot.
        d. Number of shots fired.
C. **Condition at scene and on transport.**
    1. Blood pressure.
    2. Pulse.
    3. Respiration/airway.
    4. Level of consciousness.

VI.   RE–EVALUATE THE PATIENT

VII. RECORDS AND LEGAL CONSIDERATIONS

A. Records — meticulous record keeping is essential both for optimal care and medico–legal considerations.

B. Consent for treatment — obtain if possible, but don't delay emergency treatment.

SPECIFIC INJURIES AND PROTOCOLS

I.   **THORACIC TRAUMA**

Responsible for 1 out of 4 trauma deaths. Less than 15% of these injuries require surgical intervention. Early and appropriate intervention are mandatory.

A. **Life–threatening chest injuries** identified in the primary survey.

1. Airway obstruction — see section II-A above.

2. **Tension pneumothorax.**

a. Pathophysiology — one–way valve air leak from lung or chest wall allows air to be forced into thoracic cavity (pleural space) without means of escape → collapse of affected lung → displacement of mediastinum and trachea to opposite side → kinking of SVC/IVC and impaired venous return to heart, compression of contralateral lung → hypotension, hypoxia.

b. Causes — mechanical ventilation with PEEP and air leak, ruptured emphysematous bullae, blunt chest trauma with unsealed parenchymal lung injury, penetrating thoracic injury.

c. Diagnosis — tracheal deviation, respiratory distress, unilateral absence of breath sounds, distended neck veins, cyanosis (late), hypertympanic on ipsilateral chest. It is a clinical, not radiographic, diagnosis. Do *not* wait for chest x–ray to diagnose and treat.

d. Management — initially by inserting large–bore needle (14 or 16 gauge angiocath) into chest via 2nd intercostal space in midclavicular line (diagnosis confirmed by rush of air) to relieve tension, then insert chest tube.

3. **Open pneumothorax.**

a. Pathophysiology — large chest defects often remain open causing a "sucking chest wound" → intrathoracic pressure equilibrates with atmospheric pressure; if chest wall opening is two–thirds the diameter of the trachea → air passes preferentially through the chest defect with each inspiratory effort (it is path of least resistance) → impairment of effective ventilation → hypoxia.

    b. Causes — penetrating injury to the thorax that results in a large defect.

    c. Diagnosis — presence of sucking chest wound, hypoxia, hypoventilation.

    d. Management — prompt closure of defect with sterile occlusive dressing taped on 3 sides (provides a flutter valve effect that prevents further air from entering), place chest tube in area remote from wound, surgical closure of defect is usually required.

4. **Massive hemothorax.**

    a. Pathophysiology — blood loss of 1500 ml into the chest cavity → compression/collapse of ipsilateral lung → hypoxia.

    b. Causes — usually due to penetrating thoracic injury that disrupts systemic or pulmonary vessels, can also result from blunt chest trauma. One must also consider a ruptured hemidiaphragm with intra–abdominal injury.

    c. Diagnosis — hypoxia, hypoventilation, ipsilateral chest is dull to percussion, absent/decreased breath sounds, hypotension, chest x-ray not essential, equivocal neck veins.

    d. Management — restoration of volume deficit (crystalloid and blood, often type-specific) and evacuation/decompression of chest cavity (36 or 40 Fr. chest tube), most will require surgical intervention, emergency thoracotomy rarely needed in ER.

5. **Flail chest.**

    a. Pathophysiology — occurs when a segment of chest wall does not have bony continuity with the rest of the thoracic cage, usually secondary to multiple rib fractures → paradoxical motion of the chest wall (flail segment sinks in during inspiration). Hypoxia results from injury to underlying lung, i.e., pulmonary contusion, and associated bony pain which hinders respiratory effort.

    b. Causes — severe blunt thoracic trauma, usually MVA.

    c. Diagnosis — usually apparent on visual examination of patient's chest and inspiratory pattern, may not be initially seen due to splinting, flail segment and rib fractures may be palpated, rib fractures and pulmonary contusion may be seen on chest x-ray, respiratory failure with hypoxia in severe cases.

    d. Management — initially involves adequate ventilation, O_2 therapy and avoidance of overhydration; stabilization of the chest wall defect is unimportant; definitive treatment is re-expansion of lung and maintaining adequate oxygenation; intubation and mechanical ventilation is needed in severe cases (CPAP mask use may preclude intubation); adequate pain control (best achieved with thoracic epidural, PCA or scheduled systemic analgesics also effective) is essential to allow for good ventilatory effort and respiratory care.

6. **Cardiac tamponade.**
   a. Pathophysiology — the pericardial sac is a fixed fibrous structure, and only a small amount of blood is required in an acute setting to severely restrict cardiac activity. Pericardial blood → impaired venous filling → signs of venous hypertension and systemic hypotension due to poor cardiac output.
   b. Causes — vast majority are penetrating injuries, rarely due to blunt trauma.
   c. Diagnosis — the diagnosis should be suspected in any patient who presents with penetrating injury (knife, bullet) to the anterior chest between the nipples or a transmediastinal missile path. Beck's classic triad of distended neck veins, hypotension, and muffled heart sounds is uncommon. Other signs/symptoms include pulsus paradoxus and mental anxiety/agitation. Diagnosis confirmed by pericardiocentesis or subxyphoid pericardial window (Trinkle window, performed in OR).
   d. Management — immediate removal of pericardial blood via pericardiocentesis may be life-saving, use of a plastic catheter that can be left in place allows repeated aspiration if necessary. Positive pericardiocentesis mandates emergent median–sternotomy and inspection/repair of heart. False negatives and positives do occur. Subxyphoid pericardial window is suitable for patients with a good possibility of tamponade and who are hemodynamically stable enough to make it to the OR. Many authors prefer this approach in all patients in place of pericardiocentesis.

B. **Potentially lethal chest injuries** identified in the secondary survey.
   1. **Pulmonary contusion** with or without flail chest.
      a. General — common, potentially lethal due to gradual development of respiratory failure similar to ARDS.
      b. Clinically — presents in setting of appropriate blunt chest trauma, usually MVA related. Often with associated rib fractures. Chest x-ray may show localized infiltrate, but chest x-ray findings often lag behind or do not correlate with clinical course. Hypoxia is good indicator.
      c. Management — analgesics (intermittent or continuous parenteral morphine, PCA analgesia, thoracic epidural) and good pulmonary toilet are essential. Patients should be monitored in an ICU setting for 24-48 hours if they remain non–intubated. Selective management without intubation is suitable for many patients, CPAP mask is another measure that may preclude intubation.

    d. Factors predisposing toward intubation/mechanical ventilation.
        1) Severe contusion with hypoxia.
        2) Pre–existing chronic pulmonary disease.
        3) Impaired level of consciousness.
        4) Abdominal injury resulting in ileus or exploratory laparotomy.
        5) Skeletal injuries requiring immobilization.
        6) Renal failure.
        7) Poor cough effort, atelectasis, lobar collapse.

2. **Thoracic aortic tear/rupture.**
    a. General — most common cause of sudden death after an MVA or fall (major deceleration injury); 90% of these are fatal, either at scene or prior to arriving in ER; of the 10% who make it to a hospital, half will die each day if left untreated/unrecognized. Tear usually occurs just beyond take-off of left subclavian artery, where ligamentum arteriosum inserts.
    b. Diagnosis — a high index of suspicion, along with appropriate radiologic findings, should prompt arteriography (arch and great vessels) to rule in or out the diagnosis. About 10% of aortograms will be positive if appropriate liberal indications are used.
    c. Chest x-ray findings associated with aortic tear.
        1) Widened mediastinum — > 8 cm, preferably on an upright PA film.
        2) Fractures of the first and second ribs.
        3) Obliteration of the aortic knob.
        4) Deviation of the trachea to the right.
        5) Presence of a pleural cap.
        6) Elevation and rightward shift of the right mainstem bronchus.
        7) Depression of the left mainstem bronchus.
        8) Obliteration of space between pulmonary artery and aorta.
        9) Deviation of the esophagus (NG tube) to the right.
    d. Management — these injuries require definitive surgical repair, either direct repair or resection with grafting.

3. **Tracheobronchial tree injuries.**
    a. Tracheal injuries — may be due to blunt or penetrating injury.
        1) Fracture of larynx — triad of hoarseness, subcutaneous emphysema and palpable fracture crepitus.
        2) Fiberoptic laryngoscopy may aid in diagnosis.
        3) Definitive surgical repair required.

   b. Bronchial injury.
      1) Clinically — unusual but potentially fatal injury, usually
         results from blunt trauma. Usually occurs about 1 inch
         from carina. May present with hemoptysis, subcutaneous
         emphysema or tension pneumothorax. Pneumothorax
         with persistent large air leak is typical. Diagnosis con-
         firmed with bronchoscopy.
      2) Management — usually requires direct repair via
         thoracotomy.
4. Esophageal trauma.
   a. General — usually caused by penetrating injury, rarely
      blunt trauma.
   b. Clinically — presents similar to Boerhaave's syndrome, left
      pneumothorax or hemothorax without a rib fracture, history
      of severe blow to lower sternum or epigastrium, pain or
      shock out of proportion to injury, particulate matter in
      chest tube drainage, chest tube that bubbles continuously
      and equally during inspiration and expiration, mediastinal
      air or empyema (usually on left side). Diagnosis confirmed
      by gastrografin swallow or esophagoscopy. Esophageal in-
      jury due to penetrating trauma usually occurs in the neck.
   c. Management — treatment of choice is wide drainage of
      the pleural space and mediastinum and direct repair of the
      injury via thoracotomy. Esophageal diversion in the neck
      and gastrostomy is sometimes required.
5. Traumatic diaphragmatic hernia.
   a. Clinically — more common on left side (liver protects right
      hemidiaphragm). Blunt trauma usually produces large dia-
      phragmatic tears with acute herniation (stomach, small bowel).
      Penetrating trauma produces small perforations that often
      take years to develop into hernias. In a small percentage
      of cases, defects are found bilaterally. High index of sus-
      picion is key to making the diagnosis, as well as careful
      exploration of diaphragm at time of exploratory laparotomy.
   b. Diagnosis — suggested by abnormal chest x-ray (elevated
      left hemidiaphragm, loculated hydropneumothorax, NG tube
      in left lower chest) in appropriate clinical setting. Gastro-
      grafin upper GI series and CT scan are sometimes helpful.
      Rarely discovered when peritoneal lavage fluid fills chest.
   c. Management — operative repair indicated. Best approached
      via abdomen in acute setting due to high incidence of
      associated intra–abdominal injuries. Approach via chest in
      delayed setting due to presence of intrathoracic adhesions
      that require lysis.
6. Myocardial contusion.
   a. Clinically — results from blunt chest trauma, usually un-
      restrained driver in head–on collision that results in bent/

crushed steering wheel column. Often associated with chest wall contusion or fractures of the sternum and/or ribs.

b. Diagnosis — an abnormal ECG (PACs, PVCs, atrial fibrillation, bundle branch block, ST segment changes) may be present. Major contusions are associated with hemodynamic instability and unexplained hypotension. Diagnosis can be confirmed with serial cardiac enzyme determinations, echocardiography or MUGA scanning (little or no role in patient who has normal ECG, no arrhythmias and is hemodynamically stable).

c. Management — due to risk of dysrhythmias, patients should be continuously monitored in ICU or monitored bed setting for 24 hours. Patients with documented contusions and hemodynamic compromise who require surgery with general anesthetic for treatment of associated injuries should undergo invasive hemodynamic monitoring (A–line, Swan–Ganz catheter) perioperatively.

C. **Serious chest injuries.**
1. **Subcutaneous emphysema.**
   a. May result from airway injury, lung injury or rarely, blast injury.
   b. A physical finding that often necessitates chest tube placement.
2. **Pneumothorax.**
   a. Pathophysiology — results from entry of air (either from lung or atmosphere) into pleural space. May result from penetrating or blunt chest trauma. Most commonly caused by lung laceration, often associated with rib fractures, in blunt trauma.
   b. Diagnosis — usually seen on chest x-ray. Typical signs (hyper–resonance, decreased breath sounds) are often difficult to detect in noisy ER, unless tension is present.
   c. Management — placement of chest tube in 4th or 5th interspace, anterior to mid–axillary line. Initially place tube to suction and confirm placement and lung re–expansion with repeat chest x-ray. Patients at risk for pneumothorax (rib fractures, significant blunt chest injury) should have chest tubes placed prophylactically prior to undergoing a general anesthetic for management of associated injuries.
3. **Hemothorax.**
   a. Pathophysiology — due to lung laceration or laceration of an intercostal vessel or internal mammary artery, seen in penetrating or blunt trauma.
   b. Diagnosis — effusion seen on chest x-ray, diminished breath sounds.

  c. Management — any hemothorax sufficient to appear on chest x-ray requires placement of large caliber chest tube. This provides immediate drainage to prevent a clotted hemothorax or fibrothorax with associated restrictive pulmonary function. Chest tube also provides a monitoring method to assess severity of injury ... initial drainage of ~ 1000 cc blood followed by hourly output of ≥ 200 cc or initial drainage of ≥ 1500 cc are indications for exploratory thoracotomy.   Most hemothoraces, however, require chest tube placement only.

4. **Rib fractures.**
  a. Pathophysiology — pain on motion results in splinting of thorax → impaired ventilation, poor clearance of secretions → atelectasis, pneumonia. Due to greater flexibility of chest in youth, rib fractures in young patients imply greater thoracic impact.
  b. Clinically — upper ribs (1–3) are well protected and their fracture implies major impact, often with associated head, neck, spinal cord, lung or great vessel injury. Middle ribs (5–9) are the most commonly injured, often associated with pneumothorax, hydrothorax, pulmonary contusion, or flail chest.
  c. Diagnosis — localized pain, tenderness on palpation, crepitus, palpable or visible deformity. Chest x-ray important to exclude other intrathoracic injuries.
  d. Management — adequate analgesia and pulmonary toilet, intercostal blocks or intra–pleural analgesia are helpful. Splinting or taping is of no value.

5. **Indications for chest tube insertion.**
  a. Pneumothorax.
  b. Hemothorax.
  c. Selected cases, suspected severe lung injury.
  d. Prophylaxis.

D. **Emergency Department thoracotomy.**
1. General — survival of trauma patients arriving in the ER in full cardiac arrest is not enhanced by ED thoracotomy.
2. Indications.
  a. Patients in full arrest with penetrating chest or high epigastric wounds.
  b. Patients (blunt or penetrating) who arrest (witnessed) during initial evaluation and resuscitation.
3. Technique.
  a. Anterolateral thoracotomy, 4th–5th intercostal space (inframammary), left side (some recommend side of wound), incision may be extended across midline if needed.

b. Incise pericardium with scissors along full longitudinal axis of heart anterior to phrenic nerve, evacuate hemopericardium.

c. If hemopericardium present, visualize and control cardiac wounds (finger, hand, Foley catheter).

d. Look for ruptured thoracic aorta (subadventitial hematoma).

e. Cross–clamp descending thoracic aorta.

f. Begin cardiac massage.

g. Transport to OR for definitive care.

II. ABDOMINAL TRAUMA

A. Assessment — the determination that an intra–abdominal injury exists that requires operative intervention is critical, not its specific diagnosis.

1. **Look** — examine anterior and posterior walls of abdomen, flanks, lower chest, buttocks, and perineum. Look for contusions, abrasions, lacerations and penetrating wounds.

2. **Listen** — absence of bowel sounds may indicate ileus or early peritoneal irritation (blood, bacteria, GI secretions). Ileus also associated with extra–abdominal injuries (thoracic/lumbar spine fractures, burns).

3. **Feel** — palpate anterior abdominal wall, intra–abdominal contents and posterior abdomen. Feel for early signs of peritoneal irritation:
   a. Muscle guarding.
   b. Percussion tenderness.

4. Areas of the abdomen for evaluation.
   a. Intrathoracic abdomen — portion of abdomen protected by bony thorax (costal margins up to nipples); contains spleen, stomach, liver and diaphragm. Injured by blows to lower thorax and abdomen (sometimes associated with seat belts). Diagnostic modalities include: chest x-ray, gastrografin swallow, DPL, CT scanning. Penetrating wounds of thorax below nipples may injure subdiaphragmatic organs; therefore, evaluate with DPL or abdominal exploration.
   b. True abdomen — contains small and large bowel, bladder, uterus, fallopian tubes and ovaries. More readily accessible to examination. Injuries diagnosed by increasing abdominal pain, decreasing bowel sounds, positive DPL, free air on upright chest x-ray or left lateral decubitus abdominal x-ray, blood on rectal exam, peritoneal penetration, evisceration.
   c. Retroperitoneal abdomen — difficult to evaluate and diagnose injuries in this area, DPL often falsely negative (not surprising). High index of suspicion is essential to avoid missing injuries here. Involved organs include: kidneys, ureters, duodenum, pancreas and retroperitoneal vascular

structures (IVC, aorta, iliac vessels). Diagnostic modalities include: IVP, abdominal x-rays (para–duodenal air), gastrografin swallow, CT scan, elevated serum or DPL fluid amylase.

    d. Rectal examination — look at perineum, feel sphincter tone, feel rectal wall integrity, feel prostate position and mobility, look for gross and occult blood.

    e. Vaginal examination — pelvic exam required in all female trauma patients. Look and feel for lacerations. Injuries often associated with pelvic fractures.

B. Types of injuries.

  1. Penetrating wounds.

    a. Injury results in hemorrhage from penetration of a major vessel or solid organ and perforation of a segment of bowel. Bleeding is manifest early by increasing abdominal distention, rigidity, a quiet abdomen, and varying degrees of shock. Bowel perforation is slower to manifest physical findings as peritonitis develops.

    b. Impaled objects should only be removed in OR since hemorrhage may ensue.

    c. Once a penetrating wound of the abdomen is identified, the patient should undergo abdominal exploration (see below for possible exceptions).

    d. Small bowel and colon are most commonly injured organs.

  2. Blunt trauma.

    a. Injury is produced by compression of the abdominal contents against the vertebral column, by direct transfer of energy to an organ or by rapid deceleration with resulting tears of the structures.

    b. Spleen and liver are most commonly injured organs.

    c. DPL is key diagnostic aid in identifying patients who require exploration.

C. Management of abdominal injuries.

  1. Venous access — at least two large-bore IVs.

  2. Placement of NG tube — see section III. E. above.

  3. Placement of Foley catheter — see section III. D. above.

    a. Diagnostic value includes assessment for gross or microscopic hematuria and means to perform cysto–urethrogram or IVP if indicated.

    b. Percutaneous suprapubic cystostomy is an alternate to urethral catheterization in selected cases.

  4. X-rays.

    a. Upright chest x-ray, left lateral decubitus — to look for free air in selected patients.

    b. Urologic x-rays — see below.

D. Diagnostic peritoneal lavage (DPL).
  1. General considerations.
     a. Mainstay of evaluation of blunt abdominal trauma and selected cases of penetrating trauma.
     b. Should be performed by the surgeon caring for the patient since it is a surgical procedure that alters subsequent examination of the patient.
     c. Small, but real (1–2%) incidence of complications (local or intra–peritoneal hematoma, peritonitis, bladder laceration, abdominal wall bleeding resulting in false–positive exam, perforation of intra–abdominal or retroperitoneal organs, injury to retroperitoneal vessels, evisceration, wound infection).
     d. Unreliable in assessment of retroperitoneal injuries.
     e. Usually performed early in patient evaluation, typically during secondary survey. If free intra–peritoneal air is suspected, perform abdominal films prior to DPL (DPL can introduce air).
  2. Indications.
     a. History of blunt abdominal trauma and . . .
        1) Depressed sensorium or altered pain response leading to possible false–negative physical examination (ethanol intoxication, head injury, drug abuse, spinal cord injury).
        2) Manifestations of hypovolemia — hypotension, tachycardia.
        3) Equivocal abdominal findings — often a result of lower rib fractures, pelvic fractures, and lumbar spine fractures. Nearly half of patients with hemoperitoneum will not have positive abdominal findings.
        4) Positive abdominal findings — peritonitis, localized tenderness.
        5) Unavailability of patient for continued monitoring — patient undergoing general anesthetic for other injuries, DPL needed to definitively clear abdomen.
        6) Low rib fractures, particularly on left side.
     b. Penetrating injury to surrounding areas.
        1) Lower chest — below nipples or 4th intercostal space.
        2) Flank.
        3) Buttocks and perineum.
     c. Abdominal stab wounds with negative physical signs — controversial; we explore most of these wounds unless local exploration clearly precludes fascial/peritoneal penetration.
  3. Contraindications.
     a. Absolute contraindications.
        1) Multiple abdominal operations or midline scars — appendectomy scar alone does not preclude DPL.
        2) Obvious indications for exploratory laparotomy — free air, peritonitis, penetrating trauma.

  b. Relative contraindications.
    1) Gravid uterus — use supra–umbilical open technique.
    2) Inability to decompress bladder — use supra–umbilical open technique.
    3) Inability to decompress stomach — use infra–umbilical open technique.
    4) Pelvic fracture with possible hematoma — use supra–umbilical open technique to avoid false–positive results.
4. Technique — see "Diagnostic Peritoneal Lavage"
5. Interpretation: positive lavage.
  a. Grossly positive — 5–10 cc of blood on initial aspirate (we use 10 cc as positive).
  b. Positive on lavage (blunt trauma).
    1) ≥ 100,000 RBC/mm^3 (97% sensitivity, 99.6% specificity) (≥ 1,000–20,000 for penetrating trauma).
    2) ≥ 500 WBC/mm^3 (≥ 25–100 for penetrating trauma).
    3) Presence of particulate (fecal, vegetable) matter.
    4) Presence of bacteria on gram stain.
    5) Elevated amylase, bilirubin.
E. CT scanning.
  1. Indications.
    a. To evaluate abdomen when DPL contraindicated or ineffective.
    b. To evaluate retroperitoneum — pancreas, kidneys, retroperitoneal soft tissues.
  2. Limitations — requires expertise in evaluation, time consuming, costly.
F. Specific abdominal injuries.
  1. Stomach — usually injured by penetrating trauma, repair requires debridement and primary repair.
  2. Duodenum.
    a. Duodenal hematoma — may be managed expectantly if patient not explored for other reasons; if found upon exploration → mobilize duodenum, evacuate hematoma, achieve hemostasis, rule out mucosal perforation.
    b. Duodenal injuries — most managed by primary closure; more severe injuries require resection, serosal patching, pyloric exclusion or duodenal fistulization.
  3. Pancreas.
    a. No ductal involvement — adequate drainage +/− suture repair.
    b. Ductal involvement — distal pancreatectomy for injuries of body or tail, some advocate Roux–en–Y drainage or ductal repair; injuries in head may be drained alone with resultant fistula.

     c. Combined pancreatic/duodenal injuries — severe injuries require pancreaticoduodenectomy or duodenal diverticularization.

4. Small bowel — injuries require primary repair or resection and anastomosis.

5. Large bowel — most injuries can be managed by primary repair or resection and anastomosis. Colostomy usually only required for left-sided injuries with significant fecal contamination, associated injuries and the presence of shock.

6. Spleen — injuries usually result from blunt trauma and range from minimal capsular tears to diffuse fractures with hilar involvement. Management may consist of hemostatic control, splenorrhaphy, partial splenectomy or splenectomy. Recent trend is toward splenic salvage procedures.

7. Liver — usually injured from blunt trauma; injuries include capsular tears, simple lacerations, stellate lacerations, stellate lacerations with crush injury, and retrohepatic venous injuries. Management consists of simple repair with/without drainage, direct suture of bleeding vessels, debridement of devitalized tissue, lobectomy or temporary packing. Adjuncts to management include the Pringle maneuver, placement of atrial–caval shunt or hepatic artery ligation.

8. Diaphragm — traumatic rupture may be associated with blunt or penetrating trauma.

G. Genitourinary injuries.

1. History.

    a. Blunt trauma to abdomen, lower chest, flank, genitalia or perineum associated with hematuria, diminished urinary output, abdominal or flank mass or swelling of the genitalia.

    b. Penetrating wounds of the abdomen, flank, genitalia or pelvis (20% of such injuries do not have gross hematuria).

    c. Deceleration injuries (fall, MVA) — prone to arterial intimal tears and subsequent thrombosis, ureteral avulsion).

2. Physical findings.

    a. Hematoma over fractured ribs #10 to 12.

    b. Discoloration, penetrating wound or mass in flank.

    c. Lower abdominal mass or tenderness.

    d. Genital swelling or discoloration.

    e. Inability to void following trauma.

    f. Blood at urethral meatus.

    g. Gross hematuria — requires full GU work-up.

    h. Microscopic hematuria — get IVP (low yield in blunt trauma) if RBC > 25.

3. X-ray studies.

    a. IVP — single, 5-minute film when time is of the essence, look for presence of bilateral nephrograms.

    b. Cystogram — full and post-drainage films.

       c. Retrograde urethrogram.
- 4. Specific injuries.
  - a. Renal contusion — common, microscopic hematuria, resolves spontaneously.
  - b. Renal laceration.
  - c. Perinephric hematoma — do not explore if IVP normal.
  - d. Renal artery/vein tear and thrombosis.
  - e. Ureteral transection/avulsion.
  - f. Bladder rupture (extraperitoneal, intraperitoneal, combined) — usually associated with pelvic fractures.
  - g. Urethral disruption.

H. Pelvic fractures.

1. Major problem is bleeding from complex pelvic fractures. External fixation and MAST trousers may help, occasionally selective embolization is needed.
2. Open pelvic fractures carry a high mortality. Usually require fecal diversion (colostomy, irrigation of defunctionalized segment) and urinary diversion (suprapubic cystostomy), especially if associated with perineal injuries.

III. PENETRATING ABDOMINAL INJURIES

A. General considerations.

1. The limits of the abdomen are the nipples superiorly, the perineum and gluteal folds inferiorly and the posterior axillary lines laterally.
2. Gunshot wounds of the abdomen carry a 95% probability of significant visceral injury.
3. Stab wounds of the abdomen — only two–thirds penetrate the peritoneal cavity, of these only half cause significant visceral injury that requires surgical repair.

B. Management.

1. Gunshot wounds — exploratory laparotomy is mandatory.
2. Stab wounds.
   - a. Shock — exploratory laparotomy.
   - b. Hemodynamically stable, positive physical findings — exploratory laparotomy.
   - c. Hemodynamically stable, negative physical findings ... options include:
     1) Non–directed selective management — observation and serial examinations.
     2) Directed selective management — decision to explore based on results of diagnostic procedures.
        - a) Local wound exploration — should be performed formally with sterile prep, adequate local anesthesia and extension of skin wound; do *not* probe wound with blunt object; if wound exploration indicates

penetration of peritoneal cavity → observation, DPL or mandatory exploration.
  b) DPL — positive lavage limits lowered to 1,000-20,000 RBC, 25-100 WBC (penetrating criteria).
  3) Mandatory exploration — especially if local wound exploration indicates peritoneal penetration.

IV. HEAD TRAUMA (see "Neurosurgical Emergencies")

V. SPINE AND SPINAL CORD TRAUMA
(see "Neurosurgical Emergencies")

VI. EXTREMITY TRAUMA
A. General considerations.
  1. Extremity trauma is rarely life–threatening; however, if not properly managed, permanent disability may occur.
  2. Except for direct control of bleeding, which includes maintaining traction on extremities with obvious or suspected fractures, the extremities receive little specific attention during the primary survey.
B. Extremity assessment — occurs during secondary survey.
  1. History — mechanism of injury, environment, predisposing factors, findings at the accident scene, pre–hospital care, status of tetanus prophylaxis.
  2. Physical examination.
    a. Look — deformities, angulation, shortening, swelling, discoloration, bruising, muscle spasm, wounds, color and perfusion of the extremity.
    b. Feel — tenderness, crepitation, pulse (Doppler signal), capillary filling, sensation, warmth.
    c. Movement — active motion, passive motion (not of an obvious fracture).
  3. Fracture assessment — fractures are either closed or open (associated with break in skin).
    a. Life-threatening extremity injuries.
      1) Massive, open fractures with ragged, dirty wounds.
      2) Bilateral femoral shaft fractures — open or closed.
      3) Vascular injuries, with or without fractures, proximal to the knee or elbow.
      4) Crush injuries of the abdomen and pelvis, major pelvic fractures.
      5) Traumatic amputations of the arm or leg.
    b. Limb–threatening injuries.
      1) Fracture–dislocation of the ankle with or without vascular compromise.
      2) Tibial fractures with vascular impairment.
      3) Dislocation of the knee or hip.

      4) Wrist and forearm fractures with circulatory interruption.
      5) Fractures or dislocations about the elbow.
      6) Crush injury.
      7) Amputations, complete or incomplete.
      8) Open fractures.
   c. Associated fractures or dislocations — certain injuries, because of a common mechanism, are often associated with a second injury that is not immediately apparent; such as knee contusions that may be a clue to patellar or supra-condylar fractures of the femur in patients with posterior dislocations of the hip.
   d. Occult fractures — beware of fractures in the multiple-injured patient with life-threatening injuries.

4. Blood loss assessment.
   a. Closed injury — closed femur fractures can result in 2–3 units of blood loss, closed pelvic fractures can cause hypovolemic shock.
   b. Open injury — blood loss from open fractures is usually far greater than estimated.

5. Dislocation and fracture–dislocation assessment — x-rays required for differentiation. Dislocations produce neurovascular stress that can be limb–threatening. Dislocations should be reduced as soon as possible.

6. Assessment of neurovascular bundle injury.
   a. Vascular injuries — can result in bleeding or thrombosis with impairment of distal circulation and ischemia. Often suggested by brisk bleeding from wound, although complete arterial tears bleed less than partial tears. A large hematoma or injuries to adjacent neural strictures are also suggestive. Examination of distal pulses is crucial, although the presence of a pulse does not rule out vascular injury. All pulse abnormalities must be evaluated, as well as proximity wounds, with angiography.
   b. Nerve injuries — may be complete disruption or contusion/stretch injury.

7. Vascular impairment (extremity ischemia).
   a. Signs of vascular injury.
      1) Bleeding.
      2) Hematoma–expanding.
      3) Bruit.
      4) Abnormal pulses.
      5) Impaired distal circulation.
   b. Arterial intimal tears are often not immediately recognized, although they can rapidly lead to thrombosis.
   c. Checklist for suspected vascular injury.
      1) Check immobilization device.

2) Assess fracture alignment.
3) Re–assess distal perfusion, doppler signals.
4) Consider compartment syndrome.
5) Obtain surgical consultation.

  d. Arteriogram.
  e. Goal of management is to identify vascular injuries prior to the development of ischemia (six P's — pain, paresthesias, paralysis, pallor, pulselessness, poikilothermia).

8. Compartment syndrome — can occur in lower leg or arm since neurovascular bundle is enveloped within the fascial planes. Associated with compartmental hemorrhage and edema, often associated with fractures and crush injuries.

9. Amputation — preserve amputated parts for possible reimplantation or use of skin/soft tissue for grafts to treat other injuries.

C. **Extremity trauma management** (consult orthopedic surgeon).

1. Fractures.
   a. Open fractures — remove gross contamination, culture, align with splinting techniques, cover wound with sterile dressing. Operative repair consists of internal or external fixation, wound management.
   b. Immobilization — done for pain control and prevention of further injury. Obtain x-rays and arteriograms only after extremity is splinted and dressed.

2. Joint injuries — reduce all dislocations, manage associated fractures appropriately.

3. Antibiotics — broad–spectrum antibiotic coverage for 48 hrs.

4. Compartment syndrome — measured compartment pressures of ≥ 30 mm Hg indicate need for emergent fasciotomy.

5. Tetanus prophylaxis:

TABLE 2
Tetanus Prophylaxis for the Wounded Patient

History of Tetanus Immunization (doses)	Clean, Minor Wounds		Tetanus–Prone Wounds	
	TD[1]	TIG	TD[1]	TIG[2]
Uncertain	Yes	No	Yes	Yes
0-1	Yes	No	Yes	Yes
2	Yes	No	Yes	No[3]
3 or more	No[4]	No	No[5]	No

KEY:
1 TD = 0.5 ml absorbed toxoid. For children less than 7 years old, DPT (DT, if pertussis vaccine is contraindicated) is preferred to tetanus toxoid alone. For persons 7 years old and older, TD is preferred to tetanus toxoid alone.
2 TIG = 250 units tetanus immune globulin, human. When TIG and TD are given concurrently, separate syringes and separate sites should be used.
3 Yes, if wound is more than 24 hours old.
4 Yes, if more than 10 years since last dose.
5 Yes, if more than 5 years since last dose. (More frequent boosters are not needed and can accentuate side-effects.)

VII. PENETRATING NECK INJURY
A. **Zones of the neck** (see Fig. 1).

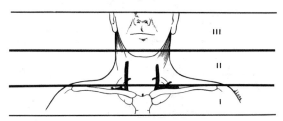

FIGURE 1
Zones of the Neck

1. **Zone I** (base of neck) — from the suprasternal notch or cricoid cartilage and inferiorly, includes great vessels, difficult exposure and control.
2. **Zone II** (neck) — between zones I and III, easy exposure and control.
3. **Zone III** (base of skull) — from the angle of the mandible and superiorly, difficult exposure and control.
B. **Management.**
   1. Surgical exploration indicated for the following signs/symptoms:
      a. Penetration of platysma (Zone II) — never probe defect.
      b. Subcutaneous or retropharyngeal air on examination or plain films.
      c. Hoarseness or stridor.
      d. Active external or oropharyngeal hemorrhage.
      e. Expanding or pulsatile hematoma.
      f. Sucking neck wound.
      g. Absent carotid pulse.
      h. Bruit or thrill suggesting intimal flap or arteriovenous fistula.
      i. Neurologic deficit.
   2. Zone I injuries — selective management.
   3. Zone II injuries — mandatory exploration.
   4. Zone III injuries — selective management.
   5. Diagnostic modalities for selective management.
      a. Arteriography — arch, great vessels, carotids, and vertebrals.
      b. Laryngoscopy, bronchoscopy — flexible and rigid.
      c. Esophagoscopy, contrast esophagography.

VIII. TRAUMA IN PREGNANCY

A. Diagnosis and management.

1. Initial assessment.
   a. Patient position — keep patient on left side (unless spinal injury suspected) to avoid IVC compression by gravid uterus; if patient is supine ... elevate right hip and manually displace uterus to left.
   b. Primary survey — support physiologic hypervolemia liberally with crystalloid and blood administration (the pregnant patient can lose up to 35% of her blood volume before tachycardia, hypotension, and other signs of hypovolemia occur; thus, the fetus may be in severe jeopardy while the mother appears stable); vasopressors should be avoided.

2. Secondary assessment.
   a. Assessment of uterine irritability, fundal height and tenderness, fetal heart tones, fetal movement.
   b. Uterine contractions, vaginal bleeding.
   c. Ruptured membranes suggested by fluid in vagina with pH of 7.0 to 7.5.
   d. Cervical effacement and dilatation, fetal presentation, station.

3. Monitoring.
   a. Patient — monitor while on left side.
   b. Fetus — continuous monitoring with ultrasonic doppler cardioscope to diagnose fetal distress (inadequate accelerations, late decelerations).
   c. Routine x-rays of mother should be performed — fetal survival depends on maternal well–being.

4. Definitive care.
   a. Initial management directed at resuscitation and stabilization of the pregnant patient — the fetus' life is totally dependent on the integrity of the mother's.
   b. DPL — open technique, above uterus.

B. Specific injuries.

1. Uterine rupture — uterus is protected during first trimester but thereafter becomes progressively more vulnerable; may present with minimal symptoms or with shock; x-ray evidence includes extended fetal extremities, abnormal fetal position, free intraperitoneal air; suspicion mandates surgical exploration.

2. Abruptio placenta (placental separation from uterine wall) — leading cause of fetal death after blunt trauma; presents with vaginal bleeding, premature labor, fetal distress and demise, abdominal pain, uterine tenderness and rigidity, expanding fundal height, maternal shock, DIC.

3. Pelvic fractures — additional hemorrhagic complications due to engorged pelvic veins.

IX. PEDIATRIC TRAUMA

A. Special considerations.

1. Airway — young infants are obligate nose breathers (clear nasal obstruction), trachea is short (avoid bronchial intubation), trachea is small (intubate with uncuffed tubes of appropriate size), cricothyroidotomy almost never indicated (use needle jet insufflation if needed).

2. Shock.

   a. Recognition of shock (normal vitals are age-related).
      1) Tachycardia — ≥ 120–160.
      2) Cool extremities.
      3) Hypotension — SBP < 80–100.

   b. Fluid replacement.
      1) Initial bolus of LR — 20 cc/kg over 10 min, may repeat once.
      2) Blood — give 20 cc/kg whole blood or 10 cc/kg PRBC after above measures fail.

   c. Acid–base disturbances — usually can be corrected with ventilation, give bicarb for pH < 7.2.

   d. Venous access — after percutaneous lines placed; cutdown options are saphenous, cephalic (elbow and upper arm), external jugular.

   e. Thermoregulation — maintain temp at 36–37°C by use of overhead heaters and thermal blankets.

B. Chest trauma.

1. Pneumothorax/hemothorax — poorly tolerated.
2. Flail chest — especially sensitive.
3. Bronchial injuries, diaphagmatic rupture — more prone.
4. Great vessel injury — less prone.

C. Abdominal trauma.

1. DPL — much less frequently used, replaced by CT scanning.
   a. Indications — hemodynamic instability, especially if unconscious; abdominal clearance for general anesthesia to care for other injuries.
   b. Technique — use 10 cc/kg of LR for lavage.

2. Spleen and liver injuries — most can be managed non-operatively after diagnosis by CT scanning, surgery indicated for hemodynamic instability.

D. Extremity trauma — potential for injury to growth plate.

E. The battered, abused child.

X. COMMON COMPLEX SCENARIOS IN TRAUMA MANAGEMENT

A. Blunt abdominal trauma and closed head injury.

1. Primary survey.

2. Resuscitation.
3. X-rays — C–spine, chest, pelvis.
4. DPL.
   a. If grossly positive → OR for exploratory laparotomy, neuro-surgeons to place prophylactic burr holes or interventricular catheter in OR, head CT scan after OR, back to OR, if further neurosurgical intervention needed.
   b. If grossly negative → to radiology for head CT scan, complete lavage during head CT, if lavage or head CT scan positive → to OR for exploratory laparotomy or neurosurgical procedure, if both negative → back to ER to complete evaluation.
B. **Blunt abdominal trauma and widened mediastinum** (rule out thoracic aortic tear).
   1. DPL.
      a. If positive → to OR for exploratory laparotomy, then to radiology for aortography, if aortography positive → back to OR for thoracotomy.
      b. If negative → to radiology for aortography.
C. **Penetrating thoracic trauma** (precordial) with negative work–up (rule out pericardial tamponade).
   1. Patient is hemodynamically stable, no signs or symptoms of cardiac tamponade.
   2. Do not admit for observation only. If one is worried enough to admit the patient, one should obtain some diagnostic work–up.
   3. Diagnostic options.
      a. Subxiphoid pericardial window.
      b. Echocardiography.
      c. CT scan.

TRAUMA APPENDIX

I. PENETRATING CHEST TRAUMA

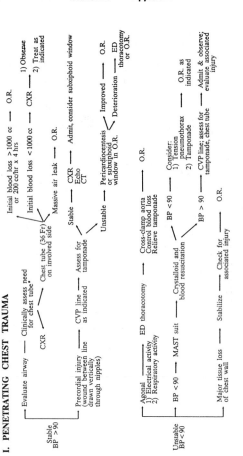

* 1) Tension pneumothorax; 2) Sucking chest wound; 3) Hemothorax

II. BLUNT CHEST TRAUMA

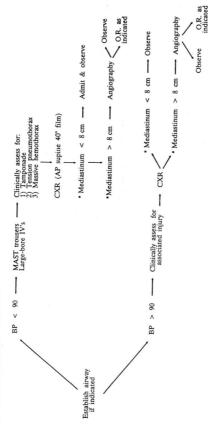

Establish airway
if indicated

BP < 90 —— MAST trousers —— Clinically assess for:
Large-bore IV's   1) Tamponade
                       2) Tension pneumothorax
                       3) Massive hemothorax

CXR (AP supine 40" film)

* Mediastinum < 8 cm —— Admit & observe

* Mediastinum > 8 cm —— Angiography ⟨ Observe
                                      O.R. as indicated

BP > 90 —— Clinically assess for
            associated injury —— CXR

* Mediastinum < 8 cm —— Observe

* Mediastinum > 8 cm —— Angiography ⟨ Observe
                                      O.R. as indicated

* See above for complete list of chest radiographic signs that are indications for angiography.

III. PENETRATING ABDOMINAL TRAUMA

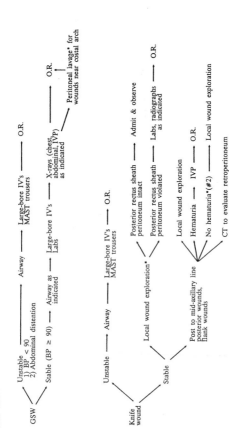

* Consider peritoneal lavage:
1) For wounds near costal arch below 4th ICS.
2) In lieu of exploration.

IV. BLUNT ABDOMINAL TRAUMA

No vital signs on admission ——— No further treatment

Agonal ——— Airway ——— Large-bore IV's ——— O.R.
1) Electrical activity
2) Respirations present

BP < 90 ——— Airway as ——— MAST suit ——— Large-bore IV's
indicated

           BP > 90 ——— Labs, X-rays, ——— Observe
                            lavage*   O.R.

           BP < 90 ——— O.R.

BP > 90 ——— Airway as ——— Large-bore IV's ——— Labs, X-rays, lavage* ——— Observe
indicated   O.R.

*Indications:
1) ETOH intoxication
2) Drug intoxication
3) Head injury
4) Cord injury
5) Equivocal exam
6) Significant trauma on both sides of diaphragm

V. PENETRATING EXTREMITY TRAUMA

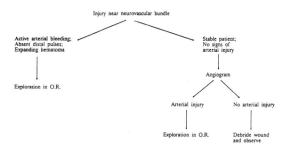

VI. PENETRATING NECK TRAUMA

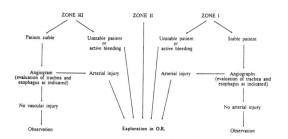

VII. BLUNT NECK TRAUMA

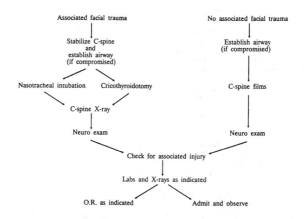

MAXILLOFACIAL TRAUMA

I. INITIAL EVALUATION
Refer to "Trauma" chapter for general initial assessment and resuscitation. Beware of causes of sudden death or permanent disability.

A. Cervical spine fractures — present in 2–4% of cases when facial fractures are present.

B. Laryngeal fractures.
  1. Symptoms.
     a. Laryngeal pain.
     b. Dysphonia or aphonia.
     c. Hemoptysis.
     d. Stridor.
     e. Dysphagia.
  2. Physical findings.
     a. Distortion of normal external landmarks.
     b. Cervical ecchymosis.
     c. Subcutaneous emphysema.
     d. Air or salivary leakage from lacerations.
  3. Treatment.
     a. Do not attempt endotracheal intubation.
     b. Early tracheostomy under optimum conditions at 3rd or 4th tracheal ring.
     c. **Open reduction with internal fixation (ORIF).**

II. HISTORY
A. Important to note both pre-injury and post-injury visual acuity and occlusion.

B. Also note special pre-injury problems, i.e., hearing deficits, nasal airway obstruction, or missing teeth.

III. PHYSICAL EXAMINATION
A. Note and diagram any lacerations or abrasions — photographs are best; determine if tissue loss is present.

B. Eye exam.
  1. Visual acuity.
  2. Extraocular muscle function.
  3. Fundi.
  4. Eyelids and conjunctiva.
  5. Fluorescein exam if corneal abrasion is suspected.
  6. Raccoon's eyes indicates basilar skull fracture until proven otherwise.
  7. Ophthalmology consult for suspected globe injury.

C. **Ear exam.**
   1. Look for distortion of normal landmarks on the external ear indicating hematoma.
   2. Otoscopic exam for foreign body, hemotympanum.
   3. Hemotympanum or CSF leak — imply basilar skull fracture.
D. **Nose exam.**
   1. Palpation for fracture — x-rays play little or no role in establishing or excluding the diagnosis of nasal fracture.
   2. Check for septal hematoma.
   3. CSF rhinorrhea — basilar skull fracture.
E. **Mouth exam.**
   1. Check occlusion.
   2. Look for loose or missing teeth — if teeth missing, check posterior pharynx or chest x-ray for aspiration.
   3. Intra-oral laceration or ecchymosis.
F. **Facial skeleton** — bimanual exam of all facial bones to assess tenderness and/or motion.

IV. **RADIOLOGIC EVALUATION**
A. **C–spine.**
B. **Reverse Waters view** for suspected zygomatic / maxillary complex fracture — may be done in E.R.
C. **Panorex** for patients with malocclusion or suspected mandibular fracture — patient needs to be able to sit up and be cooperative.
D. **CT scan** — patient should be stable hemodynamically and co-operative.
   1. Axial — good detail of zygomatic arches.
   2. Coronal/sagittal cuts — give excellent orbital detail; need clear C–spine.
   3. 3–D reconstructions not generally necessary.

V. **TREATMENT**
A. **Soft tissue.**
   1. Anesthesia.
      a. Local with 1 : 200,000 epinephrine is helpful to control hemorrhage and prolong anesthetic effect.
      b. Nerve blocks will diminish volume required and minimize distortion (Fig. 1).
      c. Mark normal landmarks before infiltration, i.e. lip vermillion.
   2. Cleansing — large–volume high–pressure irrigation, mild detergent soap.
   3. Sharp debridement.
      a. All foreign material.
      b. Any unequivocally dead tissue.

c. Preserve all viable tissue — narrowly based flaps on the face will survive because of its excellent blood supply.
d. Black powder tattoos should go to the O.R. for debridement under general anesthesia as soon as possible.
e. Drain any significant hematoma.

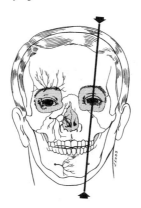

FIGURE 1
Facial Nerve Blocks

4. Reapproximation of normal landmarks.
5. Any residual soft tissue defect can be managed acutely by moist saline dressings and referral.
6. In the case of eyelid avulsion, keep the eye well lubricated with bland ophthalmic ointment and patch coverage; immediate referral.
7. Special cases.
   a. Suspected laceration of **Stensen's (parotid) duct.**
      1) Location (Fig. 2).
      2) Cannulation of duct for suspected injury.
      3) Treatment — repair soft tissue over stent with drain.

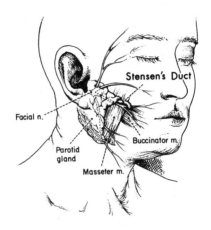

FIGURE 2

Ref: Schultz RC: *Facial Injuries*, 2nd Ed. Chicago: Year Book Medical Publishers, 1977, p. 150, with permission.

    b. Lacrimal duct laceration.
       1) Location — laceration through lid margin medial to punta or through medial canthus.
       2) Treatment — referral for cannulation of duct and repair of laceration over stent.
    c. Facial nerve injury.
       1) Note functional defect and location of lesion.
       2) Those lateral to canthus should be repaired with the microscope.

B. Facial fracture management — general considerations.
    1. Restore facial height and projection.
    2. Reestablish pre–traumatic occlusion.
    3. Wide exposure — through laceration or incisions: intra-oral, lower lid, coronal incision.
    4. Thorough debridement.
    5. Meticulous reduction and fixation.
    6. Specific approach based on anatomic diagnosis.

7. In complex cases:
   a. Restore mandibular relation to cranial base.
   b. Restore occlusion.
   c. Reconstruct midface.
C. Facial **fracture management based on diagnosis.**
   1. **Upper third** — supraorbital ridge, orbital roof, frontal sinus, naso-orbitoethmoid.
      a. Frontal sinus.
         1) Exam — pain, tenderness, edema, ecchymosis, palpable fracture; look for associated injuries.
         2) Treatment.
            a) Posterior table intact, anterior table depressed.
               (1) Duct open — ORIF of anterior table.
               (2) Duct injured — obliterate sinus or fix duct, then ORIF.
            b) Posterior table not intact.
               (1) Neurosurgery evaluation.
               (2) Nondisplaced — see (a).
               (3) Displaced — cranialization vs. obliteration.
         3) Complications — meningitis, CSF leaks, sinusitis, residual deformity.
   2. **Middle third** — maxilla, zygoma, orbit, nose.
      a. Nasal bones.
         1) Symptoms — epistaxis, pain, nasal congestion.
         2) Exam — tenderness, edema, ecchymosis, displacement, instability, crepitance.
         3) Treatment — drain septal hematoma if present.
            a) Closed reduction and splint.
            b) May require revision.
      b. Maxilla (see Fig. 3) — pass nasogastric tube via oral route if maxillofacial fracture suspected.
         1) **LeFort I** — transverse.
         2) **LeFort II** — pyramidal.
         3) **LeFort III** — craniofacial dysjunction.
         4) On exam will likely have impressive facial swelling.
         5) Midface will be unstable to bimanual exam.
         6) Treatment — ORIF within 7–14 days.
         7) Complications.
            a) Maxillary retrusion (LeFort I).
            b) "Dish face" deformity (LeFort II/III).
            c) Malocclusion.
      c. Zygoma.
         1) On exam — periorbital edema and ecchymosis, depressed cheek, tenderness, step off, proptosis or enophthalmos, infra–orbital nerve hypesthesia, trismus.

2) Treatment.
   a) Non–displaced — no treatment.
   b) Displaced — comminution or ZF suture separation.
     (1) Present — ORIF.
     (2) Absent — reduction only.
3) Complications — sinusitis, diplopia, enophthalmos, blindness, superior orbital fissure syndrome (compromise CN III, IV, VI), orbital apex syndrome (compromise CN II, III, IV, VI), persistent infra–orbital nerve anesthesia.

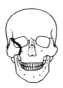

Fracture of Zygomatic Complex

LeFort I	**LeFort II**	**LeFort III**
(Transverse fracture)	(Pyramidal fracture)	(Craniofacial disjunction)

FIGURE 3

Ref: Plastic Surgery Educational Foundation: *Plastic and Reconstructive Surgery: Essentials for Students*, 3rd Ed. Chicago: Plastic Surgery Educational Foundation, 1987, p. 39, with permission.

   d. Orbital.
    1) Exam — diplopia, enophthalmos, periorbital edema, ecchymosis, infraorbital nerve hypesthesia.
    2) Treatment: to correct entrapment, prevent enophthalmos — ORIF +/– bone grafting.
    3) Operative complications — visual loss (rare), orbital hemorrhage (1%), infection (3-4%), infra–orbital neuralgia (rare), ectropion (1%), persistent diplopia (2-50%), persistent enophthalmos (15-22%).

3. **Lower third** — mandible.
   a. Symptoms — malocclusion, trismus, pain.
   b. Exam — tenderness, edema, ecchymosis, laceration, displacement, instability on bimanual exam, mental nerve hypesthesia.
   c. Panorex.
   d. Management — as soon as conveniently possible.
      1) Closed reduction.
         a) **Maxillomandibular fixation (MMF)** — 85-95% may be treated in this way.
         b) External fixation rare.
      2) ORIF — helps minimize time in MMF.
   e. Complications.
      1) Malocclusion.
      2) TMJ pain.
      3) Nonunion.
   f. Complications of MMF.
      1) Weight loss and feeding problems.
      2) Airway compromise and poor pulmonary toilet.
      3) Poor oral hygiene.
      4) Social and communication problems.
   g. Special cases.
      1) Children — avoid open reduction and internal fixation — tooth buds; early mobilization important, especially for condylar fractures.
      2) Endentulous mandible.
         a) Thin mandible with no teeth make accurate reduction, fixation and subsequent bony union a challenge.
         b) May do closed reduction with splints and MMF.
         c) ORIF may be necessary.

BURN INJURY

I. **INITIAL MANAGEMENT**

The initial management of the burn–injured patient is directed toward resuscitation, stabilization, and evaluation of injuries. In the first few hours post–injury, the burn wound itself is of secondary importance.

A. **Airway, breathing, circulation – first priority.** Ensure an adequate airway. Early endotracheal intubation is mandatory for inhalation injury, deep facial burns, supraglottic obstruction, severe facial fractures, and closed head injury with unconsciousness (see IV: Inhalation Injury). Provide humidified oxygen or assisted ventilation as indicated. Establish IV access, using 18 gauge or larger catheters. Avoid placing in burned areas, if possible.

B. **Expose** patient, and examine – be aware of associated injuries such as long–bone fractures, intra–abdominal or intrathoracic injury, spinal injuries, or closed–head injury.

C. Obtain **history.**

1. Good sources: EMT personnel, rescue record, and witnesses.
2. Identify treatment administered in field, vital signs during transport.
3. Identify the burn agent; closed *vs.* open space injury.
4. Pertinent past medical history, including allergies, immunization status, current medications, etc.

D. Perform **burn evaluation** (see III: Burn Evaluation).

E. Place NG tube – for burns > 25% total body surface area (TBSA), adynamic ileus is common and can lead to gastric aspiration.

F. Place Foley catheter – essential for monitoring urine output as an indicator of adequate resuscitation. Obtain urinalysis and check for myoglobin or hemoglobin.

G. **Analgesia** – use IV route. Morphine sulfate 2–5 mg q 2 h prn.

H. Obtain baseline body weight.

I. Obtain initial blood tests including CBC, renal profile, and arterial blood gas, alcohol level and toxin screen. Obtain blood for carboxyhemoglobin level if inhalation injury is suspected. Obtain CXR and other x-rays as indicated by injuries, as well as EKG.

J. Lavage all burned areas to remove foreign material (see VI: Burn Wound Care).

1. Chemical burns should be lavaged copiously with water to dilute agent. For specific neutralizing agents, see Table 1.
2. Asphalt burns – ice may be applied to enhance separation.

K. **Escharotomy** – perform early for circumferential burns to extremities and chest to prevent circulatory and respiratory compromise.

L. Initial medications.

1. Tetanus prophylaxis — see "Trauma" page 163.
2. Acid prophylaxis — use H_2 blocker (ranitidine 50 mg IV q8h; or cimetidine 300 mg IV q6h). Use antacids 30 cc q 2-4 h per NG to titrate gastric pH > 5.0.
3. Antifungal prophylaxis — nystatin 15 cc oral swab and 15 cc per NG tid.
4. Multivitamins one ampule in IV fluids qd.
5. Treat hemoglobinuria/myoglobinuria — furosemide 40 mg IV, mannitol 25 g IV, and alkalinize urine $NaHCO_3$ one ampule in IVF to keep urine pH > 7.0.

TABLE 1
Treatment of Chemical "Burns"

Agent	Initial Therapy	Special Considerations
Muriatic acid (HCl) Sulfuric acid (H_2SO_4) Nitric acid (HNO_3)	Soap	Then cover with Mg (OH_2) or Mg trisilicate
Oxalic acid [$2H_2O$ $(COOH)_2$] Hydrofluoric acid (HF)	$NaHCO_3$ wash, then 0.2% hyamine in ice-alcohol	Inject Ca gluconate into area for residual pain
Chromic acid (H_2CrO_4)	Dilute Na hyposulfite wash	
Sodium hypochlorite (NaClO) [Clorox, other disinfectants, bleaches, deodorizers with chlorine]	Water wash, then 1% Na thiosulfate	
Phenol (C_6H_5OH) and creosols [sanitizers, disinfectants]	10% Ethanol	Then cover with olive, castor, or vegetable oils
Lyes (metal hydroxides), Na metal, lithium hydroxide	Dilute vinegar	Alternate with lemon juice, then cover with oil
Dichromate salts Alkyl mercury salts	2% Hyposulfite Debride blisters and remove fluid	Then apply balm
White phosphorus	1:5000 $KMnO_4$	Then cover with oil
Tar	Clean with surgical antiseptic Cover with Neo-Polycin® ointment	Wash off dissolved tar at 24 and 48 hours

Ref: Hardy JD. *Hardy's Textbook of Surgery.* Philadelphia: JB Lippincott Co., 1983, p. 189. Reproduced by permission.

II. INDICATIONS FOR HOSPITAL ADMISSION

A. Some burn injuries may be managed on an outpatient basis. The following guidelines are based upon the American Burn Association Injury Severity Grading System.

B. Admission to hospital is indicated in the following situations:
   1. Full–thickness burn of > 2% TBSA.
   2. Partial–thickness burn > 15% in an adult; > 10% in a child.
   3. Involvement of the face, hands, feet, or perineum.
   4. Electrical, chemical or inhalation injury is present.
   5. High–risk patient – age > 65, < 3 years; pre–existing medical problems, multitrauma.
   6. Suspicion of abuse or neglect.

III. BURN EVALUATION – REMOVE ALL CLOTHING

A. Depth.
   1. 1st degree – epidermal; painful; pink to red.
   2. 2nd degree – partial dermal; painful; white to pink; blebs and blisters.
   3. 3rd degree – full dermal; all dermal appendages are destroyed; hypesthetic; dry and leathery, inelastic.
   4. 4th degree – underlying adipose, fascia, muscle, bone.
B. Size estimation.
   1. **Rule of nines** – 9% head and neck, 9% each upper extremity, 18% each lower extremity and each hemithorax.
   2. **Lund–Browder chart** (see Fig. 1).
   3. Total body surface area (TBSA) = 71.84 x weight (kg) x height (cm).

IV. INHALATION INJURY

A. Single most important injury that contributes to human mortality. Early intubation is mandatory for suspected or documented inhalation injury and burns involving head and neck.
B. Inhalation injury results from exposure to carbon monoxide, chemical irritants, and toxic gases. Rarely due to thermal injury (exception is injury due to superheated steam). Suspect inhalation injury if:
   1. Closed space injury (e.g., house fire).
   2. Presence of facial burns, singed nasal hairs, bronchorrhea, carbonaceous sputum, wheezing and rales, tachypnea, progressive hoarseness, and difficulty clearing secretions.
C. Upper airway – obstruction may occur within the ensuing 48 hrs (maximal edema approximately 12 hrs).
D. Lower airway – pulmonary edema and chemical tracheobronchitis due to noxious gases.
E. Diagnosis.
   1. Upper – **direct laryngoscopy.** Look for carbon deposits, airway edema.
   2. Lower – **fiberoptic bronchoscopy.** Findings of airway edema, carbon deposits in tracheobronchial tree, and mucosal necrosis.

3. **¹³³Xenon scan** — evaluates lower respiratory tract by washout of radioisotope. Incomplete washout by 90 seconds indicates lower airway involvement.
F. **Treatment** — O₂ supplementation, ventilatory assistance, bronchio-alveolar lavage to remove debris. Systemic corticosteroids are *contraindicated*.

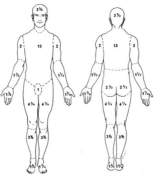

AREA	AGE: Birth-1	1-4	5-9	10-14	15	Adult	Partial thickness 2°	Full thickness 3°	Total
Head	19	17	13	11	9	7			
Neck	2	2	2	2	2	2			
Anterior trunk	13	13	13	13	13	13			
Posterior trunk	13	13	13	13	13	13			
Right buttock	2₁/2	2₁/2	2₁/2	2₁/2	2₁/2	2₁/2			
Left buttock	2₁/2	2₁/2	2₁/2	2₁/2	2₁/2	2₁/2			
Genitalia	1	1	1	1	1	1			
Right upper arm	4	4	4	4	4	4			
Left upper arm	4	4	4	4	4	4			
Right lower arm	3	3	3	3	3	3			
Left lower arm	3	3	3	3	3	3			
Right hand	2₁/2	2₁/2	2₁/2	2₁/2	2₁/2	2₁/2			
Left hand	2₁/2	2₁/2	2₁/2	2₁/2	2₁/2	2₁/2			
Right thigh	5₁/2	6₁/2	8	8₁/2	9	9₁/2			
Left thigh	5₁/2	6₁/2	8	8₁/2	9	9₁/2			
Right leg	5	5	5₁/2	6	6₁/2	7			
Left leg	5	5	5₁/2	6	6₁/2	8			
Right foot	3₁/2	3₁/2	3₁/2	3₁/2	3₁/2	3₁/2			
Left foot	3₁/2	3₁/2	3₁/2	3₁/2	3₁/2				

FIGURE 1
Lund–Browder Burn Estimate

G. **Carbon monoxide (CO) poisoning** — CO displaces oxygen, binds hemoglobin forming carboxyhemoglobin. Hypoxemia results; carboxyhemoglobin levels > 50% are potentially lethal.
   1. **Diagnosis** — signs/symptoms of hypoxia; serum carboxyhemoglobin level > 10% (non-smoker) or > 20% (smoker) is diagnostic.
   2. **Treatment** — 100% O_2 reduces $T_{1/2}$ of CO from 250 min to 50 min. Follow with carboxyhemoglobin levels, continue to treat until level 10–15%. A persistent metabolic acidosis (with adequate volume resuscitation) implies CO poisoning of cellular respiration.

V. FLUID RESUSCITATION

A. Various resuscitation formulas exist (see Table 2). In our institution, the Parkland formula is generally used. Large–bore IV access is used. CVP and pulmonary catheter monitoring is used in patients with significant cardiac or pulmonary disease.
B. Goals of therapy:
   1. Adequate urine output — adult > 30 cc/hr; child > 1 cc/kg/hr.
   2. Pulse < 120/min.
   3. Normal mentation, well–perfused extremities.
   4. Normal arterial blood pH, mixed venous oxygen saturation.

VI. BURN WOUND CARE

A. The goals of wound management are prevention of infection and debridement of necrotic tissue to allow healing either by secondary intention or by excision and skin grafting. Mortality from burn wound sepsis has been significantly reduced by use of topical antimicrobial agents.
B. **Topical agents.**
   1. **Mafenide acetate** [Sulfamylon®] — broad spectrum, but little fungicidal activity. Penetrates eschar well, but pain on application. Carbonic anhydrase inhibitor, absorption can cause hyperchloremic metabolic acidosis. Apply bid.
   2. **Silver sulfadiazine** [Silvadene®] — broad spectrum, including *Candida*. Intermediate eschar penetration but less than mafenide acetate. Non-painful on application. May cause transient leukopenia. Apply bid. *Contraindicated* in patients with glucose–6–phosphate dehydrogenase deficiency.
   3. **Silver nitrate 0.5%** — applied as wet dressing, good eschar penetration. May result in Na and Cl depletion. May cause methemoglobinemia.
   4. **Bacitracin ointment** — useful for superficial partial–thickness burns.
C. **Local care.**
   1. **First–degree burns** — minor care, symptomatic pain control.

TABLE 2
Fluid Resuscitation Formulas

	Evans	Brooke	Parkland	Modified Brooke	Hypertonic Resuscitation
Day 1					
Colloid	1 ml/kg/% burn	0.5 ml/kg/% burn	None	None	None
Crystalloid	Lactated Ringer's solution, 1 ml/kg/% burn	Lactated Ringer's solution, 1.5 mg/kg/% burn	Lactated Ringer's solution, 4 ml/kg/% burn	Lactated Ringer's solution, 2 ml/kg/% burn (adult), 3 ml/kg/% burn (child)	250 mEq Na/L, 150 mEq lactate, 100 mEq chlorine; titrate to urine flow
5% DW	2000 ml/meter^2	2000 ml/meter^2	None	None	"Liberal" free water by mouth
Urine	30-50 ml/hr (adult)	30-50 ml/hr (adult)	50-70 ml/hr (adult)	30-50 ml/hr (adult), 1 ml/kg/hr (child)	30-50 ml/hr (adult)
Rate	1/2 total first 8 hr, 1/4 total next 8 hr, 1/4 total next 8 hr	1/2 total first 8 hr, 1/4 total next 8 hr, 1/4 total next 8 hr	1/2 total first 8 hr, 1/4 total next 8 hr, 1/4 total next 8 hr	Same as Brooke	Infuse constantly
Calculation of volume	Use burn area up to a total of 50% TBSA; > 50% TBSA burn, calculate as 50% burn	Same as Evans	Use total burn area for all sizes of burns	Same as Parkland	Titrate to urine production, not burn size
Day 2					
Colloid	0.5 ml/kg/% burn	0.25 ml/kg/% burn	700-2000 ml (adult) as required to maintain urine	0.3-0.5 ml/kg/% burn	—
Crystalloid	Lactated Ringer's solution, 0.5 ml/kg/% burn	Lactated Ringer's solution, 0.75 mg/kg/% burn	None	None	—
5% DW	1500-2000 ml	1500-2000 ml	Sufficient to maintain urine	Sufficient to maintain urine	—

2. Partial–thickness burns — initial wash with antiseptic soap (e.g., chlorhexidine gluconate), remove debris, unroof vesicles. Apply topical agent.

3. Deep partial–thickness, full–thickness burns — initially treat as for partial–thicknesss burns. Eschar separation may be managed expectantly, although we advocate early excision and grafting.

D. Early excision and grafting — popularized by Janzekovic (1970). Excise eschar tangentially to point of capillary bleeding; perform within 2–7 days of admission for deep 2nd and 3rd degree burns. Graft immediately or cover temporarily with homograft or biologic dressing.

1. Advantages — early removal of eschar and coverage. Improved joint function. Shortened hospitalization. Earlier mobilization and rehabilitation.

2. Disadvantages — major procedure with significant blood loss in critically ill patient. Excision time should not exceed 2 hrs. Blood loss should not exceed 50% of total blood volume.

E. Grafting procedures.

1. Autograft = same individual; allograft = homograft = same species (e.g., cadaver); xenograft = heterograft = different species (e.g., porcine).

2. Indications for homografting.
   a. Insufficient autologous skin available.
   b. Temporary wound coverage prior to autologous skin grafting.
   c. Speeds epithelialization, prevents infection in large intra-dermal wounds.

3. Mesh grafts — not optimal for cosmetic appearance. Does expand to cover large surface area (11/2:1 to 4:1). Allows for application to less than ideal recipient beds.

4. **Skin substitutes.**
   a. Temporary — eliminate wound exudate, maximize epithelialization and new tissue formation. Material must be permeable to water vapor and oxygen, flexible, and without risk of disease transmission.
      1) Biologic materials (cadaver skin, pigskin, amnion) — short shelf–life and can transmit disease.
      2) Synthetic materials — long shelf–life, no disease transmission (e.g., **Biobrane®** — outer layer of silicone and inner layer bound with collagen).
   b. Permanent — wound closure and control of scarring possible.
      1) Cultured skin — epidermal cells only. No dermis restored; dense scar formation still occurs. Must be applied to fascial bed.
      2) Bilayer material — epidermal cells plus artificial dermal layer (collagen latticework) bound with glycosaminoglycan gel (**experimental**).

VII. MANAGEMENT OF INFECTION IN BURN INJURY

A. Pathogenesis — In untreated burn wound, surface bacteria proliferate, migrate through nonviable tissue, pause at subeschar space and, when microbial invasiveness "outweighs" host defense capability, invades viable tissue with microvascular involvement and systemic dissemination (burn wound sepsis). Avascularity and ischemia of full–thickness burn wound allows microbial proliferation and prevents delivery of systemic antibiotics and cellular components of host defense.

B. Clinical signs.
   1. Conversion from a partial to full-thickness injury, or rapidly spreading ischemic necrosis.
   2. Hemorrhage in subcutaneous tissue generally good indication of invasive infection.

C. **Invasive burn wound sepsis.**
   1. Cultures of burn wound surface do *not* accurately predict progressive bacterial colonization or incipient burn wound sepsis. Qualitative and quantitative correlation are poor between flora on the surface of the burn wound and bacterial colonization of the deep layers of the eschar.
   2. Bacterial growth is best monitored by semiquantitative **burn wound biopsy** — calculate precise number of organisms per gram of tissue. If biopsy cultures reveal $> 10^5$ organisms/g tissue or if there is 100–fold increase in the concentration of organisms/g tissue within a 48–hour period, then the organisms have escaped effective control by the topical chemotherapeutic agent, and burn wound sepsis is incipient. (Note: false–positive results often occur.)
   3. Wound colonization of dead tissue must be differentiated from invasion into viable tissue.
      a. Best evaluated on biopsy — finding organisms in viable tissue on histologic examination.
      b. Microvascular invasion connotes possible hematogenous dissemination and mandates systemic antibiotic therapy.
   4. Wound — often dry, crusted, black or violaceous color. May be unchanged.
   5. Clinical picture — fever, hypoxia, mental status changes, leukocytosis, new onset ileus, tachypnea, thrombocytopenia, hypotension, oliguria, acidosis, tachycardia, and hyperglycemia. Bacteremia is a late phenomenon in burn sepsis.

D. **Bacteriology of nosocomial burn infection.**
   1. Know your hospital's flora and be aware of sensitivities of species.
   2. Most common pathogens — *Staphylococcus aureus*, Group A streptococcus, *Pseudomonas aeruginosa*, other gram–negative rods, *Enterococcus*, *Candida albicans*.

E. **Prevention of burn infection.**
   1. Dressing change bid or tid and topical agents.
   2. Environmental controls.
      a. Strict patient isolation.
      b. Strict handwashing.
      c. Laminar air–flow isolation — usually not available.
F. **Treatment of burn infection.**
   1. Remove *all* devitalized tissue.
   2. Surgically drain closed–space abscesses.
   3. Apply diffusible topical agent.
   4. Empiric antibiotic therapy — broad spectrum (1st generation cephalosporin– or penicillinase–resistant penicillin plus aminoglycoside). Rarely needs anaerobic coverage. Specific antibiotic therapy upon bacteriologic identification.
G. **Nonbacterial infection.**
   1. Viral infection — usually heals with time. Virucidal agent recommended for systemic involvement.
   2. Fungal infection — topical application of clotrimazole or miconazole effectively clears fungi and yeast, but does not change ultimate outcome. Amphotericin B for systemic involvement. Severe fungal infection may require aggressive debridement or amputation.

VIII. ELECTRICAL INJURIES

A. Tissue destruction is most severe at the points of entry and exit (the points at which the electrical current is most concentrated). Deep tissue damage often greatly exceeds skin injury — usually not obvious at the time of initial injury. Resistance of tissues (increasing order) — nerve, blood and blood vessel, muscle, skin, tendon, fat, bone.
B. **Treatment.**
   1. CPR — high–voltage currents usually cause cardiac standstill, whereas low voltage (< 440 volts) usually produces ventricular fibrillation.
   2. Protection against neurologic damage caused by fractures of the spine — place in C–spine collar and on long–back board in order to immobilize entire spine.
   3. Fluid resuscitation — cannot be calculated from % of skin burns. Give sufficient volume to restore BP and pulse to normal, establish urine output of 1.5 cc/kg/hr.
      a. High incidence of muscular and blood injury causes hemoglobinuria/myoglobinuria. Hence, larger fluid requirements followed by mannitol (25 g/hr) and $NaHCO_3$ is necessary to prevent precipitation of myoglobin/hemoglobin in the renal tubules. Mannitol is continued until the urine clears.

    b. Progressively severe metabolic acidosis occurs with electrical injuries and massive tissue destruction. Use IV sodium bicarbonate to correct base deficit.

  4. Early debridement of grossly necrotic tissue.

  5. Requirement for extremity fasciotomy, check compartment pressures.

  6. Tetanic contraction of muscle may cause fractures of cervical and lumbosacral spine and long bones; therefore, perform screening x-rays.

C. Complications — dependent upon location of contact points and path of current through the body.

  1. Compartment syndromes and myonecrosis requiring fasciotomy, extensive debridement, and amputation.

  2. High incidence of hemoglobinuria/myoglobinuria.

  3. Spine and long–bone fractures may result from tetanic contraction.

  4. Delayed cataract formation — 4–12 months post–injury (late).

  5. Progressive peripheral neuropathy (late).

  6. Delayed spinal cord injury with progressive transverse myelitis (late).

IX. SUPPORTIVE CARE IN BURN INJURY

A. Nutrition — start early. Metabolic rate is proportional to burn size up to 40–50% TBSA burn. Total body O_2 consumption and water loss proportional to burn size.

  1. Nutrient needs.

    a. Calories.

      1) Adult — 25 kcal/kg BW + 40 kcal/% burn.

      2) Child — 35 kcal/kg BW + 60 kcal/% burn.

    b. Protein — 1.6–3.2 g N_2/kg BW.

    c. Keep calorie/nitrogen ratio 100:1 – 150:1 (*vs.* normal 150:1).

  2. Route.

    a. Enteral (nasoduodenal) preferred, start during 1st 12 hours post–injury — decreased infection, decreased cost, decreased complication.

    b. If intravenous, *must* change IV site every 48–72 hours. Catheter is used for all infusions including TPN.

B. Physical and occupational therapy (PT/OT) — aggressive PT/OT is necessary to prevent contractures, and maintain function.

  1. Positioning of limbs and joints begins **Day 1.**

  2. Splinting required to prevent contractures.

  3. Active exercise program with stretching greatly superior to passive range of motion.

  4. Involve OT early for long–term rehabilitation planning.

C. Burn treatment requires team approach — MD's, nursing care is *paramount*, PT/OT, dietary, psychiatry, social work, ministry.

X. COMPLICATIONS OF BURN INJURY

A. Gastrointestinal.

1. **Adynamic ileus** — especially large burns. Gastric and colonic involvement. Generally resolves within 24 hrs with IV hydration and NG suction. May be early sign of sepsis.

2. Ulcers — **Curling's ulcers:** Anywhere in the GI tract, mostly stomach, duodenum, jejunum: multiple sites. Etiology unknown, not necessarily related to burn size. Incidence decreased with early antacids and H_2 blockers. Approximately 12% of burn patients develop upper GI tract hemorrhage from stress ulceration. Perforation occurs in approximately 10% of patients with Curling's ulcers. Initial non–operative management and indications for surgical intervention are essentially the same as those for hemorrhage from peptic ulcer disease (see "GI Bleeding").

3. **Acalculous cholecystitis** — diagnose with HIDA scan or ultrasound. Treat accordingly.

B. Ocular.

1. **Corneal scarring** — associated with facial burns. Treatment includes topical antibiotics, and release and grafting of ectropion.

2. **Cataracts** (especially with electrical injury).

C. Cutaneous.

1. **Wound contracture.**

2. **Keloid.**

3. **Hypertrophic scar.**

   a. Increased incidence with deep burns and extended exposure of ungrafted burn wound. Commonly occurs over joints, eyelids, neck, lips, axilla, and palms, with maximal scarring at 3–6 months after injury.

   b. Treatment — Z–plasty to reclose scar; cosmetic treatment (often disappointing); fitted pressure masks, garments, etc., used for 1st year to reduce scar formation.

D. Miscellaneous.

1. **Heterotopic calcification.**

2. **Chondritis** — secondary to *Staph.* ear and joint infections.

3. Hyperpigmentation — avoid sun exposure for at least 1 year. Use sun–blocking agents.

ACUTE ABDOMEN

I. **PRINCIPLES OF DIAGNOSIS**

A. **Philosophy** — The importance of making an *early* accurate diagnosis cannot be overemphasized. The recovery rate from acute abdominal disease decreases proportionately with delay in diagnosis and treatment. In practice, analgesics and antibiotics should be withheld at least until a presumptive diagnosis has been made.

B. **Anatomy and physiology of abdominal pain** — results from the stimulation of somatic and visceral afferent fibers. Somatic innervation follows a segmental pattern, while visceral is primarily autonomic with a more diffuse distribution.

1. Abdominal pain secondary to peritoneal irritation is perceived through segmental somatic fibers. Pain may be felt in other areas innervated by nerves from the same segment; known as "referred pain," i.e., diaphragmatic irritation is referred to the distribution of the C4 and may be felt at the tip of the scapula. Reflex involuntary muscle wall rigidity may result from irritation of segmental sensory nerves. In addition, increased sensation (hyperaesthesia) of the skin may result from ipsilateral peritoneal irritation.

2. Visceral pain is more diffuse and ill–defined than somatic pain. Pain from stimulation of visceral afferents (e.g., bowel) results from contraction or spasm, stretching or distention against resistance, and chemical irritation.

   a. Visceral pain may be referred to a body region, e.g., small intestine to epigastric or periumbilical region, large intestine to hypogastrium, biliary tree to right upper quadrant, kidney to the ipsilateral groin.

   b. Visceral pain is also frequently associated with autonomic responses producing diaphonesis, nausea, vomiting and reflex hypotension. Severe somatic pain may produce autonomic responses as well.

   c. Visceral organs may be burned, crushed, or cut without eliciting pain.

3. Generalized pain — sudden flooding of peritoneal cavity by blood, pus or acrid fluid.

4. Epigastric and umbilical pain — small intestinal origin, appendicitis.

5. Precipitating factors — exertion, laxatives.

6. Acuteness of pain — sudden acute onset often associated with fainting or collapse; seen with an ulcer perforation, viscus perforation, ruptured ectopic pregnancy, ruptured aortic aneurysm.

7. Location of pain.

8. Character of pain — sharp, dull, heavy, burning, squeezing, achy.

9. Intensity of pain — nagging, mild, severe, "worst ever".
10. Radiation of pain — back, flank, shoulder, hip, groin.
    a. Biliary colic — to right scapula.
    b. Renal colic — to ipsilateral testicle.
11. Time course of pain — constant, intermittent, increasing, decreasing, and how long for each.
12. Relation to exacerbating and ameliorating factors — food, position, medications, vomiting, defecation, cough, activity.
13. Associated complaints — respiratory, GI, genitourinary.
14. Special varieties of pain.
    a. Pain during micturition — urinary source, pelvic abscess, appendicitis (inflammation near right ureter).
    b. Testicular pain — renal colic, appendicitis, ruptured abdominal aortic aneurysm.
    c. Worsening with reclining, relieved when upright — retroperitoneal origin (pancreatitis).

C. **Nausea and vomiting.**
    1. Causes.
        a. Severe irritation of the nerves of the peritoneum or mesentery — ulcer perforation, gangrenous appendicitis, ovarian cyst torsion, pancreatitis (celiac plexus involvement), intestinal strangulation.
        b. Obstruction of an involuntary muscular tube — biliary duct, ureter, uterine canal, intestine, appendix. Secondary to peristaltic contraction and muscle stretching; hence colic comes in spasms with vomiting at its peak.
        c. Action of absorbed toxins on medullary centers — may contribute to vomiting in intestinal obstruction or pancreatitis.
    2. Relationship of pain to vomiting — in acute appendicitis, nausea and vomiting rarely occurs before the onset of pain.
    3. Frequency of vomiting — in intestinal obstruction, frequency of vomiting is related to the site of obstruction. The more proximal the obstruction, the more frequent the vomiting.
    4. Character of vomitus.
        a. Bilious — nonspecific.
        b. Food — upper obstruction.
        c. Retching — torsion of viscus.
        d. Feculent — pathognomonic of intestinal obstruction (unusual in colonic obstruction).

D. **Anorexia.**
    1. May have same etiology as nausea and vomiting.
    2. Common complaint.
    3. Acute appetite loss — frequently significant, important complaint in acute appendicitis.

E. **Bowel function** — diarrhea, constipation, obstipation.
    1. Recent changes in pattern.

    2. Several small loose stools — appendicitis in children.

    3. Hypogastric pain/diarrhea, then tenderness/constipation — suspect pelvic abscess.

    4. Blood/mucus — intussusception in children; colitis, proctitis in adults.

F. Menstruation.

    1. Regularity.

    2. Timing in relation to pain — ruptured follicular or corpus luteum cyst, ruptured ectopic pregnancy, pelvic infection.

G. Thorough review of systems.

H. Past history — ask "Have you ever had a pain like this before?"

    1. Prior operations, GI complaints, endocrine disorders, urologic symptoms, hematologic disorders, gynecologic symptoms, cardiovascular complaints.

    2. Drugs — digoxin, theophylline, steroids, analgesics, antipyretics, antiemetics, barbiturates (porphyria), drugs for Parkinson's disease, diuretics (cause decreased K^+ → ileus).

II. METHOD OF DIAGNOSIS: PHYSICAL EXAMINATION

A. General appearance.

B. Attitude in bed — restless (colic) vs. stillness (peritonitis).

C. Pulse.

    1. Tachycardia is common and may be due to fever, hemorrhage, dehydration, pain, anxiety.

    2. Bradycardia can be seen with advanced sepsis or metabolic disturbances (i.e., hypothyroidism).

D. Respiratory rate.

    1. Tachypnea is common.

    2. Respiratory alkalosis can be present as early finding in sepsis.

E. Temperature.

    1. A subnormal, normal, or elevated temperature can accompany an acute abdomen.

    2. 95–96°F (core) — severe shock or toxemia.

    3. Normal temperature — common in non–inflammatory process. Does *not* rule out inflammatory processes.

    4. 99–100°F (oral) — early inflammatory process, usual finding with acute appendicitis.

    5. 104–105°F — suspect intra–abdominal collection, kidney as source.

F. Blood pressure.

G. Cardiopulmonary exam.

    1. Cardiac murmur, rub or gallops may be significant in cardiac disease presenting as abdominal pain (MI, CHF, etc.).

    2. Pulmonary consolidation, effusion, pleural rub may be significant in pulmonary disease presenting as abdominal pain (pneumonia, pleuritis, infarct, etc.).

H. Abdominal examination.
  1. Observation, inspection.
    a. Scaphoid, flat, obese, distended.
    b. Movement with respiration — note limitation of movement indicating rigidity of the abdominal muscles or diaphragm.
    c. Have patient indicate the exact point of maximal pain.
    d. Inspect all potential sites for hernias, especially the inguinal and femoral region.
  2. Auscultation — bowel sounds: absent, present, rushes, high-pitched, abdominal bruits.
    a. **Rule** (many exceptions): quiet abdomen — peritonitis; borborygmi — intestinal obstruction.
    b. The absence of a bruit never excludes the presence of an aortic aneurysm.
  3. Palpation/percussion — gentleness is essential.
    a. Evaluate presence and extent of muscular rigidity.
    b. Palpate four quadrants of abdomen, costovertebral angles (CVA) to assess tenderness (mild, moderate, severe), abdominal masses, abnormal pulsations, hernial orifices. Begin *away* from point of maximal pain. Have patient's legs flexed and relaxed.
    c. Signs of peritoneal irritation.
      1) Percussion ("**rebound**") tenderness.
      2) Pain with coughing or valsalva.
      3) Rigidity — "**involuntary guarding.**"
        a) Pain worsens when rigidity is overcome in abdominal disease.
        b) Muscular rigidity/resistance may be slight, even in the presence of serious peritonitis — fat, flabby abdominal wall; severe toxemia; elderly patients.
      4) "**Obturator sign**" — pain with flexion and internal rotation of the hip. Positive with inflammation of obturator internus muscle (e.g., appendicitis).
      5) "**Psoas Sign**" — iliopsoas rigidity.
        a) Pain on passive extension of hip (stretching the psoas muscle), may perform with the patient in decubitus position and moving thigh.
        b) Positive with irritation of psoas/iliopsoas muscle.
      6) **Cutaneous hyperaesthesia** — may be tested by pin–stroke or light touch. Nearly always indicates parietal peritoneal inflammation. Most commonly caused by appendicitis; occurs in lower abdominal wall.
      7) Unimanual and bimanual palpation of the flank to detect renal disease (perinephric abscess, inflamed kidney) or retrocecal appendix (both affect quadratus lumborum muscle).
      8) Liver dullness.

       a) Normal dullness is detected from the 5th rib to the costal margin along the right vertical nipple line and from the 7th to 11th rib in the midaxillary line.

       b) Loss of liver dullness (with new resonance) occurs with free air in the peritoneum (must be in the absence of abdominal distention).

   9) Free fluid.

       a) Most commonly presents with ascites from liver disease.

       b) Of some value in intestinal obstruction, to detect fluid–filled bowel.

I. Examination of the pelvic cavity.

  1. Suprapelvic palpation and percussion.

  2. Rectal examination — extremely important and informative.

    a. Look for localized tenderness, fluctuance, induration, mass, occult or gross blood.

    b. Include bimanual, recto–abdominal, vaginoabdominal exams.

    c. Include digital examination of stomas (colostomy, ileostomy).

  3. **Pelvic examination (bimanual)** — assess for bleeding, discharge, cervical motion tenderness, adnexal tenderness or mass. Look for signs of pregnancy — cyanosis of cervix, uterine size.

  4. Check for bladder distention — percuss bladder size, catheterize if necessary to confirm bladder empty in older patients.

III. METHOD OF DIAGNOSIS: LABORATORY EXAMINATION

A. WBC — degree of leukocytosis and **differential**. <u>Note</u>: The absence of leukocytosis *never* excludes an inflammatory abdominal diagnosis.

B. Hematocrit.

C. Platelet count — thrombocytopenia consistent with severe sepsis.

D. Electrolytes — hypokalemia is common with prolonged vomiting or diarrhea; glucose is elevated (plus ketones) in diabetic ketoacidosis (DKA).

E. Arterial blood gas (ABG) — metabolic acidosis or alkalosis.

F. Urinalysis.

G. Serum BHCG — mandatory in all women of child-bearing age to 40; ruptured ectopic pregnancy.

H. Liver function tests.

I. Amylase.

J. Upright CXR — pneumonia, free air.

K. Abdominal flat and upright (or left lateral decubitus) x-ray — bowel obstruction, ileus, free air, abnormal calcifications.

L. EKG — acute MI, ischemia, arrhythmias.

M. Paracentesis of the abdominal cavity (peritoneal lavage) — may be helpful if a diagnosis remains in doubt; critical with abdominal injury in unconscious patient (see "Diagnostic Peritoneal Lavage").

N. Culdocentesis in suspected ruptured ectopic pregnancy.

IV. **METHOD OF DIAGNOSIS: GROUPING OF SYMPTOMS AND SIGNS**
A. Abdominal pain by itself.
   1. Appendicitis — initial pain is epigastric or umbilical.
   2. Transverse colon obstruction — lower abdominal pain (hypogastrium).
   3. Renal colic — one-sided abdominal, back, flank, or CVA pain radiating to ipsilateral groin/scrotum.
   4. Biliary colic —epigastric and right hypochondrium pain radiating to subscapular region.
B. Abdominal pain followed by nausea and vomiting — appendicitis, intestinal obstruction, gastroenteritis, pancreatitis.
C. Mid–abdominal pain.
   1. Intestinal colic.
   2. Acute appendicitis.
   3. Mesenteric thrombosis.
   4. Extra–abdominal causes.
      a. Tabes dorsalis.
      b. Herpes zoster.
      c. Coronary thrombosis.
      d. DKA.
      e. Uremic crises.
      f. Acute glaucoma.
   5. Follow–up examination is key to diagnosis.
D. Right upper quadrant pain, radiation to back and/or scapula; intermittent, often after fatty meals, accompanied by nausea or vomiting — biliary colic and/or chronic cholecystitis; persistence of symptoms suggests acute cholecystitis if fever and leukocytosis present.
E. Severe mid–abdominal pain with severe shock.
   1. Acute pancreatitis.
   2. Ruptured aortic aneurysm.
   3. Dissecting aneurysm.
   4. Mesenteric thrombosis.
   5. Coronary thrombosis.
   6. Internal hemorrhage (aneurysm, splenic rupture, ectopic gestation).
F. Severe subjective symptoms with minimal findings — suspect vascular accident (see "Mesenteric Ischemia").
G. Pain with vomiting and increasing distention, but no rigidity — intestinal obstruction.
H. Abdominal pain with constipation, increasing distention, with or without vomiting.
   1. Large bowel obstruction (usually sigmoid) — vomiting would imply ileocecal valve incompetence.
      a. Volvulus — rapid onset, often in the elderly patient.

  b. Rule out uremia (can cause abdominal distention and vomiting) due to renal failure (prostatic obstruction, polycystic kidneys, calculous pyonephrosis).

 2. Congenital small bowel obstruction in newborns.

 3. Intussusception.

  a. Infants, age 6–18 months, usually male.

  b. Pain, screaming attack, sausage–shaped abdominal mass, bloody (currant jelly) stool.

I. Severe abdominal pain with generalized rigidity of the abdominal wall.

 1. Perforated viscus.

  a. Patient may be able to relate *exact* time of onset of pain of perforation.

  b. Initial collapse, then improvement for several hours, then peritonitis.

 2. Bilateral pleuropneumonia.

 3. Localized tenderness suggests anatomic etiology.

  a. Right hypochondriac pain and rigidity.

   1) Acute cholecystitis.

   2) Leaking duodenal ulcer.

   3) Appendicitis with high appendix.

   4) Amebic hepatitis, hydatid liver disease.

  b. Left hypochondriac pain and rigidity.

   1) Acute pancreatitis.

   2) Perforated gastric ulcer localized by adhesions.

   3) Ruptured jejunal diverticulum.

   4) Leakage of splenic artery aneurysm.

   5) Spontaneous splenic rupture (leukemia).

   6) Acute pyelonephritis, perinephric abscess.

  c. Right iliac pain, tenderness and rigidity.

   1) Acute appendicitis.

   2) Pancreatic disease.

   3) Cholecystitis (low gallbladder), biliary peritonitis.

   4) Leaking duodenal ulcer.

   5) Diverticulitis — redundant sigmoid to right of midline.

   6) Pyelonephritis.

   7) Regional ileitis.

   8) Meckel's diverticulitis.

   9) Retained testis.

   10) Fallopian tube/ovarian disease.

  d. Left iliac pain, tenderness, with/without rigidity.

   1) Diverticulitis (sigmoid) — with/without mass, slight fever, no vomiting.

   2) Colon carcinoma.

   3) Acute pyelonephritis (low–lying left kidney).

   e. Hypogastric pain and rigidity.
      1) Perforated appendix in young or middle–aged person.
      2) Perforated diverticulum in older person.
      3) Uterine, fallopian or ovarian disease.

V. CONDITIONS PRESENTING WITH ACUTE SYMPTOMS
A. Inflammatory.
  1. Perforated viscus.
    a. Stomach, duodenum — ulcer.
    b. Bowel — diverticulum, appendix, carcinoma, traumatic small bowel injury.
    c. Gallbladder.
  2. Ruptured ovarian cyst (menstrual history).
  3. Primary peritonitis (peritonitis without obvious etiology).
    a. Gram–positive organisms (*Pneumococcus*, *Streptococcus*) formerly most common; gram–negatives are increasing, especially in females.
    b. Tuberculosis — "doughy" abdomen.
    c. Cirrhotics — signs minimal.
  4. Gastroenteritis, colitis — viral or bacterial.
  5. Inflammatory bowel disease.
  6. Diverticulitis.
  7. Meckel's diverticulitis.
  8. Pancreatitis — alcoholic, biliary, viral, thiazide–induced, steroid–related, hyperlipidemia, hypercalcemia.
  9. Hepatitis.
    a. Viral — mimics cholecystitis.
    b. Alcoholic.
  10. Hepatic abscess — look for other primary septic focus.
  11. Splenic abscess.
  12. Mesenteric lymphadenitis.
  13. Foreign body perforation of bowel.
  14. Pelvic inflammatory disease.
    a. Unilateral or bilateral lower quadrant (above groin crease) pain and tenderness on abdominal and pelvic exam.
    b. Cervical motion tenderness.
    c. *Neisseria gonorrhoea*, *Chlamydia*, and *Hemophilus* most common pathogens.
    d. Difficult to distinguish right–sided salpingitis from appendicitis.
    e. Tubo–ovarian abscess — palpable mass on pelvic and/or rectal exam, fever, leukocytosis.
  15. Endometritis.
    a. Menstrual irregularity, postmenstrual staining.
    b. Inflammation of stroma of endometrium.

        c. Treat with antibiotics and curettage.

        d. History of IUD.

    16. Toxic shock syndrome.

B. Mechanical.

    1. Intestinal obstruction.

        a. Small bowel — adhesions, hernia, neoplasm, volvulus, intus- suception, gallstone ileus, Meckel's band.

        b. Gastric outlet obstruction — peptic ulcer disease (pyloric channel), gastric carcinoma.

        c. Colon — neoplasm, hernia, diverticulitis, volvulus.

    2. Biliary obstruction.

        a. Cholelithiasis with impacted or "ball–valve" cystic duct stone.

        b. Choledocholithiasis.

        c. Cholangitis.

            1) Neoplasm.

            2) Choledochal cyst.

            3) Stone.

        d. Hematobilia.

            1) Free communication between blood vessel and biliary tree.

            2) Triad of abdominal injury, subsequent GI hemorrhage, colicky pain — may have jaundice.

            3) Days or weeks after injury; multiple episodes.

            4) Confirm and possibly treat with angiography.

    3. Solid viscera (rare).

        a. Acute splenomegaly — various hematologic disorders.

        b. Acute hepatomegaly — pericarditis, CHF, Budd–Chiari.

    4. Omental torsion — rare.

    5. Torsion of ovarian cyst.

    6. Torsion of uterine fibroid — rare.

    7. Ectopic pregnancy.

        a. Symptoms of early pregnancy — delayed menses, nausea, vomiting, breast tenderness.

        b. Increased uterine size, but less than anticipated by dates.

        c. Pain and cramping.

        d. Adnexal mass, cervical motion tenderness.

        e. BHCG may not be positive.

        f. Rupture or extrusion from tube shows signs of localized peritonitis due to presence of blood.

        g. Hypovolemic shock due to hemorrhage in 10%.

C. Vascular.

    1. Intraperitoneal bleeding.

        a. Traumatic rupture of liver, spleen, mesentery.

        b. Delayed splenic rupture.

        c. Ruptured ectopic pregnancy.

    d. Ruptured abdominal aortic aneurysm — sudden onset of new back pain in an individual with atherosclerotic risk factors.

    e. Ruptured splenic or hepatic aneurysm — rare.

    f. Bleeding hepatic adenoma — associated with estrogen ingestion.

  2. Ischemia.

    a. Mesenteric thrombosis or embolus.

      1) Usually see other signs of peripheral atherosclerosis.

      2) Atrial fibrillation, cardiac valvular disease, history of MI predispose to embolization.

      3) Severe pain, benign abdominal exam and leukocytosis should arouse suspicion.

      4) Metabolic acidosis is a late finding and usually indicates gangrene.

      5) Short segment involvement may result in self–limiting episodes and late stricture.

  3. Splenic infarction — common in sickle cell.

D. Other gynecologic conditions.

  1. Endometriosis.

    a. Endometrial implants outside the uterus.

    b. Undergo cyclic change (pain) with menses.

    c. Implants on the bowel can cause cyclic lower GI bleeding.

  2. Fitz–Hugh–Curtis syndrome (gonococcal perihepatitis).

    a. History of gonococcal pelvic inflammatory disease.

    b. Pain and tenderness over the liver.

VI. COMMON CONDITIONS MIMICKING THE ACUTE ABDOMEN

A. Pneumonia — may be localized RUQ or LUQ if lower lobes involved.

B. Angina or myocardial infarction — epigastric pain, "heart burn".

C. Obstructive uropathy (urethral and prostatic).

D. Acute hepatitis.

E. Cardiac involvement by scarlet fever.

F. Sickle cell crisis — diffuse pain.

G. Leukemia — diffuse pain.

H. Radiculopathy from spinal cord tumors, compression fracture of spine, fracture of hip.

I. Cystitis — suprapubic pain and tenderness.

J. Prostatitis — rectal and buttock pain.

K. Pyelonephritis — CVA tenderness.

L. Ureteral obstruction.

  1. Calculus or neoplasm.

  2. Pain, nausea, vomiting out of proportion to exam.

M. Toxins — lead poisoning, venoms, tetanus, petroleum distillates, aspirin in children.

N. Abdominal wall hematoma — swimmers, gymnasts, or following severe effort.
O. Psychogenic — may have ingested foreign body causing psychogenic pain without trauma to the GI tract, or may have true perforation, hemorrhage, or obstruction.
P. Pericarditis.
Q. Herpes zoster (shingles).
R. Diabetic ketoacidosis.
S. Systemic lupus erythematosus (SLE).
T. Uremia.
U. Lead poisoning.
V. Torsion of the testes.
W. Acute intermittent porphyria — Watson–Schwartz urine test, urine for porphobilinogen.

VII. INITIAL TREATMENT GUIDELINES

A. Plan on prompt, timely work–up in first 4–6 hrs.
B. Decide on: (1) operation, (2) no operation, (3) admit & observe.
C. Diet — NPO until diagnosis is firm and treatment plan formulated.
D. IV fluids; base on expected fluid losses; may require large volumes with hemodynamic monitoring.
E. Nasogastric intubation for vomiting, bleeding, signs of obstruction.
F. Foley catheter to monitor fluid resuscitation.
G. Serial examinations every 2–4 hrs during the first 12–24 hrs in cases without definite diagnosis; minimal narcotics and sedatives are mandatory to avoid masking physical signs and symptoms; monitor vital signs frequently.
H. Serial lab exams may be useful; repeat CBC every 4–6 hrs.
I. Maintenance of critical medications in IM, IV or suppository form, e.g., antihypertensives, theophylline, steroids, insulin.

VIII. USEFUL DIAGNOSTIC STUDIES

A. **Ultrasound.**
   1. Right upper quadrant and upper abdomen if symptoms suggest gallstones, common duct obstruction, pancreatitis.
   2. Kidney — perinephric abscess, hydronephrosis.
   3. Lower abdomen, pelvis — symptoms of appendicitis, diverticulitis, pelvic inflammation (TOA, torsion of ovarian cyst, etc.).
B. Upper GI with water–soluble contrast for suspected upper GI perforation. **Note:** Diagnosis can usually be made clinically; upper GI only for equivocal cases.
C. If colon obstruction suspected, careful diagnostic enema — no barium if any chance of colon perforation.
D. Emergency excretory urogram (IVP) without compression if urinary pathology suspected.
E. Peritoneal lavage if intraperitoneal trauma or bleeding suspected.

GI BLEEDING

I. INITIAL MANAGEMENT

A. Assess magnitude of hemorrhage.
1. Class I — < 15% loss of blood volume. Normal exam.
2. Class II — 20–25% loss of blood volume: P > 100, R > 25, decreased pulse pressure, patient thirsty and anxious.
3. Class III — 30–35% loss of blood volume: P > 120, R > 30, decreased systolic and pulse pressure, decreased urine output, confusion.
4. Class IV — 40–50% blood volume loss: P > 140, SBP < 50, R > 35, virtually no urine output, severe confusion, lethargy or coma.

B. Stabilize hemodynamic status.
1. Two large–bore IVs (14–16 gauge if possible).
2. Crystalloid resuscitation.
3. Place foley catheter.
4. Type and crossmatch for 6 units PRBC.
5. Blood replacement (packed cells) when it becomes available. O–negative or type-specific blood in extreme situations.
6. Endotracheal intubation if marked hypotension is present.

C. Monitor for continued blood loss (admit to ICU).
1. Frequent vital signs.
2. Frequent labs.
   a. Assess the adequacy of transfusion and correction of coagulopathy.
   b. Maintain HCT > 30.
3. Monitor urine output.
4. CVP/Swan–Ganz if unstable or poor–risk patient.

D. Place NG tube — this will help determine an UGI *vs.* LGI source of bleeding. If bright–red blood returns from the NG tube, saline lavage should be used to remove clots from the stomach. Use a large bore (Ewald) tube if gastric lavage is required. If the patient remains unstable, or gastric contents do not lavage to light pink in a short time, there may be rapid bleeding requiring urgent intervention (see VI: Treatment).

II. HISTORY

A. Presentation of bleeding.
1. **Hematemesis** (bright red or coffee–grounds material) — upper GI source proximal to the ligament of Treitz.
2. **Hematochezia** (bloody stool or blood covering stool) — usually lower GI bleeding (i.e., distal to the ligament of Treitz), but can occur with brisk upper GI source.

    3. Melena (black tarry stools) — frequently upper GI source.
    4. No obvious bleeding but occult blood in stool — either upper or lower source.
B. Try to estimate the volume and duration of bleeding.
C. **Associated abdominal pain** (localized or diffuse).
    1. Acute, chronic ulcer or reflux symptomatology.
    2. Crampy abdominal pain may be associated with diverticulitis, inflammatory bowel disease, or infections.
    3. Painless bleeding is the most common presentation and may be associated with varices, ulcer disease, angiodysplasia, or diverticulosis.
    4. Pain out of proportion to abdominal tenderness associated with hematochezia or guaiac positive stools — consider ischemic bowel.
    5. Severe acute, sudden onset of pain — consider perforated viscus. (Perforated duodenal ulcers rarely present with concomitant bleeding.)
    6. RUQ pain with bleeding — consider ulcers, hemobilia (rare).
D. **Precipitating factors.**
    1. Ulcerogenic drugs or agents such as aspirin or salicylates, non-steroidal anti–inflammatory agents, steroids, alcohol, cigarettes.
    2. Severe stress such as burn or major trauma.
    3. GI instrumentation such as nasogastric intubation, esophago-gastroduodenoscopy or colonoscopy.
    4. Severe vomiting or retching (Mallory–Weiss tear of the G–E junction).
    5. Significant blunt or penetrating trauma.
E. **Systemic complaints.**
    1. Fever and chills may be associated with an inflammatory or infectious etiology.
    2. A history of unintentional weight loss may signal the presence of a neoplasm.
    3. The history of a change in bowel habits or character of stool may help pinpoint the source of bleeding. Painful bowel movement suggests anal fissure.
F. **Significant past history.**
    1. Prior GI bleed.
    2. Prior surgery, either GI, vascular or ENT (rule out unrecognized posterior nose bleed).
    3. Previous GI complaints, including previous work–ups.
    4. Significant medical history, including cardiac, vascular, pulmonary, DM, blood dyscrasias, cirrhosis, anticoagulant therapy.
G. **Social history.**
    1. Drug and alcohol use.
    2. Psychiatric history — consider ingestion of caustic agent or possibly malingering.

III. PHYSICAL EXAM

A. **General appearance** — may be pale, diaphoretic, or anxious, with moderate to severe hemorrhage.

B. **Vital signs.**

1. BP — hypotensive or orthostasis (postural drop in systolic BP of > 20 mm Hg).
2. Pulse — tachycardia or orthostasis (postural increase of > 10 bpm).
3. Respirations — may be shallow and rapid with significant volume loss.
4. Temperature — normal or elevated with an infectious process.

C. **Skin** — jaundice, spider angiomata, and palmar erythema may be signs of cirrhosis and portal hypertension with variceal bleeding. Petechiae or purpura may be signs of a contributing coagulopathy or thrombocytopenia.

D. **HEENT** — look for pale/dry mucous membranes, ENT lesions or bleeding; oral or pharyngeal burns; and adenopathy.

E. **Abdomen** — look for distention, dilated veins, ascites, hyper- or hypoactive bowel sounds, mass, hepatosplenomegaly, tenderness, rebound or rigidity.

F. **Rectal** — melena, hematochezia, occult blood, mass, hemorrhoids, fistula, or tenderness.

G. **Other signs of cirrhosis and possible portal hypertension** — gynecomastia, atrophic testicles, mental status change of encephalopathy, Dupuytren's contracture.

IV. LABORATORY EVALUATION

A. **CBC** — the Hct and Hgb do not accurately reflect magnitude of acute blood loss. They usually underestimate loss because hemodilution takes time. Hypochromia and microcytosis suggest a source of chronic blood loss.

B. **Platelet count** — thrombocytopenia is the usual defect present in coagulopathies secondary to massive hemorrhage.

C. **PT/PTT** — screen for coagulation defects. Fibrinogen and fibrin split products to identify a consumptive coagulopathy after massive transfusion.

D. **Renal profile** — may identify renal failure, electrolyte disturbance secondary to volume loss or emesis. Increased BUN can be due to the increased protein absorbed from blood in the GI tract as well as hydration. BUN > 100 is associated with poor platelet function.

E. **Liver function studies** — screen for hepatic dysfunction.

F. **Serum calcium** — may fall with bleeding. Citrate toxicity and excessive binding of ionized calcium have been blamed as possible etiologies. If multiple transfusions are given rapidly (over less than 4 hours), 1 g of calcium chloride (37% Ca by weight) or 4 g of

Ca gluconate (9% Ca by weight) should be administered for every 3–5 units of whole blood or 5–8 units of packed cells transfused.
G. **Chest x-ray and abdominal films** — check for free air, pulmonary infiltrate, and splenic or hepatic enlargement.

V. DIAGNOSTIC PROCEDURES — UPPER GI
A. **NG tube.**
   1. Check for bright–red blood *vs.* coffee grounds.
      a. False–negative (1%) if duodenal source with pylorospasm. Aspirated material will usually be non–bilious.
      b. False–positive (7%) if trauma secondary to NG tube placement. Blood loss from NG trauma should be minimal.
B. **EGD** (esophophagogastroduodenoscopy).
   1. Requires thorough gastric lavage with large (Ewald) tube prior to exam.
   2. 95% diagnostic accuracy if used in the first 24 hours.
   3. May be used therapeutically for cauterization or sclerotherapy.
C. **Angiography.**
   1. Diagnostic — requires brisk bleeding to identify the source ($\geq$ 0.5–1 cc/min).
   2. Therapeutic — may be used for selective embolization. Selective arterial vasopressin may also decrease blood loss (gastritis, Mallory–Weiss tear).
   3. Contraindicated if the patient is hemodynamically unstable. It is technically not possible if a recent enteric contrast study has been performed.
D. **Labeled red cell scan** — less invasive, fewer complications than angiography. Also more sensitive, detects bleeding if $\geq$ 0.2 cc/min; however, far less specific than angiography. Useful for slower cryptic bleeding problems. May be performed with a portable camera in the ICU.
E. **Upper GI** — rarely useful in acute setting. Has a poor yield and interferes with ability to perform EGD or angiography.

VI. TREATMENT — UPPER GI BLEEDING
A. **Peptic ulcer disease.**
   1. Surgery if there is exsanguinating hemorrhage, > 5 unit transfusion/24 hrs, or rebleed during the same hospitalization while on optimum medical management.
   2. Older patients and those with multiple medical problems should have *early* surgical intervention prior to the onset of hemodynamic instability, development of a coagulopathy, etc.
   3. If bleeding appears to be slowing or stopping:
      a. H2 blockers, antacids, NG suction, gastric pH monitoring (keep pH > 5).

    b. Iced saline lavage — helps remove clots from stomach and aids in evaluating continuation of bleeding, but is of little value in actually stopping the bleeding.

    c. EGD laser or electrocautery, or injection sclerotherapy, especially in high–risk patients.

    d. Vasopressin may be of benefit, especially in high–risk patients, but is contraindicated in patients with significant atherosclerotic coronary artery disease or recent MI.

B. Stress ulceration.

  1. Etiology not clear — it is thought that gastric mucosal ischemia is the initial insult with bile reflux and intraluminal acid acting on the injured mucosa.

  2. Superficial mucosal erosions — occur predominantly in the proximal acid– and pepsin–producing portion of the stomach.

  3. Prophylaxis is necessary in high–risk situations (trauma, burn, sepsis, etc.).

    a. Gastric pH monitoring — maintain pH > 5.0

    b. H2 receptor antagonists — administered alone at a fixed rate, is not as effective as antacids in controlling intragastric pH (and does little to control established bleeding).

    c. Antacids — 15–30 cc PO or per rectum q 2–4 h, titrate by gastric pH.

  4. Non-operative treatment of bleeding stress ulcerations.

    a. Treat underlying cause of illness (e.g., sepsis).

    b. Saline lavage.

    c. Antacids to maintain gastric pH > 5.0.

    d. Selective intra–arterial vasopressin infusion.

      1) Begin at 0.2 U/min.

      2) If evidence of constriction of distal arterial bed, or cessation of bleeding, vasopressin is continued for an additional 24 hrs at this rate, then tapered over the next 12 hrs.

      3) If bleeding continues, the rate may be increased at increments of 0.1 U/min up to a maximum of 0.5 U/min.

      4) Effective therapy in ≥ 50% of patients.

      5) Contraindicated if recent MI or significant CAD.

    e. Operative treatment — overall success of non–operative treatment is 75%. If bleeding is not controlled by vigorous non–operative measures, surgical intervention may be required. Choice of operation is controversial.

      1) Truncal vagotomy and pyloroplasty with oversewing discrete bleeding point(s) — rebleeding can occur in 30% – 100%.

      2) Gastric resections and total gastrectomy have lower incidences of rebleeding, but are more radical procedures in desperately ill patients.

C. **Esophageal varices** (in order of priority) (also see "Cirrhosis").
   1. Peripheral administration of vasopressin (IV) decreases portal pressure (begin at 0.4 U/min – 0.9 U/min maximum). Contraindicated in significant CAD.
   2. Addition of nitroglycerin by continuous infusion may improve efficacy of vasopressin while decreasing some of the end–organ ischemia.
   3. Sengstaken–Blakemore tube (initially gastric balloon only; esophageal balloon if needed; maintain for 24 hrs if effective).
   4. Endoscopic sclerotherapy.
   5. Portosystemic shunt or other surgical intervention for better-risk patients.
D. **Aortoenteric fistula.**
   1. Suspect this cause in all patients with history of abdominal vascular procedures.
   2. Aggressive work–up with EGD to 4th portion duodenum, angiography if active bleeding, and/or abdominal CT scan.
   3. Immediate surgery if unstable or work–up positive.
E. **Mallory–Weiss syndrome.**
   1. Mucosal tear at GE junction.
   2. Frequent history of violent retching and vomiting.
   3. Treatment.
      a. Supportive – the majority stop bleeding spontaneously.
      b. Sengstaken–Blakemore or Linton tube may be effective.
      c. Endoscopy and bipolar or laser coagulation.
      d. Direct suture if bleeding persists.
F. **Other** – esophagitis, esophageal or gastric carcinoma, telangiectasias.

VII. DIAGNOSTIC PROCEDURES – LOWER GI
A. **NG** – rule out rapid transit UGI bleed.
B. **Anoscopy/sigmoidoscopy/colonoscopy.**
   1. Identify obvious lesions if bleeding permits adequate exam.
   2. Therapeutic intervention with cautery and/or laser.
   3. Preparation difficult. If bleeding is heavy, this is usually futile and may delay definitive diagnosis.
C. **Technetium–labeled RBC scan.**
   1. Extremely sensitive (can visualize bleed of 0.2 ml/min).
   2. Can usually identify site but not cause – diverticular *vs.* angiodysplasia.
D. **Angiography.**
   1. Requires brisk bleed ($> .5–1$ cc/min).
   2. Therapeutic intervention with arterial vasopressin or embolization may be of benefit in high–risk patients.
   3. May define non–bleeding angiodysplasia.

E. **Barium enema.**
  1. Identify mass lesions, diverticuli, "thumb–printing" (ischemic colitis), etc.
  2. Interferes with subsequent endoscopic/angiographic procedures.
  3. May tamponade bleeding secondary to diverticulosis. Effect may be due to astringent agent given with enema.

VIII. **LOWER GI SOURCES OF BLEEDING — TREATMENT**
A. **Diverticulosis** (70% of significant lower GI bleeds).
  1. 60% stop spontaneously; therefore, monitor/transfuse.
  2. 40% continue to bleed or re–bleed, necessitating surgery.
  3. Vasopressin may control bleeding.
  4. Identify right *vs.* left colon source prior to surgery (if the patient is stable). The most common location is hepatic flexure.
  5. Operative procedure of choice in majority of patients remains a subtotal colectomy with ileoproctostomy. Hemicolectomy may be considered if bleeding point is unequivocally identified.
B. **Angiodysplasia** (right colon more common than left colon).
  1. Acute/significant bleed — supportive care, identify right *vs.* left colon, surgery if persists.
  2. Chronic/intermittent bleed — elective surgery.
C. **Carcinoma** — elective surgery with good prep whenever patient can be stabilized.
D. **Other** — polyps, inflammatory bowel disease, ischemic bowel, trauma, anal or rectal varices with portal hypertension.

INTESTINAL OBSTRUCTION

I. DEFINITIONS

A. **Ileus** — intestinal obstruction from *any* cause, mechanical or functional; most common usage of the word is to connote failure of aboral passage of bowel contents due to dysfunctional motility of the bowel, as in "adynamic ileus".

B. **Mechanical obstruction** — actual blockage of the intestinal lumen.

C. **Closed loop obstruction** — both the afferent and efferent limbs of bowel are occluded, as in a volvulus; may be accompanied by strangulation.

D. **Strangulation** — occlusion of the blood supply to a segment of bowel.

II. ETIOLOGY

A. **Small bowel obstruction (SBO).**

1. Adhesions — the *most common* cause of SBO. Approximately 90% of SBO's in patients with prior abdominal surgery are due to adhesions or internal herniation through a surgically created defect.

2. Hernias — the second most common cause of obstruction overall, but the *most common* cause in patients without prior abdominal surgery.

3. Other causes of SBO.

   a. Extrinsic.

      1) Carcinomatosis or tumor encasement from non-small bowel source.

      2) Intra-abdominal abscess.

      3) Hematoma.

      4) Malrotation with Ladd's bands or midgut volvulus.

      5) Annular pancreas (duodenal obstruction).

      6) Endometriosis.

      7) Superior mesenteric artery syndrome(SMA syndrome) — compression of third portion of the duodenum by the SMA in patients with severe acute weight loss.

   b. Intrinsic.

      1) Small bowel neoplasms.

      2) Congenital lesions.

         a) Small bowel atresia, stenosis or webs.

         b) Small bowel duplications, or mesenteric cysts.

         c) Meckel's diverticulum or other remnants of the omphalomesenteric duct.

      3) Inflammatory lesions.

         a) Regional enteritis, Crohn's disease.

         b) Radiation enteritis, stricture.

    c. Intraluminal obstruction.
      1) Meconium ileus.
      2) Gallstone ileus.
      3) Intussusception.
      4) Foreign bodies — bezoars, barium, worms.
  4. Other conditions that mimic the clinical picture of SBO.
    a. Colonic obstruction — right colonic obstruction may be indistinguishable from SBO.
    b. Adynamic ileus (see II. C. below).
    c. Vascular insufficiency.
      1) Mesenteric embolism.
      2) Mesenteric ischemia — secondary to hypoperfusion.
      3) Mesenteric thrombosis — due to severe dehydration, DIC, polycythemia (see pages 405–406).
    d. Hirschsprung's disease involving small bowel.

B. Colonic obstruction.
  1. Extrinsic.
    a. Adhesions.
    b. Hernia — particularly sliding type.
    c. Volvulus — sigmoid approximately 80%; cecal approximately 20%.
    d. Endometriosis.
  2. Intrinsic.
    a. Carcinoma of colon — most common cause (60%) of colonic obstruction.
    b. Congenital lesions — imperforate anus.
    c. Inflammatory lesions.
      1) Ulcerative colitis.
      2) Diverticulitis.
      3) Radiation enteritis.
  3. Intraluminal obstruction.
    a. Meconium ileus.
    b. Intussusception.
    c. Fecal impaction, foreign bodies, barium.
  4. Other conditions that may mimic colonic obstruction.
    a. Adynamic ileus — see below.
    b. Hirschsprung's disease.
    c. Focal ischemic colitis.

C. Adynamic ileus.
  1. Metabolic.
    a. Hypokalemia.
    b. Hypomagnesemia.
    c. Hyponatremia.
    d. Ketoacidosis.
    e. Uremia.
    f. Porphyria.

    g. Heavy metal poisoning.
2. Response to localized inflammatory process within peritoneal cavity — appendicitis, cholecystitis, diverticulitis, abscess.
3. Diffuse peritonitis — bacterial or chemical.
4. Retroperitoneal process.
    a. Retroperitoneal hematoma.
    b. Pancreatitis.
    c. Spinal or pelvic fracture.
5. Drugs.
    a. Narcotics.
    b. Antipsychotics.
    c. Anticholinergics.
    d. Ganglionic blockers.
    e. Agents used to treat Parkinson's disease.
6. Neuropathic disorders.
    a. Diabetes.
    b. Multiple sclerosis.
    c. Scleroderma.
    d. Lupus erythematosis.
    e. Hirschsprung's disease.
7. Postoperative ileus following intra–abdominal surgery.
    a. Small bowel motility usually returns within 24–48 hours.
    b. Gastric motility usually returns by 48 hours.
    c. Return of colonic motility may take 3–5 days.
8. **Ogilvie's syndrome.**
    a. Colonic pseudo–obstruction of uncertain etiology.
    b. Associated with pelvic retroperitoneal processes, long–term debilitation, chronic disease, immobility, prolonged bedrest and polypharmacy.
    c. Usually manifested by moderate to marked segmental cecal dilatation. Cecal diameter $\leq$ 12 cm significantly increases risk of perforation.
    d. Treatment of choice is decompression with gentle enemas. If unsuccessful, or marked cecal dilatation is already present, colonoscopic decompression is indicated. Rarely, cecostomy or right hemicolectomy is needed for perforation, ischemia, or unsuccessful colonoscopic decompression.

III. DIAGNOSIS OF INTESTINAL OBSTRUCTION
A. History.
1. Age.
    a. Neonate — consider congenital etiology, meconium ileus, Hirschsprung's disease.
    b. 2–24 months — consider congenital, intussusception, Hirschsprung's disease.
    c. Young adults — consider hernia, inflammatory bowel disease.
    d. Adults — hernia, neoplasms, diverticular disease.

      e. Elderly — consider hernia, neoplasms, diverticular disease, Ogilvie's syndrome.

2. Nausea, vomiting, obstipation. In *proximal* obstruction, bilious vomiting may occur early and the patient may have little abdominal distention. He may continue to pass stool and flatus as the bowel distal to the obstruction is evacuated. In *distal* bowel obstruction, the patient may initially complain of obstipation and distention prior to the onset of vomiting feculent material (secondary to bacterial overgrowth of small bowel contents).

3. Pain. In *proximal* obstruction, colicky pain is referred primarily to the periumbilical region and is due to distention of the bowel lumen secondary to continued peristalsis against the obstruction. In *distal* obstruction, pain is usually referred to the lower abdomen. If there is immediate torsion and vascular compromise of a bowel segment, obstruction and ischemia can occur early. Pain may be very severe and continuous due to ischemia or perforation.

4. Past surgical history. Prior operative procedures, particularly pelvic and lower abdominal procedures, implicate adhesions or internal herniation as the cause of the obstruction. Sudden cessation of colostomy or ileostomy output signals mechanical obstruction.

5. Past medical history.
      a. History of severe atherosclerosis, cardiac arrhythmias, prior MI, chronic congestive cardiac failure and use of digitalis may suggest intestinal ischemia.
      b. Previous history of inflammatory bowel disease or diverticulitis may suggest a mechanical obstruction.
      c. Gallstone ileus should be considered in a patient with known gallstones or history of recurrent biliary colic.

6. Medications.
      a. Digitalis — possible intestinal ischemia.
      b. Narcotics — adynamic ileus.
      c. Anticholinergics, ganglion blockers, antipsychotics, drugs for Parkinson's disease — suggest adynamic ileus.
      d. Diuretics — consider hypokalemia as the source of adynamic ileus.
      e. Polypharmacy — consider Ogilvie's syndrome (see above).

7. Review of systems.
      a. Recent weight loss — consider neoplasm.
      b. If severe acute weight loss from other cause, consider SMA syndrome (see above).

B. Physical exam.
  1. Vital signs.
      a. Fever — usually absent in uncomplicated obstruction; if present, consider inflammatory process or strangulation.

    b. Tachycardia — may be secondary to dehydration and hypovolemia, but if associated with leukocytosis and localized tenderness, it is one of the cardinal signs of strangulation.

    c. Orthostatic hypotension — often associated with dehydration and "third space" losses as fluid is sequestered in the obstructed bowel.

  2. Abdominal exam.

    a. Bowel sounds —initially active with intermittent **rushes** and borborygmus, but as fatigue occurs they may become decreased. In adynamic ileus, bowel sounds are usually absent.

    b. Mass — may be palpable due to a fixed distended loop of bowel or due to a carcinoma or inflammatory mass that is the cause of the obstruction. A careful exam for the presence of an inguinal, femoral, umbilical, or incisional hernia is mandatory.

    c. The presence of surgical scars from prior operations should always be noted.

    d. Peritoneal signs will be present with inflammatory processes, perforation, or strangulation.

  3. Rectal exam.

    a. Rectal vault is usually empty with established obstruction.

    b. Fecal impaction can be ruled out.

    c. Guaiac positive stool makes the diagnosis of carcinoma more likely.

    d. Extrinsic masses as well as intrinsic colon lesions can be diagnosed.

C. Laboratory evaluation.

  1. WBC — usually normal in uncomplicated SBO. Elevated with strangulation or if the source of obstruction is inflammatory. Markedly elevated later in mesenteric infarction.

  2. Hematocrit — is often increased due to hemoconcentration. Anemia in the presence of clinical low SBO or colonic obstruction often is characteristic of colon carcinoma.

  3. Electrolyte abnormalities — especially hypokalemia (see above).

  4. Alkalosis — usually develops in proximal SBO or pyloric obstruction because vomiting results in loss of chloride via gastric acid and fluid.

  5. Acidosis — usually occurs late in the course of **bowel infarction**; a normal pH does not rule out bowel infarction.

  6. Amylase may or may not be elevated in SBO.

D. Radiographs.

  1. Upright CXR — most sensitive for detection of free air under the diaphragm (perforation of an obstructed loop of bowel).

  2. Abdominal flat and upright (left lateral decubitus if the patient is unable to stand) — the characteristic features of intestinal obstruction are dilated bowel loops usually containing air–fluid levels proximal to the point of obstruction with little or no gas distally. Air fluid levels are not normally seen in an upright x-ray of the abdomen in persons with normal bowel motility. Gas may still be visualized distally with a partial obstruction, early in the course of complete obstruction, or if air has been introduced from below during rectal exam or enema.

   a. Small bowel can be distinguished from large bowel by the presence of **valvulae conniventes** (also known as plicae circulares) which traverse the entire diameter of the bowel as opposed to haustral markings of the colon which only extend 1/2 to 2/3 the diameter of the bowel.

   b. Air fluid levels in the upright projection can be seen with both ileus and obstruction. In obstruction they are usually more pronounced and a "step–ladder" pattern is often seen progressing down the abdomen.

   c. Fluid-filled loops of bowel appear as areas of increased density without gas and *can easily be overlooked.*

   d. In colonic obstruction or ileus, if the cecal diameter is **> 12 cm**, the patient is at increased risk of perforation; emergency decompression of the colon should be considered. When the cecum is acutely dilated to 12–14 cm, the wall tension exceeds perfusion pressure, and focal areas of necrosis may occur. These may progress even though the cecum is decompressed by non–operative means.

   e. **Sigmoid volvulus** appears as a large dilated loop of bowel which resembles a "bent inner tube", "coffee bean" or the symbol "omega" with the apex in the LLQ and the convexity in the RUQ.

   f. **Cecal volvulus** — a large, dilated, ovoid, air–filled cecum is usually visualized in the upper abdomen as the hyper-mobile cecum has rotated upward and to the left around the ileocolic vessels.

3. Contrast enema — most commonly used to rule out obstruction of the colon.

   a. Useful when the diagnosis is uncertain.

   b. Must be done with low pressure. The objective is identifying the site of obstruction, not defining mucosal detail. Free barium in the peritoneum from perforation of the colon has a very high mortality. If any question of a perforation exists, use **water–soluble contrast,** but omit the exam unless absolutely necessary.

   c. Will show the point of colonic obstruction, but care must be taken not to force barium beyond a partial obstruction and thereby create a complete obstruction (controversial).

   d. In unclear cases of suspected distal SBO, barium enema should be done prior to upper GI series:

      1) To rule out colonic obstruction with a fluid-filled proximal colon indistinguishable from SBO on plain radiographs.

        2) Reflux through the ileocecal valve will often visualize a collapsed terminal ileum, confirming diagnosis of SBO.
- **e.** Hydrostatic barium enema may be used if intussusception is suspected, to make the diagnosis, and to attempt a reduction. Up to 60–70% of children with intussusception will reduce with enema alone. Hydrostatic reduction should *not* be attempted in adults.
- **f.** In sigmoid or cecal volvulus, a "birds–beak" pattern is demonstrated at the site of the volvulus.
4. Upper GI series with small bowel follow–through.
- **a.** Useful if the diagnosis is uncertain or for demonstrating a partially obstructing lesion.
- **b.** In cases of uncertain diagnosis, barium enema should be done first.

VI. TREATMENT

A. Resuscitation.
1. Rehydration — rapid volume repletion with normal saline until adequate urine output (1/2 cc per kg body weight) is established.
2. Correction of electrolyte abnormalities — patients often have hypochloremic, hypokalemic metabolic alkalosis (see "Fluids and Electrolytes") and NS with added KCl is the fluid of choice. (KCl is added only after urine output is established.)
3. Foley catheter to monitor urine output.

B. Nasogastric suction — to prevent vomiting with aspiration.
1. Prevents further gaseous distention and partially decompresses the bowel.
2. The stomach must be empty in preparation for and during induction of anesthesia. Anesthesia relaxes the esophageal sphincters, allowing free regurgitation. Small bowel contents may rapidly refill the stomach.

C. Small bowel intubation — with "long tube" (i.e., Miller–Abbott or Cantor tube). Use of long tube as therapy for mechanical intestinal obstruction is generally inappropriate, because it may delay operation for a complete mechanical obstruction. The only major indications for long–tube therapy are:
1. Resolving partial obstruction.
2. Partial obstruction in the immediate postoperative period — about 50–60% of cases will resolve with a long tube.
3. Partial small bowel obstruction or obstruction due to inflammation which is expected to resolve with non–operative therapy, or due to carcinomatosis or radiation enteritis — these seldom strangulate and are often very difficult operative procedures, with high complications and recurrence rates.

D. Perioperative antibiotics — coverage of gram–negative aerobes and anaerobes is indicated because of bacterial overgrowth in the obstructed lumen and the possibility of small or large bowel

resection. If necrotic bowel or abscess is found, a full treatment course rather than perioperative prophylaxis is given.

E. **Operative treatment of SBO** — SBO is a surgical emergency and should be treated by laparotomy with few exceptions.

1. Patients with **localized peritoneal signs, leukocytosis** and **tachycardia** with SBO should be assumed to have ischemic or necrotic bowel and should be taken to the O.R. as soon as they are hemodynamically stable.

2. Patients with **complete obstruction** but without signs of vascular compromise should be resuscitated and operated upon urgently (as soon as possible within 6–8 hours of admission).

3. Patients with an uncertain diagnosis or those who continue to pass flatus or stool, indicating either a very early complete obstruction or a partial obstruction, can be treated conservatively while a diagnostic evaluation is in progress.

4. Lysis of all adhesions or resection of the involved segment of bowel is recommended. Intestinal bypass may be necessary in cases of advanced malignancy. This carries the risk of creating a blind loop with bacterial overgrowth in the bypassed segment of bowel, resulting in chronic diarrhea and malabsorption.

5. In obstruction due to radiation injury, lysis of adhesions should be limited. Radiation–injured bowel may be "revascularized" through adhesions.

6. Intraoperative tube decompression of the small bowel is frequently necessary to facilitate closure of the abdomen in cases of extreme bowel distention (see "GI Intubation"). Oral passage of a decompressive tube is much more desirable than an operative enterotomy, which is associated with a high likelihood of fecal contamination, late leakage, abscess, etc.

F. **Operative treatment of colonic obstruction.**

1. Obstructing carcinoma.

a. Right colonic obstruction — usually treated by resection and primary anastomosis when there is no gross contamination and when the bowel is not massively edematous.

b. Left colonic obstruction.

1) Primary resection with creation of colostomy and mucous fistula or Hartman's pouch (**2-stage procedure**) is usually indicated. In extremely debilitated/unstable patients without perforation or abscess, an initial diverting colostomy allows decompression & stabilization prior to resection and colostomy closure at later dates (**3-stage procedure**). [Mucous fistula is the term used to describe a stoma created from the proximal end of the remaining distal bowel after a segment has been resected. A **Hartman's pouch** is created by closing distal divided end of recto-sigmoid and leaving it within the abdomen after sigmoid resection. This procedure is done if there is insufficient length to bring the bowel out as a mucous fistula.]

   2) Some surgeons recommend resection with primary anastomosis, but this is uncommon because of the high risk of leakage and sepsis in obstructed, unprepared bowel.
  c. Patients with peritonitis secondary to an ischemic colon should be treated with resection of the involved bowel, end colostomy and mucous fistula or Hartman's pouch.
 2. Obstructing diverticulitis — see "Colonic Diverticulosis", page 293.
 3 Sigmoid volvulus.
  a. Initial treatment is non-operative decompression via sigmoidoscopy and placement of a long, soft, well-lubricated rectal tube past the point of obstruction. This usually results in the reduction (80% of cases) of the volvulus with immediate passage of stool and flatus. Mucosal inspection is then done to evaluate bowel viability.
  b. Because of the high frequency of recurrence ($\geq$ 50% in the first year), many authors recommend surgical resection after the first episode if the patient is a reasonable operative risk.
  c. After bowel preparation, resection of the redundant loop with primary anastomosis is performed.
  d. If volvulus cannot be reduced, strangulation should be suspected and immediate resection carried out.
 4. Cecal volvulus — always treated operatively. Resection is indicated for vascular compromise, but cecopexy or cecostomy is adequate in remaining cases.

V. RESULTS OF SURGICAL TREATMENT OF BOWEL OBSTRUCTION

A. Recurrent SBO will occur in 10% of patients treated by enterolysis and this incidence increases with each subsequent enterolysis.
B. Patients who have had multiple enterolysis may benefit from plication of the bowel in an organized position to promote the formation of adhesions in a non–obstructed pattern.
 1. **Transmesenteric plication** — seromuscular stitches are used to plicate adjacent bowel loops.
 2. Intraoperative oral placement of a Leonard tube or a Baker tube through a gastrostomy or high jejunostomy. This tube is left in place 12–14 days and is stiff enough to hold bowel in position until adhesions can form.
C. **Mortality of operation.**
 1. SBO — 0–5%.
 2. Colonic obstruction.
  a. 1-5% in diverticulitis.
  b. 5–10% in carcinoma.
  c. 40–50% if bowel necrosis has occurred with volvulus.

JAUNDICE

Through history, physical examination, laboratory and diagnostic studies, one must identify causes of jaundice which are surgically correctable.

I. GENERAL CONSIDERATIONS
A. Bilirubin metabolism.
1. Hemoglobin (Hgb), myoglobin → biliverdin → bilirubin.
2. 70–90% from Hgb, RBC breakdown.
3. 10–30% from myoglobin breakdown, liver enzymes, non–Hgb heme and non–Hgb porphyrin.
4. Indirect – bilirubin complexed with albumin; water insoluble (unconjugated).
5. Direct – bilirubin conjugated with glucuronide; water soluble (conjugated).
   a. Conjugation occurs in the liver.
   b. Diglucuronide – normal.
   c. Monoglucuronide – present in hepatocyte injury; may react as "direct".
B. Enterohepatic circulation – conjugated bilirubin excreted by liver → biliary system → duodenum. Bilirubin reduced to urobilinogen by small intestine bacteria. Terminal ileum: 10–20% absorbed and re-excreted by the liver and kidneys.
C. Clinical jaundice – evident when total bilirubin > 2 mg/dl.

II. LABORATORY TESTS
A. Bilirubin:

	Normals (mg/dl)	Hemolysis	Hepatocellular disease	Bile duct obstruction
Serum bilirubin:				
Indirect	0.2–1.3	Increased	Increased	Normal
Direct	0–0.3	Normal	Increased	Increased
Urine:				
Urobilinogen	2–4	Increased	Increased	Absent
Bilirubin	Negative	Negative	Positive	Positive
Fecal:				
Urobilinogen	40–280	Increased	Decreased	Absent

(**Pearls:** In jaundice of hemolysis and hepatocellular disease, indirect bilirubin makes up 90–95% of total. In obstructive jaundice, direct bilirubin makes up **greater than 50%** of total bilirubin.)

B. CBC.
1. Microcytic anemia with increased reticulocyte count suggests hemolysis. Peripheral smear will reveal sickle cells, spherocytes, target cells.

      2. Increased WBC is consistent with ascending cholangitis, but is non-specific.

C. **Transaminases** — increased with hepatocellular injury (viral, alcoholic, or drug-induced hepatitis).
    1. Serum glutamic-pyruvic transaminase (SGPT) or alanine serum transaminase (ALT) — more specific for liver than SGOT.
    2. Serum glutamic-oxaloacetic transaminase (SGOT) or aspartate serum transaminase (AST) — found in liver, heart, skeletal muscle, kidney, pancreas.

D. **Alkaline phosphatase** — increased production by proliferating terminal biliary ductules in response to intrahepatic or extrahepatic obstruction.
    1. Sources: liver, bone, placenta, kidney, WBCs, intestine.
    2. Increased level may also be due to hepatic infiltrative diseases (TB, sarcoid, lymphoma), space-occupying lesions (abscess, neoplasm), bone disease, pregnancy.

E. **5'-Nucleotidase** — comparable sensitivity to alkaline phosphatase, but with increased specificity. Sources: liver (bile canaliculi and sinusoidal membranes), intestine, heart, brain, blood vessels, endocrine pancreas (also increase during third trimester of pregnancy).

F. **Gamma glutamyl transferase (GGT)** — sensitivity and specificity greater than alkaline phosphatase.

G. **Prothrombin time (PT).**
    1. Dependent upon hepatic synthesis of factors V, VII and X, prothrombin and fibrinogen, and intestinal absorption of vitamin K.
    2. Helpful in assessment of hepatic reserve.
    3. If PT > 3 sec above control, treat with vitamin K 10 mg SQ or IV.
       a. Corrects within 48 hours if due to cholestasis or deficiency.
       b. Remains prolonged if due to hepatocellular insufficiency.

H. **Albumin.**
    1. Reflection of hepatic synthetic function and nutritional status.
    2. Half-life of approximately 15–20 days; not as valuable in detecting acute liver injury; short-turnover proteins (retinol binding protein, etc.) are more indicative of current synthetic status.

I. **Urobilinogen** — total absence from urine and feces indicates complete biliary obstruction.

J. **Hepatitis serology.**
    1. Hepatitis A.
       a. IgM — acute and transient.
       b. IgG — appears during recovery and persists.
    2. Hepatitis B (Fig. 1).
       a. HBsAg — surface antigen; first marker to appear; absent by 3 months.
       b. HBsAb — surface antibody; appearance variable but usually persists for life.

c. HBcAb — core antibody; present during "window" when HBsAG and HBsAB are too low to measure.

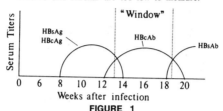

FIGURE 1

Interpretation of Test Results

HBsAg	anti–HBcIgM	anti–HAVIgM	Interpretation
−	−	+	Recent acute hepatitis A infection.
+	+	−	Acute hepatitis B infection.
+	−	−	Early acute hepatitis B infection or chronic hepatitis B.
−	+	−	Confirms acute or recent infection with hepatitis B virus.
−	−	−	Possible non–A, non–B hepatitis, other viral infection, or liver toxin.
+	+	+	Recent probable hepatitis A infection and superimposed acute hepatitis B infection (uncommon profile).

Ref: Abbott Laboratories. *Perspectives on Viral Hepatitis.* North Chicago: Abbott Laboratories, 1983, with permission.

III. DIAGNOSTIC STUDIES
A. Abdominal flat plate.
1. Gallstones — 15% are radiopaque.
2. Gas in biliary tree — seen in fistulas and surgical anastomoses with intestinal tract, cholangitis with gas–producing organism.

3. Emphysematous cholecystitis — extremely rare; seen in presence of infection, especially in diabetics.

B. **Ultrasonography.**
   1. Accuracy > 90% for cholelithiasis.
   2. Can identify dilated intra– and extrahepatic ducts, common duct stones, hepatic and pancreatic masses.
   3. Accuracy affected by obesity, ascites, bowel gas, skill of technician and radiologist.

C. **Nuclear biliary scan** (HIDA, etc.).
   1. Unreliable if bilirubin > 20 mg/dl. (Hepatic secretion of agent decreases as serum bilirubin exceeds 5 mg/dl.)
   2. Visualization of bile ducts but not GB suggests cystic duct obstruction; 95% sensitive for acute cholecystitis.
   3. Visualization of the duodenum rules out *complete* common duct obstruction.

D. **Oral cholecystogram (OCG).**
   1. Dependent upon intestinal absorption, hepatic uptake, conjugation and secretion, patency of cystic duct, and patient compliance.
   2. Unreliable when total bilirubin exceeds 2 mg/dl.

E. **Liver scan** — reveals liver and spleen size, masses (> 2 cm), and parenchymal disease better than HIDA scan.

F. **Computed tomography** — most effective in identifying liver and pancreatic masses and level of extrahepatic biliary obstruction.

G. **Percutaneous transhepatic cholangiography (PTC).**
   1. Identifies cause, site, extent of obstruction prior to surgery.
   2. Obtainable in 95% of patients with dilated ducts secondary to extrahepatic biliary obstruction.
   3. Contraindications.
      a. Coagulopathy — prolonged PT, PTT; platelets < 40,000.
      b. Ascites — unable to tamponade liver puncture.
      c. Peri– or intrahepatic sepsis.
      d. Disease of right lower lung or pleura.
   4. Complications — bile peritonitis, bilothorax, sepsis, hemobilia, bleeding.

H. **Endoscopic retrograde cholangiopancreatography (ERCP)** (see "GI Endoscopy").
   1. Visualization of UGI tract, ampullary region, biliary and pancreatic ducts.
   2. Allows collection of cytology and biopsy specimens.
   3. Complications — traumatic pancreatitis (1–2%), pancreatic or biliary sepsis (pre-procedure coverage with broad–spectrum antibiotic indicated).

I. **Percutaneous liver biopsy.**
   1. Evaluation of liver parenchyma.
   2. Contraindications — see PTC above.

IV. DIFFERENTIAL DIAGNOSIS OF JAUNDICE
A. **Prehepatic jaundice.**
1. **Hemolysis.**
    a. Increased indirect bilirubin; unconjugated bilirubin is bound with albumin and cannot be excreted renally.
    b. Production of bile pigments can raise total bilirubin by only 3 mg/dl (total bilirubin > 5 mg/dl indicates associated liver disease or biliary obstruction).
2. **Gilbert's disease** — defect in hepatocyte uptake of indirect bilirubin.
3. **Crigler–Najjar** (type I & II) — decreased conjugation secondary to impaired enzyme production or function.
B. **Hepatic jaundice.**
1. Viral hepatitis.
    a. Insidious onset of anorexia, malaise, fever, nausea, arthralgias, myalgias, headache, photophobia, pharyngitis, cough, coryza, and low–grade fever precede abdominal pain.
    b. Tender enlarged liver.
    c. Serologic markers (see section II–J above) — CMV titers.
    d. Non–A, non–B hepatitis is a diagnosis of exclusion.
2. Alcoholic hepatitis — long history of alcohol overuse.
3. Drug–induced hepatitis — acetaminophen, halothane, erythromycin, isoniazid, chlorpromazine, valproic acid, phenytoin, oral contraceptives, 17,α-alkyl, substituted anabolic steroids, chlorpropamide, methimazole.
4. Cirrhosis (see "Cirrhosis").
5. **Dubin–Johnson syndrome** — impaired hepatic excretion of conjugated bilirubin.
C. **Posthepatic/obstructive jaundice.**
1. General considerations.
    a. Increased total bilirubin, bilirubin present in urine (dark–colored, "Coca–Cola" urine), clay–colored stool.
    b. When total bilirubin > 3 mg/dl, both direct and indirect fractions increased.
    c. Abdominal pain usually precedes symptoms of systemic disease.
    d. Painless jaundice with palpable gallbladder suggests cancer distal to the cystic duct (Courvoisier's Law).
    e. **Charcot's triad** — fever, RUQ pain, jaundice; suggests extra-hepatic obstruction with ascending cholangitis; a surgical emergency.
    f. **Reynolds' pentad** — Charcot's triad, shock, mental obtundation.
2. Choledocholithiasis (see "Gallbladder" section III).
3. Cholangitis (see "Gallbladder" section IV).

4. **Sclerosing cholangitis.**
   a. Non–bacterial inflammatory narrowing of bile ducts — predominantly men ages 20–50; etiology unknown.
   b. Present with fatigue, weight loss, anorexia, insidious development of jaundice and pruritis, intermittent RUQ pain.
   c. Estimated that 50% of patients with sclerosing cholangitis have or will develop frank ulcerative colitis.
   d. ERCP and biopsy used for diagnosis — rule out malignancy.
   e. Treatment.
      1) Medical — corticosteroids, long–term antibiotics to prevent cholangitis, immunosuppression, bile–acid binding agents, penicillamine.
      2) Surgical — T–tube, transhepatic stent, other decompressive procedure.
   f. May progress to secondary biliary cirrhosis with ascites, varices, and hepatic failure requiring transplantation.
5. **Benign biliary stricture.**
   a. 95% caused by surgical trauma, 5% caused by abdominal trauma, chronic pancreatitis or impacted stone.
   b. Presents with intermittent cholangitis, jaundice.
   c. Diagnosis with PTC or ERCP: stricture usually within 2 cm of bifurcation.
   d. Treatment.
      1) Antibiotics for cholangitis.
      2) Surgical repair with tension-free anastomosis and mucosal apposition — choledochoduodenostomy, choledochojejunostomy, or end–to–end bile duct anastomosis.
   e. Complications (if untreated):
      1) Infection — cholangitis, abscess, sepsis.
      2) Liver disease — cirrhosis, portal hypertension.
6. **Carcinoma of the bile ducts.**
   a. Diagnosis usually made in 7th decade — commonly metastatic at presentation.
   b. Associated conditions — ulcerative colitis (incidence unaffected by colectomy), *Clonorchis senensis* infection (oriental liver fluke), chronic typhoid carrier state, choledochal cyst, sclerosing cholangitis.
   c. Presentation includes insidious onset of jaundice, pruritus, anorexia, pain, and possible cholangitis.
   d. Diagnosis — PTC or ERCP associated with CT scan.
   e. Therapy.
      1) Curative resection (rarely possible) — wide resection and reconstruction of biliary tree.
      2) Palliative resection — cholecystojejunostomy, choledochojejunostomy, U–tube or other stent.
      3) Postoperative radiation may prolong life.
   f. Prognosis — 5–year survival 10–15%.

7. **Carcinoma of the head of pancreas.**
   a. Peak age 5th and 6th decade — increasing in incidence.
   b. 80% are ductal adenocarcinomas, 2/3 in head.
   c. Symptoms — weight loss, obstructive jaundice, deep–seated vague abdominal or back pain.
   d. Courvoisier's Law — painless jaundice with palpable gall-bladder.
   e. Diagnosis — CT scan (ERCP and PTC may be helpful).
   f. Treatment.
      1) Pancreaticoduodenectomy (Whipple procedure) — resect head of pancreas or total pancreatectomy, duodenum, gastric antrum, gallbladder, and distal common bile duct. Only 10% have disease confined to area of Whipple resection at time of exploration.
      2) If unresectable (majority of patients explored):
         a) Choledochojejunostomy or cholecystojejunostomy and gastrojejunostomy for palliation (up to 40% may develop duodenal obstruction).
         b) Consider radiation therapy plus chemotherapy (5-FU).
   g. Prognosis.
      1) Operative mortality (for Whipple procedure) should be < 5%.
      2) Resection of carcinoma of the head of the pancreas for cure (10% of patients) — 14% 5–year survival.
      3) Nonresectable or palliative resection — mean survival 6 months.
      4) Carcinoma of body or tail of pancreas — essentially no survivors due to late presentation.
8. **Carcinoma of the Ampulla of Vater.**
   a. 10% of obstructing tumors of common duct.
   b. Presentation — early jaundice, occult blood in stool.
   c. Diagnosis with CT and biopsy during ERCP.
   d. Spread locally with slow rate of metastasis.
   e. Therapy — pancreaticoduodenectomy.
      1) 5–10% operative mortality.
      2) Prognosis — 5–year survival 39%.
9. **Choledochal cyst** — congenital cyst of the extrahepatic biliary tree.
   a. Classic triad consists of RUQ mass, jaundice, pain.
   b. 4 times more common in females.
   c. One–third diagnosed before age 10.
   d. Three subtypes (Alonso–Lej classification):
      1) Type A — cystic dilation of entire common hepatic and common bile duct.
      2) Type B — diverticulum of common bile duct.
      3) Type C — cystic dilation of the distal common bile duct (choledochocele).

   e. Natural history — if left untreated, may progress to complete biliary obstruction, cholangitis, secondary biliary cirrhosis, spontaneous rupture (frequently occurs during pregnancy), or carcinoma.

   f. Treatment.

      1) Procedure of choice — excision of cyst with Roux–en–Y hepaticodochojejunostomy.

      2) Roux–en–Y cystojejunostomy.

         a) High incidence of postoperative cholangitis.

         b) Late malignancy.

SURGICAL ENDOSCOPY

I. INTRODUCTION
A. Endoscopy provides a non–invasive view of the GI tract.
B. The advances in fiberoptics have enhanced the capabilities of diagnosis and treatment of GI tract disorders.

II. INSTRUMENTATION AND TECHNIQUES
A. The basic instrument has a head with an eyepiece and controls, a variable length shaft, and a maneuverable tip (Fig. 1).

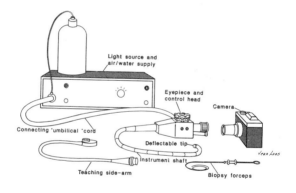

FIGURE 1

B. Centrally–located flexible fiberoptic light and viewing bundles allow for maneuverability of instrument while providing a clear image.
C. The fiberoptics are arranged so that the scope may be either forward viewing or side viewing.
D. The flexibility of the tip allows for up and down and side–to–side deflection of > 180°.
E. Shaft is torque–stable, allowing rotary movements to be transmitted the length of the scope.
F. Keeping the shaft of the instrument relatively straight allows rotatory movements to be transmitted to the tip.

G. The scope has 2 or more channels for the passage of instruments, and introduction of air and water (Fig. 2).

H. The light source is attached to the scope via an "umbilical cord." An air pump, water pump, and suction are frequently built into the light source, and their channels pass through the umbilical cord.

I. The instrument can be controlled with one hand.

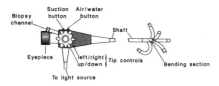

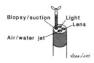

FIGURE 2

J. After introduction of the scope, orientation is maintained by use of marker at the 12 o'clock position in the field of view, with upward deflection being toward the mark (Fig. 3).

FIGURE 3

K. **Important rules for endoscopic examination.**
1. Prepare patient.
2. **Do not advance without vision.**
3. If in doubt, withdraw.
4. Tissue can be obtained for histologic and cytologic exam during most of the multiple endoscopic procedures.
5. Biopsies should be taken from multiple areas of the suspected pathology (all specimens should be placed in formalin).

    6. Most common complications are perforation and bleeding.

III. ESOPHAGOGASTRODUODENOSCOPY (EGD)
    Used for evaluation and selective treatment of diseases of the esophagus, stomach, and proximal duodenum.

A. Indications.
    1. Rule out malignancy.
    2. Evaluate source of bleeding (higher yield in first 24 hours).
    3. Evaluate abnormalities found by radiographic study.
    4. Dysphagia.
    5. Evaluate and treat esophageal varices.
    6. Diagnosis of ill–defined or atypical upper abdominal complaints or chest pain.
    7. Rule out new, persistent, or recurrent ulcers and tumors.
    8. Gastric ulcer by radiologic diagnosis.

B. Preparation.
    1. Fast for 4–6 hours prior to study.
    2. Urgent EGD may require prior gastric lavage and decompression.
    3. Ensure airway is protected.
    4. IV sedation is recommended (e.g., midazolam 1 mg IVP).
    5. Topical anesthesia for pharynx (e.g., Cetacaine® spray).

C. Technique.
    1. A 120 cm **forward–viewing** scope is used.
    2. The patient is placed in a left lateral decubitus position.
    3. The instrument may be introduced manually or by having the patient swallow the scope.
    4. The instrument is further safety enhanced under direct vision of the lumen through the esophagus into the stomach and duodenum.
    5. Important landmarks are the cricopharyngeal sphincter, LES, incisura, pylorus, and superior duodenal angle. The distance from the incisors for each landmark should be noted in report.
    6. Careful inspection of the upper GI tract is done both upon insertion and withdrawal of the instrument.
    7. Retroflexion of scope is performed to inspect the incisura, cardia and the esophageal hiatus (gastric side).
    8. The "pinch line" (corresponds to diaphragmatic crus) may be visualized by having the patient sniff with the scope in the lower esophagus. The "Z–line" (squamo-columnar junction) can be visually identified.
    9. The vocal cords should be seen on withdrawal through the hypopharynx.

D. Contraindications.
    1. Uncooperative or combative patient.

2. Acute corrosive or phlegmonous esophagitis.
3. Relative contraindications.
   a. Pulsion diverticulum.
   b. Bleeding diathesis.
   c. Aneurysm of ascending aorta.
   d. Large goiter.
   e. Large cervical osteophytes (increases risk of esophageal perforation).
E. **Complications** – risk of occurrence is approximately 0.2%.
   1. Perforation – most commonly at level of pharynx, cervical esophagus, cardia, or superior duodenal angle.
   2. Bleeding.
   3. Aspiration.
   4. Vasovagal response – associated bradycardia and hypotension.
   5. Cardiac arrhythmias.
   6. Transmission of infection (no documented instances).
   7. Mortality 0.02% – cardiac dysrhythmias are the most common cause of EGD–associated deaths.

IV. ENDOSCOPIC RETROGRADE CHOLANGIO–PANCREATOGRAPHY (ERCP)

Used for evaluation and treatment of pancreaticobiliary disorders.

A. **Preparation** – same as for EGD. Addition of prophylactic antibiotics covering enteric organisms may be necessary.
B. **Technique.**
   1. The 120 cm **side–viewing** scope is used.
   2. Introduction of the instrument is the same as for EGD, except scope is passed relatively blindly through the cricopharyngeus due to its side–viewing nature.
   3. The instrument is passed into the second portion of the duodenum until the ampulla of Vater is identified.
   4. The ampulla is cannulated and dye is injected under fluoroscopic control. Subsequently, radiographs of the biliary and pancreatic systems are obtained. Attention to radiologic detail is critical.
C. **Indications.**
   1. Suspected abnormality of ampulla, biliary, or pancreatic system.
   2. Biliary obstruction.
   3. Chronic/recurrent pancreatitis.
   4. Atypical abdominal pain (low–yield study).
D. **Contraindications.**
   1. Same as for EGD.
   2. Acute pancreatitis – relative. Currently recommended for severe biliary pancreatitis.

E. **Adjunct techniques.**
1. Common duct stone extraction — procedure of choice following cholecystectomy.
2. Sphincterotomy.
3. Placement of nasobiliary stent for ampullary obstruction.

F. **Complications** — complication rate 0.8%, mortality rate 0.05%.
1. Pancreatitis.
2. Perforation.
3. Cholangitis.
4. Infection of pseudocyst.

V. **COLONOSCOPY**
Allows for diagnostic evaluation of the colon and terminal ileum. Most accurate diagnostic modality available for the lower GI tract. Allows for early detection of colorectal carcinoma.

A. **Preparation.**
1. Mechanical bowel prep prior to procedure (e.g., Golytely® 4 L over 4 hours at least 12 hours prior to study).
2. Clear liquids for 24–48 hours prior to procedure.
3. NPO for 6 hours preceding procedure.
4. Normal coagulation profile.
5. Should be preceded by anoscopy.

B. **Technique.**
1. The 140–180 cm **forward–viewing** scope is used.
2. The patient is placed in left lateral decubitus position with knees flexed and the instrument is introduced through the anus.
3. The instrument is passed under direct visualization until the cecum/terminal ileum is reached.
   a. Endoscopically the lumen of the ascending colon is circular and the lumen of the transverse colon is triangular.
   b. Splenic and hepatic flexures may be identified by the extra-luminal bluish hue of the spleen and liver.
   c. The appendiceal orifice may be identified as the point of fusion of the tinea.
4. As with EGD, careful inspection is performed upon withdrawal of the scope.
5. Adequate insufflation of the colon must be maintained in order to completely evaluate all mucosal surfaces.

C. **Indications.**
1. Hemoccult positive stool.
2. Lower GI bleed.
3. Rule out synchronous colon carcinoma.
4. High–risk group for colon carcinoma (familial polyposis, ulcerative colitis, etc.).
5. F/U previously treated polyps or colon carcinoma.

6. Abnormal radiologic findings on barium enema.
7. Persistent diarrhea.

D. Contraindications.
1. Acute inflammatory disease of colon/rectum — relative.
2. Toxic megacolon.
3. Peritonitis.
4. S/P recent myocardial infarction.
5. 1st trimester of pregnancy.

E. Complications — complication rate is approximately 0.14%.
1. Perforation.
2. Cardiac dysrhythmias.
3. Vasovagal response.
4. Mesenteric hematoma.
5. Splenic injury.
6. Bleeding.

VI. PROCTOSIGMOIDOSCOPY

Allows visualization of the anal canal, rectum, and proximal portion
of sigmoid colon from 30–60 cm.

A. Preparation.
1. (2) Fleet® enemas prior to procedure.
2. Adequate rectal exam.
3. Anoscopy can be performed to evaluate the anal canal and
   distal rectum.

B. Technique.
1. A 30 cm rigid or 30–60 cm flexible scope can be used.
2. The longer flexible scope affords better visualization and a
   higher yield, as well as greater patient comfort.
3. The procedure can be performed with the patient in the lateral
   decubitus position with knees flexed, lithotomy, or knee–chest
   (genupectoral) position.
4. The instrument is passed per rectum under direct vision.

C. Indications.
1. Hematochezia.
2. Anorectal symptoms.
3. Change in bowel habits.
4. Routine exam for population > 40. ACS recommendations:
   a. Rectal exam every year > 40.
   b. Sigmoidoscopy every year > 50; if two successive exams
      are negative, then repeat every 3–5 years.
5. Approximately 30% of colorectal carcinoma can be detected by
   rigid sigmoidoscopy (50–60% by lower flexible sigmoidoscopy).
6. Serves as a good screening tool, since approximately 60–80%
   of all colorectal tumors occur within 30 cm of the anal verge.

D. **Contraindications** (relative).
1. Fulminant colitis.
2. Diverticulitis.
3. Uncooperative patient.
4. Toxic megacolon.
5. Peritonitis.
E. **Complications** — lowest risk of any endoscopic diagnostic procedure.
1. Perforation.
2. Bleeding.
3. Mesosigmoid hematoma.
4. Cardiac dysrhythmias.

VII. EMERGENCY ENDOSCOPY
A. Most commonly done for GI bleeding.
B. 85% of all acute bleeding episodes from the GI tract originate proximal to the ligament of Treitz.
C. Allows early identification of the bleeding source with the capacity for therapeutic intervention.
1. Approximately 80% of all GI bleeding stops spontaneously.
2. Emergent endoscopy has not been proven to improve mortality, the incidence of recurrence, transfusion requirements, or the length of hospital stay.
D. **Preparation.**
1. Protect airway.
2. Volume resuscitation.
3. Hemodynamic stabilization.
4. Rule out bleeding diathesis or coagulopathy.
5. Lavage stomach clear prior to EGD, if possible.
6. Cleansing enemas or mechanical prep prior to colonoscopy (blood itself is an excellent cathartic).
7. Anoscopy and sigmoidoscopy should be performed if the patient is passing bright–red blood per rectum.
E. **Technique** — as previously stated for each diagnostic procedure. Remember position–changes to move a pool of blood to a different side of the stomach.
F. **Indications** — all patients with evidence of acute GI bleeding.
G. **Contraindications.**
1. Refractory hemorrhagic shock.
2. Do *not* biopsy in the presence of a coagulation abnormality.
H. **Complications.**
1. Same as for individual diagnostic procedures. Significant increased (x 100) incidence of complications compared to elective.
2. Reactivation/exacerbation of the bleeding source.

VIII. THERAPEUTIC ENDOSCOPY

A. Endoscopy has evolved to the point that many therapeutic interventions can be carried out via the scope, thus avoiding more invasive therapy.

B. Often palliative measures may be performed, allowing surgery to be performed under more optimal conditions, or in lieu of surgery.

C. Therapeutic endoscopy is relatively less invasive than surgery and usually has a more rapid recovery.

D. Preparation.

1. Same as for the individual diagnostic procedures.

2. Rule out coagulopathy. **Note:** Check coagulation status prior to planned endosphincterotomy; type and screen for possible transfusion.

3. Administration of antibiotics is recommended prior to ERCP to decrease the incidence of biliary sepsis. Use for active or recent cholangitis, planned endo–stent insertion, planned endosphincterotomy and stone removal with gallbladder *in situ*, acute pancreatitis.

E. Technique.

1. Same basic techniques are used as for diagnostic procedure. Endoscopic biliary and pancreatic therapy often utilizes guide–wire based techniques with exchanges over guide–wire.

2. Instrument introduction and manipulation is through the instrument port of the scope.

3. All manipulations and procedures are carried out under direct visualization.

4. Some of the procedures require fluoroscopic assistance.

F. Indications.

1. When surgery would be more hazardous or has known poor results.

2. Lesion must be intraluminal and within reach of the endoscope.

Indication	Therapy
Foreign body (unable to pass)	Extraction
GI polyp	Polypectomy
Stenosis/obstruction of ampulla	Sphincterotomy
Severe biliary pancreatitis	Sphincterotomy (controversial)
Choledocholithiasis	Sphincterotomy and/or endoscopic/ intraoperative extraction
Suppurative cholangitis	Sphincterotomy and nasobiliary tube/stent
Esophageal varices	Sclerotherapy
Stenosis	Dilatation/stent
Unresectable tumor	Dilatation/stent
Gastric emptying disorder — Inability to take P.O.	Intubation of GI tract with feeding tube and/or drainage tube
GI bleeding	Cautery (laser/electric); sclerotherapy
Pseudocolonic obstruction	Colonoscopic decompression

G. Contraindications.
1. Same as for the corresponding diagnostic procedure (e.g., hemodynamic instability).
2. Anatomic inaccessibility.
3. For removal of a foreign body from GI tract:
    a. Demonstrate passage.
    b. Development of abdominal pain, obstruction, ileus, fever, abscess, fistula — all are indications for surgical intervention.
4. Polypectomy — multiple polyposis syndrome, inflammatory polyp, wide base/sessile polyp, unprepared colon.
5. Sphincterotomy — where surgery clearly indicated, unfavorable anatomy, i.e., inability to deeply cannulate (BD), acute pancreatitis (except severe biliary), coagulopathy.
6. Sclerotherapy.
7. Cautery — rapid bleeding impairing visualization, poorly prepped colon.
8. Colonic decompression — peritonitis, pneumoperitoneum.
9. Stent/dilatation — complicated strictures.

H. Complications.
1. Same as for the corresponding diagnostic procedure.
2. Removal of foreign body — laceration of bowel or GE junction, aspiration of foreign body, erosion into mesentery, obstruction.
3. **Polypectomy.**
    a. Explosion.
    b. Full–thickness burn — perforation.
    c. Complication rate 2%.
4. **Sphincterotomy.**
    a. Bleeding (most common), perforation, pancreatitis, cholangitis, recurrent stone, restenosis.
    b. Complication rate approximately 7–10%.
    c. Mortality rate 1.1%.
5. **Sclerotherapy** — ulcerations, gastric variceal bleeding, pulmonary changes, esophageal stricture, pyrexia, dysphagia.
6. **Intubation** — displacement, obstruction, tube blockage, erosion, leakage, knotting, local infection, gastrocolic fistula.
7. **Cautery** — perforation, rebleeding.
    a. Failure of hemostasis.
    b. Explosion.
    c. Ulcerations.
    d. Intra–abdominal bleeding.
    e. Complication rate 1.8%.
    f. Mortality rate 0.5%.

8. **Stent/dilatation** — in biliary stenting, most common complication is clogging of stent with secondary cholangitis.
   a. Reflux.
   b. Obstruction.
   c. Migration of stent.
   d. Perforation.

ESOPHAGUS

I. ANATOMY

A. A muscular tube 25 cm long, lined by mucosa, extending from the cricopharyngeus (15 cm from the incisor teeth) to the ill–defined gastroesophageal junction (40 cm from the incisor teeth). Three anatomic areas of narrowing: the **cervical, bronchoaortic,** and **diaphragmatic** constrictions. The distal 2–3 cm of esophagus is intra–abdominal.

B. Mucosa — squamous changing to columnar at the GE junction.

C. Submucosa.
   1. Glands, arteries, Meissner's neural plexus.
   2. Lymphatics — extensive longitudinal network (submucosal spread of cancer may extend 4–6 cm from tumor).
   3. Veins — may become varices with portal hypertension.

D. Muscle — inner circular and outer longitudinal layers with blood vessels and neural plexuses between layers.

E. No serosa — lack of serosa contributes to the increased potential for anastamotic leakage and early mediastinal invasion by cancer.

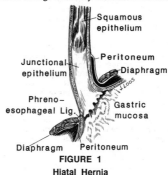

FIGURE 1

Hiatal Hernia

II. GASTROESOPHAGEAL REFLUX AND HIATAL HERNIA

A. **Anatomy and physiology.**
   1. **Lower esophageal sphincter (LES).**
      a. A functional high–pressure zone.
      b. 3–5 cm long, 10–20 mm Hg gradient.

      c. Regulated by autonomic innervation, gut hormones (gastrin) and smooth muscle tone.

      d. Abdominal pressure transmitted to the intra–abdominal esophagus helps maintain LES competence.

   2. Acid protection mechanisms.

      a. A competent LES preventing reflux.

      b. Peristalsis clearing esophageal contents.

      c. Bicarbonate rich saliva (1000–1500 ml/day, 30 mEq/L).

   3. Etiology of reflux.

      a. Decreased LES tone.

      b. Delayed gastric emptying.

      c. Increased intra–abdominal pressure due to obesity, tight garments, large meals.

      d. Motor failure of esophagus with loss of peristalsis and LES tone, such as with systemic collagen disease (e.g., scleroderma).

      e. Iatrogenic — LES destroyed or bypassed.

B. Reflux esophagitis.

   1. Corrosive injury to mucosa.

   2. Grades (assessed via EGD):

      a. Grade I — mucosal erythema.

      b. Grade II — superficial ulceration.

      c. Grade III — ulceration, transmural fibrosis, dilatable stricture.

      d. Grade IV — non–dilatable stricture.

   3. Symptoms.

      a. Heartburn — retrosternal pyrosis.

      b. Regurgitation of bitter or sour liquids.

      c. Recurrent nocturnal aspiration.

      d. Dysphagia implies obstruction, motility disorder.

      e. Symptoms exacerbated by recumbency, large meal, any increase in intra–abdominal pressure.

   4. Diagnosis.

      a. UGI series.

         1) May demonstrate reflux in the absence of symptoms.

         2) May document an ulcer or stricture.

      b. Esophagoscopy with mucosal brushings and biopsy essential to diagnosis.

      c. Esophageal pH probe.

         1) Accurate documentation of magnitude and duration of reflux.

         2) Acid reflux test (sensitive for reflux).

            a) HCl is placed in stomach, and the pH electrode is placed proximal to manometrically defined LES.

            b) Esophageal pH monitored while intragastric pressure is increased. A decrease in pH to < 4 is evidence of gastroesophageal reflux.

    d. Esophageal manometry.
        1) Does not test for reflux, although reflux is more frequent in the presence of lower LES pressure (< 6 mm).
        2) May identify a predisposing motility disorder.
    e. Bernstein test — reproduces symptoms by midesophageal HCl instillation.
        1) A positive test results when symptoms occur only with acid, but not saline or alkali instillation.
        2) Differentiates esophagitis from other causes of substernal pain.
C. Esophageal hiatal hernia (incidence 5/1000).
    1. Type I — sliding (Fig. 2).
        a. GE junction migrates above diaphragm.
        b. Most common (90%) hiatal hernia.
        c. Etiology.
            1) Chronically increased intra–abdominal pressure, including obesity.
            2) Weakness of supporting structures at esophageal hiatus.
        d. Significant only if contributing to reflux or symptoms.

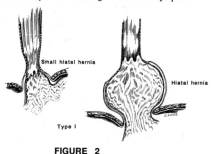

FIGURE 2

Type I (Sliding) Hiatal Hernia

    2. Type II — paraesophageal (Fig. 3).
        a. Gastric fundus herniates alongside esophagus, while the GE junction remains in normal position with an intact phreno-esophageal ligament.
        b. May incarcerate or strangulate, resulting in a surgical emergency. Should be repaired electively if possible.
        c. "Pure" Type II hernia is rare.
    3. Type III — combined Type I and II. Type III represents most "paraesophageal hernias".

4. Type IV — contains organs other than stomach.
5. Reflux and hiatal hernia — most patients with reflux have an associated sliding hiatal hernia; the converse is not true.

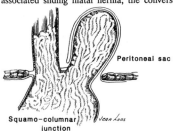

Type II

FIGURE 3

Type II (Paraesophageal) Hiatal Hernia

D. **Medical management of GE reflux.**
 1. Dietary.
  a. Avoid substances that decrease LES tone (alcohol, tobacco and caffeine).
  b. No oral intake 2 hrs before sleep.
 2. Avoid anticholinergics, tranquilizers, muscle relaxants.
 3. Weight reduction if obese.
 4. Elevate head of bed 6".
 5. Increase LES pressure.
  a. Metoclopramide (Reglan®) 10 mg q 8 h.
  b. Bethanechol 10–50 mg PO tid or qid.
 6. Decrease gastric acid.
  a. Antacids.
  b. H_2 blockers.
  c. Omeprazole.
 7. Most *compliant* patients respond to medical management.
E. **Complications of reflux esophagitis.**
 1. Intractable subjective distress.
 2. Bleeding.
 3. Esophageal stricture.
  a. Dilatable — 78% of strictures do not recur after dilation if compliant with medical therapy.
  b. Non–dilatable.

      c. Rule out malignancy by endoscopy with brush and biopsy.
  4. Shortening of esophagus.
  5. Ulceration (with perforation).
  6. Barrett's esophagus.
      a. Columnar mucosa in distal esophagus.
      b. Etiology — most often attributed to reflux; almost always associated with hiatal herna, but may be secondary to congenital rests of gastric mucosa.
      c. Associated with an increased risk (10–15%) of developing adenocarcinoma of the esophagus.
      d. Correction of reflux does not prevent malignant transformation; close follow–up required.
  7. Dysmotility.
  8. Schatzki's ring — constrictive band at squamocolumnar junction composed of mucosa and submucosa; usually asymptomatic unless ring is < 12 mm.
  9. Respiratory aspiration — may result in recurrent lower lobe pneumonias.
F. Surgical therapy — antireflux procedures.
  1. Indications.
      a. Failure of adequate medical therapy.
      b. Grade II–IV esophagitis.
      c. Complications of reflux esophagitis.
      d. Presence of type II, III, IV hernias.
  2. Principles of repair.
      a. Secure an intra–abdominal length of esophagus.
      b. Restore high pressure zone.
      c. Narrow the hiatus.
  3. Techniques:

Procedure	Approach	Wrap	Features
Hill	Abdomen	180°	Phrenoesophageal ligament anchored to median arcuate ligament of diaphragm.
Belsey	Chest	270°	Exaggerated G–E angle, stomach anchored below diaphragm.
Nissen	Either	360°	Fundus wrapped completely around the esophagus.
Angelchik®	Abdomen	—	Silicone prosthesis placed around the esophagus below diaphragm.
Collis gastroplasty	Abdomen	—	Lengthens foreshortened esophagus by creating a "tube" of gastric mucosa.

  4. Complications.
      a. Mortality/morbidity (T = total; S = splenectomy).
         1) Hill — 4.3%/8.7% (T and S).

2) Belsey — 0.5%/14.3% (T); 7.3% (S).
3) Nissen — 1.2%/24.1% (T); 16.8% (S).
b. Excessively tight repair — dysphagia.
c. Excessively loose or short wrap — persistent reflux.
d. "Slipped Nissen" — wrap slides down, GE junction retracts into chest, and the stomach is partitioned.
e. "Gas–bloat syndrome" — difficulty with eructation due to a restored competent LES in a patient who swallows air. Can be avoided by repair over larger dialator (54–60 Fr).
f. The Angelchik® prosthesis has an excessive incidence of complications secondary to migration and erosion. It is not generally considered a valid repair.

G. Long–standing disease with stricture or Barrett's esophagus may necessitate esophageal resection.

III. DYSPHAGIA

A. **Motility disorders — oropharyngeal.**
1. Cricopharyngeal achalasia.
   a. Upper esophageal sphincter dysfunction (cricopharyngeus).
   b. Abnormal muscle contracture or delayed relaxation contributes to the development of a **Zenker's diverticulum.**
2. Pharyngoesophageal diverticulum (Zenker's diverticulum).
   a. Most common esophageal diverticulum.
   b. Rare before age of 50.
   c. Located in posterior midline between the oblique fibers of the inferior pharyngeal constrictor and the transverse cricopharyngeus muscles (Killian's triangle).
   d. Can result in regurgitation of undigested foods or in recurrent aspiration.
   e. Diverticulectomy with myotomy of cricopharyngeus usually curative with low (1.2%) mortality and recurrences (4%).
3. Neuromuscular diseases — CVA, ALS, Parkinson's, myesthesia, thyrotoxicosis, hypothyroidism.

B. **Primary esophageal dysmotility.**
1. **Achalasia.**
   a. Absence or destruction of Auerbach's plexus results in abnormal peristalsis and failure of LES to relax.
   b. Barium swallow demonstrates "bird's beak" narrowing of distal esophagus with proximal dilatation.
   c. Preoperative work–up includes manometry to exclude other motility disorders and endoscopy to rule out stricture and tumor.
   d. Controversy as to whether dilatation or operation is best form of therapy.
   e. Longitudinal (Heller) myotomy of distal esophagus improves symptoms.

   2. **Diffuse esophageal spasm.**
      a. Pain is a more pronounced symptom than dysphagia.
      b. Hyperperistaltic, uncoordinated contractions.
      c. Diagnosis by motility studies.
      d. Treatment — small, soft meals; Ca^{++} channel blockers; extended esophagomyotomy.
   3. **Scleroderma.**
      a. Esophageal muscular atrophy and fibrosis results in a rigid esophagus with poor contractility.
      b. Treatment — medical/surgical antireflux therapy to control esophagitis.
   4. Esophageal reflux (see Section II) — symptoms of reflux esophagitis are usually more prominent than dysphagia.
   5. Epiphrenic diverticula.
      a. Sensation of post-prandial pressure in epigastrium.
      b. Symptoms may be due to the associated motility disorder, rather than the diverticulum.
      c. Treatment — usually none. If large, diverticulectomy and distal esophageal myotomy.
   6. Parabronchial (midesophageal) diverticulum.
      a. "Traction" diverticulum (as opposed to "pulsion" diverticulae like Zenker's and epiphrenic).
      b. Usually due to previous inflammation involving mediastinal lymph nodes which adhere to the esophagus.
      c. Rarely symptomatic.
      d. Tracheoesophageal fistula may develop, requiring surgery.
C. Mechanical obstruction — oropharyneal tumors.
D. **Mechanical obstruction — esophagus.**
   1. Esophagitis with strictures.
   2. Tumor.
   3. Proximal esophageal web (Plummer–Vinson syndrome).
   4. Schatzki's ring.
   5. Congenital vascular rings.
   6. Foreign body.
   7. Mediastinal mass with extrinsic compression.
E. **History.**
   1. Dysphagia with liquids more than solids suggests a motility disorder.
   2. Dysphagia progressive from solids to liquids suggests a mechanical obstruction.
   3. Odynophagia suggests spasm or esophagitis. Increased pain with cold liquids is suggestive of spasm.
   4. Difficulty with swallowing or nasopharyngeal reflux suggests a neurologic or muscular disorder.
   5. Symptoms of reflux.

    6. Gurgling with swallowing, regurgitation suggest a Zenker's diverticulum.
    7. Duration of symptoms.
    8. Hematemesis, weight loss, alcohol and tobacco use should be questioned.
F. Diagnostic studies.
    1. Physical exam.
    2. Chest x-ray.
    3. Barium swallow with cinefluoroscopy.
    4. Esophagoscopy with biopsy and brushings.
    5. Esophageal manometry.
        a. Decreased LES pressure — reflux.
        b. Increased LES pressure — achalasia.
        c. Normal LES pressure, uncoordinated contraction — spasm.
    6. Methacholine infusion.
        a. High pressure generated — achalasia.
        b. Low pressure remains — scleroderma.

IV. BENIGN TUMORS OF THE ESOPHAGUS

A. Incidence — rare lesions. Most common are leiomyomas (75%). Others: cysts, polyps, lypoma, hemangioma.
B. Leiomyoma.
    1. Less common in esophagus than in stomach and small bowel.
    2. Most esophageal leiomyomas are in the distal two–thirds.
    3. Less than 5 cm lesions are asymptomatic.
    4. Most (97%) are intramural in the circular muscle layer.
    5. Symptoms.
        a. Progressive intermittent dysphagia most common symptom.
        b. Vague, retrosternal achy pain.
        c. Heartburn.
    6. Diagnosis by chest x-ray, barium swallow, endoscopy.
    7. Treatment.
        a. Enucleation through a thoracotomy (mortality < 2%).
        b. Those tumors not amenable to enucleation (10%) may require esophageal resection (mortality 10%).

V. ESOPHAGEAL CARCINOMA

A. Incidence.
    1. Male : female = 3:1.
    2. Black : white = 4:1.
    3. Peak incidence 50–70 years old.
B. Risk factors.
    1. Alcohol and tobacco use.
    2. Diet.

3. Lower socioeconomic status.
4. History of caustic ingestion (1–5% incidence with mean delay of 40 years).
5. Achalasia — 2–8% incidence of squamous cell carcinoma (SCCA).
6. **Plummer–Vinson syndrome** — esophageal webs, anemia, brittle nails, glossitis.
7. Vitamin and mineral deficiencies.
8. Barrett's esophagus — approximately 10% incidence of adeno-carcinoma. Progression toward malignancy seems irreversible and is not arrested by an antireflux operation.

C. Pathology.
1. 90% are squamous cell carcinomas (SCCA).
2. Adenocarcinomas arise from the gastric cardia or Barrett's esophagus.
3. Incidence by location.
   a. 35% distal 1/3.
   b. 50% middle 1/3.
   c. 15% upper 1/3.
4. The tumor spreads circumferentially and longitudinally via the lymphatics, vascular invasion and direct extension.
5. Usually extramural spread or mediastinal metastasis are present at the time of diagnosis; common distant metastases are to liver, lungs and bone.
6. Tumor length, lymphatic spread, and depth of invasion are important prognostic factors.
7. A fungating mass is the most common appearance, followed by polipoid and less often superficial spreading.

D. Staging (Thompson's based on American Joint Committee).
1. Tumor (T).
   a. T_0 — no demonstrable tumor.
   b. T_{is} — carcinoma *in situ*.
   c. T_1 — length ≤ 5 cm, no obstruction, not circumferential, no extra–esophageal spread.
   d. T_2 — length > 5 cm with obstruction and circumferential, but no extra–esophageal spread.
   e. T_3 — tumor into mediastinal structures.
2. Lymph nodes (N) — cervical esophagus (neck nodes).
   a. N_0 — no nodal metastases.
   b. N_1 — unilateral movable nodes.
   c. N_2 — bilateral movable nodes.
   d. N_3 — fixed nodes.
3. Distant metastases (M).
   a. M_0 — none.
   b. M_1 — metastases present (includes neck and abdominal nodes for thoracic tumor).

4. Stages.
   a. Stage 1 — T_{is} or $T_1N_0M_0$.
   b. Stage 2 — T_1, $T_2N_1N_2M_0$.
   c. Stage 3.
      1) Any T_3N_3 (cervical and primary).
      2) Any N_1 (thoracic primary).
      3) Any M_1.
E. **Clinical presentation.**
   1. Dysphagia, progressive from solids to liquids ($> 80\%$ of cases); any patient older than 40 years with the complaint of dysphagia should be evaluated.
   2. Weight loss (with dysphagia $> 90\%$).
   3. Odynophagia.
   4. Regurgitation.
   5. Anemia.
   6. Vocal cord paralysis (left $>$ right).
   7. Aspiration pneumonia.
   8. Tracheoesophageal or bronchoesophageal fistula.
   9. Pain is a late symptom indicating extraesophageal involvement.
F. **Diagnosis.**
   1. Barium swallow — 92% accuracy.
      a. Abnormal peristalsis with mucosal irregularity.
      b. Annular constriction.
   2. Fiberoptic endoscopy with biopsy and brushings (confirmatory $94–96\%$ of the time).
   3. Bronchoscopy with biopsy to rule out involvement of bronchus for upper 2/3 tumors and a synchronous lung primary.
   4. Nasopharyngoscopy and direct laryngoscopy to rule out a synchronous head and neck lesion (vocal cord involvement).
   5. CT scan of chest and upper abdomen — assess direct extention, mediastinal nodal involvement and evidence of metastases.
G. **Management.**
   1. Principles.
      a. The majority of patients have advanced disease at presentation and are incurable.
      b. Approximately 50% are resectable at presentation; preoperative chemotherapy increases operability rates.
      c. Best results are with early tumors; numbers detected may be increased by screening populations at risk.
      d. Successful palliation is goal of treatment for most patients.
   2. Surgery.
      a. Treatment for early cancers, part of a multimodality approach to more advanced cancers, provides the most successful long–term palliation.

    b. **Esophagectomy techniques.**
       1) Ivor–Lewis — thoracotomy (right for upper 2/3, left for lower 1/3) and abdominal incisions. Esophagectomy, gastric mobilization, G–E anastomosis in chest or neck.
       2) Transhiatal — neck and abdominal incisions. Blunt esophagectomy, gastric mobilization, G–E anastomosis in neck.
       3) Esophageal reconstruction can also be achieved with a colon interposition, jejunal interposition or free graft.
    c. Surgical mortality rates are from 5–30%.
3. Radiotherapy.
    a. Dose range from 4000–6000 cGy to mediastinum.
    b. Primary treatment for poor-risk patient, especially for tumors of upper 1/3.
    c. Palliation for unresectable lesions.
    d. Preoperative radiotherapy failed to show an advantage over surgery alone at the cost of pulmonary injury.
    e. May have a value when given postoperatively for residual mediastinal disease.
    f. Radiation–only 5–year survival slightly worse than surgery–alone 5–year survival.
4. Chemotherapy.
    a. Current regimen 5–FU and cisplatinum.
    b. Increased disease–free and long–term survival when given pre-op, then post-op for responding tumors.
    c. May increase resectability rates by decreasing tumor mass when given preoperatively.
5. Multimodality.
    a. Preoperative chemotherapy, esophagectomy, then post-op chemotherapy for responding tumors and radiotherapy for residual mediastinal disease current treatment of choice.
    b. This combination has increased 5–year survival in early, non–randomized trials.
6. Palliation.
    a. Palliative resection or esophageal bypass provides the best "long–term" palliation.
    b. Successful chemotherapy may obviate the need for surgical palliation.
    c. Laser fulgeration successful for rapidly relieving obstruction.
    d. Repeated dilation, pulsion placement of endoprosthesis is an unfavorable treatment reserved for poor–risk, short–term patients.
7. Prognosis.
    a. Radiotherapy — 4–25%, average 6%.
    b. Surgery — 2–24%, average 10%.
    c. Multimodality — pending.

VI. ESOPHAGEAL RUPTURE AND PERFORATION

A. **Etiology.**
   1. Iatrogenic (most common).
      a. Endoscopy — direct injury or during removal of foreign body. More common with rigid than flexible esophagoscope.
      b. Dilation.
      c. Biopsy.
      d. Intubation (esophageal, endotracheal).
   2. Non–iatrogenic.
      a. Barogenic trauma.
         1) Postemetic — transmural tear following forceful vomiting (**Boerhaave syndrome**); usually associated with gluttony, bulemia, alcohol binge.
         2) Blunt chest or abdominal trauma.
         3) Other (labor, convulsions, defecation, etc.).
      b. Penetrating neck, chest, or abdominal trauma.
      c. Postoperative.
         1) Anastomotic disruption.
         2) Devascularization following pulmonary resection, vagotomy, or repair of hiatus hernia.
      d. Corrosive injuries (acid or alkali).
      e. Erosion by adjacent inflammation.
      f. Carcinoma.

B. **Clinical presentation** — dysphagia, neck or chest pain, fever, tenderness, subcutaneous emphysema, pneumothorax. **Note:** These symptoms and signs following esophageal instrumentation or operation must be attributed to a leak until ruled out with an esophagiogram.

C. **Diagnostic studies.**
   1. Chest x-ray — pneumothorax, pneumomediastinum, pleural effusion, subdiaphragmatic air.
   2. Lateral neck x-ray.
   3. Water soluble contrast study to localize perforation.
   4. If suspicion of leak is high, and water soluble study is negative, dilute barium swallow may identify perforation. The complications of barium mediastinitis are less than that of a missed perforation.

D. **Treatment.**
   1. Early recognition and treatment are essential to survival.
      a. NPO.
      b. Fluid resuscitation.
      c. Broad–spectrum antibiotics.
   2. Non–operative.
      a. Controversial and only applicable in specific situations of a small perforation with minimal contamination, or a "contained" leak in setting of pre–existing periesophageal and mediastinal fibrosis.

    b. NG suction, IV antibiotics, close observation.
3. Operative — repair of perforation with drainage and antibiotics is the preferred treatment.
    a. If perforation is associated with distal obstruction (i.e., stricture or carcinoma), esophageal resection with/without primary anastomosis is appropriate. Reconstruction may have to be delayed.
    b. If a major perforation of lower esophagus:
        1) Wide (frequently bilateral) drainage of chest and mediastinum.
        2) Reconstruction created to prevent G–E reflux.
        3) Divert or collect salivary stream.
        4) Establish access for enteral feeding.
E. **Complications** of esophageal perforation — sepsis, abscess, fistula, empyema.

GASTRIC CANCER

I. EPIDEMIOLOGY
A. Steadily declining death rates due to decreased incidence worldwide.
B. Male:female ratio 2:1.
C. 70% of patients > 50 years old.
D. Highest incidence and mortality in Orient (Japan), most likely due to dietary factors.

II. ETIOLOGIC RISK FACTORS
A. Environment.
   1. Diet — smoked, pickled, salted foods; nitrosoamine compounds.
   2. Local soil factors.
   3. Cigarette smoking, alcohol intake.
B. Genetic.
   1. Increased in type A blood groups.
   2. More common in some families (2–6 x increased risk); however, the inheritance pattern is unknown.
C. Pernicious anemia.
   1. Due to its association with achlorhydria.
   2. 10% of patients with pernicious anemia may develop gastric carcinoma (controversial).
   3. Questionable increased risk from achlorhydria secondary to chronic H_2 blockers.
D. Previous gastric surgery.
   1. Most cases following Billroth II reconstruction > 20 years after the original procedure.
   2. Chronic bile reflux gastritis following pyloric resection/bypass may be an etiologic factor.
E. Polyps.
   1. Approximately 5% are malignant.
   2. Incidence of cancer greatest in polyps ≥ 2 cm. Polyps should be removed for biopsy; polyps < 2 cm can be removed endoscopically, > 2 cm may require wedge gastrectomy.
F. Chronic atrophic gastritis.
G. Hypertrophic gastropathy (Menetrier's disease); up to 10% risk.

III. PATHOLOGY
A. Gastric malignancies.
   1. Carcinoma 90–95%.
   2. Lymphoma 3%.
   3. Leiomyosarcoma 2%.
B. Location of primary — Lesser curve (40%) > Anterior or posterior wall = Circumferential (25%) > Greater curve (10%).
C. Morphology (in order of worsening prognosis).

1. Superficial (6%) — Tumors are detected infrequently in this early stage of disease.
2. Polypoid (7%) — mass extends intraluminally.
3. Fungating (36%).
4. Ulcerative (25%) — 2–8 cm ulcer with a shaggy necrotic base and beaded margins overhanging crater.
5. Diffuse (26%) — "**Linitis plastica**" ("leather bottle").
   a. Diffuse thickening of nondistensible gastric wall.
   b. Worst prognosis of all gross pathologies.

D. Patterns of invasion.
1. Direct extension to adjacent organs.
2. Peritoneal seeding — omentum, parietal peritoneum, ovaries (**Krukenberg's tumors**), cul–de–sac (**Blumer's Shelf**).
3. Hematogenous via the portal or sytemic circulation.
4. Lymphatic.
   a. Regional nodes — greater, lesser curve, celiac axis.
   b. Supraclavicular (**Virchow's**); umbilical (**Sister Mary Joseph's**) nodes — later spread.

IV. DIAGNOSIS

A. Symptoms are rarely present with early gastric carcinoma; patients are usually asymptomatic until the tumor is locally advanced.
1. Pain (96%).
2. Anorexia with weight loss (> 95%).
3. Palpable abdominal mass (50%).
4. Nausea and vomiting (40%).
5. Dysphagia (15%).
6. Ascites, pleural effusions, anemia from metastasis.
7. Hematemesis is rare; however, occult blood in stool is common.
8. Average duration of symptoms to diagnosis is 8 months.
9. Symptoms of fatigue, weight loss, anemia, or indigestion in patients > 40 years old need to be evaluated to rule out gastric carcinoma.

B. Radiology.
1. Barium upper GI series, preferably air contrast.
2. Characteristics of malignant ulcer.
   a. Ulcer in a mass where ulcer bed does not extend outside gastric wall.
   b. Mucosal folds do not radiate from ulcer (they do with benign gastric ulcers).
   c. Ulcers are usually larger than 1 cm.

C. Endoscopy.
1. 90% accurate in diagnosing advanced cancers.
2. Combination of endoscopy, directed biopsy, brushing and lavage cytology improve accuracy.

3. Yearly surveillance gastroscopy recommended for high–risk groups (see section II above).

D. Abdominal CT scan or ultrasound (high resolution/endoscopic) for preoperative staging.

E. Overall, of 100 patients in the U.S. with gastric cancer:
    1. 85–90 are operable.
    2. 60–70 undergo gastrectomy.
    3. 40 will have a resection for cure.
    4. 10 will survive 5 years.
    5. For those patients who are found to have an early superficial lesion, 70–90% 5–year survival following resection is possible.
    6. The two major factors affecting survival following curative resection are **extent of spread** through stomach wall and **involvement of regional lymph nodes.**

V. T–N–M CLASSIFICATION

Primary Tumor (T)

T_1 Tumor limited to mucosa and submucosa regardless of its extent or location.

T_2 Tumor involves the mucosa, the submucosa (including muscularis propria), and extends to or into the serosa, but does not penetrate through the serosa.

T_3 Tumor penetrates through the serosa without invading contiguous structures.

T_4 Tumor penetrates through the serosa and invades the contiguous structures.

Nodal Involvement (N)

N_0 No metastases to regional lymph nodes.

N_1 Involvement of perigastric lymph nodes within 3 cm of the primary tumor along the lesser or greater curvature.

N_2 Involvement of the regional lymph nodes, more than 3 cm from the primary tumor, which are removable at operation, including those located along the left gastric, splenic, celiac, and common hepatic arteries.

N_3 Involvement of other intra–abdominal lymph nodes that are not removable at operation, such as the para–aortic, hepatoduodenal, retropancreatic, and mesenteric nodes.

Distant Metastasis (M)

M_0 No (known) distant metastasis.

M_1 Distant metastasis present.

Surgical Results (R)

R_0 No residual tumor.

R_1 Microscopic residual tumor.

R_2 Macroscopic residual tumor.

VI. TREATMENT
A. **Surgical resection.**
   1. Indicated for both curative intent and palliation. Quality of life is improved following resection for advanced tumors.
   2. Extent of resection and procedure determined by site and extent of tumor, presence of regional or distal disease.
   3. **Curative resection** — 33% of laparotomies with curative intent.
      a. Carcinoma of antrum and pylorus — subtotal gastrectomy (to GE junction on lesser curve and short gastric vessels on greater curve), lesser and greater omentectomy, and division of left gastric artery at celiac axis. Reconstruction optimally by ante–colic gastrojejunostomy.
      b. Carcinoma of cardia, fundus, proximal body — total gastrectomy including regional lymph nodes, lesser and greater omentectomy. Reconstruction with Roux–en–Y esophago-jejunostomy.
   4. **Palliation.**
      a. Usually can be achieved with a subtotal gastrectomy, rarely with gastrojejunostomy or gastrostomy tube.
      b. Surgical palliation should be attempted whenever possible.
      c. Total gastrectomy usually is *not* appropriate for palliation.
   5. **Chemotherapy.**
      a. Therapy with 5–FU, adriamycin, mitomycin, or methyl–CCNU (FAM).
      b. Tolerated in outpatient setting.
      c. 33% response rate, median response 9 months.
      d. Usefulness as an adjunct to surgery is under study.
   6. Radiotherapy — marginal response with external beam irradiation.

VII. LYMPHOMA
A. 2% of all non–Hodgkin's lymphomas, **most common extranodal lymphoma.** Predominant histology is lymphosarcoma or histiocytic lymphoma.
B. Clinical presentation similar to adenocarcinoma.
C. Treatment of choice is **subtotal gastrectomy** followed by external beam radiotherapy and/or chemotherapy — 40% to 90% 5–year survival. The combination chemotherapy used for diffuse non–Hodgkin's lymphoma has been used as an adjunct to resection in patients with greater control of recurrences (especially extra–abdominal recurrences) than irradiation.

VIII. LEIOMYOSARCOMA
A. Rare gastric malignancy.
B. Present usually as bulky intraluminal tumors, with characteristic necrosis of center of tumor, resulting in a large ulcerated lesion.
C. 70% 5–year survival following resection.

PEPTIC ULCER DISEASE

The use of H_2 blockers, surface protectants, and prostaglandins has decreased the need for surgical treatment of peptic ulcer disease. However, specific indications for peptic ulcer surgery remain. Emergency surgery is common for the complications of bleeding and perforation.

I. DUODENAL ULCER (DU)

A. Pathogenesis.
   1. Relative or absolute excess of acidic gastric and peptic secretions.
      a. Increased acid delivery into duodenum.
      b. Impaired neutralization or mucosal defense mechanisms are probably *contributory* but not causative.
   2. Higher rates of gastric acid secretion (basal and stimulated) in 40% of patients.
   3. Increased number of parietal cells.
   4. Increased sensitivity of parietal cells to gastrin.
   5. Increased serum pepsinogen I, reflecting increased acid secretory potential.
   6. Increased vagal tone and gastrin secretion, at least in part secondary to impaired negative feedback loop on gastrin release.
   7. Local infection (e.g., *Campylobacter pylori*).

B. Epidemiology.
   1. DU 10 times more prevalent than gastric ulcer.
   2. Overall incidence is *decreasing* in the U.S. (1.7 / 1000).
   3. Male > female.
   4. 25–35 year age group most commonly affected.
   5. Genetic factor is present — higher incidence in monozygous male twins and O^+ blood type.

C. Pathology.
   1. Rarely malignant.
   2. Usually within 1–2 cm distal to pyloric sphincter.
   3. Equal frequency anterior and posterior walls.
   4. Ulcers that are *multiple* or in the *second and third portion* of the duodenum should arouse suspicion of Zollinger–Ellison (Z–E) syndrome or ulcerations secondary to drug ingestion.

D. Clinical presentation.
   1. Most common symptom — pain is perceived as a "gnawing" or burning sensation when the stomach is empty (hours after eating), and is usually relieved by eating.
   2. DU should be suspected if patient is awakened by pain (1–2 a.m.) and can go back to sleep following relief by eating or antacids.

3. Epigastric tenderness on exam may be present.

E. **Diagnosis and laboratory findings.**

1. **Stool guaiac** — if positive, rule out LGI cause as well.

2. **UGI series** is 75–80% accurate for diagnosis. Positive findings include ulcer crater in duodenal bulb, edema, spasm, duodenal deformity.

3. **Endoscopy** is 95% accurate for diagnosis and may also detect lesions in esophagus, stomach, duodenum (including ampulla). The advantage over UGI is that it can detect bleeding.

4. **Gastric acid analysis** — performed by placing an NG tube, collecting 4 samples at 15–min intervals [**basal acid output (BAO)**] and injecting pentagastrin, histamine or betazole, and collecting 4 samples at 15–min intervals [**maximal acid output (MAO)**].

   a. BAO — upper limit of normal = 5 mEq/hr.

   b. MAO — upper limit of normal = 30 mEq/hr.

   c. Vagotomy decreases maximal acid output by 50%, antrectomy decreases output by 40%, and combined operation (V & A) decreases output by 90%.

   d. This test lacks precise correlation with ulcer disease and is not normally part of the preoperative evaluation for DU.

   e. Can be used to test for the completeness of vagotomy following surgery.

   f. An hourly BAO > 15 mEq/L in the intact stomach or > 5 mEq/L after partial gastrectomy, a 12–hr nocturnal secretion > 1000 ml or 100 mEq and a ratio of BAO to MAO > 0.6 are diagnostic for Z–E syndrome.

   g. Also useful for evaluation of achlorhydria with gastric ulcer. Low/no acid and ulcer should alert to the possibility of gastric carcinoma.

5. **Serum gastrin.**

   a. Not indicated for routine ulcer patient; it is indicated for non-responders to conventional treatment, associated endocrine disorders (rule out MEN–I), recurrent ulcers, or patients with early onset or aggressive ulcer diathesis.

   b. Obtain in fasting state. Value of > 1000 pg/ml strongly suggestive of gastrinoma. Since basal levels may be highly variable in Z–E (200–800 pg/ml), at least 3 fasting levels should be obtained before definitively making the diagnosis of Z–E syndrome.

   c. Must withhold H_2 blockers for at least 24 hrs prior to assay.

   d. Elevated levels (> 200 pg/ml) seen in variety of disorders.

      1) High gastric acid — gastrinoma, retained antrum, gastric outlet obstruction, renal failure, short bowel syndrome.

      2) Low gastric acid — pernicious anemia, chronic gastritis, gastric carcinoma, S/P vagotomy, pheochromocytoma.

6. Amylase may be elevated in posterior penetrating ulcers with pancreatitis or free anterior perforation with spillage of duodenal contents.

F. **Medical treatment.**
  1. Goal of medical therapy is reduction of both acid secretion and activation of pepsinogen; 75% of duodenal ulcers will heal following 6 weeks of adequate therapy; however, long term the disease may be chronic with recurrences requiring medical management or surgery.
  2. Discontinuation of habits and medications associated with DU — alcohol, smoking, aspirin, coffee, all xanthines including tea and chocolate, spices, steroids. Reduce stress if possible.
  3. Antacids.
     a. Magnesium–containing tend to cause diarrhea.
     b. Aluminum–containing tend to cause constipation.
     c. Alternating the two types may be optimal, or use of mixed preparation (e.g., Maalox®).
     d. Calcium–containing antacids may stimulate acid secretion.
     e. Full regimen — 30 ml PO 1 hr and 3 hrs after meals and at bedtime.
  4. H_2 receptor antagonists.
     a. **Cimetidine** [Tagamet®] (300 mg PO p.c. and qhs) — significant side–effects (impotence, confusion, gynecomastia).
     b. **Ranitidine** [Zantac®] (150 mg PO bid) — may have less side–effects and improved compliance.
     c. **Famotidine** [Pepcid®] — 5–10 mg PO bid.
     d. A single higher bedtime dose may be as effective as divided doses.
     e. Yearly relapse rate is 30% if, after complete healing, H_2 blockers are continued at bedtime (ranitidine 150 mg PO qhs).
  5. **Sucralfate** [Carafate®] — 1 g PO 1 hr prior to meals and at bedtime.
     a. Basic aluminum sucrose sulfate which is dissociated in an acid medium (pH < 3–4) and forms a negatively charged polymerized molecule that adheres to the proteinaceous exudate (positive–charge proteins: albumin, fibrinogen, and damaged or dead cells) found within the ulcer.
     b. Binding lasts up to 6 hours with little (3–5%) systemic absorption.
     c. Healing action thought to be a result of a physical barrier that prevents acid and pepsin from acting further on the ulcer. Also produces a 30% inhibition of pepsin activity and adsorption of surface–active bile salts.
     d. Minimal acid–neutralizing capacity.
     e. Useful in treatment of active duodenal and gastric ulcers. A good protectant against the disruptive effects of alcohol or non–steroidal anti–inflammatory drugs.

    f. Requires an acid medium. Should be taken on an empty stomach and antacids should be avoided.

    g. Comparable to cimetidine in efficacy in the healing of duodenal ulcers.

    h. Most noticeable side–effect is constipation.

  6. Omeprazole (Losec®), a parietal cell proton pump blocker, reduces acid secretion by 99%. Hypergastrinemia is a side-effect.

  7. Synthetic prostaglandins of the E series (arbaprostil, misoprostol, enprostil) have been shown to be effective in healing duodenal and gastric ulcers in clinical studies. Their major mechanism of action is uncertain (have anti–secretory as well as cyto-protective effect).

  8. Anticholinergics – pirenzepine may be helpful as an adjunct to H_2 blockers for resistant ulcers.

  9. Mild sedation – especially in stressful situations (i.e., Ativan® 1 mg, Valium® 2.5 mg PO q6h meal).

 10. Following diagnosis, the patient should undergo a 6–week course of therapy with H_2 blockers and/or antacids. At 6 weeks, patients are re–studied; those that have not healed may be changed to sucralfate. If ulcer is still active at 12 weeks, then surgery is recommended.

 11. Ulcer relapse after healing may be decreased by single nocturnal dose of H_2 blockers – ranitidine 150 mg PO qhs or cimetidine 400 mg PO qhs.

G. Surgical treatment.

  1. Indications.

    a. Intractability – persistent demonstrable ulcer despite adequate medical therapy or ulcer recurrences resulting in disability, interference in patient's lifestyle.

    b. Hemorrhage – see "GI Bleeding".

    c. Gastric outlet obstruction – definite indication.

    d. Perforation into the peritoneal cavity or adjacent organs – definite indication.

  2. Preoperative evaluation.

    a. UGI barium study and/or fiberoptic endoscopy (preferably performed or attended by the operating surgeon) mandatory for intractability, hemorrhage, or obstruction.

    b. In suspected perforation, rigid abdomen, and appropriate history are sufficient indications for exploration. Free air under the diaphragm is best seen on upright CXR, present in 75% of perforations. Barium studies are contraindicated; use water soluble contrast if suspect perforation.

    c. Gastric analysis and serum gastrin as indicated.

  3. Procedures.

    a. Resections.

1) **Subtotal gastrectomy (SG)** — mortality 1–3%, recurrence 4%. No longer commonly done because of increased postoperative problems and no demonstrable superiority over lesser procedures.
2) **Truncal vagotomy and antrectomy (V & A)** — mortality 1–3%, recurrence 1%.
3) **Truncal vagotomy and drainage (V & D)** — mortality < 1%, recurrence 6–7%.

b. Reconstruction.
1) **Billroth I** — gastroduodenostomy (Fig. 1).
2) **Billroth II** — closure of duodenal stump and gastro-jejunostomy (Fig. 2).
3) **Roux–en–Y gastrojejunostomy.**

FIGURE 1
Billroth I

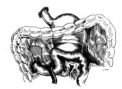

FIGURE 2
Retrocolic Billroth II

c. **Selective vagotomy** — denervates entire stomach, but preserves innervation to liver and biliary tree and to the celiac ganglia so as to minimize post–vagotomy diarrhea and gallstones. Because entire stomach is denervated, antral stasis may occur (10-20% of cases); thus some type of drainage procedure is generally performed along with selective vagotomy.

    d. Proximal gastric vagotomy (PGV) — also known as parietal cell vagotomy, highly selective vagotomy, and superselective vagotomy.

      1) Mortality < 1%.

      2) Recurrence variable due to variable technical expertise; long-term recurrence at least 10%, but increases linearly with time.

      3) 90% of recurrences respond to H_2–blockers post PGV.

      4) Antrum and pylorus is not denervated; therefore, a drainage procedure is not necessary.

H. Selection of operation for peptic ulcer disease.

  1. No one operation is best — clinical and intraoperative findings must dictate which to perform (i.e., thin woman with nutritional problems, you would tend to avoid resective procedures; for an alcoholic with intractable disease or a person needing to take aspirin or non-steroid anti-inflammatory agents, you would probably pick antrectomy and vagotomy).

  2. Secretory levels (BAO and MAO) are *no guide* to operation.

  3. V & A definitely has lowest recurrence, but has a significant incidence of dumping and complications. Resections are poorly tolerated by middle–aged females, especially asthenic females.

  4. PGV technically difficult, thus higher recurrence, but very low incidence of side–effects or operative morbidity.

  5. Surgical approach to duodenal ulcer disease depends upon indications for surgery, patient's general medical condition, and findings at laparotomy.

    a. Intractability — if no evidence of pyloric obstruction or history of life-threatening complication in past (i.e., bleeding or perforation), proximal gastric vagotomy (PGV) should be considered. Trade-off and long-term morbidity for higher recurrence rate. Recurrences refractory to medical therapy following PGV should undergo V & A.

    b. Perforation — if patient is stable and there is minimal peritoneal soilage, perforation should be closed or patched and a proximal gastric vagotomy performed. If patient is unstable or there is long–standing purulent peritonitis, the perforation should be closed or patched and the patient should be treated with antacids and/or H_2 blockers. Some surgeons recommend this approach when perforation is first manifestation of PUD (30% will have no further manifestations).

    c. Bleeding — these patients have the most life–threatening complication and therefore deserve the most definitive procedure possible. If stable, truncal V & A is procedure of choice. If unstable, bleeding point should be oversewn and truncal V & D (pyloroplasty or gastrojejunostomy) should be performed.

      d. Obstruction — the obstruction generally involves the pylorus and thus must be either resected or bypassed (gastro-enterostomy, pyloroplasty) along with a truncal vagotomy.

I. **Complications — early.**

  1. **Duodenal stump leakage** — breakdown of duodenal stump following a Billroth II reconstruction.

      a. Usually results following closure of a badly scarred or inflamed duodenum.

      b. Presents as severe epigastric or RUQ pain, fever and leukocytosis on the 3rd–6th post–op day.

      c. Immediate reoperation and drainage of stump is essential.

      d. Breakdown is minimized by use of tube duodenostomy at initial procedure if duodenal stump intensity is questioned.

  2. **Gastric stasis** — loss of coordinated gastric contractility usually secondary to a vagotomy.

J. **Complications — late.**

  1. **Dumping syndrome** — distention of jejunum by transudation of extracellular fluid into bowel lumen due to rapid gastric emptying of hypertonic chyme. Neuroendocrine response of the small bowel with secretion of gut hormones may mediate some of the systemic effects.

      a. Incidence — SG 36%, V & A 29%, V & D 25%, PGV < 5%. Incidence is much higher with resection, bypass or disruption of pylorus.

      b. Manifested by nausea, weakness, sweating, cramps, oligemia, hypotension, vertigo, tachycardia, palpitations, diarrhea occurring after eating (especially high carbohydrate).

      c. Most patients experience some degree of dumping early postoperatively, but symptoms subside in time or with dietary modification.

      d. Treatment — initially, use conservative measures.

        1) High protein/fat, low carbohydrate diet. Reduce the load of simple sugars and starches (candy, sugar, ice cream, jams, jellies, bread, pasta).

        2) Avoid liquids with meals — take fluids between meals.

        3) Frequent small feedings.

        4) Lie down for 20–30 minutes after meals (slows gastric emptying).

        5) Antispasmodic drugs.

        6) Psychotherapy and hypnosis helpful in a select few.

      e. Surgical treatment — indicated for disabling symptoms. Interposition of reversed jejunal segment between gastric remnant and duodenum is most common procedure.

  2. **Afferent loop syndrome** — due to chronic partial obstruction of proximal loop of a gastrojejunostomy. Symptoms are post-prandial distention, usually RUQ pain and nausea relieved by sudden vomiting of pure bile (no food).

   a. If the problem is minimal and if it occurs in immediate post-op period, wait for anastomosis edema to subside; maintain on conservative treatment. Occasionally the obstruction is near total in post–op period and requires urgent operation. The most severe form may result in **acute necrosis** of the afferent loop and **fulminant pancreatitis**, with a high mortality.

   b. If chronic, requires surgical decompression by afferent-efferent jejunojejunostomy (Fig. 3) or revision of gastrojejunostomy to Roux–en–Y or gastroduodenostomy.

   c. The problem can be minimized at initial operation by taking down the duodenal redundancy at the ligament of Treitz and being certain that the retrocolic gastrojejunostomy is below the opening in the mesocolon.

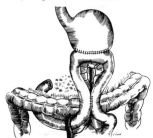

FIGURE 3
Afferent – Efferent Jejunojejunostomy

3. **Marginal ulceration** — recurrent ulcer occurring at the anastomotic site following gastrojejunostomy.
   a. Pain and bleeding are most common symptoms.
   b. Causes (in order of frequency):
      1) Incomplete vagotomy.
      2) Inadequate drainage.
      3) Inadequate gastric resection.
      4) Inadequate alkaline neutralization (long afferent limb after Billroth II).
      5) Drugs (alcohol, salicylates, anti–inflammatory agents, steroids, etc.).
      6) Retained antrum, particularly an antral remnant in the duodenal stump with a Billroth II.

       7) G–cell hyperplasia.

       8) Z–E syndrome.

   c. Endoscopic confirmation is mandatory because UGI only diagnostic in 50% of cases.

   d. **Treatment is surgical**, requiring **revagotomy** (if suspicion or proof of incomplete vagotomy), re-resection (if <50% resection done initially), or completion gastrectomy with esophagojejunostomy. Make certain there is no retained antrum at the duodenal suture line by reviewing pathology specimen.

   e. Medical therapy alone is usually *not* curative.

  4. **Bile reflux gastritis** — gastritis induced by reflux of bile into stomach usually after gastrojejunostomy, resulting in constant epigastric pain, nausea and vomiting, aggravated by food.

   a. Endoscopy reveals red, friable mucosa.

   b. Medical treatment using H_2 blockers or Carafate® is the first line of therapy.

   c. Use of bile salt binding agents such as cholestyramine may be attempted, but not shown to be effective.

   d. Symptoms may not correlate with degree of gastritis.

   e. Surgical treatment may be judiciously considered following thorough evaluation. Goal of surgical treatment is to divert bile so that it does not enter the stomach. Surgical revision of anastomosis usually requires Roux–en–Y gastrojejunostomy; **Tanner 19** is also useful and has the advantage of relieving unsuspected efferent loop obstruction.

  5. **Post–vagotomy diarrhea.**

   a. Increased stool frequency in a majority of patients undergoing vagotomy, usually self–limited.

   b. Diarrhea usually episodic instead of constant.

   c. Pathophysiology poorly understood.

   d. Most are treated satisfactorily with constipating agents. Severe, disabling cases may require reversed segment of jejunum or ileum to slow transit time.

K. Giant duodenal ulcer.

  1. Variant of peptic ulcer disease. Defined as a full–thickness ulceration at least 2 cm in diameter, usually involving a large portion of the duodenal bulb.

  2. Easily missed on upper GI series due to large size of the ulcer that causes it to look like a scarred duodenal bulb or duodenal diverticulum.

  3. Mortality rate variable; 7–40% reported.

  4. These patients do very poorly with medical therapy alone, and the mortality rate is increased if emergency surgery is required for perforation or acute hemorrhage.

  5. Medical therapy is useful as an adjunct to surgery.

6. **Surgical approach** — definitive acid–reduction operation is the procedure of choice.
   a. Truncal V & A whenever technically possible and the patient is stable.
   b. Size and extent of the ulcer often makes closure of the duodenal stump difficult. In these situations, a duodenostomy tube should be utilized.
   c. Truncal vagotomy and pyloroplasty or gastrojejunostomy if patient is unstable or antrectomy is not technically possible.

II. GASTRIC ULCER (GU)

The major issue with gastric ulcers is distinguishing between a benign ulcer and gastric carcinoma.

A. Pathogenesis.
1. Atrophic gastritis usually present.
2. 95% on lesser curvature, near the incisura.
3. Multiple in 2%.
4. Associated DU in 42%.
5. Type I — no history of PUD, located on lesser curvature, normal or low gastric acid output, serum gastrin may be high.
6. Type II — GU associated with DU.
7. Type III — prepyloric ulcer.
8. Types II and III — resemble DU in behavior and response to treatment. If surgery required, should be treated as a high acid duodenal ulcer.
9. In absence of specific factors (salicylates, non–steroidal anti-inflammatory drugs, alcohol), bile reflux (with pyloric sphincter dysfunction) is likely a causative factor of type I ulcers.
10. Smoking and psychologic factors also play a role.

B. Clinical findings.
1. Peak incidence 40–60 year old group.
2. Pain similar to DU.
3. Pain often 1/2–11/2 hours after eating (sooner than pain with DU).
4. Pain may be relieved by food or antacids, but may also be exacerbated by eating, especially warm liquids or alcohol.

C. Diagnosis.
1. **UGI (air contrast).**
   a. Contour important in differentiating benign and malignant. Rugal folds radiate from center of GU but not carcinoma.
   b. Benign ulcers tend to penetrate beyond the projected line of the wall of the stomach, whereas malignant ulcers more often represent an erosion into a filling defect that protrudes into the stomach.

      c. Serial exams — It is said that malignant ulcers will not heal, but they sometimes appear to. Not all non–healing ulcers are malignant, however.

  2. **Endoscopy.**
      a. Ulcerated carcinoma will appear exophytic with irregularity of surrounding mucosa.
      b. Benign appearance does not rule out neoplasm; *always* biopsy gastric ulcers.
      c. Take multiple biopsies, especially at edge (not center).

  3. **Cytology** — if properly collected and read, 95% accuracy for diagnosis of carcinoma.

  4. **Gastric analysis** — achlorhydria suggests malignancy. Type I patients have low or normal basal and Histalog or pentagastrin stimulated acid secretion.

D. Medical treatment.
  1. Elimination of exacerbating factors — tobacco, alcohol, spices, drugs, stress.
  2. H$_2$ blockers — 6–week trial warranted if biopsy is negative for malignancy.
  3. Antacids probably of no value in GU.
  4. Sucralfate — slightly inferior to cimetidine in the healing of gastric ulcer.
  5. Gastric ulcers are more difficult to heal than DU — 2–year recurrence rate after healing with medical therapy is 40%.

E. Surgical treatment — the major objective is to excise the non–healing ulcer. If type II or III, do an acid–reducing procedure.
  1. **Indications.**
      a. Absence of documented complete healing following adequate medical therapy (6–12 weeks).
      b. Bleeding, obstruction, perforation similar to DU.
  2. Elective operative mortality 0–6%.
  3. Emergency operative mortality for bleeding or perforation is as high as 34%.
  4. Type I — partial gastrectomy (antrectomy) alone has very low recurrence rate.
  5. Types II and III — standard DU (acid–reducing) operation.
  6. If ulcer is in proximal stomach, locally excise and close; consider distal gastrectomy or drainage procedure if stasis is a contributing factor. Distal gastrectomy alone usually results in healing of Type I gastric ulcer, but extensive biopsies must be taken to confirm absence of malignancy.
  7. For ulcers at or near the GE junction, consider a Pauchet gastrectomy (Fig. 4).

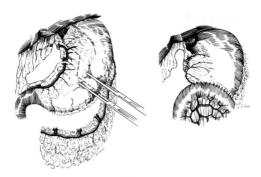

FIGURE 4
Pauchet resection of antrum and entire lesser curve
up to the GE junction

III. COMPLICATIONS OF GU AND DU

A. Perforation.

1. Usually with anterior DU or giant DU.
2. 75% have antecedent symptoms.
3. Abrupt onset of excruciating pain, often radiating to tip of scapula (diaphragmatic irritation), RLQ pain simulating appendicitis if fluid accumulates in right paracolic gutter.
4. Nausea and vomiting common, hematemesis rare.
5. Rigid abdomen.
6. Free air under diaphragm on upright CXR is sentinel finding in appropriate clinical setting (75%), but may be absent if perforation is rapidly walled off.
7. May occur into lesser sac if posterior; air–fluid level seen on upright abdominal film.
8. Perforated GU much less common, but has higher morbidity and mortality.
9. Treatment of perforated GU.
   a. Distal gastric resection incorporating ulcer.
   b. Excision and closure alone in poor–risk patients with biopsies to rule out malignancy.
10. Treatment of perforated DU (see section I–F and I–G).

B. Obstruction.

1. Usually seen with preplyoric and duodenal ulcers.

2. Incidence of obstruction less than perforation.
3. Results from edema during acute phase or from inflammation and fibrosis in chronic disease. With gastric ulcer alone, lesser curve edema and interruption of propagated lesser curve peristaltic wave may interfere with gastric emptying.
4. If seen with type I GU, probably malignant.
5. Long prior history of PUD common.
6. Abdominal pain, nausea and vomiting, early satiety.
7. On exam may have distended, palpable stomach and succusion splash.
8. Characteristic electrolyte imbalance (hypokalemic, hypochloremic, metabolic alkalosis).
9. Saline load test is diagnostic of gastric outlet obstruction.
    a. Empty stomach with NG tube.
    b. Instill 750 cc NS.
    c. Place patient in sitting position for 30 min.
    d. Aspirate contents — positive test if > 400 cc residual.
10. **Treatment.**
    a. NG suction, initiate H2 blockers.
    b. IV fluids.
    c. Start TPN early — these patients are already nutritionally deprived. A prolonged period of conservative treatment without nutritional supplementation will place a patient at greater risk should surgery become necessary.
    d. If no resolution within 3–5 days of intensive in–hospital medical treatment, operative intervention is indicated.
    e. V & A commonly employed, but V & gastroenterostomy or V & P can be performed in certain cases if resection of pylorus is too dangerous technically or if patient is a poor choice for resection.
        1) Consider gastrostomy — incidence of poor gastric emptying post–op is high, especially after vagotomy.
        2) Needle catheter or other jejunostomy useful for same reason.
    f. Massive gastric distention produces a non–contractile atonic stomach — metaclopramide (10 mg IV or PO q 6 h) may be useful postoperatively due to persistent gastric atony.
C. **Hemorrhage** — see "GI Bleeding".

IV. **ZOLLINGER–ELLISON SYNDROME**
   (see "Miscellaneous Endocrine Disorders")

V. **STRESS ULCERATION**
   (also see "GI Bleeding")
A. UGI bleeding in patients subjected to other physiologic stress.

B. Most commonly seen in ICU setting, acute burns, trauma, increased intracranial pressure (especially in neurosurgical patients with use of steroids).
   1. Overt clinically significant bleeding has decreased due to greater awareness and wide use of prophylactic measures.
   2. Endoscopic evidence can be found in up to 80% of patients with burns > 35% TBSA.
   3. 25-40% incidence in ICU patients with 7% requiring transfusion.

C. Common associated clinical factors.
   1. Uremia due to ATN.
   2. Mechanical ventilation.
   3. Hypotension.
   4. Sepsis.

D. Gastric mucosal ischemia and intraluminal acid are key pathogenetic factors.
   1. Gastric mucosa is very sensitive to periods of hypoperfusion.
   2. Patients are usually not acid hypersecretors.
   3. Increased acid back–diffusion and bile reflux may be injurious agents to compromised mucosa.

E. Best diagnostic maneuver is endoscopy.

F. Prophylaxis.
   1. Antacids are mainstay — maintain gastric pH ≥ 4.5. Increase amount and frequency of antacids as needed. If pH monitoring is unavailable or unreliable, 60 cc of antacid every 2 hours (Clamp tube 1/2 hour, to suction 1 1/2 hours) usually neutralizes acid.
   2. Antacid therapy can reduce incidence of superficial erosion to ≤ 5% and transfusable bleed rate to 1%.
   3. Usual doses of H_2 blockers alone fail to control low gastric pH in 33% of these patients.

G. Treatment — see "GI Bleeding".
   1. Non–operative treatment successful in 75%.
   2. The operation used depends on the condition of the patient.
      a. Oversewing of bleeding points and a V & P is quickly performed, but has a high re–bleed rate.
      b. V & A is a longer procedure, but more certain to prevent re–bleeding. Its use is restricted by the general poor condition of these patients.
      c. May require high subtotal gastrectomy if bleeding sites cannot be controlled by (a) or (b).

APPENDICITIS

Appendicitis is one of the common causes of abdominal pain and may be extraordinarily difficult to diagnose, especially at the extremes of age.

I. INCIDENCE
A. Incidence of acute appendicitis has declined for unclear reasons.
B. Appendicitis is rare in infants and then increases throughout childhood with peak incidence in the teens and early twenties.

II. PATHOPHYSIOLOGY
A. **Etiology** — appendicitis results from the luminal obstruction of the appendix.
   1. 60% — hyperplasia of submucosal lymphoid follicles. Most common etiology in children, teens, and young adults.
   2. 35% — fecalith. Most common in adults.
   3. 4% — foreign bodies.
   4. 1% — stricture, tumors.
   5. < 1% — parasites.
B. **Natural history.**
   1. Luminal obstruction causes mucus to accumulate and leads to distention of the appendix and bacterial overgrowth from stasis.
   2. Distention causes obstruction of lymphatic and venous drainage.
   3. A localized abscess may form at this stage — **acute focal appendicitis.**
   4. A mixed flora infection quickly progresses throughout the wall of the edematous appendix — **acute suppurative appendicitis.**
   5. Worsening edema, continued mucosal secretion, and ongoing infection finally occlude the arterial supply leading to **gangrenous appendicitis.**
   6. Persistently elevated intraluminal pressure eventually leads to perforation through a gangrenous portion of the wall — **acute perforated appendicitis.**
      a. The perforation may be walled off by omentum and surrounding small bowel, producing a localized infection. This barrier may fail if the process continues.
      b. Free spillage into abdominal cavity results in generalized peritonitis.
   7. Fecaliths are more commonly associated with progression to gangrenous perforation (90% with fecaliths) than acute simple appendicitis (40% with fecaliths) in adults.

III. DIAGNOSIS
A. A high index of suspicion and early surgical intervention are key.

B. **Symptoms** – classical presentation occurs in just over 50% of patients.
   1. Usually begins with periumbilical or crampy epigastric pain due to luminal obstruction of appendix.
   2. Anorexia, nausea, and vomiting *follow* the onset of pain. "So frequent is anorexia or nausea at least to some degree that the presence of hunger should raise serious question of the diagnosis of acute appendicitis" (Zachary Cope).
   3. Abdominal pain then becomes persistent in the RLQ due to localized parietal peritoneal inflammation.
   4. Generalized peritonitis occurs only after perforation and free contamination of the peritoneum.
   5. Alteration of bowel function (constipation, diarrhea) is not a consistent finding.
   6. **Points to remember.**
      a. Anorexia may not be present in children.
      b. Atypical presentations are more common at the extremes of age and in patients on steroids or antibiotics.
      c. The location of the appendix is highly variable (Fig. 1); 65% are found posterio–medial to the cecum; unusual locations of the appendix may lead to an atypical presentation.

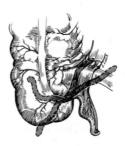

FIGURE 1

C. **Signs.**
   1. Temperature rarely is > 38° C unless there is abscess formation or generalized peritonitis.
   2. Classically, the patient is most tender at **McBurney's point**. (On an imaginary line between the umbilicus and the right anterior iliac spine, this point is at the junction of the middle and lateral thirds) (Fig. 2).

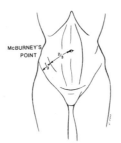

FIGURE 2
McBurney's Point

3. Localized peritonitis occurs in the RLQ with guarding, heightened sensation to touch and pinprick in the RLQ (cutaneous hyperesthesia) and referred pain in the RLQ with palpation of the LLQ (**Rovsing's sign**).
4. During rectal and/or pelvic exam, the patient may feel pain on the right. A tender mass may be present with a pelvic abscess.
5. **Iliopsoas sign** — passive extension of the right hip worsens the pain (usually with a retrocecal appendix causing retroperitoneal inflammation).
6. **Obturator sign** — pain with internal rotation of a flexed hip (usually associated with a pelvic appendix).
7. A palpable tender mass in the RLQ represents a periappendiceal abscess or phlegmon.

D. **Laboratory tests.**
   1. One-third of patients, particularly older adults, may have a normal WBC count. Even with a normal WBC count, most have an abnormal differential with a left shift. Less than 4% have a normal WBC count and differential.
   2. Urinalysis may contain protein and a few WBC's or RBC's.

E. **Radiologic studies** — no pathognomonic findings in early appendicitis.
   1. A radiopaque fecalith in the RLQ is helpful when accompanied by the appropriate signs.
   2. Absent bowel gas in the RLQ with a normal bowel gas pattern in the remainder of the abdomen.
   3. Gangrenous or perforated appendix — intramural gas in appendix, displaced cecum, gas in a RLQ abscess, or free air in the peritoneum.

    4. Loss of the right psoas shadow usually with late or complicated appendicitis and retroperitoneal inflammation.

    5. Loss of the properitoneal fat line of the right flank.

    6. **Barium enema** — may be considered for patients with increased operative risk secondary to systemic disease, patients in a high negative laparotomy group (young women), and late presentations with a possible periappendiceal abscess.

      a. Non–filling or partial filling of appendix with extrinsic compression of cecum are diagnostic.

      b. 10% false–negative rate.

    7. Introduction of graded compression ultrasonography of the cecum and appendix in the hands of experts has proven helpful in difficult cases.

    8. **Pelvic and adnexal ultrasound** may show a tubo–ovarian source of symptoms.

F. Laparoscopy may be useful in young women, but has an operative risk similar to simple appendectomy.

IV. DIFFERENTIAL DIAGNOSIS

A. Young children.

    1. Acute gastroenteritis.

    2. Mesenteric adenitis — usually preceded by URI.

    3. Meckel's diverticulitis.

    4. Intussusception — most common in children < 2.

    5. Enteric duplication.

    6. Henoch–Schoenlein purpura.

    7. Postero–basilar pneumonia.

    8. Unrecognized blunt trauma.

B. Teenagers and young adults.

    1. Females — acute cystitis, urinary tract infection, ovarian/tubal pathology, Mittleschmerz, PID, ectopic/normal pregnancy, endometriosis, ruptured ovarian cyst, ovarian torsion.

    2. Males — testicular torsion, epididymitis.

    3. Mesenteric adenitis.

    4. Regional enteritis.

    5. Right renal/ureteral calculus.

    6. Acute onset diabetes with hyperlipidemia, acidosis.

    7. Trauma.

    8. Hepatitis.

    9. Mononucleosis.

    10. Gastroenteritis.

C. Adults.

    1. Gastroenteritis.

    2. Diverticulitis.

3. Right renal/ureteral calculus.
4. Perforated duodenal/gastric ulcer.
5. Acute cholecystitis.
6. Pancreatitis.
7. Intestinal obstruction.
8. Prostatitis.
9. Colon carcinoma.
10. Perforated ileal diverticulum.
11. Mesenteric vascular occlusion.
12. Abdominal aortic aneurysm.
13. Infarct of epiploic appendage or omentum.
14. Etc., etc.

V. SPECIAL CIRCUMSTANCES

A. Infants and young children.
  1. Presentation is quite similar to acute gastroenteritis.
  2. Subsequent delay in diagnosis leads to high rate of perforation: infants approximately 100%, < 2 approximately 70%, < 5 approximately 50%.
  3. Mortality for perforated appendicitis is approximately 5%.

B. Elderly.
  1. Symptoms may be less pronounced with a delay in seeking medical treatment and a delay in diagnosis.
  2. Approximately 30% are perforated at the time of operation.
  3. Diminished physiologic reserve may also contribute to the high morbidity and mortality.
  4. Look for a concomitant carcinoma of the right colon in patients > 50.

C. Pregnancy.
  1. **Most common extrauterine abdominal procedure** performed during pregnancy.
  2. Most frequent during the initial two trimesters. Presentation and natural course similar to non-pregnant women. Operation should *not* be delayed secondary to pregnancy.
  3. Appendicitis in third trimester notable for cephalad and lateral displacement of appendix, impaired local containment of inflammation/perforation. Delay in diagnosis resulting in rupture results in an increased fetal mortality (35% *vs.* 10% non-ruptured).

VI. TREATMENT

A. If acute or perforated appendicitis is suspected, immediate exploration and appendectomy is indicated.

B. Periappendiceal abscess ("walled off" perforation) or phlegmon.
  1. Conservative treatment may be indicated. Immediate exploration has a higher incidence of intestinal fistula formation and need

for a right colectomy due to the dense inflammatory process encountered.

2. NPO until documented improvement; broad–spectrum IV antibiotics with gram–negative and anaerobic coverage; serial exams.

3. If the patient improves, continue IV antibiotics for 10 days, followed by PO antibiotics (trimethoprim–sulfamethoxazole, metronidazole).

4. Resolution of the abscess or phlegmon should be documented by serial ultrasound or abdominal CT scan. Resolution is followed by interval appendectomy 6 weeks after the original attack.

5. Adequate drainage of localized abscesses with radiologic guidance (ultrasound, CT) has been successful.

6. If pain, fever, intestinal obstruction persist or worsen, consider exploratory laprarotomy with abscess drainage and appendectomy.

C. **Negative appendectomies** are acceptable in 20% of cases. "There is only one way to have a 100% accurate diagnostic record for acute appendicitis, and that is to wait until they all rupture" (Mark Ravitch).

1. The morbidity/mortality for acute uncomplicated appendicitis is 0.6%, perforated appendix 5%.

2. When a normal appendix is encountered, the pelvic organs, cecum, terminal ileum (regional enteritis, Meckel's), gallbladder, duodenum, and stomach should be examined to rule out other causes of the patient's symptoms.

3. The excessive morbidity of perforated appendicitis justifies a relatively high incidence of negative appendectomies.

VI. APPROACH TO THE PATIENT WITH SUSPECTED ACUTE APPENDICITIS

A. Patients with minimal findings who improve rapidly under observation may be discharged without further work–up.

B. Serial exams every 2 hrs until the diagnosis is made or the patient recovers.

C. Vital signs hourly.

D. Initial labs — CBC with differential, urinalysis, electrolytes, CXR, AXR, IVP if a renal calculus is suspected. Gram stain and culture any cervical or urethral discharge.

E. Serial CBC's every 4 hours.

F. NPO, IVF.

G. I/O's.

H. Do *not* administer analgesics or antibiotics until the diagnosis is made. These may mask the signs of peritonitis.

I. The decision to operate or treat conservatively should be made within 12 hours following admission.

INFLAMMATORY BOWEL DISEASE (IBD)

IBD represents one of the more difficult problems encountered in general surgery. It is important to distinguish between the two principal diseases — Crohn's disease and ulcerative colitis. From the standpoint of the surgeon, resection for ulcerative colitis (with or without some form of continence–preserving procedure) almost always results in cure. Crohn's disease, however, is chronic and recurrent, and the surgical approach is to reserve operative therapy for the treatment of the complications and intractability.

I. DEFINITIONS

A. **IBD** usually refers to two diseases that may be difficult to differentiate on clinical grounds.
   1. **Ulcerative colitis (UC)** — a diffuse inflammatory disease limited to the mucosa of the colon and rectum. "Backwash ileitis" may be present, but resolves after colonic resection.
   2. **Crohn's disease** (regional enteritis, granulomatous colitis) — chronic, relapsing, transmural, usually segmental, and often granulomatous inflammatory disorder which can involve any portion of the GI tract.

II. ULCERATIVE COLITIS

A. **Etiology** — unknown. Multiple theories include:
   1. Infectious — viral, bacterial, mycobacterial.
   2. Autoimmune — less likely.
   3. Genetic — increased in whites, females and Jews (2–4 x); 50% less in blacks; familial predisposition.
   4. Psychological — not supported by recent studies.
   5. Environmental — diet, geographic distribution.
B. **Epidemiology.**
   1. Bimodal distribution of onset age — 15–30, 50–70.
   2. Females affected slightly more frequently than males.
   3. Family history of IBD present in 15–40% of cases.
   4. Incidence — 5–12/100,000.
C. **Clinical manifestations/evaluation.**
   1. Signs and symptoms (incidence in %):
      a. **Diarrhea** (79%), abdominal pain (71%), rectal bleeding (55%), pus and mucus in stool, weight loss (20%), tenesmus (15%), vomiting (14%), fever (11%).
      b. Onset may be insidious or acute, fulminant (15%).
      c. Abdominal tenderness present with severe disease.
      d. Extraintestinal manifestations — see II.E.1 below.
   2. Disease distribution.
      a. Confined to colon and rectum; no skip areas.

  b. 10% have "backwash" ileitis; resolves after colonic resection.
  c. Almost always involves rectum (95%); ulcerative proctitis if only rectum involved.
3. Laboratory findings.
  a. Anemia, leukocytosis, elevated ESR.
  b. Negative stool cultures for ova and parasites.
  c. Severe disease – hypoalbuminemia; water, electrolyte and vitamin depletion; steatorrhea.
4. **X-ray findings.**
  a. Plain abdominal films – follow colonic size during acute phase or if ileus–like pattern to rule out toxic megacolon.
  b. Barium enema – mucosal irregularity, ulcers, destruction of mucosal pattern, loss of haustrations, colonic narrowing and shortening, increased presacral space, stricture (rule out malignancy); ileum spared.
5. **Sigmoidoscopy.**
  a. Essential to diagnosis.
  b. Rectal mucosa – dull, hyperemic, granular, friable, edematous.
  c. Uniform disease pattern.
  d. Biopsy findings.
    1) Mucous depletion in goblet cells.
    2) Inflammatory polyps in healing stage.
6. Colonoscopy.
  a. Not necessary to establish diagnosis.
  b. Valuable for specific investigations (stricture, rule out malignancy) and for cancer surveillance in chronic disease.
D. **Differential diagnosis.**
  1. Crohn's disease – 10% of IBD cases are indeterminate.
  2. Neoplasm, diverticulitis, spastic colitis.
  3. Infectious enteritis – bacillary dysenteries (*Salmonella*, *Shigella*, *Campylobacter*, amebiasis), gonococcal proctitis, *Chlamydia trachomatis*.
  4. Pseudomembranous (antibiotic–associated) colitis.
  5. Ischemic colitis.
E. **Complications.**
  1. **Extraintestinal.**
    a. Skin – erythema nodosum, pyoderma gangrenosum, erythema multiforme, aphthous ulcers/stomatitis.
    b. Eyes – conjunctivitis, iritis (uveitis), episcleritis.
    c. Joints – arthritis, sacroileitis, ankylosing spondylitis (association of the HLA-B27 antigen with ankylosing spondylitis in patients who have ankylosing spondylitis and IBD).

      d. Hepatobiliary — fatty liver, pericholangitis, hepatitis, bile duct carcinoma; UC probably leading cause of sclerosing cholangitis.
2. Anorectal.
      a. Hemorrhoids, anal fissure, rectal stricture common.
      b. Rectovaginal fistula, fistula–in–ano, perianal/perirectal abscesses are rare; more common with Crohn's.
3. **Toxic megacolon** — leading cause of death in UC; 40% of cases are fatal.
      a. Affects 3–5% of patients.
      b. Highest risk of perforation with initial attack and toxic megacolon.
      c. Pathology — inflammation extends into muscular layers of bowel wall.
      d. May cause localized abscess or generalized peritonitis.
      e. Clinical findings — systemic toxicity, transverse colon > 6 cm in diameter.
      f. Contributing factors — hypokalemia, opiates, anti-cholinergics, recent barium enema (avoid during acute attacks).
4. Massive hemorrhage — uncommon.
5. **Carcinoma of colon/rectum.**
      a. Begins to appear after 5–10 years of active disease. More common in patients whose colitis presented before age 25.
      b. Incidence — controversial.
        1) 10 years — 5%.
        2) 20 years — 20–25%.
        3) 3% per year if disease present over 10 years.
      c. Predictors — extent of colitis, continued activity.
      d. Often multicentric; lesions are small and flat.
      e. Vigilant surveillance with colonoscopy and biopsies is mandatory. When dysplasia is present in moderate or severe degree, incidence of carcinoma increases.
      f. Strictures — 50% malignant.
      g. Overall prognosis is worse than with idiopathic colon cancer.
6. Malnutrition — with acute, severe episodes. Growth retardation in children.
F. **Medical management.**
1. Sulfasalazine (Azulfidine®) — less value in severe UC.
      a. Dose.
        1) 2–8 g/day orally during acute attacks.
        2) 2 g/day chronically to decrease relapse rate.
      b. Metabolized by bacteria to 5-amino-salicylic acid, the active component, and sulfapyridine, which is responsible for the majority of side–effects.

  c. Side–effects.
   1) Oligospermia.
   2) Inhibits folate absorption.
   3) Hemolytic anemia.
   4) Nausea, vomiting, headache, abdominal discomfort.
   5) Allergic hypersensitivity.

2. Corticosteroids.
  a. IV steroids (hydrocortisone 100–300 mg/day; prednisolone 20–80 mg/day; ACTH 20–40 U/day as continuous infusion) for severe or fulminant disease.
  b. Oral steroids (prednisone 20–60 mg/day) for less severe or improving disease.
  c. Does not prevent relapse in inactive disease.
  d. Topical retention enemas for rectal disease.
  e. Complications associated with long-term, high-dose steroids:
   1) Peptic ulcer.
   2) Psychosis.
   3) Altered healing.
   4) Immunosuppression.
   5) Cushing's syndrome.
   6) Osteoporosis, degenerate joint (hip) disease.

3. Supportive measures.
  a. Acute exacerbation — NPO; NG suction; TPN may improve overall nutritional state and may reverse growth retardation in children.
  b. During remission — diet of choice, avoid milk products, opiates; loperomide or diphenoxylate, and psyllium may control diarrhea.

G. Surgical management.

1. Indications for surgery.
  a. Severe, acute attack unresponsive to intense medical therapy.
  b. Colonic complications — perforation, toxic megacolon, massive hemorrhage, obstruction.
  c. Chronic, debilitating disease.
  d. Carcinoma or high risk for carcinoma.
  e. Growth failure in children.
  f. Severe extraintestinal complications.

2. Surgical procedures (total proctocolectomy is curative).
  a. Total proctocolectomy with standard (Brooke) ileostomy.
   1) Remains "gold standard" operation for general use.
   2) 1–3% elective operative mortality.
   3) 10–15% develop impotence.
  b. Total proctocolectomy with continent (Kock) ileostomy.
   1) Avoids need for conventional ileostomy/appliances.

        2) Major problem stability of continent nipple valve within ileal reservoir (40–50% may require re-operation).
- c. **Total abdominal colectomy, mucosal proctectomy, ileal reservoir and ileoanal anastomosis.**
  1) Eliminates all diseased mucosa; preserves rectal continence and normal defecation.
  2) Should only be performed in experienced centers.
  3) Probably will become operation of choice (Martin LW, et al. *Ann. Surg.* 203:525, 1986).
- d. **Total abdominal colectomy with ileostomy, rectal preservation.**
  1) Reserved for emergency procedures to decrease operative morbidity and mortality (3–10%).
  2) Proctectomy completed at later date as an elective procedure to control proctitis and reduce cancer risk.

H. Prognosis.
1. Initial attack.
   - a. 60% respond rapidly to medical therapy.
   - b. 15% respond slowly to medical therapy.
   - c. 25% require emergency colectomy with severe initial attack.
   - d. 1% colitis–related death rate in first year; 5% over 10 years.
2. Pancolitis.
   - a. 25% require surgery during first year.
   - b. 5% death rate over 10 years.
3. Ulcerative proctitis — only 10% develop colonic disease by 10 years.

III. CROHN'S DISEASE
A. Etiology — may be similar to those for UC. Others:
1. Infectious — possibly atypical mycobacteria.
2. Genetic — 15–20% of patients have family history of IBD.

B. Epidemiology.
1. Peak incidence between 2nd and 4th decades; late peak ages 50–60.
2. Equal sex distribution.
3. Incidence — 2–5/100,000.

C. Clinical manifestations/evaluation.
1. **Signs and symptoms.**
   - a. <u>Diarrhea</u> — 90% of patients, usually non–bloody.
   - b. <u>Recurrent abdominal pain</u> — mild colicky pain, often initiated by meals and relieved by defecation.
   - c. Abdominal symptoms and constitutional symptoms — RLQ mass often present.

   d. Anorectal lesions — chronic recurrent or non–healing anal fissures, ulcers, complex anal fistulas, perirectal abscesses (may precede bowel involvement).
   e. Malnutrition — protein–losing enteropathy, steatorrhea, mineral and vitamin deficiencies, growth retardation.
   f. Acute onset — an acute appendicitis–like presentation due to acute inflammation of the distal ileum; only 15% of these patients (with isolated terminal ileitis) develop chronic Crohn's disease. May be due to a different pathogen (i.e., *Yersinia*).
   g. Extraintestinal manifestations (see II.E.1 above).
   h. Psychological disturbances.
2. **Disease distribution.**
   a. May involve entire GI tract (from lips to anus); distal ileum is most frequently involved; skip areas found in 15% of cases.
   b. Small bowel alone — 15–30%.
   c. Distal ileum and colon — 40–60%.
   d. Colon alone — 25–30%.
   e. Duodenum — 0.5–7%.
   f. Anorectum alone — 3%.
3. **Laboratory findings** — nonspecific and varied.
   a. Anemia — iron or B$_{12}$/folate deficiency.
   b. Hypoalbuminemia and steatorrhea are common.
   c. Tests of small bowel function (D–xylose absorption, bile acid breath test) are abnormal with extensive disease.
4. **X-ray findings.**
   a. Upper GI series (usual way to establish the diagnosis) — distal ileum disease.
   b. Barium enema — thickened bowel wall, strictures ("string sign"), longitudinal ulcerations and fissures, cobblestone formation, rectal sparing.
5. **Endoscopy.**
   a. Proctosigmoidoscopy reveals a normal rectum in 50% of patients with colonic disease.
   b. Characteristic lesions (aphthous ulcers, mucosal ulcerations and fissures, cobblestoning) may be seen in colon and distal ileum.
   c. Involvement is typically patchy.
6. **Intraoperative findings.**
   a. Creeping of mesenteric fat toward antimesenteric border.
   b. Bowel wall thickening, strictures.
   c. Bowel and mesenteric foreshortening.
   d. Enlargement of mesenteric lymph nodes; nodes adjacent to bowel indicate mucosal disease.
   e. Inflammatory masses, abscesses, adherent bowel loops.

    f. Exudate.
D. Differential diagnosis.
    1. Ulcerative colitis.
    2. Acute appendicitis.
    3. Tuberculosis.
    4. Lymphoma.
    5. Miscellaneous — carcinoma, amebiasis, ischemia, diverticulitis.
E. Complications.
    1. Extraintestinal (see II.E.1 above).
        a. More common with colonic involvement.
        b. Urinary — cystitis, calculi (oxalate), ureteral obstruction.
    2. Intestinal obstruction.
    3. Abscess formation.
    4. Fistulization — internal and external.
    5. Anorectal lesions — exuberant granulomatous process.
    6. Free perforation and hemorrhage are rare.
    7. Carcinoma — much less common than in UC; usually occurs in surgically excluded bowel segments; is not associated with chronicity of disease.
    8. Toxic megacolon — occurs in 5% of patients with colonic disease; responds better to medical therapy than UC.
F. Medical management.
    1. Drug therapy.
        a. Steroids (prednisone) and sulfasalazine for acute attack. (Sulfasalazine works best for colonic involvement.)
        b. Azathioprine (2.5 mg/kg/day) in combination with above may be helpful.
        c. 6–mercaptopurine may be useful (two randomized trials demonstrated no effect).
        d. Metronidazole (Flagyl®) is often helpful, especially for anal complications; requires long–term use. Some flare–ups may be due to presence of *Clostridium difficile* which is treated with metronidazole.
    2. Supportive measures.
        a. Bedrest, relief of emotional stress.
        b. NPO, nasogastric suction as needed.
        c. Diet — low residue, milk–free, high protein.
        d. TPN for fistulas and malnutrition.
G. Surgical management — intervention necessary in 70–75% of cases. Reserved for treatment of complications of Crohn's disease.
    1. Indications for surgery.
        a. Small bowel obstruction — indication in 50% of surgical cases.
        b. Fistulas.
        c. Abscess.

        d. Perianal disease (when unresponsive to medical therapy).
  2. Surgical procedures (not curative).
      a. Conservative resection of diseased/symptomatic bowel segment, primary end–to–end anastomosis.
          1) Only resect grossly diseased area with small "normal" margins. Difficult, and unnecessary in some patients, to get histologically totally–free margins for anastomosis.
          2) Distal ileum and cecal resection with ileo–colostomy is common procedure.
          3) 60% recurrence in long–term follow–up.
      b. Exclusion bypass — to bypass unresectable inflammatory masses. Higher incidence of recurrence.
      c. Continent (Kock) ileostomy and mucosal proctectomy procedures are contraindicated.
H. Prognosis — Crohn's is a chronic disease. None of the available modes of therapy are curative.
  1. Medical therapy — does not avoid surgery.
  2. Recurrence rate 10 years after initial operation:
      a. Ileocolic disease — 50%.
      b. Small bowel disease — 50%.
      c. Colonic disease — 40–50%.
  3. Re–operation rates at 5 years:
      a. Primary resection — 20%.
      b. Bypass — 50%.
  4. 80–85% of patients who require surgery lead normal lives.
  5. Mortality rate: 15% at 30 years — disease tends to "burn out".

COLORECTAL CANCER

I. **INCIDENCE**
A. Excluding skin cancers, colorectal cancer is second in incidence only to lung cancer in males and breast cancer in females.
B. Colorectal cancer accounts for 15% of all yearly cancer deaths.
C. The peak incidence is in the 7th decade. Colon cancer has slight *female* predominance; rectal cancer has slight *male* predominance; 8% of colorectal cancers are diagnosed before the age of 40.

II. **ETIOLOGY**
A. **Environmental factors** — Western countries have higher incidence of colorectal cancer than countries in Asia and Africa. Immigrants from Asia and Africa have a higher incidence of colorectal cancer than their countrymen, suggesting an environmental etiology. The low–fiber, high–fat diet common in the West is associated with an increased exposure of the colonic mucosa to bile acids. Combined with delayed transit time, this allows for longer exposure to potential carcinogens.
B. **Genetic predisposition** — no clear evidence for inherited risk other than polyposis syndromes, although the incidence is higher within certain families. Well-described polyposis syndromes include:
1. **Familial polyposis** — adenomatous polyposis of the colon with a 100% risk of malignant degeneration. May also be associated with polyps in the proximal GI tract. Autosomal dominant inheritance.
2. **Gardner's syndrome** — polyposis associated with exostoses, soft tissue tumors, and osteomas. May be a variant of familial polyposis.
3. **Turcot's syndrome** — polyposis of the colon associated with CNS tumors. Autosomal recessive inheritance.
4. **Cronkite-Canada** — GI polyposis with alopecia, nail dystrophy, hyperpigmentation. Minimal malignant potential. No inheritance pattern.
5. **Peutz-Jeghers** — hamartomatous polyps of entire GI tract with mucocutaneous deposition of melanin in lips, oral cavity and digits. Minimal malignant potential. Autosomal dominant inheritance.
C. **Inflammatory bowel disease.**
1. Ulcerative colitis (UC) and to a lesser extent Crohn's disease are associated with increased rates of colon cancer.
2. After 10 years the risk of cancer in UC is felt to be 1-2%/year.
D. **Adenomatous polyps** — probably premalignant lesion; thought to represent an early step in transformation of normal mucosa to cancer, although a majority of polyps will not progress to carcinoma.

Increasing polyps size (≥ 2 cm) and increased number of polyps are associated with an increased risk of developing cancer.

1. **Tubular adenomas** — 65% of adenomas; 15% have cancer *in situ* or frank carcinoma.
2. **Tubulovillous adenomas** — 25% of adenomas; 19% have cancer *in situ* or frank carcinoma.
3. **Villous adenomas** — 10% of adenomas; 25% have cancer *in situ* or frank carcinoma.

E. **Summary of risk factors.**
   1. Hereditary polyp syndromes.
   2. Adenomatous polyps.
   3. Previous colorectal cancer.
   4. Ulcerative colitis.
   5. Family history.
   6. Age > 40 years.

III. DIAGNOSIS

A. A thorough history and physical remain the mainstay of diagnosis.
B. Colorectal cancer may present with different symptoms and manifestations related to the region of the bowel from which it arises.
   1. Right–sided lesions — bulky, fungating, ulcerative lesions that project into the lumen.
      a. Anemia — microcytic, secondary to chronic intermittent occult blood loss in the stools.
      b. Systemic complaints — anorexia, fatigue, weight loss, or dull persistent abdominal pain and mass in patients with more advanced tumors.
      c. Obstruction is rare, secondary to the liquid consistency of the stool and the large diameter of the bowel.
      d. **Triad — anemia, weakness, mass in RLQ.**
   2. Left–sided lesions — annular, "napkin ring" lesions that often obstruct the bowel.
      a. Change in bowel habit — obstipation, alternating constipation and diarrhea, small–caliber "pencil" stools.
      b. Obstructive symptoms are more prominent due to growth pattern of tumor, smaller caliber of bowel, and solid stool.
   3. Rectal cancer — blood streaking in stools, tenesmus. This finding must *not* be attributed to hemorrhoids without further investigation. Obstruction is uncommon, but is a poor prognostic sign when present.
C. Signs of local extension or metastases.
   1. Abnormal LFT's, jaundice or hepatomegaly.
   2. Fistula formation.
   3. **Virchow's node** — spread via lymphatics through thoracic ducts to left supraclavicular node.

D. **Diagnostic studies.**
1. **Rectal exam** — all patients undergo rectal exams unless they do not have a rectum, have unstable angina, or recent MI. Up to 25% of lesions are *palpable* on rectal exam.
2. **Stool guaiac** — up to 50% of positive tests are due to colorectal cancer. It should be repeated on at least 3 separate occasions so that an intermittently bleeding tumor will not be missed.
3. **Barium enema** or **flexible sigmoidoscopy** for routine screening in patients over 40; may substitute with colonoscopy if index of suspicion is high.
4. **Work–up for metastatic disease** in biopsy–proven cases.
a. If the diagnosis is made on sigmoidoscopy, need to visualize entire colon due to a 6% incidence of synchronous lesions.
b. Chest x–ray.
c. Liver function tests.
d. Abdominal CT/MRI (investigational).
e. Carcinoembryonic antigen (CEA).
f. IVP +/– in patients with low–lying lesions or urinary symptoms.

IV. **PATHOLOGY**
A. The majority of lesions are located in the distal colon, although recent studies have reported an *increasing incidence* of right–sided lesions.
B. **Gross descripton.**
1. **Polypoid** — sessile or pedunculated. Bulky polypoid lesions are more common in the right colon.
2. **Scirrhous** — annular ("napkin–ring", "apple–core") lesions. They are more common in the left colon.
3. **Ulcerated.**
4. **Nodular.**
C. **Histologic staging.**
1. **Duke's classification** — standard for categorizing colonic neoplasms.
a. Stage A — limited to the bowel wall.
b. Stage B — through entire bowel wall.
c. Stage C — regional node metastases.
2. There have been several modifications to Duke's original classification.
a. **Duke's modification.**
1) Stage C_1 — regional node metastases.
2) Stage C_2 — lymphatic involvement at the point of vessel ligation.
b. **Astler Coller** (1959) classification most commonly used.
1) Stage A — limited to mucosa (above lymphatic channels).

     2) Stage B_1 — into muscularis propria.

     3) Stage B_2 — through muscularis propria.

     4) Stage C_1 — limited to the bowel wall, with positive nodes.

     5) Stage C_2 — through entire bowel wall, with positive nodes.

  c. Gunderson, Sosin (1974).

     1) Stage A — limited to mucosa.

     2) Stage B_1 — through mucosa, within bowel wall.

     3) Stage B_2 — through entire bowel wall.

     4) Stage B_3 — adherent to or involving adjacent organs.

     5) Stage C_1 — limited to the bowel wall, with positive nodes.

     6) Stage C_2 — through entire bowel wall, with positive nodes.

     7) Stage C_3 — Stage B_3 with positive lymph nodes.

  d. Stage D is not part of any of these classifications. Patients are considered to have stage D disease if they have distant metastases or are unresectable.

  e. American Joint Committee for Cancer Staging and End Results TNM classification:

Stage	Tumor Penetration	Regional Nodes	Distant Metastases
0	*in situ*	−	−
I	confined	−	−
II	extended	−	−
III	any	+	−
IV	any	any	+

  f. Prognosis is related to the stage of disease, not the size of the tumor.

     1) Most studies use the **Astler Coller modification:**

       a) Stage A — 80–90% 5–year survival.

       b) Stage B_1 — 65% 5–year survival.

       c) Stage B_2 — 55% 5–year survival.

       d) Stage C_1 — 30–35% 5–year survival.

       e) Stage C_2 — 20–25% 5–year survival.

       f) Stage D — 1–2% 5–year survival. Patients with isolated hepatic metastases that are resected for cure, 15–20%.

     2) Rectal carcinoma has increased local recurrence rate and decreased 5–year survival compared to colonic tumors.

     3) Only 70% of patients who present are curable at the initial laparotomy.

       a) 10% of lesions are unresectable.

     b) 20% have distant metastases.

    4) Overall 5–year disease-free survival is ~ 50% for colon cancer and ~ 40% for rectal cancer resected for cure.

V. TREATMENT

A. An adequate cancer operation requires resection of tumor-containing bowel with **3-5 cm margins**, and resection of the mesentery at the origin of the arterial supply including the primary lymphatic drainage of the tumor. Recent studies suggest that 90% of tumors can be adequately handled by 2 cm margins. This is especially important for lesions of the lower 1/3 of the rectum which may be managed with a low anterior resection and primary anastomosis. For a few highly–selected, poor–risk patients with thin mobile rectal cancers, electrocoagulation or cone-focused irradiation may be appropriate.

B. **Preoperative bowel prep.**

    1. Mechanical cleansing to eliminate stool from the colon, and preoperative oral antibiotics have been proven to reduce wound and intra–abdominal infections.

    2. Perioperative systemic antibiotics may further decrease incidence of infectious complications.

C. **Choice of operation** (Fig. 1).

    1. Lesions of **cecum** and **ascending colon** are treated by resection of the distal ileum, cecum, and right colon to the mid-transverse colon. This includes the ileocolic and right colic vessels with accompanying mesentery. An ileo–transverse colon anastomosis is performed.

    2. Tumors in the **left transverse colon** and **splenic flexure** require resection of the transverse and proximal descending colon. The middle and left colic branches are removed.

    3. Tumors in the **descending** and **sigmoid colon** require removal from the splenic flexure to the rectosigmoid. The left colic and sigmoidal branches are removed.

    4. Tumors in the **upper 1/3** of the rectum are treated by an anterior resection and primary anastomosis.

    5. Lesions between **5-10 cm** from the **anal verge** are treated by a low anterior resection and primary anastomosis or an abdominal-sacral resection (Kraske, York–Mason).

    6. Lesions in the **lower 1/3** of the rectum (0–5 cm) usually require an abdominoperineal resection (Miles procedure) with a permanent end sigmoid colostomy; a few may be amenable to a low anterior resection with anastomosis using a stapler (EEA). At least 4 cm of rectal stump is probably necessary for maintenance of fecal continence in most patients.

    7. Direct adherence of the tumor to adjacent structures may result from inflammation rather than from tumor extension. A cure in the presence of local invasion may still be possible with resection of the involved structures.

8. The **Turnbull "no–touch" technique** of early isolation and ligation of the blood supply has *not* been proven to decrease recurrence or increase survival rates.
9. Early isolation of the tumor–involved bowel between umbilical
   tapes (for prevention of intraluminal spread) is effective in
   experimental models and may decrease suture line recurrences.
10. Electrocoagulation or wide local excision may have a role in
    poor–risk patients with small rectal lesions.
11. There is some conflicting evidence that suggests perioperative
    transfusions may increase the risk of recurrence.

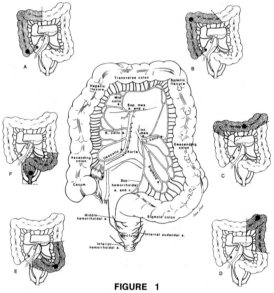

FIGURE 1

Anatomic resection commonly employed for cancer at different sites
within the large bowel: (A) right hemicolectomy; (B) extended right
hemicolectomy; (C) transverse colectomy; (D) left hemicolectomy; (E)
sigmoid colectomy; (F) abdominal perineal resection.

D. **Adjuvant therapy.**
1. **Chemotherapy** with 5-fluorouracil (5–FU) has *not* been demonstrated to produce an increase in long–term survival although it may aid in shorter term tumor control. Early studies show that a combination of **5–FU with leucovorin** or **levamisole** may increase its effectiveness.
2. Treatment of hepatic metastases with the insertion of a hepatic artery pump for direct infusion of chemotherapy has been disappointing. Although local control of hepatic metastasis was achieved, there was no long–term survival advantage due to failure at distal sites. In addition, some patients developed significant hepatotoxicity as a side–effect.
3. **Radiation therapy** has been helpful in shrinking large rectal lesions, thereby increasing resectability, although routine use of preoperative radiation therapy does not increase 5–year survival. Radiation has *not* been effective in the adjuvant treatment of colonic cancers.
4. **Bilateral oophorectomy** in female patients may be reasonable (since 10-20% of patients will have microscopic involvement of the ovaries); however, it has *not* increased 5–year survival.
5. Hepatic metastases − most common site of metastatic disease. Those with 4 or less metastases involving one lobe and who are amenable to hepatic resection have an increased 5–year survival to approximately 20%.

VI. RECURRENCE
A. Detection and treatment of recurrent disease remains problematic. Careful history, physical exam, LFT's, and CEA screening will detect greater than 90% of recurrent disease.
1. CEA helpful only if initially elevated and returns to normal post resection.
2. An increase in CEA (> 5 ng/ml) requires prompt investigation including CT, CXR, colonoscopy, and barium enema. If no abnormalities are found, some advocate a blind second–look laparotomy. Whether this results in increased 5–year survival is controversial. However, recurrences detected by frequent CEA screening alone are more frequently resectable than recurrences detected by the appearance of symptoms.
3. Other screening tests − tissue peptide antigen (TPA) and CA 19–9 are not as sensitive or specific as CEA.
B. **Treatment.**
1. Surgery is the only hope for cure.
2. Radiation treatments and chemotherapy are strictly palliative.

COLONIC DIVERTICULOSIS

I. **DEFINITION**
A. Congenital (true) diverticuli.
   1. Contains all layers of the GI tract wall.
   2. Much less common than acquired diverticuli; usually single.
   3. Predominantly located in the right colon in or near the cecum.
B. **Acquired (pseudo) diverticuli.**
   1. Most common type of diverticulum.
   2. A false diverticuli which contains only the mucosal and sub-mucosal layers of the GI tract.
   3. These diverticuli occur at weak points in the bowel wall musculature, i.e., penetration of blood vessels at the mesenteric border. Increased intraluminal pressure, probably secondary to uncoordinated contraction, produces mucosal and sub-mucosal herniation at these weak points.
   4. Diverticuli may occur throughout the GI tract, but are most common in the large bowel, especially sigmoid colon.

II. **ANATOMY**
A. Colonic diverticuli do not occur below the peritoneal reflection.
B. Sites of diverticuli:
   1. Cecal — true/pseudo; incidence 0.1%.
   2. Colon (80% in left colon) — pseudo; incidence 50–60% over age 40.

III. **COMPLICATIONS**
A. Infection (diverticulitis), perforation, bleeding, fistulization, and obstruction are potential complications, with diverticulitis being the most common complication. Incidence of both diverticuli and diverticular complications increases with age.
B. **Diverticulitis** — occurs in 20% of patients > age 40 with diverticulosis.
   1. Pathophysiology (proposed mechanism):
      a. Inspissated stool lodges in the diverticulum, producing increased intraluminal pressure with impairment of venous return. Venous hypertension with impaired capillary filling results in ischemia and mucosal injury with subsequent inflammation.
      b. Ischemia usually leads to a contained perforation into the mesentery or pericolic fat, causing focal inflammation and localized peritonitis.
      c. Approximately 10-15% of patients with diverticulitis will have free perforation producing generalized peritonitis. This is more

common in immunosuppressed patients, patients on steroids, and debilitated patients. Free perforation is associated with a greater mortality than simple diverticulitis (i.e., contained perforation).

2. Presentation.
   a. Symptoms:
      1) Most common — mild to moderate pain, usually in left lower quadrant. Pain is usually dull and achy, but may be crampy and associated with tenesmus. Location of pain *anywhere* in lower abdomen may be due to the redundancy of the sigmoid colon.
      2) Pain is generalized with free perforation and diffuse peritonitis.
      3) Fever, malaise, anorexia, nausea with/without emesis.
      4) Change in bowel habits — diarrhea, constipation, alternating diarrhea and constipation, change in stool caliber, obstipation, tenesmus.
      5) Urinary symptoms — frequency, nocturia, dysuria when inflammation is adjacent to bladder. Pneumaturia (3–5% presenting symptom) and/or polymicrobial urinary tract infections in non-catheterized patients are seen with colovesical fistulas.
   b. Physical exam.
      1) Tenderness and guarding over involved portion of bowel.
      2) Distention due to ileus or mechanical small bowel obstruction.
      3) Palpable tender mass, especially on pelvic or rectal exam.
      4) Hypoactive or absent bowel sounds with peritonitis.
      5) Hyperactive, high–pitched bowel sounds with obstruction.
      6) Guaiac positive stools.
   c. Laboratory exam.
      1) Mild to moderate leukocytosis.
      2) Previous barium enema showing diverticulosis.
3. Differential diagnosis.
   a. Acute appendicitis.
   b. Perforated colon carcinoma.
   c. Pelvic inflammatory disease, rupture or torsed ovarian cyst, endometriosis.
   d. Inflammatory bowel disease.
   e. Intestinal obstruction.
   f. Vascular insufficiency (ischemic colitis).
   g. Perforated peptic ulcer.
   h. Irritable bowel disease.
4. Diagnostic tests.
   a. Initial diagnosis is made on clinical assessment. Once acute symptoms have resolved, the diagnosis is verified. Diagnostic

studies can be carefully performed during the acute phase in difficult cases.
- **b. Flex sigmoidoscopy** with minimal insufflation.
- **c. Contrast enema.**
  1) Deferred until peritoneal signs subside (usually 2-4 weeks). If used in acute setting, use water–soluble contrast.
  2) May see spasm, external compression, or a "string sign".
- **d. CT scan.**
  1) May be performed during an acute attack with water–soluble rectal contrast.
  2) Superior to contrast enemas for defining pericolic inflammation and evaluating complications of diverticulitis.

IV. TREATMENT

A. Initial management – non–operative.
1. IV hydration.
2. NPO, NG suction (especially if ileus, small bowel obstruction, emesis).
3. **Parenteral antibiotics** – gram–negative and anaerobic coverage (e.g., an aminoglycoside and clindamycin or metronidazole). Continue until afebrile, with normal WBC and non–tender.
4. Pain control with meperidine.
5. Serial exams to detect worsening or complicated disease.
6. Use of oral antibiotics (i.e., neomycin) in addition to parenteral antibiotics is controversial.
7. **Oral antibiotics** (e.g,. trimethoprim-sulfamethoxazole plus metronidazole; or ciprofloracin) for mild attacks, or for 1-2 weeks after discontinuation of parenteral antibiotics for more severe attacks.
8. Dietary regimen of clear liquids followed by a low residue diet for 2–4 weeks after an acute attack. Patients are then placed on a high–bulk diet including psyllium that may decrease the long–term recurrence rate of further symptoms. Probably does *not* decrease incidence of further attacks of diverticulitis.

B. Surgical management.
1. About 50% of all patients admitted to the hospital resolve with conservative therapy. Only a small percentage (25%) return with a subsequent attack.
2. Of the 50% who do not respond during initial hospitalization:
   a. 30% do not resolve or recur after discontinuation of antibiotic therapy.
   b. 15% have free perforation requiring immediate surgery.
   c. 5% have urinary fistulas.
   d. 1% have a solitary right–sided diverticulum.
3. 10-20% of patients diagnosed with diverticulitis on clinical grounds are subsequently found to have carcinoma of the colon; therefore, one is *obligated to rule out carcinoma* following resolution of the acute attack.

4. **Indications for operation.**
   a. Repeated attacks (≥ 2).
   b. Failure of conservative management.
   c. Peritonitis (with or without pneumoperitoneum).
   d. Fistula formation.
   e. Colonic obstruction.
   f. Inability to rule out carcinoma.
5. **Operative procedures.**
   a. **Single–stage** – resect all diverticulum-bearing colon with a primary anastomosis; usually an elective operation on prepared bowel.
   b. **Two–stage.**
      1) First stage – primary resection of diseased colon with end colostomy and mucus fistula or Hartmann pouch.
      2) Alternative first stage – primary resection and anastomosis with a proximal diverting colostomy.
      3) Second stage – reanastomosis after 2–6 months.
      4) Used in acute inflamed bowel or an obstructed, unprepared bowel; most common operation for acute diverticulitis.
   c. **Three–stage** (rarely used).
      1) First stage – drainage of abscess and proximal diverting colostomy.
      2) Second stage – resection of involved colon with anastomosis.
      3) Third stage – closure of diverting colostomy.
      4) Employed for severe peritonitis or gross peritoneal soilage from perforation, on any unstable patient, or for a prohibitively difficult resection.

V. **RIGHT–SIDED (ISOLATED) DIVERTICULITIS**
A. May be congenital (true diverticulum) or acquired (false diverticulum). Congenital diverticuli do not increase in number with age.
B. Location.
   1. Cecum – usually congenital with approximately 0.1% incidence. Most common complication is inflammation.
   2. Ascending colon – most are acquired. Most common complication is bleeding.
C. Presentation.
   1. Usually occurs in younger (20–35) age group.
   2. Mimics appendicitis.
   3. Symptoms may be prolonged and persistent.
D. Differential diagnosis.
   1. Appendicitis.
   2. Inflammatory bowel disease.

    3. Gastroenteritis.
    4. Right colon carcinoma.
  E. Diagnosis.
    1. Barium enema, or flexible colonoscopy if no perforation.
    2. Must rule out malignancy.
    3. Usually the diagnosis is not made preoperatively.
  F. Therapy.
    1. Isolated ileo–right colectomy is usually necessary.
    2. Has a lower morbidity and mortality rate when compared to diverticulectomy.

VI. DIVERTICULAR BLEEDING (see "GI Bleeding")

Massive bleeding occurs as a complication of diverticulosis (not diverticulitis).

ANORECTAL DISORDERS

I. **ANATOMY**
A. **Rectum.**
    1. 12–15 cm in length extending from level of 3rd sacral vertebrae to the anal canal.
    2. No haustra, taenia coli or appendices epiploicae.
    3. No serosal layer (below the peritoneal reflection).
B. **Anus.**
    1. 4 cm in length.
    2. Lined by columnar epithelium above the columns of Morgagni, transitional (cuboidal) epithelium above the dentate line, and modified squamous epithelium below dentate line.
    3. Internal sphincter − thickened continuation of smooth circular muscle of rectum; involuntary control.
    4. External sphincter − three separate rings of striated muscle surrounding the anus (subcutaneous, superficial, and deep); voluntary control.

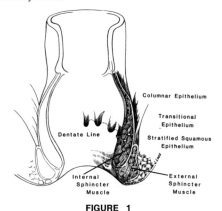

FIGURE 1
Three Zones of the Rectum

Ref: Martin LW et al. *Ann. Surg.* 203:526, 1986, with permission.

C. **Physiology of continence.**
1. **Zone I** — true anal canal below the dentate line; squamous epithelium, no hair follicles or sweat glands.
   a. Sensation is acute but meaningless, since by the time stool is appreciated it is beyond the sphincter.
   b. Acute sensation results in a great deal of pain and irritation related to disorders in this region.
2. **Zone II** — area of the columns of Morgagni above the dentate line to the tops of the columns; cuboidal epithelium (not subject to the disease of ulcerative colitis).
   a. True pain sensation is absent.
   b. Delicate proprioceptive nerve endings constitute the afferent phase of a reflex arc. This arc is responsible for constricting the sphincters and for the involuntary control of continence.
3. **Zone III** — area above the columns of Morgagni; transitional epithelium ends and the proper mucous–containing glands containing columnar epithelium begin (subject to the disease of ulcerative colitis).
   a. Proprioceptive nerve endings are present deep within muscle wall of rectum.
   b. Likely responsible for the sensation of the urge to defecate when the rectum is distended; not involved in triggering the involuntary sphincter reflex.
D. **Blood supply and lymphatic drainage.**
1. Arterial supply — segmental but with rich anastomoses.
   a. Superior hemorrhoidal — last branch of inferior mesenteric artery.
   b. Middle hemorrhoidal — arise from internal iliac arteries.
   c. Inferior hemorrhoidal — arise from internal pudendal arteries.
2. Venous drainage parallels arterial supply.
3. **Lymphatic drainage.**
   a. Superior and middle rectum eventually drains to IMA nodes.
   b. Lower rectum and upper anal canal drains to superior rectal lymphatics (leading to IMA) and to internal iliac nodes.
   c. Anal canal distal to dentate line has dual drainage to inguinal nodes as well as to IMA and internal iliac areas.

II. **HEMORRHOIDS**
A. Definitions.
1. **Internal hemorrhoids** — dilated submucous venous plexus arising proximal to the dentate line.
2. **External hemorrhoid** — dilated veins arising from inferior hemorrhoidal plexus, below the dentate line and covered with squamous epithelium.
3. **Thrombosed hemorrhoid** — one in which the blood has clotted.

B. Symptoms and signs.
   1. Pain, pruritus, rectal bleeding, perianal moistness/drainage; rarely can lead to perianal infection.
   2. Most commonly the symptoms are due to prolapsing internal hemorrhoids. External hemorrhoids are infrequently symptomatic. Perianal moisture is caused by columnar (secretory) mucosa prolapsing beyond sphincter. Moistness and maceration leads to skin irritation and *pruritis ani*.

C. **Treatment.**
   1. Initial treatment is non–operative, except with symptomatic thrombosed hemorrhoids.
      a. Sitz baths, stool softeners and bulk agents (psyllium) to minimize constipation; substitute cotton balls soaked in 1 quart water, 1 Tbsp baking soda, 1 Tbsp salt and 1 Tbsp witch hazel for toilet paper.
      b. **Rubber band ligation** of internal hemorrhoids — rubber bands must be placed above dentate line where mucosa does not have pain sensation.
      c. **Sclerotherapy** — submucosal injection of hemorrhoid with sclerosing agent. Hemorrhoid obliterated by fibrosis, with relief of symptoms.
      d. Cryotherapy commonly used in some centers.
   2. **Surgical treatment — hemorrhoidectomy.**
      a. Indicated for prolapse, pain, bleeding, or large hemorrhoids.
      b. Dissection should be carried out in no more than 3 quadrants of the anal canal to avoid stricture formation (Whitehead deformity).
      c. Typical location of hemorrhoidal tissue: right anterior, right posterior, and left lateral.
      d. Basic technique — Hemorrhoidal vein must be ligated early in dissection. Venous plexus dissected, preserving mucosa and anoderm. Suture closure of mucosa for essential hemostasis. External skin left open for drainage.
      e. Adjuncts for pain relief (optional):
         1) Partial division of external sphincter.
         2) Injection of steroid and/or long–acting local anesthetic agent (Marcaine®) in combination around sphincter.

III. ANAL FISSURE

A tear in the squamous epithelium.

A. > 90% occur in anterior or posterior midline; lateral fissures should raise suspicion of traumatic injury, inflammatory bowel disease, lymphoma, or infectious etiology.

B. Symptoms and signs — perianal pain during and after defecation, blood streaking on toilet paper, anal spasm, and "sentinel pile" (skin tag) at end of fissure. **Note:** Rectal bleeding and pain may be due to colon or rectal cancers (adults) and juvenile polyps (children). One should *never* assume that rectal blood is due to hemorrhoids or fissures without complete evaluation of the colon by sigmoidoscopy and barium enema or colonoscopy.

C. **Treatment.**
1. Non–operative — stool softeners, sitz baths; intermittent gentle dilation, local anesthetic suppositories; avoid rectal/anal trauma.
2. Operative — indicated when non–operative treatment fails.
   a. **Lateral partial internal sphincterotomy** has best results with lowest morbidity; fissurectomy may be added.
   b. **Anal dilation** — may tear sphincter more than necessary and cause hematoma formation, higher incidence of incontinence than sphincterotomy.
   c. **Fissurectomy and posterior sphincterotomy** — increased morbidity due to delayed healing of open anal wound.

IV. **ANORECTAL ABSCESSES**
A. Etiology — two theories:
1. Infections originate in blocked crypts along dentate line and then extend by fistula formation and lead to abscess cavities.
2. Discontinuous areas in anorectal mucosa are infected by fecal bacteria, leading to abscess formation.
B. Definitions.
1. **Perianal abscess** — abscess cavity is superficial and extends internally into anal canal distal to dentate line or externally to perianal skin.
2. **Ischiorectal abscess** — abscess cavity is lateral to the sphincters in the ischiorectal fossa.
3. **Intersphincteric abscess** — abscess cavity is between internal and external sphincters, and may point proximally or distally.
4. **Supralevator abscess** — abscess cavity is above levator ani and does not have any perianal signs.
5. **Horseshoe abscess** — any abscess involving both sides of the midline.
C. Signs and symptoms.
1. Progressive pain and swelling in perianal area.
2. Note: vague pain and bulging mass on rectal exam may be only evidence of supralevator abscess.
D. Treatment.
1. Surgical drainage *always* indicated — a fistulous tract to the dentate line from the abscess cavity is identified in 30% of cases.
2. Antibiotics usually indicated for diabetics, immunocompromised, or toxic patients.
3. Complicated abscesses and *all* abscesses in diabetics should be drained in the operating room.
4. Proximal fecal diversion may be required for healing of complex abscesses.

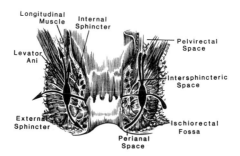

FIGURE 2
Pathways of Infection in Perianal Spaces

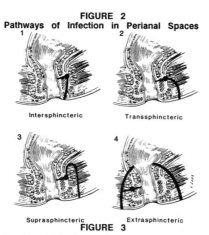

FIGURE 3
The Four Main Anatomical Types of Fistulae:
(1) Intersphincteric; (2) Transsphincteric;
(3) Suprasphincteric; (4) Extrasphincteric

V. **FISTULA–IN–ANO**

An inflammatory tract with internal (primary) opening along the dentate line and an external (secondary) opening in the perianal skin.

A. Etiology — most commonly associated with anorectal abscess, although inflammatory bowel disease also causes perirectal/anal disease.

B. **Goodsall's rule** — fistulae with external openings posterior to a transverse line through the anal opening will have internal openings on the posterior midline, and fistulae with external openings anterior to this line can have internal openings anywhere anteriorly (anterior midline is 12 o'clock and posterior mid-line 6 o'clock [by convention] for purposes of description).

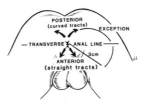

FIGURE 4
Goodsall's Rule

C. **Treatment.**

1. Careful examination and delineation of fistula tract is most important — *adequate* anesthesia necessary.

2. Operative treatment involves unroofing entire fistulous tract and curetting the lining of the tract (**fistulotomy**); alternatively, fistula tract may be excised *in toto* (fistulectomy).

3. High fistulae (supralevator) often require a 2–stage procedure (utilizing a seton) to maintain continence.

   a. Seton — heavy suture passed through the fistulous tract and secured. Healing with fibrosis around the tract (sphincters) occurs over 2–3 months. Residual tract may then be safely treated by fistulotomy.

   b. Local healing and fibrosis behind the constricting seton protects patient from becoming incontinent when the sphincter is divided during fistulotomy.

   c. Sphincters may be divided at only one site; division at more than one site invariably results in incontinence.

1.

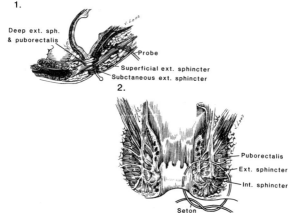

Deep ext. sph.
& puborectalis
— Probe
— Superficial ext. sphincter
— Subcutaneous ext. sphincter

2.

— Puborectalis
— Ext. sphincter
— Int. sphincter
Seton

FIGURE 5
Use of a Seton in High Fistula

VI. RECTAL PROLAPSE (Procidentia)
A. Classification.
1. **Type I** — false prolapse: a protrusion of redundant rectal mucosa, usually associated with hemorrhoids. Forms a spherical mass with *longitudinal* furrows radiating from the center of the anal canal. Distinguished from complete (true) prolapse where the mass is lined by *circumferential* furrows.

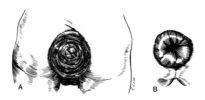

A   B

FIGURE 6
Differential Diagnosis of True Rectal Prolapse (A)
vs. Type I Mucosal Prolapse (B)

   2. **Type II** — rectal intussusception without associated cul-de-sac sliding hernia.
   3. **Type III** (most common) — complete prolapse with a sliding hernia of the cul-de-sac.
B. Clinical features.
   1. 85% of patients are female with maximal incidence in 5th and subsequent decades. Disproportionately frequent in nulliparous women and in women who have had prior gynecologic surgery.
   2. In men, the incidence is evenly distributed throughout the age range.
   3. High incidence of associated chronic neurologic or psychiatric disorders.
   4. Presenting complaints may be related to the prolapse itself, or to the disturbance of anal continence that frequently co-exists.
      a. Extrusion of mass with defecation, exertion, coughing, sneezing, etc.
      b. Difficulty in bowel regulation —tenesmus, constipation, fecal incontinence.
      c. Florid form —permanently extruded rectum, excoriated and ulcerated.
      d. Associated urinary incontinence, uterine prolapse.
   5. Physical findings.
      a. Demonstrate prolapse by having patient bear down.
      b. Absent/diminished external sphincter contraction.
      c. Excoriated or inflamed circumferential region in the mid-rectum on anoscopy.
C. Evaluation.
   1. Replace prolapse, if possible, and perform sigmoidoscopic exam to determine the condition of the bowel and the presence or absence of any pathologic lesion (e.g., carcinoma).
   2. Assess sphincter tone and degree of fecal continence by exam. Many patients with prolapse have poor sphincter tone.
   3. Barium enema; IVP — ureters may be distracted along with rectum into the sliding hernia.
   4. Radiographs of lumbar spine and pelvis — rule out possible neurological disease.
   5. Cineradiography — demonstration of occult prolapse.
   6. Anorectal manometry and electromyography may be used for early diagnosis.
D. Treatment of Type I prolapse — depends on disease severity and age of the patient.
   1. Very young children — non–surgical treatment is usually successful. Gently replace protrusion after each defecation, place gauze pad against anus, and tape buttocks together until next defecation. If conservative therapy fails, submucosal injection (phenol or alcohol) may be employed to fix the lax mucosa to the underlying muscle coat (rarely necessary).

2. Adults — hemorrhoidectomy with excision of redundant mucosa or band ligation of hemorrhoids is frequently therapeutic.

E. Treatment of Type II, Type III prolapse — multiple procedures are advocated.

    1. Basic features of the corrective operations include correction of:

        a. Abnormally deep or wide cul-de-sac.

        b. Weak pelvic floor with diastasis of levators.

        c. Patulous anal sphincter.

        d. Redundant rectosigmoid.

        e. Lack of fixation of the rectum to the sacral hollow with abnormal mobility and loss of the normal horizontal position of the lower rectum.

        f. Anorectal hyposensitivity.

    2. Abdominal approaches — most popular operation currently is a posterior rectopexy.

        a. **Ripstein procedure** — popular in the U.S. Involves full mobilization of rectum down to coccyx; then rectum is fixed to presacral fascia with Teflon or Marlex wrap and perineal defect is closed. Recurrence 2.3%; overall morbidity 16.5%.

        b. **Ivalon sponge wrap** — popular in U.K. Similar to Ripstein procedure, except Ivalon sponge is sutured to sacral hollow and to posterior rectum.

        c. **Abdominal proctopexy** and sigmoid resection — lateral rectal stalks sutured to sacral periosteum and cul-de-sac is obliterated by suture of the endopelvic fascia anteriorly. Recurrence 1.9%.

    3. Perineal approach.

        a. **Thiersch operation** — simple palliative procedure, wire or Teflon circlage of anus. May be performed under local anesthesia. Does not cure problem; complicated by fecal impaction, breakage of wire. (Recommended only for short-term palliation or very old and very debilitated patients.)

        b. **Perineal rectosigmoidectomy** with obliteration of hernia sac by high ligation, approximation of levator ani muscles, and resection of the prolapsing and redundant bowel with primary end-to-end anastomosis (AltemeierProcedure) — well tolerated even by high-risk patients; may be performed under spinal or epidural anesthesia; minimal operative trauma. Recurrence 3%.

VII. CONDYLOMA ACUMINATUM (Venereal Warts)

Multiple, cauliflower-like excrescences may occur on perianal skin, anal or rectal mucosa, vulva, vaginal wall, and penis. Usually benign, these lesions are difficult to eradicate.

A. Pathophysiology — papillomatous hyperplasia of the squamous epithelium in response to the **papilloma virus**. Condylomata arise in the papillary junction of the dermis and epidermis. Frequently begin as small, pointed projection which multiplies, forming large vegetating clusters. Characterized by hyperkeratosis, acanthosis, papillomatosis.

B. **Treatment** — combination of local ablation of lesions with improved perianal hygiene and treatment/control of sexual contact(s). Genital lesions should be treated *concurrently*.

1. **Podophyllin resin** — 25% solution in mineral oil or tincture of benzoin for small, scattered lesions and limited perianal involvement. Initial treatment of choice.
   a. Apply with care — caustic to normal tissue. Apply small amounts with cotton–tipped or wooden applicator.
   b. Protect surrounding skin with petroleum jelly or benzoin.
   c. Local chemical coagulation of lesions: ideally resolves in 3-5 days with sloughing of the lesions and subsequent healing of the underlying skin. Multiple applications often required.

2. **Fulguration** with electrocautery or laser photocoagulation is often the most effective treatment for patients with extensive disease.

3. Local **surgical excision** of large polypoid lesions alone or in combination with podophyllin or fulguration.

C. Regardless of the method of treatment, short- and long-term recurrence rates remain high, often requiring multiple ablative treatments. This is partially due to a high reinfection rate and continued poor hygiene.

D. In those lesions with florid acanthosis, differentiation from squamous cell carcinoma may be somewhat difficult; however, malignant transformation and other serious sequalae, such as stricture formation, are uncommon.

VIII. ANAL CANCER

A. **Epidermoid carcinoma** (1–2% of all colorectal carcinomas).

1. Two cell types — squamous cell and transitional cell (cloacogenic).

2. Tend to invade sphincteric muscles early and may extend 5–8 cm submucosally upward into rectal wall.

3. Rectal pain and bleeding are the most common presenting symptoms.

4. Treatment — abdominoperineal (AP) resection formerly the "gold standard." Chemotherapy (Mitomycin–C and 5–FU) combined with radiation after wide excision is now recommended as the initial mode of therapy. AP resection for residual tumor may still be necessary following chemotherapy and radiation. Inguinal node dissection is reserved for nodes clinically involved with neoplasm.

5. Survival — 40–70% (55% mean) 5-year survival for operative treatment. Combination of chemotherapy, radiotherapy and surgery may yield improved survival. Some series of highly-

selected patients with advanced lesions have reported lower survival rates.

B. Malignant melanoma (0.5–1.0% of malignant anal tumors).
   1. Anal canal is third most common site for melanoma occurrence (following skin and eyes).
   2. Most common symptom is bleeding.
   3. Most lesions are amelanotic (non–pigmented) and thus misdiagnosed.
   4. AP resection is only treatment option.
   5. Five–year prognosis is < 15% survival.

IX. ANOSCOPY

For examination of lesions of lower rectum and anal canal.

A. **Materials needed:**
   1. Examination gloves.
   2. Lubrication jelly.
   3. Gooseneck lamp.
   4. Cotton–tipped rectal swabs.
   5. Examination table.
   6. 4 x 8 inch gauze packs.
   7. Anoscope (tubular or bivalvular).

B. **Patient preparation** — none. Fleet enema is desirable, but not essential.

C. **Technique.**
   1. Position patient in either right or left lateral decubitus position with hips and knees flexed.
   2. Inspection — note presence or absence of fissures, external hemorrhoids, skin tags, etc., as well as blood or pus.
   3. **Palpation.**
      a. Adjust light to ensure proper illumination.
      b. Important to perform digital rectal exam *prior* to introduction of anoscope.
      c. Note presence or absence of masses, induration, sphincter spasm, tenderness, or discharge.
      d. Palpate normal structures such as prostate, seminal vesicles, anal intersphincteric groove, anorectal ring (posteriorly).
      e. Inspect exam finger following removal from rectum for blood, pus, stool, mucus.
   4. Anoscopy.
      a. Lubricate anoscope generously and insert obturator.
      b. Introduce anoscope into anus and point in direction of umbilicus. Once upper end of rectal canal is reached, direct anoscope posteriorly toward sacral hollow.
      c. When entire anoscope inserted, remove obturator and direct light into lumen of scope.

d. Have cotton-tipped rectal swabs on hand to swab away fecal debris, blood, pus, mucus, etc.

e. Note character of anal **mucosa** (e.g., friable, bleeding), presence of **masses** (polyp, tumor) or foreign body.

f. Slowly withdraw anoscope. At level of the anorectal ring, mucosa will close over lumen of rectum seen through scope. Internal hemorrhoids are noted at this level.

g. Never reinsert obturator into anoscope while scope is in anal canal, as the mucosa will invariably be pinched, causing pain and/or bleeding.

h. If necessary to reinsert scope, remove completely, reinsert obturator into scope, and then proceed with reinsertion of anoscope.

X. RIGID SIGMOIDOSCOPY

A. **Rigid** sigmoidoscopy will reach to 25–30 cm (lower rectum).

B. Materials needed — same as anoscopy procedure, but in addition:
1. Sigmoidoscope and insufflator (light source built into shaft of scope).
2. Suction with long sigmoidoscopic suction tip.
3. Biopsy forceps (if necessary).

C. Patient preparation.
1. Evening before procedure:
   a. Milk of Magnesia (30 cc P.O.) or Castor oil (30 cc P.O.).
   b. N.P.O. after midnight.
2. Morning of procedure — single Fleet® enema.

D. **Technique.**
1. Whenever possible, use a proctology table. Position patient either in right or left lateral decubitus position with knees and hips flexed, or kneeling on special sigmoidoscopy table in elbow/chest position.
2. Inspect perianal region as in anoscopy procedure, and perform digital rectal exam.
3. Connect light source to sigmoidoscope and insert obturator. Lubricate sigmoidoscope.
4. Insert sigmoidoscope into anus in direction of umbilicus.
5. As soon as rectum is entered, remove obturator and close window over end of sigmoidoscope. Further advancement of sigmoidoscope **should** **not** be done **without visualization of lumen**. If unable to visualize lumen, insufflate with small amounts of air to distend bowel. Do not use large amounts of air, as this will create severe discomfort.
6. Slowly advance sigmoidoscope through the lumen of the bowel. Generally, movements are initially upward and backward (into sacral hollow) until rectosigmoid junction is reached (12-15 cm) at which point direction will change anteriorly to patient's left. Further insufflation of air will enable entering of sigmoid colon.

7. When entire sigmoidoscope has been inserted (25-30 cm), **slowly** withdraw instrument in circular fashion, examining all mucosa.
8. Whenever necessary, window at proximal end of sigmoidoscope may be opened `o use cotton–tipped rectal swab or suction to remove any fecal material, mucus, blood, etc. Additionally, gaseous distention may be relieved.
9. If biopsy is to be performed, this is done at end of entire exam, as resultant bleeding may interfere with remainder of the exam.
10. Precise description of lesions should be recorded as:
    a. Distance from anus.
    b. Location of lesion on bowel wall (anterior, posterior, left or right lateral).
    c. Size of lesion.
    d. Fixed or mobile.

E. **Flexible scopes.**
   1. Flexible fiberoptic sigmoidoscopes are 35 cm and 60 cm long.
   2. Higher patient acceptance and comfort with the flexible scopes.
   3. Higher cost, slightly shorter exam time.
   4. Higher yield of polyps and cancer.

ACUTE PANCREATITIS

Acute pancreatitis involves a broad spectrum of pathologic changes, ranging from mild edema to fulminant hemorrhagic necrosis. Eighty percent of patients experience a mild self–limiting illness and recover fully with only supportive care. However, about 10–15% will develop acute hemorrhagic or necrotizing pancreatitis. Over the past 25 years, mortality from acute pancreatitis has decreased from 25% to 5%. This most likely reflects improved supportive care, better awareness, and earlier recognition of complications.

I. **ETIOLOGY**
A. Gallstones and alcohol are the most common etiologies (> 90%).
B. Toxic.
    1. Alcoholic (most common).
    2. Hyperlipidemia.
        a. Types I and V associated with triglyceride elevation and may cause pancreatitis.
        b. Hyperlipemic abdominal crisis must be differentiated from pancreatitis.
            1) Triglycerides 2000–5000 mg/dl — mild to moderate pain.
            2) Triglycerides > 6000 mg/dl — severe pain.
            3) Usually resolves within 48 hours.
            4) Associated with diabetic ketoacidosis.
    3. Hyperparathyroidism — ? role of Ca^{++}.
    4. **Drugs** — azathioprine, sulfonamides, thiazides, furosemide, estrogen contraceptives, tetracycline, steroids.
    5. Post–renal transplant — probably drug–related.
C. Obstructive — gallstones, ampullary stenosis, accessory papilla (pancreas divisum — controversial), duodenal diverticulum, tumor.
D. Infection — **viral** (mumps, hepatitis B, CMV), mycoplasmal, ascariasis (mechanical).
E. Trauma — external (penetrating and blunt), post–op (usually after common duct exploration, cholangiography, pancreatic procedures, gastroduodenal procedures, splenectomy, rarely after operations remote from pancreas), pancreatography.
F. Ischemia — circulatory shock, emboli, vasculitis, hypothermia, aortic graft, polyarteritis nodosum.
G. Other — penetrating peptic ulcer, pregnancy, scorpion envenomation.
H. Idiopathic.
I. Familial.

II. **CLINICAL PRESENTATION**
     First episode usually most severe.

A. **Symptoms** — epigastric pain, usually rapid onset in 90% of patients. Onset often follows heavy meal or alcohol consumption. Half experience radiation to back. Alleviated by sitting upright, aggravated by movement. Nausea, vomiting, and anorexia are common.

B. **Signs** — low–grade fever, tachycardia.
   1. Epigastric or diffuse abdominal tenderness with peritoneal signs; RLQ tenderness may be present. Bowel sounds diminished or absent.
   2. Flank ecchymosis (**Grey–Turner's sign**) and periumbilical ecchymosis (**Cullen's sign**) occur in 1% of cases and suggests severe hemorrhagic pancreatitis.

III. DIAGNOSIS

A. Usually based on clinical impression supported by lab and radiologic evaluation.

B. **Lab tests.**
   1. CBC with platelets, PT,PTT, electrolytes, Ca^{++} glucose, amylase, lipase, BUN, creatinine, bilirubin, SGOT, SGPT, LDH, alkaline phosphatase, GGT, arterial blood gases, urinalysis, triglycerides.
   2. EKG — exclude MI.
   3. **Serum amylase** — elevated in 80–90% of cases. Degree of elevation does *not* correlate with severity of attack, nor does it predict clinical course. Increased amylase is *not specific* for pancreatitis. **Other causes for hyperamylasemia:**
      a. Pancreatic — trauma, carcinoma, abscess, pseudocyst, ascites.
      b. Intra–abdominal disorders — biliary tract disease, intestinal obstruction, mesenteric infarction, ruptured aortic aneurysm, perforated ulcer, peritonitis, acute appendicitis, ruptured ectopic pregnancy salpingitis, ruptured graafian follicle.
      c. Salivary gland disorders — mumps, parotitis, trauma (amylase isoenzymes help differentiate).
      d. Impaired amylase excretion: renal failure, **macroamylasemia**.
      e. Miscellaneous — severe burns, DKA, pregnancy, cerebral trauma, drugs, pneumonia, liver disease.
   4. **Amylase–creatinine ratio** (urinary amylase is very sensitive):

   $$\frac{\text{Urine amylase}}{\text{Serum amylase}} \quad x \quad \frac{\text{Serum creatinine}}{\text{Urine creatinine}} \quad x \quad 100$$

   Normal range 1–9; > 6 has been considered diagnostic of acute pancreatitis; normal ratio rules out pancreatitis; can be elevated in other conditions besides acute pancreatitis.
   5. **Serum lipase** — remains elevated longer than amylase. More specific. May be elevated in acute cholecystitis, perforated ulcer, intestinal infarction.

C. **Radiologic procedures.**
   1. CXR — rule out **pneumoperitoneum**; pleural effusion, atelectasis, pneumonia, baseline in case of respiratory deterioration.

2. Flat and upright AXR — ileus, **"sentinel loop"**, **"colon cut–off"**.
3. Ultrasound — in first 48 hrs to evaluate pancreas and rule out cholelithiasis or pseudocyst.
4. CT scan — more sensitive and specific than ultrasound for pancreatic abnormalities, but not cholelithiasis.
5. ERCP — contraindicated for diagnosis; indicated after resolution, for recurrent disease, or if anatomic abnormality suspected.

IV. PROGNOSIS
A. 10–15% of patients develop severe prolonged illness, with a high incidence of morbidity and 25–50% mortality.
B. **Ranson's criteria** for identifying high–risk patients.
   1. At admission:
      a. Age > 55.
      b. WBC > 16,000/mm^3.
      c. Glucose > 200 mg/dl.
      d. LDH > 350 IU/L.
      e. SGOT > 250 U/dl.
   2. During initial 48 hours:
      a. Hematocrit decrease > 10%.
      b. BUN increase > 5 mg/dl.
      c. Ca^{++} decrease > 8 mg/dl.
      d. PO$_2$ < 60 mm Hg.
      e. Base deficit > 4 mEq/L.
      f. Fluid sequestration > 6 L.
   3. Mortality — correlates with incidence of peripancreatic sepsis.
      a. < 3 signs = 1%.
      b. 3–4 signs = 16%.
      c. 5–6 signs = 40%.
      d. > 7 signs = approximately 100%.

Ref: Ranson JHC, et al. *Surg. Gynecol. Obstet.* 138:69, 1974.

V. THERAPY
A. Fluid and electrolyte replacement — cornerstone of therapy; use Ringer's lactate or normal saline to maintain urine output of 0.5–1 cc/kg/hr.
B. Foley catheter — facilitates accurate I's and O's.
C. NG suction — indicated if severe vomiting persists. Has not been shown to alter clinical course in mild disease by randomized, prospective trials.
D. Diet — NPO until abdominal pain, tenderness, ileus have resolved, and amylase is normal or near normal.
E. TPN — indicated in cases of severe pancreatitis or when patient expected to be NPO > 7 days. Incidence of severe complications

and overall mortality *not* affected. Administration of lipid preparation is controversial.

F. Antibiotics — not indicated in uncomplicated pancreatitis, but may be in severe disease.

G. Serial labs — close monitoring of CBC, electrolytes including Mg, Ca^{++}.

H. Respiratory monitoring — respiratory complications occur 15–55% of cases. Requires careful monitoring of ABG's.

I. ICU monitoring — indicated in severe cases or high–risk patients (Ranson's criteria).

J. Peritoneal dialysis — may decrease early mortality, but late mortality is unchanged.

K. Histamine H_2 blockers —no beneficial effect in treatment of acute pancreatitis, but may be indicated in critically ill patients as prophylaxis or treatment of associated upper GI disease.

L. Inhibition of pancreatic enzymes — no evidence to support the use of specific enzyme inhibitors.

M. Analgesia — meperidine preferred; thought to have less effect on sphincter of Oddi.

N. Alcohol withdrawal prophylaxis — scheduled dose of benzodiazepine, thiamine 100 mg IM qd x 3d; folate 1 mg IM qd x 3d; MVI.

O. **Surgical management.**
   1. Indicated when diagnosis is uncertain to rule out other intra-abdominal process.
   2. Progressive clinical deterioration despite optimal supportive care.
   3. Treatment of complications (abscess, pseudocyst).
   4. **Treatment of biliary pancreatitis.**
      a. Surgery indicated after acute attack has subsided (during same hospitalization).
      b. If patient is worsening with aggressive supportive therapy, consider endoscopic sphincterotomy.
      c. Early surgery — within 48 hours of **onset of symptoms** (controversial).
      d. 30% recurrence rate if surgery delayed 4–6 weeks.

VI. COMPLICATIONS

A. **Pancreatic sepsis** — may present as an acute fulminant event (**infected necrosis**) or an indolent course after a period of well-being (**pneumatic abscess**); incidence of 1–9%.
   1. **Organisms** — *E. coli, Klebsiella, Proteus, Enterobacter, Pseudomonas,* enterococcus, *Staphylococcus, Streptococcus, Candida*; 50% are polymicrobial.
   2. Diagnosis — usually in 1st to 4th week of hospitalization.
      a. Abdominal pain, distention, tenderness.
      b. Spiking or low–grade fever.
      c. Persistent amylase elevation.

        d. CT most accurate mode for diagnosis.
    3. **Treatment** — surgical drainage, broad–spectrum antibiotics.
B. **Pseudocyst** — forms in 2–10% of patients with acute pancreatitis.
    1. Signs and symptoms — abdominal pain, nausea, vomiting, epigastric tenderness, abdominal mass, persistent hyperamylasemia.
    2. Diagnosis — CT and ultrasound each 90% accuracy; ERCP to demonstrate **site of duct disruption** and/or multiple cysts or ductal anatomy.
    3. Complications — occur in 30–55%.
    4. **Treatment** — 8–40% resolve spontaneously.
        a. Expectant management for 6–8 weeks until thick reactive wall is present and cyst remains unchanged; then internal drainage is treatment of choice via **cystogastrostomy, cystojejunostomy,** or **cystoduodenostomy.** *Always biopsy* pseudocyst wall to rule out malignancy.
        b. External drainage if cyst infected or wall immature.
        c. Occasionally, small pseudocysts in tail may be resected by distal pancreatectomy.
        d. Late, isolated collections may be amenable to percutaneous CT–guided drainage.
C. **Hemorrhage.**
    1. Usually due to pseudoaneurysm secondary to pseudocyst, abscess, or necrotizing pancreatitis. May be gastrointestinal, retroperitoneal due to splenic artery erosion, or intraperitoneal. Incidence up to 10% with pseudocysts.
    2. Symptoms and signs — pain, increased size of abdominal mass, hypotension, decreased hematocrit.
    3. Diagnosis — angiography and treatment if stable, to localize.
    4. Therapy — surgery if uncontrolled or unstable.
D. **Pancreatic ascites.**
    1. Secondary to ductal or pseudocyst disruption.
    2. High amylase and protein > 2.5 g/dl in peritoneal fluid.
    3. **Treatment** — NPO, hyperalimentation. Surgery if no resolution; perform internal drainage; identify ductal disruption via Greep procedure.

CIRRHOSIS

Cirrhosis represents the sixth leading cause of death in the U.S. and the fourth leading cause in persons over 40 years old. Few patients require more time and medical resources than the patient with complications of cirrhosis. These complications include variceal bleeding, liver failure, hepatic encephalopathy, renal insufficiency, and infection.

I. GENERAL CONCEPTS

A. Etiologic classification.

1. Alcohol is implicated in over 70% of cases of cirrhosis in the U.S. Up to 30% of chronic alcoholics have clinical or morphologic evidence of cirrhosis.
2. Post–necrotic cirrhosis is seen in viral, toxic, infectious and metabolic disorders as well as advanced alcoholic cirrhosis.
3. Biliary cirrhosis usually seen in long-standing biliary obstruction.
4. Hemochromatosis.
5. Chronic congestive heart failure.
6. Idiopathic.

B. Natural history.

1. Most series suggest that alcoholic cirrhosis has a worse prognosis than non–alcoholic cirrhosis. Patients with cirrhosis who **abstain** from alcohol have a 5–year survival of **about 60%**, versus 40% in those who continue to drink.
2. Early aggressive medical care improves survival with decreased morbidity.
3. Primary causes of death from cirrhosis include hemorrhage (34%), liver failure (34%), renal failure (11%) and infection (9%).

C. Symptoms —pruritis, fatigue, malaise, anorexia, nausea, weight loss, epistaxis, confusion, forgetfulness, dysmenorrhea and amenorrhea.

D. Signs — jaundice, dark urine, muscle wasting, ascites, peripheral edema, purpura, mental status changes, splenomegaly, spider angiomata, caput medusa, asterixis, gynecomastia, testicular atrophy, palmar erythema, loss of body hair, and Dupuytren's contractures.

E. Laboratory abnormalities include both biochemical (hyperbilirubinemia, hypoalbuminemia) and hematologic (prolonged PT and PTT, leukopenia, and thrombocytopenia). Diagnosis is further suggested by characteristic findings on liver/spleen scan, computed tomography, and ultrasound. Liver biopsy is diagnostic and allows histologic classification.

F. Child's classification — an assessment of hepatic reserve originally used as a predictor of early mortality in patients undergoing shunt procedures. Since then it has been expanded for use as a general measure of liver function and in classifying groups in study protocols.

Child's Classification

	A	B	C
Ascites	none	controlled	uncontrolled
Bilirubin	< 2.0	2.0-2.5	> 3.0
Encephalopathy	none	minimal	advanced
Nutritional status	excellent	good	poor
Albumin	> 3.5	3.0-3.5	< 3.0
Operative mortality (portacaval shunt)	2%	10%	50%

II. PORTAL HYPERTENSION

A. Portal hypertension exists when portal vein pressure exceeds 15 mm Hg (20 cm H_2O). Leads to dilation of portosystemic collateral veins termed **varices**. These include esophageal, gastric, abdominal wall, and hemorrhoidal varices.

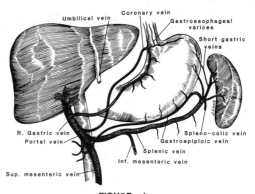

FIGURE 1

Portal Venous Anatomy

B. Portal hypertension is commonly classified by the level of venous obstruction.
  1. Pre-sinusoidal — portal vein occlusion, schistosomiasis, primary biliary cirrhosis.
  2. Sinusoidal — alcoholic and post-necrotic viral cirrhosis.
  3. Post-sinusoidal — Budd-Chiari syndrome (hepatic vein occlusion).

C. **Diagnosis.**
  1. Portal venography — allows assessment of size and position of portal and splenic veins and provides a qualitative estimate of hepatic portal perfusion. It may be done directly at operation or via splenoportography, transhepatic cannulation, or umbilical vein catheterization. The study may also be done indirectly with "venous phase imaging" by obtaining delayed films during superior mesenteric and splenic arteriograms.
  2. Portal pressure — can be measured directly or indirectly. Direct portal vein pressure **> 15 mmHg** is indicative of portal hypertension. Portal pressures may be approximated by the hepatic vein pressure gradient (HVPG), provided that no pre–hepatic occlusion is present. This is obtained by directly measuring wedged hepatic venous pressure (WHVP) and free hepatic vein pressure (FHVP). HVPG is then calculated by subtracting FHVP from WHVP (HVPG = WHVP – FHVP).

III. ESOPHAGEAL VARICES

A. Incidence and natural history of variceal bleeding.
  1. Esophageal varices are present in 15–30% of cirrhotics, but less than 50% of patients with esophageal varices will bleed from the varices.
  2. Mortality from the initial hemorrhage ranges from 20–50% or more. Within one year of the initial hemorrhage, mortality becomes 60–70%.
  3. Recurrence rate of variceal hemorrhage can exceed 70%; two–year recurrence varies from 30–70%.
  4. Incidence of variceal hemorrhage is related to the **size** of varices and not to the degree of portal hypertension (e.g., larger varices are more likely to bleed).
B. Differential diagnosis of UGI bleeding in cirrhotics.
  1. Diagnosis initially made by history and physical, then established by endoscopy.
  2. Historically, about 50% of UGI bleeds in cirrhotics are due to variceal hemorrhage. More recent studies implicate varices in 50–90% of cases.
  3. Hemorrhagic gastritis/esophagitis, Mallory-Weiss syndrome, peptic ulcer, and gastric or esophageal neoplasm account for the remaining 10-15%.
C. **Emergency treatment of variceal bleeding** (see also "GI Bleeding").
  1. Resuscitation.
    a. ABC's (airway, breathing, circulation).
    b. Volume resuscitation with blood and blood products. Maintain hematocrit above 30%.
    c. Monitor in ICU with foley catheter and NG tube in all patients; consider invasive hemodynamic monitoring in any unstable patient.

  d. Correct coagulopathy with blood products (fresh–frozen plasma, cryoprecipitate and platelets as appropriate).
  e. IV hydration with D10W plus vitamins B, K and C. *Avoid* sodium–containing solutions.
  f. Cautious sedation, e.g., small doses of midazolam (Versed®).
  g. Encephalopathy prophylaxis and treatment — in conscious patient use lactulose syrup (30 cc PO/NG q2h until bowel movement) and PO cathartics, and in unconscious patient use neomycin (500 mg PO q6h) or lactulose enemas (200 cc PR bid).
  h. Correct any electrolyte abnormalities.
2. Medical measures to control hemorrhage.
  a. Gastric lavage.
  b. Intravenous vasopressin.
    1) Potent vasoconstrictor that decreases splanchnic blood flow; provides initial control in over 75% of patients, but re–bleeding is common within several hours after discontinuation.
    2) Administration is by continuous IV infusion at 0.4 U/min. May begin with an IV bolus of 20 U/100 ml D5W over 20 min before beginning infusion. Wean by 0.1 U/min increments over 6–12 hours after bleeding ceases.
    3) Side–effects — **cardiac ischemia**, decreased cardiac output, stroke, hyponatremia and water retention. Contraindicated in patients with coronary artery disease. Numerous fatalities have been reported.
    4) Recent controlled studies reported that vasopressin in combination with nitroglycerin (50 μg/min IV drip starting dose) is more effective and associated with fewer complications than vasopressin alone.
  c. Esophageal balloon tamponade (e.g, Sengstaken–Blakemore or Linton/Nachlas tubes).
    1) Requires ICU monitoring and strict adherence to protocol, including consideration of prophylactic endotracheal intubation.
    2) Effective in 75–90% of patients for initial temporary control of hemorrhage. However, 20–50% of patients rebleed soon after deflation; therefore, definitive therapy should be planned during tamponade period.
    3) Significant complication rate with potentially fatal outcome. Complications include esophageal perforation, esophageal pressure necrosis, asphyxiation and aspiration pneumonitis.
  d. Emergency endoscopic sclerotherapy.
    1) First line therapy at many institutions. Emergency control of bleeding varices is accomplished in 80–90% of cases with a hospital mortality of approximately 20–30%. After initial control is established, sclerotherapy should be repeated every 3–4 days until varices obliterated. Patients

who require more than 2 sclerotherapy sessions during a
single hospitalization have a higher mortality, and should
be considered for surgical therapy.

2) Sclerosing agents most commonly used — ethanolamine
oleate is the agent of choice (other agents that are less
effective are sodium morrhuate and sodium tetradecyl
sulfate); administered either intravariceal, paravariceal or
both, with similar results. Flexible and rigid endoscopy
have equivalent efficacy. The flexible scopes are easier
to use and are generally preferred.

3) Complications — esophageal perforation, esophageal
stricture, aspiration, and worsening of hemorrhage.

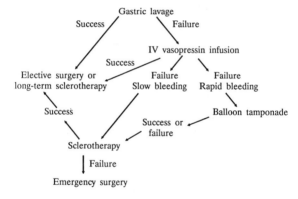

FIGURE 2

Treatment of acute variceal hemorrhage

Ref: Rikkers LF: Bleeding esophageal varices. *Surg. Clin. N. Am.*
67:475, 1987, with permission.

3. Emergency surgical measures to control hemorrhage.
   a. **Portacaval shunt** — used primarily when bleeding is not controlled by medical means. Operative mortality may exceed
   40–50%. Five–year survival *not* significantly different than
   emergency sclerotherapy. Risk of rebleeding *is* significantly
   less than with sclerotherapy.

b. **Esophageal transection** and reanastomosis with EEA stapling device (includes ligation of coronary vein) — Japanese results good; these have yet to be confirmed in Western studies. Used occasionally when sclerotherapy fails *and* a shunt is not feasible. Addition of distal esophageal devascularization is known as the **Sugiura procedure.** Most experience is in Japanese patients with non-alcoholic liver disease. In the U.S. literature, significant mortality and re-bleeding have been reported using this procedure.

D. **Therapeutic options** in prevention of recurrent variceal hemorrhage.
   1. Pharmacologic therapy — beta blockers, nitrates, and calcium channel blockers are currently under study; unlikely that they will have any significant benefit.
   2. Endoscopic sclerotherapy.
      a. Decreases the frequency of recurrent variceal hemorrhage (48–58%) when compared to conventional medical management. Improved survival has been demonstrated in a recent study.
      b. Injection sclerotherapy should be performed until all varices are eradicated. Despite complete eradication, varices have been shown to recur at a mean interval of 1 to 2 years. Rebleeding rate is about 15% per year after obliteration of varices achieved.
      c. Patients with gastric varices, or whose varices are difficult to eradicate or have recurrent bleeding during therapy, should have early consideration for surgery.
   3. **Non–selective (total) portosystemic shunts.**
      a. **Portacaval shunt** — end-to-side (Eck fistula) and side-to-side portacaval shunts are the "gold standard" by which other shunts are evaluated.
         1) Prospective, randomized trials have failed to show any survival benefit compared to conventional medical therapy. When data from these trials are combined, however, some survival benefit is probable.
         2) Very effective in preventing recurrent variceal hemorrhage (> 90%). **Hepatic encephalopathy** occurs in about 15–30% of cases, while **hepatic failure** is a major cause of post–shunt mortality (13–18%).
         3) The failure to show significant survival benefit has significantly decreased use of total portosystemic shunts. At present the most common indications include the use of an end-to-side shunt in acute variceal hemorrhage and a side-to-side shunt in the prevention of post-op ascites.
      b. **Interposition H–graft shunts** — mesocaval, portacaval and mesorenal.
         1) Grafts > 10 mm diameter are generally considered total shunts.

2) Increased frequency of late thrombosis compared to conventional portacaval shunts.
3) Useful in patients who are transplant candidates.
c. **Proximal splenorenal shunt (Linton shunt).**
1) Includes splenectomy with anastomosis of portal side of splenic vein to the left renal vein.
2) Physiologically and hemodynamically becomes a total portosystemic shunt with time.
3) Results similar to portacaval shunts, but probably has a higher thrombosis rate.

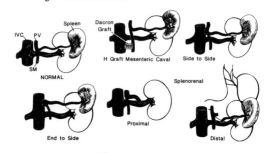

FIGURE 3

Types of Portosystemic Shunts

4. Selective portosystemic shunts.
   a. **Distal splenorenal (Warren–Zeppa) shunt.**
      1) Most commonly employed selective shunt used in U.S. Splenic vein is divided and splenic side is anastomosed end-to-side to left renal vein. Spleen remains *in situ* and the coronary vein is ligated.
      2) Varices are decompressed via the short gastric veins. Decompresses the varices while maintaining portal perfusion in about 90% of patients.
      3) Operative mortality (7–10%) and long–term survival are similar to non–selective shunts in patients with alcoholic cirrhosis. Survival seems to be improved in patients with non–alcoholic cirrhosis.
      4) Possibly lower incidence of late hepatic failure and encephalopathy compared to non–selective shunts (in 3 of 6 studies).
      5) Long–term survival (60% 5-year survival) following distal splenorenal shunt is similar to that of endoscopic sclerotherapy. Rate of rebleeding is higher in sclerotherapy,

while shunting may lead to progression of liver dysfunction.

   6) Splenic vein must be ≥ **7 mm** in diameter and ascites must be absent or medically controlled.

   b. Small–bore (8-10 mm) portacaval H–grafts — may be effective in controlling rebleeding with less post–shunt encephalopathy.

   c. Left gastric–venacaval shunt — not used much in U.S.

5. **Orthotopic liver transplantation.**

   a. Only therapy that treats both the portal hypertension and the underlying liver disease. May become the treatment of choice in advanced cirrhotics with a history of variceal bleeding. Limited availability of donor organs is a major obstacle preventing routine use of liver transplantation.

   b. Approximately 70% 5-year survival in large centers using study groups of predominantly non-alcoholic cirrhotics. Alcoholics who continue to drink are poor transplant candidates.

   c. **Avoid portacaval shunt** in potential transplant recipients. Endoscopic sclerotherapy, mesocaval shunt, or esophageal transection preferred if treatment is necessary for acute bleed while awaiting transplant.

6. Esophageal transection and devascularization procedures (see III.C.3 above) — limited use in U.S. Esophageal transection alone is not advocated for long–term management.

7. Optimal therapy for recurrent variceal hemorrhage is controversial. Endoscopic sclerotherapy and distal splenorenal shunt are currently the most utilized. Trials comparing the two modalities are in progress; preliminary data have failed to clearly demonstrate superiority of one method over the other.

IV. ASCITES SECONDARY TO CIRRHOSIS

A. General characteristics.

   1. Pathogenesis is thought to be due to the interaction of portal and sinusoidal hypertension, hypoalbuminemia, and alterations of sodium and water excretion by the kidneys.

   2. Most important feature is sodium retention by the kidney.

      a. Sodium retention due to a combination of secondary hyperaldosteronism and the deficiency of a proposed natriuretic factor, which normally blocks sodium absorption in the proximal tubule during salt overload.

      b. Renal redistribution of blood flow and decreased perfusion of the renal cortex leads to release of large amounts of renin, angiotensin and aldosterone.

      c. Water retention is due to sodium retention and impaired free–water clearance secondary to an increase in ADH.

      d. Decreased effective extracellular fluid volume decreases renal perfusion.

    3. Clinically detectable at > 500 cc.
    4. Associated with variceal hemorrhage, hepatorenal syndrome and spontaneous bacterial peritonitis.
B. **Medical therapy** — effective in 90–95% of cases.
    1. Goal is to mobilize not more than 1 kg of ascites/day. More rapid mobilization of ascites may result in hypotension.
    2. Bed rest.
    3. Sodium restriction — 400 mg/day (30 mEq/day).
    4. Fluid restriction — controversial, only really necessary for hyponatremia. Usually restrict intake to 1000–1500 cc/day.
    5. Spironolactone (Aldactone®) — 25-50 mg q6h; delayed onset of action in 3–4 days. Gradually increase dose until therapeutic effect noted up to 400 mg/day.
    6. Add lasix or thiazide diuretics if inadequate response to spironolactone. Careful monitoring of fluids and electrolytes required.
    7. Paracentesis — indicated only for respiratory compromise and diagnosis of spontaneous bacterial peritonitis.
C. **Surgical therapy** — indicated in the 5–10% of cases of intractable ascites.
    1. **Peritoneovenous shunt** (LeVeen and Denver shunts) [Fig. 4].
        a. Consists of silastic tubing with a pressure–sensitive one–way valve implanted into the abdominal wall. Tubing drains peritoneal cavity fluid into the superior vena cava via the internal jugular vein. One–way valve opens when the intra-peritoneal pressure exceeds 3 cm H_2O.
        b. When combined with diuretics, results in striking natriuresis, diuresis, mobilization of ascites, and an increase in effective circulating blood volume.
        c. Possible improved survival and decreased incidence of the hepatorenal syndrome.
        d. **Denver shunt** — incorporates a subcutaneously implanted pump which prevents clogging by active pumping.
        e. Complications — include infection, sepsis, CHF, DIC, hypokalemia, variceal bleeding, infection, shunt malfunction, air embolism, and superior vena cava thrombosis.
        f. Post-op, monitor for DIC for several days with serial fibrinogen, fibrin degradation products and platelet counts. If suspect DIC, shunt may be temporarily ligated until DIC resolves.

V. HEPATORENAL SYNDROME

A. Spontaneous renal failure associated with hepatic decompensation in cirrhotics. Usually associated with the accumulation of ascites, leading to a decreased plasma volume, inadequate glomerular perfusion, and a diminished glomerular filtration rate (GFR).
B. Often precipitated by bleeding varices, overly vigorous diuresis, excessive paracentesis, surgery, or progression of jaundice.

C. Azotemia without marked oliguria (until very late) despite kidneys with normal histology.
D. Characteristic pattern differentiates it from acute tubular necrosis and CHF:
   1. Elevated BUN and creatinine.
   2. Specific gravity of urine 1.016 – 1.020.
   3. Urine sodium < 10 mEq/liter (usually > 3 mEq/liter).
   4. Urine osmolality : plasma osmolality > 1.
   5. Urine creatinine : plasma creatinine > 30:1.
   6. Unremarkable urine sediment.
E. Mortality exceeds 70%.
F. No specific treatment, other than attempting to reverse liver dysfunction. Diuretics may aggravate renal insufficiency; hemodialysis has not proven useful.
G. Many patients thought to have this syndrome have good return of renal function when adequate plasma volume and GFR are restored by peritoneovenous shunt.
   1. The best candidate for peritoneovenous shunting is the stable cirrhotic with tense ascites and effective hypovolemia. Paracentesis with intravenous re–infusion may predict response to peritoneovenous shunting. Improved hemodynamics with an increase in urine output is considered a positive response.
   2. Survival of decompensated patients with bilirubin > 5 mg/dl is very rare.

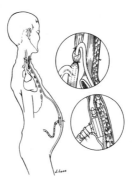

FIGURE 4
Peritoneovenous Shunt

VI. HEPATIC ENCEPHALOPATHY (HEPATIC COMA)

A. The most common terminal event in cirrhosis.

B. Etiology — severe hepatocellular dysfunction or portosystemic shunt.

C. Pathogenesis — not clearly established; likely a complex combination of factors.
   1. Ammonia (NH_3) intoxication.
      a. Most likely cause in those patients with surgical portosystemic shunt.
      b. A significant number of patients in hepatic coma have a normal serum NH_3.
      c. CSF glutamine correlates better with coma than blood NH_3 levels.
   2. False neurotransmitters.
      a. Decreased ratio of branched–chain amino acids to aromatic amino acids gives rise to increased octopamine and tyramine, and decreased levels of dopamine and norepinephrine in CNS.
      b. Act as weak inhibitory neurotransmitters.

D. Precipitating factors.
   1. Gastrointestinal hemorrhage — increased nitrogen absorption from gut.
   2. Post–portosystemic shunt procedure.
   3. Excessive diuretic administration — hypokalemia, hyponatremia, azotemia.
   4. Infection — increased catabolism and nitrogen load.
   5. Narcotics, sedatives — poor hepatic clearance.
   6. Excessive dietary protein.
   7. Constipation — increased contact time between bacteria and nitrogenous substances in the intestine.

E. Diagnosis.
   1. Presence of advanced liver disease.
   2. Change in mental status — subtle changes may be detected by Number Connection Test ("Trail Test").
   3. Fluctuating neurologic findings: rigidity, hyperreflexia, Babinski's sign, asterixis ("liver flap").
   4. Bilaterally synchronous high voltage, low frequency EEG waves.

F. Therapy.
   1. Eliminate precipitating factors.
      a. Diagnosis and treatment of infection.
      b. Resuscitation and treatment of acute GI bleeding.
      c. Reduce dietary protein (e.g,. 40-60 g/day for mild encephalopathy).
      d. Correct fluid and electrolyte abnormalities.
      e. Discontinue sedatives, tranquilizers, and analgesics. If required, give in reduced dosages and frequency.

2. Decreased NH₃ production and absorption in GI tract.
   a. Neomycin 0.5–1 g q6h for reduction in bacteria count; *avoid* in patients with compromised renal function.
   b. Lactulose 50 ml PO q6h until bowel movement (titrate dose to produce 2-3 soft stools each day) or PR via retention enema (500 ml syrup + 500 ml water) for comatose patients.
3. Consider hyperalimentation —patients with encephalopathy will tolerate parenteral nitrogen better than enteral nitrogen.
   a. Standard amino acid solution diluted to reduce nitrogen concentration is most commonly used.
   b. High BCAA solutions are available; as effective as standard therapy in resolving coma; possibly improves survival (see "Nutrition").

GALLBLADDER AND BILIARY TREE

I. CHOLELITHIASIS AND CHRONIC CHOLECYSTITIS
A. Incidence.
  1. 15–20% of adults have gallstones.
  2. Incidence increases with age; 50% by age 75.
  3. Predisposing factors include obesity, pregnancy, diabetes mellitus, cirrhosis, pancreatitis, chronic hemolytic states and certain racial/genetic factors (i.e., Pima Indians).
B. Etiology — the most important factor is composition of bile, having three major constituents:
  1. Bile salts.
  2. Phospholipids (90% lecithin).
  3. Cholesterol — although insoluble, both lecithin and cholesterol are incorporated along with bile salts into more soluble mixed micelles.
     a. Conditions that affect the relative concentrations of these components give rise to lithogenic bile.
     b. Bile containing **excess cholesterol** relative to bile salts and lecithin predispose to gallstone formation.
C. Types of gallstones.
  1. Mixed (80%).
     a. Most common; usually multiple.
     b. Cholesterol makes up at least 70% of the content.
     c. 15–20% may ultimately calcify and, therefore, become radiopaque. (**Note:** calcification usually occurs *late* in the natural history of gallstones.)
  2. Pure cholesterol (10%).
     a. Often solitary with large (> 2.5 cm) round configuration.
     b. Usually not calcified, or calcify late.
  3. Pigment (10%).
     a. Composed of unconjugated bilirubin, Ca^{++} and variable amounts of organic material.
     b. 50% radiopaque.
     c. Forms in conditions that produce excess unconjugated bilirubin (i.e., hemolytic states).
D. Natural history.
  1. 80% of gallstones are asymptomatic. Each year about 2% of patients with asymptomatic stones will develop symptoms, most (75%) commonly biliary colic.
  2. Incidence of development of symptoms in patients with asymptomatic gallstones is approximately 15–30% over 15 years.
  3. Elective cholecystectomy is recommended whenever symptoms attributable to cholelithiasis develop.

E. **Biliary colic** — pain arising from gallbladder without established gallbladder infection. Often difficult to differentiate between colic and intermittent smoldering cholecystitis.
   1. Etiology — thought to be transient gallstone obstruction of the cystic duct.
   2. History.
      a. Pain — generally presents with moderate intermittent RUQ and epigastric pain.
         1) May radiate to back or below right scapula.
         2) Pain usually begins abruptly and subsides gradually, lasting from minutes to hours.
         3) Pain of biliary colic is usually steady, not undulating like that of renal colic.
      b. Nausea.
         1) May have history of fatty food intolerance, intermittent nausea or anorexia (not a reliable symptom).
         2) Episodes of pain frequently associated with vomiting.
   3. Physical exam.
      a. No associated fever.
      b. May have some mild epigastric or RUQ tenderness, or palpable gallbladder.
   4. Differential diagnosis — pancreatitis, peptic ulcer disease (PUD), hiatal hernia with reflux, gastritis, nervous dyspepsia, carcinoma of hepatic flexure, carcinoma of liver or gallbladder, cardiopulmonary disease.
   5. Complications.
      a. Prolonged cystic duct obstruction may allow bacterial growth and progress to acute cholecystitis.
      b. Stones may pass into common duct and produce obstruction.
F. **Diagnosis** (see also "Jaundice" section II).
   1. Lab findings.
      a. None are diagnostic.
      b. Liver function tests, amylase and WBC should be obtained.
      c. Elevation of alkaline phosphatase is common in biliary disease.
   2. 10–25% of all gallstones are radiopaque and evident on plain films of the abdomen.
   3. **Oral cholecystogram (OCG)** — evaluates presence of gallstones as well as gallbladder function.
      a. 3 g of iopanoic acid (Telepaque®) is ingested at bedtime. The radiopaque material is absorbed by the GI tract, taken up by the hepatocyte, excreted into the biliary system, stored and concentrated by the gallbladder. If the gallbladder is not visualized, a second dose is given ("double dose") and the x-rays repeated.
      b. Single–dose study diagnostic in 75% of cases. Persistent non–opacification with double–dose indicates gallbladder disease with approximately 98% accuracy.

    c. OCG is unreliable if bilirubin > 2, the contrast is not ingested or absorbed, and during acute cholecystitis.

4. **Ultrasound.**
   a. Has become the diagnostic procedure of choice. Identifies stones, determines wall thickness, presence of masses, ductal dilatation and fluid collection, and examines the pancreas.
   b. Technical difficulties include obese patients, bowel gas, and technician skill.
   c. Sensitivity 95%, with overall specificity approximately 90%.

5. **Radionuclide scan (HIDA).**
   a. Diagnoses **acute cholecystitis** (up to 95% accuracy) if gallbladder does not visualize within 4 hours of injection and the radioisotope is excreted in the common bile duct.
   b. Reliable with a bilirubin up to 20, but is unreliable if the patient has been NPO ≥ 48 hours.

G. **Treatment** — cholecystectomy should be performed in most patients with symptoms and demonstrable stones. Common bile duct is examined for presence of stones by palpation and intraoperative cholangiogram (see Acute Cholecystitis below).

1. Early postoperative complications.
   a. Post–op fever — most commonly due to RLL atelectasis.
   b. Bile leakage may lead to bile peritonitis (about 1%) or subphrenic abscess.
   c. Wound infections.
   d. Hemorrhage.
   e. Postoperative pancreatitis.
   f. Bacterial pneumonia and urinary tract infection.

2. Prognosis — operative mortality for elective surgery < 0.1% in patients under 50 years old and 0.5% if over 50 years old.

H. **Management of asymptomatic stones.**

1. Truly **asymptomatic** patients do *not* require cholecystectomy unless it can be performed safely at the time of an operation for another condition.

2. Prophylactic cholecystectomy should be considered in asymptomatic patients with the following conditions:
   a. Diabetics may have an increased frequency of serious complications (empyema or emphysematous cholecystitis) and increased mortality.
   b. The patient with a non–functioning gallbladder or oral cholecystogram.
   c. The patient with a calcified "porcelain" gallbladder. Cancer is found in 25–30%.
   d. Any patient that has experienced biliary pancreatitis.

II. ACUTE CHOLECYSTITIS

A. **General considerations** — 95% of cases of acute cholecystitis are associated with obstruction of the cystic duct by a gallstone.

Approximately 30% of patients with biliary colic will develop acute cholecystitis within 2 years.

B. **Symptoms** – constant severe pain in the RUQ and/or the epigastrium that may radiate to infrascapular region. Anorexia, nausea, and vomiting are common.

C. **Physical exam.**
   1. RUQ tenderness on palpation. Signs of peritoneal irritation may be present.
   2. **Murphy's sign** – the examiner palpates the RUQ and asks the patient to inspire deeply. The diaphragm descends and pushes the inflamed gallbladder against examiner's fingertips, causing enough pain that the patient arrests his inspiration.
   3. Low–grade fever of 99–101°F.
   4. Palpable gallbladder.

D. **Lab findings.**
   a. Moderate leukocytosis (10–20,000).
   b. Frequent mild elevation of bilirubin (**elevation > 4 mg/dl is unusual** in simple cholecystitis and suggests choledocholithiasis).
   c. Frequent elevation of alkaline phosphatase.
   d. Transaminases may be elevated.

E. **Differential diagnosis** – acute PUD with or without perforation, acute pancreatitis, acute appendicitis, cecal volvulus, pneumonia, acute myocardial infarction (MI), liver congestion, acute gonorrheal peri-hepatitis (FitzHugh–Curtis syndrome), acute viral or alcoholic hepatitis.

F. **Complications.**
   1. **Perforation** – may be localized, leading to abscess that is confined by the omentum, or free perforation may occur, leading to generalized peritonitis and sepsis (mortality is 30–50%). Emergency laparotomy is indicated.
   2. **Empyema** of the gallbladder (suppurative cholecystitis) – a condition in which the gallbladder contains frank pus. The patient is often toxic and urgent surgery is required.
   3. **Cholecystenteric fistula.**
      a. Duodenum, colon, and stomach, in decreasing order of frequency.
      b. Air is present in the biliary tree in 40% of cases.
      c. May not cause symptoms unless the gallbladder is partially obstructed by stones or scarring.
      d. Symptomatic cholecystenteric fistulas should be treated with cholecystectomy and closure of the fistula.
   4. **Gallstone ileus** – gallstones causing the cholecystenteric fistula pass into the gut lumen.
      a. Symptoms of acute cholecystitis immediately preceding onset of gallstone ileus is **uncommon** (25–30%).

    b. Stones < 2–3 cm usually pass spontaneously and do not cause bowel obstruction.

    c. Terminal ileum is most common site of obstruction.

    d. Causes 1–2% of mechanical SBO.

    e. Mortality 10–15% (elderly patients).

    f. Small bowel enterotomy proximal to point of obstruction is usually required to remove stone; fistula usually does not require immediate cholecystectomy and repair.

G. Treatment of acute cholecystitis.

    1. The preferred treatment is cholecystectomy within 3 days of the onset of symptoms. Conservative treatment with IV fluids and antibiotics (1st or 2nd generation cephalosporin) may be justified in some high–risk patients in order to convert an emergency to an elective situation. In some high–risk situations, immediate operative therapy is indicated (e.g., diabetes, steroids). Lack of noticeable improvement with 1–2 days of conservative therapy suggests possible **complicated** acute cholecystitis necessitating surgery. In extremely high–risk patients, some authors advocate cholecystostomy and drainage to stabilize the patient prior to elective cholecystectomy. This may be done under local anesthesia.

    2. The risk of gangrene and perforation is relatively low during the first 3 days after onset of symptoms. After this period, the incidence **increases** to approximately 10%.

    3. Advantages of early cholecystectomy.

        a. Decreased duration of illness and hospitalization.

        b. Cholecystectomy may be technically easier to perform.

        c. Slightly decreased mortality.

    4. Microbiology and antibiotics.

        a. *E. coli*, *Klebsiella*, enterococcus and *Enterobacter* account for 80% of infections.

        b. 1st or 2nd generation cephalosporins are first choice.

        c. Broader spectrum antibiotics are used, depending on the severity of infection and patient response. Ampicillin, aminoglycosides, and clindamycin or metronidazole are useful in septic patients.

H. Acalculous cholecystitis — 5% of cases occur in the **absence** of cholelithiasis; 50–80% present in an advanced state (gangrene, perforation, abscess).

    1. Acalculous cholecystitis is primarily seen as a complication of prolonged fasting after an unrelated operation or trauma (e.g., acute burns, thoracic or cardiovascular surgery). Etiologies are believed to include:

        a. Bile stasis results from a lack of cholecystokinin–stimulated contraction.

        b. Dehydration leads to formation of an extremely viscous bile which may obstruct or irritate the gallbladder.

    c. Bacteremia may result in seeding of the stagnant bile.

    d. Sepsis with resultant mucosal hypoperfusion may promote gallbladder wall invasion.

    e. Ischemia of gallbladder during episode of trauma, hypoperfusion, etc.

    f. May be associated with large amounts of parenterally administered narcotics with resultant spasm of the sphincter of Oddi.

  2. Acalculous cholecystitis may also be due to cystic duct obstruction by another process such as malignant tumor, lymph nodes.

  3. The diagnosis may be difficult and often delayed because patients are often in the intensive care setting with multiple medical problems.

  4. Diagnosis is by HIDA scan; **treatment** is cholecystectomy.

III. CHOLEDOCHOLITHIASIS

A. General considerations.

  1. Approximately 10–15% of patients with gallstones also have stones in their common bile duct (CBD). Most CBD stones arise from the gallbladder, but may also form *de novo* in the CBD (primary common duct stones). As many as 50% of patients may remain asymptomatic.

  2. Complications include biliary colic, cholangitis, jaundice, pancreatitis, or late benign stricture.

B. Diagnosis.

  1. Ultrasound is 95% accurate in detecting dilated ducts which are often present when choledocholithiasis causes partial or complete obstruction; 25% of patients with CBD stones have **normal** size ducts.

  2. Cholangiography.

    a. Can be done intraoperatively at time of cholecystectomy.

    b. Percutaneous transhepatic cholangiography (PTC) is the diagnostic procedure of choice for patients in whom abdominal exploration is not anticipated.

    c. ERCP is useful in those patients in whom a CBD stone is suspected but ducts are not dilated on ultrasound exam.

  3. CT scan *may* help visualize the site and cause of obstruction, but is not as valuable as the above.

C. Treatment — surgical treatment of stones within the biliary tree requires opening the CBD with removal of all stones and debris and establishment of free flow of bile into the GI tract. When all debris is removed, the CBD is closed, leaving a T–tube in the duct to drain externally.

  1. Indications for mandatory cholangiography (stones present in only 20% of cases) include obstructive jaundice, a history of biliary pancreatitis, small stones in the gallbladder with a wide cystic duct, and a single faceted stone in the gallbladder.

2. **Absolute indications** for common bile duct exploration:
   a. Palpable stones in the CBD (99% reliable).
   b. Jaundice with acute suppurative cholangitis (97% reliable).
   c. Proven presence of CBD stones by preoperative imaging (ultrasound, CT scan, ERCP, PTC) or by intraoperative cholangiography (85% reliable).
3. Strong indications for common bile duct exploration:
   a. Dilated CBD over 15 cm (35% reliable).
   b. Bilirubin > 8 mg/dl.
4. **Technique of common duct exploration.**
   a. The duodenum is mobilized with a Kocher maneuver and the anterior surface of the CBD is identified.
   b. The duct is opened longitudinally, with stones and/or sludge removed by means of irrigation and a Fogarty (balloon) catheter. Stone forceps and biliary spoons may be used with **caution.** Choledochoscopy is recommended.
   c. Pass a #5 pediatric tube into the duodenum. After this, a T–tube is placed into the CBD with the choledochotomy closed around the tube. The T–tube is brought out lateral to the incision.
   d. In an uncomplicated course, the T–tube may be removed 10–14 days postoperatively when a stable tract has formed and a **normal** T–tube cholangiogram has been obtained. Much argument about timing of this; some prefer to leave T–tube for 6 weeks.

D. **Retained common duct stones** — found in up to 5% of patients undergoing CBD exploration and 1–9% of simple cholecystectomy patients.
   1. Patients with a T–tube in place — two alternatives:
      a. Remove stones using a "basket" passed through the T–tube tract utilizing fluoroscopic control (> 90% success rate). T–tubes greater than **14 French** facilitate removal through the tract. Smaller tracts may be dilated to allow passage of the basket.
      b. Dissolve stones using a litholytic agent (e.g., monooctanoin) administered via the T–tube.
         1) Of radiolucent stones 25% will dissolve, 25% will decrease in size, 50% have no response.
         2) Radiopaque stones do not dissolve.
   2. Patients without a T–tube.
      a. Endoscopic papillotomy and "basket" removal of stones trans-duodenally.
      b. Percutaneous transhepatic biliary (PTC) catheter placement with stone dissolution using a litholytic agent.
      c. Re–operation.
      d. Extracorporeal shock wave lithotripsy (ESWL).

IV. **CHOLANGITIS**
A. General considerations.
   1. A life–threatening disease that requires prompt recognition and treatment.
   2. Caused by obstruction of the biliary tract and biliary stasis leading to bacterial overgrowth, suppuration, and subsequent infection under pressure.
B. **Etiology.**
   1. Benign postoperative strictures (36%).
   2. Common bile duct stones (30%).
   3. Pancreatic or biliary neoplasm (8%).
   4. Miscellaneous causes (25%).
C. **Clinical findings.**
   1. **Charcot's triad** — RUQ pain, jaundice, fever and chills. The classic Charcot's triad is only seen in 50–70% of cases.
   2. In advanced cases, **Reynold's pentad** — Charcot's triad plus shock and mental obtundation.
D. **Diagnosis.**
   1. Initial study should be RUQ ultrasound; presence of ductal dilatation and presence of gallstones is suggestive. Thickening of bile duct walls, a liver abscess, or gas in the biliary tree is helpful.
   2. Leukocytosis, hyperbilirubinemia, and elevated liver function studies are often present.
E. **Management** — the goal is to decompress the biliary tree. The method by which this is accomplished must be tailored to fit each individual's clinical situation.
   1. Initially, antibiotics, IV fluids, and electrolyte repletion are necessary.
   2. The toxic patient is readied for the O.R. and immediate drainage.
   3. Patients with protracted course usually have more complicated obstruction and may require percutaneous cholangiography or ERCP. PTC may be therapeutic in the acute situation by decompressing the biliary tree.
   4. ERCP may be effective in decompressing the biliary tree by papillotomy, depending upon the source of obstruction, but has considerable risks.

V. **CARCINOMA OF THE GALLBLADDER**
A. General considerations.
   1. Associated with gallstones in 90% of cases.
   2. Increased incidence in patients with diffuse gallbladder wall calcification ("porcelain gallbladder").
   3. Male : female ratio = 1 : 2.
   4. Adenocarcinoma is most common.
B. **Presentation.**

1. Commonly found incidentally at the time of elective chole-cystectomy. A loss of clear dissection planes in the gallbladder bed or near the hilum is common.
2. Symptoms include RUQ pain, jaundice and those secondary to metastasis.

C. **Operative approach.**
   1. Cholecystectomy with wedge resection of adjacent liver (direct invasion of the hepatic parenchyma is common), and regional lymphadenectomy. This rarely results in cure.
   2. Relieve ductal obstruction if present.

D. Adjuvant therapy of chemotherapy or radiation therapy is largely ineffective.

E. Prognosis is poor: 90% mortality at 1 year.

VI. NON–SURGICAL TREATMENT OF GALLSTONES

A. **Bile acid dissolution therapy.**
   1. Chenodeoxycholic acid and ursodeoxycholate are the currently available agents. Ursodeoxycholic acid requires a smaller dose and causes fewer side–effects. Investigators have now shown that a combination of the two agents may be more effective than either agent alone. Adverse effects include either diarrhea (40%) and abnormal liver function tests (15–20%).
   2. Proper selection of patients is essential. They must exhibit good gallbladder function and have cholesterol stones (radio-lucent), optimally < 2 cm in diameter. Unfortunately, 30–40% of patients with gallstones that do not show up on plain film still contain significant amounts of calcium and/or pigment that will decrease efficacy of the dissolution therapy.
   3. Recurrence is 10% per year **after discontinuation** of therapy.
   4. Dissolution may take up to 2 years at a cost of $1000 – $1500 per year.
   5. Results — early data shows complete dissolution in only 13.5% of patients on high–dose chenodeoxycholic acid and partial dis-solution in another 27.3%. Further studies utilizing ursodeoxy-cholic acid in combination show improved results.

B. **Contact dissolution** by ether solvents.
   1. Patient selection is the same as for bile salt therapy, i.e., pure cholesterol stones. A percutaneous cholecystostomy is placed under local anesthesia. Methyl tert–butyl ether is injected and allowed to remain for several minutes and then aspirated. These injections continue until the stones are no longer seen on fluor-oscopy. Therapy may take up to 2 days.
   2. Sedation, transient pain, foul odor, and hemolysis are major problems; if the ether is accidentally injected intravenously or into liver parenchyma, hemolysis or hepatic necrosis may occur.
   3. Early studies suggest that total to partial dissolution is possible in 85–95% of cases.

    4. Follow–up has been short, but it can be theorized that recurrence will approach that of bile acid dissolution therapy (50% in 5 years).

C. **Extracorporeal shock wave lithotripsy (ESWL)** — fragmentation of gallstones.

    1. Selection of patients is strict:

        a. Symptomatic disease.

        b. Stones < 2.5 cm in diameter.

        c. Absence of calcified stones.

        d. Less than 3 stones.

        e. Functioning gallbladder.

    2. Nearly all patients will receive concomitant oral bile salt therapy starting one week prior to lithotripsy and continue for 3 months after.

    3. Adverse effects — cutaneous petechiae in 14% and transient hematuria in 3%. Biliary colic occurred in 30% of patients up to 18 months and then disappeared completely.

    4. **Results** — 93% of patients were free of stones 18–24 months after treatment.

    5. Recurrence of stones after discontinuation of bile salt adjuvant therapy can be expected to be the same as reported for bile salt therapy alone (50% recurrence in 5 years).

    6. Summary — Only about one–third of all symptomatic gallstone patients meet the requirements to be treated by lithotripsy and bile salt therapy. Recurrence is high without long–term bile salt therapy.

ABDOMINAL WALL HERNIAS

It has only been within the past century, with an improved understanding of inguinal anatomy, aseptic technique and improvements in suture material, that significant improvements in hernia management have occurred.

I. TERMINOLOGY

A. **Hernia** — a potential weakness or abnormal opening, with or without a protrusion, in an enclosing layer.
B. Reducibility — contents can be restored to their anatomic location.
C. Incarceration — an irreducible hernia; may be acute and painful or chronic and asymptomatic.
D. **Strangulation** — an incarcerated hernia with vascular compromise of the herniated contents.
E. **Sliding hernia** (Fig. 1) — a portion of the hernial sac composed of a wall of a viscus (frequently cecum or sigmoid colon).
F. **Richter's hernia** (Fig. 2) — only one wall of a viscus lies within the hernial sac (i.e., a "knuckle" of small bowel); may incarcerate or strangulate without obstructing.

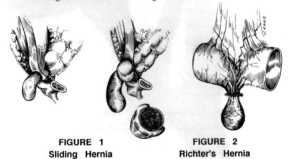

FIGURE 1
Sliding Hernia

FIGURE 2
Richter's Hernia

II. INCIDENCE

A. Male : female = 9 : 1.
B. Lifetime risk of developing a hernia — males 5%, females 1%.
C. **Most common surgical disease of males.**
D. Most common groin hernia in either sex is **indirect inguinal hernia**; however, femoral hernias are more common in females.

III. ANATOMICAL CONSIDERATIONS

A. Layers of the abdominal wall — skin, subcutaneous fat, Scarpa's fascia, external oblique, internal oblique, transversus abdominus, transversalis fascia, peritoneum.

B. **Hesselbach's triangle** — bordered by lateral edge of rectus sheath, inferior epigastric vessels and inguinal ligament.

C. **Inguinal ligament** — runs from anterior superior iliac spine to the pubic tubercle.

D. **Lacunar ligament** — inguinal ligament reflected from the pubic tubercle onto the iliopectineal line of the pubic ramus.

E. **Cooper's ligament** — a strong fibrous band on the iliopectineal line of the superior pubic ramus.

F. **External ring** — opening in external oblique aponeurosis through which the ilioinguinal nerve and spermatic cord or round ligament pass.

G. **Internal ring** — bordered superiorly by internal oblique muscle, and inferomedially by inferior epigastric vessels and transversalis fascia.

H. **Processus vaginalis** — a diverticulum of parietal peritoneum which descends from the abdomen along with the testicle and comes to lie adjacent to the spermatic cord. There is subsequent obliteration of its lumen in normal individuals.

I. **Femoral canal** — bordered by inguinal ligament, lacunar ligament, Cooper's ligament, and femoral sheath.

IV. CLASSIFICATION OF HERNIAS

A. **Groin hernias** (Fig. 3).

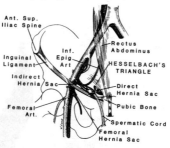

FIGURE 3
Groin Hernias

   1. **Indirect inguinal hernia** — sac lies anteromedial to cord exiting through the internal ring; lateral to inferior epigastric artery; most common inguinal hernia in either sex.
   2. **Direct inguinal hernia** — passes through Hesselbach's triangle (medial to inferior epigastric artery).
   3. **Pantaloon hernia** — components of both direct and indirect inguinal hernias.
   4. **Femoral hernia** — passes through femoral canal, medial to femoral vein.
B. **Ventral hernias.**
   1. **Umbilical hernia** — congenital or acquired.
   2. **Incisional hernia** — develops in previous fascial closure.
   3. **Epigastric hernia** — defect in linea alba above the umbilicus.
C. Miscellaneous hernias.
   1. **Littre's hernia** — inguinal hernia sac contains Meckel's diverticulum.
   2. **Spigelian hernia.**
      a. Ventral hernia occurring at the semilunar line (lateral edge of rectus).
      b. Usually occurs where semilunar line and semicircular line intersect and rectus sheath becomes completely anterior.
   3. **Petit's hernia** — through lumbar triangle.
   4. **Obturator hernia** — through obturator foramen.
   5. **Perineal hernia** — defect occurs in the muscular floor of the pelvis; anterior, posterior, or complete rectal prolapse.
   6. **Sciatic hernia** — rarest of all hernias; sac exits through the greater or lesser sacrosciatic foramen.

V. ETIOLOGY

A. **Indirect inguinal** — congenital patency of processus vaginalis; herniation through internal ring facilitated by a weak inguinal floor.
B. **Direct inguinal** — acquired weakness in the floor of Hesselbach's triangle.
C. Contributing factors — obesity, chronic cough, pregnancy, constipation, straining on urination, ascites, previous surgery.

VI. DIAGNOSIS

A. History of a palpable, soft mass that increases with straining; may reduce spontaneously or manually; there may be pain with straining. In children, the physician may have to take the parent's word for it.
B. **Examination** — palpable mass which increases in size while the patient strains. Examine patient when upright and supine.
   1. Femoral hernia may reflect superiorly over the inguinal ligament presenting in the inguinal region.
   2. Obesity may make identification of small hernias difficult.

3. Obturator, lumbar, sciatic, and even femoral hernias may be easily missed by physical exam.
4. Abdominal x-rays or CT scan may demonstrate hernias not detectable by physical exam.

C. Small bowel obstruction — may be first manifestation of a hernia.

VII. REPAIR OF HERNIAS

A. **Inguinal hernias** — need to repair defect in transversalis fascia.
   1. High ligation of sac — in children, where only defect is patent processus vaginalis; repair usually added.
   2. Bassini — transversalis fascia and conjoined tendon are approximated to the shelving edge of inguinal ligament. Can be done in 2 layers:
      a. Transversalis repair.
      b. Conjoined tendon to inguinal ligament.
   3. McVay (Cooper's ligament repair) — conjoined tendon approximated to Cooper's ligament; must use relaxing incision in rectus sheath.
   4. Halsted I — Bassini–type repair except the imbricated external oblique reinforces the repair beneath the spermatic cord which lies in the subcutaneous tissue.
   5. Ferguson — Bassini–type repair; however, spermatic cord lies beneath reconstructed inguinal floor.
   6. Preperitoneal — expose hernial defect from beneath fascia. Useful approach for repair of recurrent hernia.
   7. Shouldice — multilayer fascial closure with running suture.

B. **Femoral hernias** — require a Cooper's ligament repair (McVay). Many large direct hernias are also repaired in this manner.

C. **Ventral hernias** — wide mobilization, primary repair of fascial defect if able; often requires Marlex® mesh.

VIII. POSTOPERATIVE COMPLICATIONS

A. Scrotal hematoma — from blunt dissection and inadequate hemostasis.
B. Deep bleeding will enter the retroperitoneal space and may not be apparent initially. Suspect this with hypotension, orthostasis or tachycardia.
C. Difficulty voiding — more common in elderly males.
D. Painful scrotal swelling from compromised venous return of testes.

IX. RECURRENCE

A. 2–3% with indirect inguinal hernias; some recur as direct hernias.
B. Higher with direct hernias and when the underlying process (chronic cough, constipation, urinary obstruction) causing increased intra-abdominal pressure has not been corrected.

C. **Technical errors.**
1. Excessive tension on suture line.
2. Internal ring too loose.
3. Indirect hernia sac not identified at the time of operation.
4. Inadequate tissue strength despite adequate reconstruction. (Requires Marlex® or other reinforcement.)
5. Failure to identify concomitant femoral hernia at time of repair of inguinal hernia.

X. MISCELLANEOUS

A. Marlex® (polypropylene) mesh placed over the fascial defect may be used if the defect cannot be closed due to inadequate tissue or excessive tension. Often used to reinforce repairs.
B. Repair of bilateral inguinal hernias recommended only in children and occasionally in adults with small indirect inguinal hernias, due to the increased risk of recurrence in bilateral repair.
C. Consider orchiectomy in elderly males with multiple recurrences.
D. **Reduction of incarcerated hernia.**
1. Trendelenburg position, sedation, and gentle continuous compression may allow reduction of a recently incarcerated hernia.
2. Significant tenderness, induration, erythema or leukocytosis suggest possible strangulation, and necessitate immediate surgical exploration. (**No reduction should be attempted!**)
3. Use of a truss can result in distortion of anatomy, due to fibrosis of the inguinal canal, complicating and delaying the required surgery; a truss should be avoided in all but extremely high-risk patients.

BREAST DISEASE

The primary problem encountered by the surgeon is distinguishing benign breast disease from malignancy. Evaluation of breast masses is a frequent occurrence in surgical practice.

I. ANATOMIC AND PHYSIOLOGIC CONSIDERATIONS

A. Relevant anatomy.

1. Modified sweat gland enveloped by superficial and deep layers of superficial fascia of chest wall.
2. Suspended from chest wall. Fibrous septae (Cooper's ligaments) extend from the pectoral fascia to the dermis.
3. Medial border = lateral edge of sternum; lateral border = anterior axillary line.
4. Divided into 4 quadrants — upper outer (OUQ); lower outer (LOQ); upper inner (UIQ); and lower inner (LIQ).

B. Arterial supply — branches of internal mammary artery, axillary artery, and acromiothoracic trunk.

C. Venous drainage.

1. Predominant drainage parallels the arterial supply to the internal mammary and axillary veins.
2. Posterior branches of intercostal veins drain via Batson's plexus to the vertebral veins (may account for relatively higher incidence of vertebral metastases than other carcinomas).

D. Lymphatic drainage — of importance during mastectomy and axillary node sampling.

1. **Axillary nodes** — 65% of drainage from ipsilateral breast; contains ~ 40–50 nodes. Drains nipple, UOQ and LOQ. Axillary nodes secondarily drain to supraclavicular and jugular nodes.
2. Levels of axillary nodes.
   a. **Level I** — lateral group, located lateral to border of pectoralis minor.
   b. **Level II** — deep to the insertion of pectoralis minor on coracoid process.
   c. **Level III** — medial to pectoralis minor.
3. **Internal mammary nodes** — accounts for 25% of drainage; contains 3-4 nodes per side. Located in first three interspaces and drains UIQ and LIQ.
4. Interpectoral (**Rotter's**) nodes — approximately 10% of drainage from various areas of ipsilateral breast and axilla.

E. Associated nerves (surgical importance).

1. **Intercostobrachial nerve** traverses the axilla from chest wall to innervate upper medial arm. Sacrificing nerve results in hypoesthesia or anesthesia of inner upper arm.
2. **Long thoracic nerve** — courses along lateral chest wall and innervates serratus anterior muscle. Injury results in a "winged" scapula with posteriorly directed force to shoulder.

    3. **Thoracodorsal nerve** — courses through posterior axilla to innervate latissimus dorsi muscle. Injury results in loss of forced adduction of arm.

    4. **Lateral pectoral nerve** — penetrates the pectoralis minor and innervates both pectoralis major and minor muscles. Injury results in atrophy of pectoralis minor and lateral border of pectoralis major.

F. **Physiology.**

    1. Pregnancy and lactation — 2–3 x size increase. At 6 months colostrum formation begins. Post–partum, acini begin milk formation which continues as long as suckling occurs.

    2. Menopause —involution of breast tissue with atrophy of lobules, loss of stroma and replacement with fatty tissue.

II. HISTORY (Consider the following during evaluation)

A. **Age.**

    1. Age < 30 years — consider fibrodenoma, papillomatosis, breast abscesses (especially during lactation), fat necrosis. While uncommon, breast cancer can still occur in this age group.

    2. Age 30–50 years — consider fibrocystic disease, breast cancer, fat necrosis, and cystosarcoma phyllodes.

    3. Age > 50 years — majority of breast cancers occur in this age group.

B. **Mass** — determine when first noted, tenderness, size change.

C. **Nipple discharge** — assess whether unilateral or bilateral, clear or bloody, and associated with mass.

    1. Bloody — intraductal papilloma or cancer.

    2. Milky — lactation, acromegaly, cancer.

    3. Clear — normal menstrual cycle.

    4. Yellow — galactocoele.

D. **Gynecologic history** (factors associated with increased risk of breast cancer).

    1. Age at menarche (early menarche).

    2. Menstrual pattern — fibrocystic disease and premenstrual pain often cyclic and related to menstrual cycle.

    3. Age at menopause (late menopause).

    4. Parity; age at first delivery (nulliparity; > 25 years).

    5. Use of oral contraceptives.

E. **Past medical history.**

    1. Previous breast cancer.

    2. Previous benign breast disease (e.g., fibrocystic disease).

    3. Prior breast radiation exposure.

F. **Family history of breast disease.**

III. PHYSICAL EXAMINATION

A. **Inspection** — evaluate with patient seated with arms at side; seated with arms raised over head; seated with arms pressed on hips; trunk bent forward, and supine. Note breast size, shape, contour, skin coloration, venous pattern, skin dimpling ("peau d'orange"), and nipple inversion or excoriation.

B. **Palpation** — examine with patient supine with arms at side and above head.
   1. Identify mass (es), noting location, size, consistency, tenderness, skin dimpling, and mobility.
   2. Palpate nipple, check for discharge.
   3. Examine axilla, supraclavicular fossae, and cervical region for adenopathy. Note node size and mobility.

C. *Emphasize* **breast self–examination (BSE)**. Instruct patient by demonstration. (Booklet, audiovisual materials are available from local American Cancer Society chapter).

D. **Recommended follow–up.**
   1. BSE on monthly basis beginning at age 20–25. The majority of breast masses are found by patients themselves.
   2. Physician exam every 1–3 years depending upon risk factors.

IV. RADIOGRAPHIC STUDIES

A. **Indications for mammography.**
   1. Screening (current American Cancer Society recommendations).
      a. Baseline mammogram for women ages 35–39 years.
      b. Mammogram every other year for ages 40–50 years. If risk factors present, mammogram yearly.
      c. Annual mammogram for age > 50 years.
   2. Follow–up.
      a. Serial examination of large, difficult–to–examine breasts.
      b. Follow–up of ipsilateral breast following breast–conserving surgery for cancer, contralateral breast following mastectomy.
      c. Follow–up of fibrocystic disease.
   3. Metastatic adenocarcinoma without known primary.
   4. Nipple discharge without palpable mass.

B. **Mammographic findings** suggestive of malignancy (false–positive $\sim 11\%$, false–negative $\sim 6\%$).
   1. Stippled calcification, either focal or diffuse.
   2. Stellate or discrete masses.
   3. Assymetric localized fibrosis.
   4. Increased vascularity.
   5. Altered subareolar duct pattern.

C. **Xerography** — similar to conventional mammography, but uses slightly higher radiation dose. Demonstration of microcalcifications is poorer, although method is less expensive.

D. **Thermography** — thermogram illustrates relative heat radiation in various breast areas (malignancy → increased vascularity → in-

creased heat). Questionable reliability, true–positive rate 29%, false–negative rate 54%.
E. **Ultrasonography** — useful for distinguishing between cystic and solid masses. Effective for lesions > 0.5 cm in diameter.
F. No current clinical role for CT scanning, MRI, or subtraction angiography. Currently under investigation.

V. EVALUATION OF BREAST MASS

Most lesions present as palpable lesions. However, with the widespread use of screening mammography, the evaluation of non-palpable lesions is becoming more common.

A. **Needle aspiration** — use for palpable cystic lesions; 18 or 20 gauge needle with or without local anesthetic. Send fluid for cytology.
   1. Greenish, turbid fluid, and disappearance of mass; follow–up for recurrence. If recurs, excisional biopsy indicated.
   2. Bloody fluid or no fluid; if mass remains, then excisional biopsy should be performed.
B. **Needle aspiration biopsy** — performed using 20 or 22 gauge needle and 10 cc syringe under local anesthesia. Use multiple passes at different angles through the mass while aspirating on syringe. Immediately rinse material in fixative solution.
   1. Negative result — excisional biopsy.
   2. Positive result — discuss cancer treatment options. Still needs confirmation excisional biopsy prior to starting treatment.
C. **Excisional biopsy** — *definitive* method for tissue diagnosis. Majority of procedures performed on outpatients, usually under local anesthesia.
   1. Non–palpable lesions — requires prior radiographic localization and marking with needles or dye.
   2. Biopsy incisions should be placed with deliberation. Subsequent mastectomy should be able to incorporate biopsy incisions.
   3. Specimen should be removed with **complete uninvolved** margins, and sent fresh (unfixed). If histologic exam reveals malignancy, fresh tissue will be available for estrogen (ER) and progesterone (PR) receptors and flow cytometry.
   4. If no malignancy, routine follow–up (see previous section).

VI. DEVELOPMENTAL BREAST LESIONS

A. **Supranumerary breast/nipples** — congenital lesion, localization of breast tissue along "milk line".
B. **Hypoplastic breasts** — associated with Poland's syndrome.
C. **Virginal hypertrophy** — pronounced breast enlargement with pubertal growth. May be symptomatic, occasionally leads to reduction mammoplasty.

VII. BENIGN BREAST DISEASE

A. **Fibrocystic disease** (chronic cystic mastitis). Not true inflammatory disease. Wide spectrum of disease ranging from large cysts to diffuse nodularity to indurated nodules.
   1. Incidence greatest around age 30–40 years, but persists into eighth decade.
   2. Presentation — usually presents with breast pain or mass (or both). Lesions frequently are bilateral; size and pain may vary with menstrual cycle.
   3. Variants.
      a. **Schimmelbusch's disease** — diffuse multiple cysts, rubber consistency. Large "blue–domed" cysts (**Bloodgood cyst**) may be present.
      b. Cystic hyperplasia — similar to above.
      c. **Sclerosing adenosis** — indurated areas of fibrosis present. May be difficult to differentiate from scirrhous carcinoma. Increased risk (~ 3 x) for development of cancer.
   4. **Treatment.**
      a. Rule out carcinoma by aspiration or excisional biopsy of discrete masses.
      b. Frequent examinations (BSE and physician).
      c. Avoid xanthine products (e.g., coffee, tea, chocolate, cola beverages).
      d. Annual mammograms for age > 40.
      e. **Danacrine** (Danazol®) 100 mg PO qid for severe disease. Pain relief within 1 month; decreased nodularity in 2-6 months; 50% recurrence within 1 year of discontinuing drug.
B. **Fibroadenoma.**
   1. Most common breast lesion in women under 25.
   2. Most common in the second or third decade.
   3. Often lobular, firm, rubbery, well circumscribed and mobile.
   4. Treatment — excision.
C. **Intraductal papilloma.**
   1. Presents with bloody nipple discharge in premenopausal women.
   2. 30% are associated with a small, painful subareolar nodule.
   3. Differential diagnosis — Paget's disease, adenoma of nipple, carcinoma.
   4. Treatment — exploration of involved duct and wedge excision of duct.
D. **Fat necrosis.**
   1. Often impossible to differentiate from carcinoma by exam.
   2. History of trauma in 50%, pain characteristic.
   3. Treatment — symptomatic, may need biopsy to rule out carcinoma.
E. **Cystosarcoma phyllodes** — rare variant of fibroadenoma.
   1. Presents as a large bulky mass, overlying skin is red, warm and shiny, with venous engorgement.

   2. Some consider this a low–grade malignancy.

   3. Approximately 10% develop into sarcoma with local invasion or metastases.

   4. Poorly encapsulated, often recurs after excision or enucleation.

   5. Treatment — simple mastectomy.

F. Mammary duct ectasia.

   1. Presents as a diffuse mass, nipple retraction and axillary nodes.

   2. Occurs around menopause, history of difficult nursing.

   3. Subacute inflammation of ductal system.

   4. Excisional biopsy to rule out carcinoma.

G. Galactocele.

   1. Occurs after the cessation of lactation secondary to obstructed lactiferous ducts distended with milk and epithelial cells.

   2. Often presents as a subareolaer mass, yellow nipple discharge.

   3. Treatment — excision.

H. Granular cell myoblastoma (a benign tumor despite its ominous name) — presents like carcinoma; therefore must prove diagnosis on biopsy.

I. Mastitis/abscess.

   1. Commonly occurs in lactating females. Suckling leads to nipple excorciation and secondary infection.

   2. Common organsisms — *Staphylococci* and *Streptococcus.*

   3. Treatment — discontinue nursing. Antibiotics followed by incision and drainage. Multiple incisions may be required due to septae.

J. Mondor's disease (superficial vein thrombophlebitis of breast).

   1. Presents with acute pain often related to trauma.

   2. Must differentiate from other mass lesions.

   3. Treatment is heat and analgesics.

K. Gynecomastia — breast enlargement in males.

   1. Physiologic.

     a. Newborns — due to exposure to maternal estrogens.

     b. Adolescents — often asymmetric, resolves spontaneously.

     c. Elderly — relative estrogen increase in elderly males.

   2. Drug–induced — associated with estrogens, spironolactone, digitalis, resperine, methyldopa, isoniazid, griseofulvin, cimetidine, and marijuana. Treatment is primarily discontinuing drug.

   3. Pathologic.

     a. Deficient production/action of testosterone (e.g., Klinefelter's syndrome).

     b. Increased estrogen levels from testicular tumors, hermaphroditism, adrenal dysfunction, cirrhosis, thyrotoxicosis.

   4. Carcinoma of the breast may present as gynecomastia. Unilateral gynecomastia needs to be evaluated with excisional biopsy to rule out carcinoma.

BREAST CANCER

I. EPIDEMIOLOGY

A. Most common non–skin cancer in U.S. women – 1 in 10.
B. Second leading cause of cancer deaths in U.S. women and the leading cause of death in U.S. women 35–54 years of age.
C. Higher mortality in developed countries (except Japan) and higher socioeconomic groups.
D. Increasing incidence after age 20, with slight plateau during menopausal period (ages 45–55).

II. RISK FACTORS

A. Mother/sister with breast cancer – 2–3 x increased risk.
B. Family disease of premenopausal or bilateral disease – 50 x increased risk.
C. Previous history of breast cancer – 5 x increased risk in contralateral breast.
D. Fibrocystic breast disease – probably only certain types, e.g., sclerosing adenosis; 2.6 x increased risk.
E. Early menarche (< 12 years of age); prolonged menstrual activity (> 30 years) (? increased estrogen exposure) – 1.5 x increased risk.
F. Early menopause (< 45 years of age); castration (by age 35–40) – 1/3 to 1/2 **decreased** risk.
G. Age of patient at 1st delivery.
   1. > 25 years old – 2 x increased risk *vs.* those < 25 years old.
   2. > 31 years old – 3 x increased risk *vs.* those < 21 years old.
H. Radiation – linear dose–response relationship.
I. Cancer of ovary, uterus, or colon – possible increased risk.

III. CLINICAL PRESENTATION

A. Non–palpable lesion on screening mammogram – requires needle localization biopsy.
B. **Palpable mass** – 40–50% upper–outer quadrant; 70-80% scirrhous; majority patient–detected; 15–40% multicentric; bilateral masses up to 30% with lobular carcinoma.
   1. Adenopathy – axillary, supraclavicular, cervical.
   2. Skin changes – dimpling (Cooper's ligament retraction); *"peau d'orange"* (dermal lymphatic invasion); ulceration; inflammation (nipple eczema with Paget's, diffuse skin involvement with inflammatory cancer).
   3. **Nipple retraction.**
   4. Pain – late symptom.
   5. Nipple discharge – bloody; uncommon.

C. Distant metastatic disease.

1. Bone pain/pathologic fracture — bone metastasis. } 55-65% of
2. Malignant pleural effusion — lung metastasis. } metastases
3. Liver metastasis.

IV. STAGING — TNM CLASSIFICATION

Stage	T	N	M
T_{IS}	*in situ*	–	–
I	T_1 (< 2 cm)	N_0 (no nodes)	M_0 (no metastasis)
II	T_0 (mammographically) or T_1	N_1 (any nodes)	M_0
II	T_2 (2–5 cm)	N_0 or N_1	M_0
IIIa	T_0, T_1, or T_2	N_2 (fixed nodes)	M_0
IIIa	T_3 (> 5 cm)	Any	M_0
IIIb	Any	N_3 (supraclavicular or other nodes)	M_0
IIIb	T_4 (chest wall fixation, peau d'orange, ulceration)	Any	M_0
IV	Any	Any	M_1 (distant mets)

V. PATHOLOGY

A. Growth patterns.

1. Ductal — from epithelium of large or intermediate ducts.
2. Lobular — from epithelium of terminal ducts.
3. Ductal or lobular may be either *in situ* (noninvasive) or invasive.

B. Histology.

Type	% Occurrence
Infiltrating ductal (not otherwise specified)	70 – 80
Medullary	5 – 8
Colloid	2 – 4
Tubular	1 – 2
Papillary	1 – 2
Invasive lobular	6 – 8
Noninvasive	4 – 6
Ductal carcinoma *in situ* (DCIS)	2 – 3
Lobular carcinoma *in situ* (LCIS)	2 – 3
Rare types: juvenile; adenoid cystic; epidermoid; sudiferous	< 1
Paget's disease of the nipple	1

C. **Staging** more important than histology in determining prognosis.

D. 1–3% of patients with DCIS have foci of invasive cancer of any type elsewhere in ipsilateral breast.

E. **LCIS** — up to 30% have bilateral involvement; progression to invasive lobular carcinoma in up to 30%; biopsy of the contralateral breast is positive in 15% even if no mass palpated.

F. Total DNA content determined by flow cytometry may be best indicator of prognosis. Aneuploidy associated with more aggressive tumors and poorer prognosis.

VI. SURGICAL TREATMENT OPTIONS

A. **Wide local excision (WLE)/lumpectomy/segmental mastectomy.**
   1. Complete excision, with adequate margins, is important.
   2. May be done with or without axillary node dissection.
   3. May be done with or without radiotherapy (XRT).
   4. Advantages — reconstruction not needed; cosmetic results are generally good.

B. **Subcutaneous mastectomy.**
   1. Removes breast tissue only, sparing nipple/areola, skin, and nodes.
   2. Not a cancer operation — leaves behind 1–2% of breast tissue.
   3. May be indicated for LCIS or prophylaxis for contralateral breast at high risk.

C. **Simple mastectomy** (total mastectomy) — breast, skin, nipple/areola removal.
   1. No nodal dissection performed.
   2. Advantage — amenable to reconstruction.

D. **Modified radical mastectomy (MRM).**
   1. Removes breast, skin, nipple/areola, and Level I & II axillary nodes, sparing pectoralis muscles.
      a. "Patey" modification — spares pectoralis major (remove pectoralis minor and nodes).
      b. "Madden" modification — spares pectoralis major and pectoralis minor.
   2. Advantage — amenable to reconstruction.

E. **Radical mastectomy (Halsted).**
   1. Removes breast, skin, nipple/areola, both pectoral muscles, and axillary nodes.
   2. Cosmetic/functional results are often suboptimal, frequently requiring skin grafting. Largely abandoned.

F. **Extended radical mastectomy (Urban).**
   1. As for radical mastectomy, but also removes internal mammary nodes with medial costal cartilages and part of sternum.
   2. Disfiguring and no improvement in survival; thus, has been largely abandoned.

VII. SURGICAL TREATMENT BY STAGE, AND OUTCOME

A. **Stage TIS (controversial).**
 1. **DCIS** — WLE and XRT or MRM.
 2. **LCIS** — MRM *vs.* close follow-up with or without mirror image biopsy — controversial, as 1/3 will become invasive and 1/3 are bilateral.
 3. **Paget's disease** — MRM *vs.* WLE and AND with or without mirror image biopsy.
 4. **Results** — > 90% 5–year survival (**Note:** *not* 100%).

B. **Stages I & II** — represents approximately 80% of breast cancers.

| Treatment Group | 8–Year Survival (%) (n = 1843) | | |
	DFS	DDFS	Overall Survival
All Patients			
MRM	67	74	82
WLE + XRT	71	74	84
Node–Negative			
MRM	65.5	73.8	78.7
WLE + XRT	65.6	70.7	82.9
Node–Positive#			
MRM	44.5	50.7	59.9
WLE + XRT	46.6	53.1	68.3

DFS = disease–free survival (local/regional recurrence).
DDSF = distant disease–free survival (metastasis).
All groups received **axillary node dissection.**
#All node–positive patients received chemotherapy.

C. **Current recommendations.**
 1. WLE plus XRT, with chemotherapy if node (+), is appropriate therapy for Stage I and II if specimen margins are free of tumor.
 2. WLE plus XRT in terms of disease–free survival, distant disease–free survival, and overall survival do not differ from those for MRM. WLE plus XRT allows breast conservation with similar results.
 3. Addition of XRT to WLE improves disease–free survival (i.e., decreased local/regional recurrence), but does not improve distant disease–free survival or overall survival in node (–) patients (not shown by data above).
 4. Hence, for Stage I or II, current recommendations are MRM or WLE with axillary node dissection plus XRT. Depends upon patient's wishes and the ability to closely follow patient.
 5. Addition of XRT to WLE with axillary node dissection significantly reduces recurrence in ipsilateral breast, even in node (–)

patients who receive chemotherapy (from 37% to 12% in node–negative and from 43% to 6% in node–positive).
6. MRM is as effective as radical mastectomy at 10 years in terms of survival, DFS, and DDFS (for both node–positive and node–negative).
7. WLE (with XRT) and mastectomy are used *only* to provide **local** control of the disease in node (+) patients. Chemotherapy is needed to provide **systemic** control.

D. **Stages III & IV** — represents approximately 20% of breast cancers.
1. Goals of therapy — control of local disease and improved quality of life, as almost all of these patients will die of distant metastases.
2. Surgical therapy must be individualized from "toilet" simple mastectomy to aggressive surgery (radical mastectomy) for deeply invasive tumors (to control ulceration, etc.).
3. Mainstay of therapy — palliation with chemotherapy, radiotherapy.
4. Survival — 10% 5–year survival.

VIII. RADIOTHERAPY

A. Rarely used as single modality except for palliation in extremely debilitated patients.
B. Improves 8–year disease–free survival when added to local excision with axillary node dissection in node (–) patients with Stage I or II disease, but does not improve distant disease–free survival or overall survival.
C. Decreases local/regional recurrence after local excision with axillary node dissection, even in node (–) patients.
D. Local excision with axillary node dissection plus radiotherapy provides survival as good as mastectomy, and allows breast conservation.
E. Possible complications — breast atrophy/fibrosis; rib fracture; pneumonitis; pericarditis; dermatitis; skin ulceration; edema of arm/breast especially when combined with axillary node dissection.
F. Dose — generally 5,000 RAD external beam, fractionated. An axillary boost is probably not indicated if adequate axillary node dissection has been performed (no decrease in recurrence but increased arm edema).

IX. DRUG THERAPY

A. Rationale.
1. Natural history of breast cancer suggests multicentricity (15–40%) and/or slow tumor growth, but with early subclinical metastasis (e.g., late recurrences following adequate therapy for small tumor with negative nodes and < 100% survival after treatment for C.I.S.).
2. Patients at highest risk of treatment failure.
   a. Premenopausal women, especially node (+).

    b. > 3 positive axillary nodes.
    c. High tumor grade and size if node (+).
    d. ER/PR (–) tumors.
    e. Even Stage I/II node (–) patients have 15% mortality with metastatic disease 5 years after treatment.
    f. High DNA content (?).
3. Therefore: Systemic therapy to control systemic disease, with surgery/radiotherapy for loco–regional control.
4. Categories.
    a. Hormonal — anti–estrogen; additive; ablation (medical or surgical).
    b. Cytotoxic — especially for node (+) patients.
5. **Adjuvant drug therapy for primary breast cancer.**

Menopausal Status	Nodal Status	ER/PR Status*	Therapy
Post	(+)	(+)	Tamoxifen® (or DES or aminoglutethimide)
Post	(–)/(+)	(–)	? Chemotherapy
Pre	(–)	(+)	Tamoxifen®
Pre	(–)	(–)	Chemotherapy
Pre	(+)	(–)/(+)	Chemotherapy

    *(+) ER is ≥ 10 fmol/mg cytosol protein

6. **Adjuvant drug therapy for recurrence.**

Menopausal Status	ER/PR Status*	Therapy	% Response	Second Line
Post	(+)	Tamoxifen®	60	DES, aminoglutethimide
Pre	(+)	Oophorectomy	60	Tamoxifen®; estrogen/ progesterone
Post/Pre	(–)	Chemotherapy	60	

    * Receptor status of recurrence is often (although not always) similar to that of primary tumor.

B. Hormonal manipulation.
    1. Anti–estrogen — Tamoxifen®; DES; aminoglutethimide ("medical adrenalectomy").
        a. Tamoxifen® significantly reduces mortality in women > 50.
        b. As good or better than chemotherapy for ER (+) post–menopause.

      c. Increased disease–free survival in both pre– and post–meno-
pausal patients with (–) nodes and ER (+) tumors (4–year
follow–up).
  2. "Additive" high–dose estrogen/progesterone.
      a. Equivalent response (~ 60%) to surgery or Tamoxifen® in
pre–menopausal patients with ER (+) recurrence.
      b. Side–effects are major — thus, rarely used.
  3. Ablative.
      a. Oophorectomy for pre–menopausal women with ER (+) re-
currence — response (~ 60%) equivalent to Tamoxifen®.
      b. Adrenalectomy — currently less popular than Tamoxifen®
and aminoglutethimide ("medical adrenalectomy") for post–
menopausal women with ER (+) recurrent disease.
C. **Cytotoxic chemotherapy** — currently multi–agent.
  1. CMF and CMFVP — high toxicity secondary to alkylating
agents.
  2. **Methotrexate and 5–FU** — probably less toxicity, especially for
node (–), ER (–) tumors; increased disease–free survival, but
no increase in overall survival (4–year follow–up).
  3. **PFT** (L–PAM®, 5–FU + Tamoxifen®) — increases disease–
free survival in post–menopausal, node (+), ER (+) women.
  4. Chemotherapy better than no chemotherapy in node (+). Not
enough data to judge in node (–).
  5. Multi–agent chemotherapy better than single agent, especially
for women < 50 years old.
  6. If node (–), no increased survival for women > 50 years old,
but chemotherapy *does* decrease recurrence in both pre– and
post–menopausal women.
D. Controversies and studies ongoing at present.
  1. Chemotherapy for node (–), ER (+) — is DNA flow cytometry analysis able to identify patients at risk?
  2. Tamoxifen® for node (–), ER (+) — NSABP B–14 protocol.
  3. Chemotherapy for node (–), ER (–) — duration, drugs? —
NSABP B–13 protocol.
  4. Risk of later malignancy following aggressive chemotherapy.

X. CANCER OF THE MALE BREAST
A. About 1% of breast cancer occurs in males.
B. Presents as gynecomastia, biopsy needed to rule out cancer.
C. Worse prognosis than female patients because of early and diffuse
lymphatic involvement.
D. Prompt excision of gynecomastia will help improve survival.

THYROID

I. THYROID NODULE
A. Overview.
1. Estimated 4% of U.S. population have clinically palpable thyroid nodules.
2. 85% of thyroid nodules are benign (colloid) nodules that can usually be managed non–operatively.
3. Of the 15% of nodules surgically managed, only 5–8% are thyroid carcinomas.
4. Women have 4 times the incidence of thyroid nodules, but the incidence of cancer is equal in men and women. Therefore, the incidence of a nodule being cancerous is greater for men.
5. Increased risk of malignancy in nodules arising before age 30 or after age 60.

B. **High–risk groups.**
1. Patients with prior history of low–dose radiation to head and neck region (acne, tonsillitis, thymic enlargement).
   a. 30% of patients with prior cervical irradiation develop nodules.
   b. About 30% of these nodules will be malignant.
2. Family history of medullary thyroid cancer or multiple endocrine neoplasia (MEN) — transmitted as autosomal dominant trait, thus 50% of offspring would be expected to have this disease.
3. Single nodule increases chance of neoplasm (benign or malignant).
4. Enlarging nodule on thyroid hormone suppression.

C. **History.**
1. Weight loss, irritability, intolerance to heat, thinning of hair, softening of the skin, palpitations and tachycardia suggest hyperthyroidism.
2. Weight gain, lethargy, coarseness of hair, thickened skin, and intolerance to cold suggest hypothyroidism.
3. Rate of growth of nodule — more rapid growth suggests malignancy. Nodule present for several years — less chance of carcinoma.
4. Dysphagia, dyspnea, hoarseness, vocal cord paralysis, Horner's syndrome, other neck masses or adenopathy suggest malignancy within the thyroid nodule, other head and neck malignancy or lymphoma.

D. **Physical exam.**
1. Palpate the thyroid from behind the patient with the head upright but relaxed.
2. A normal thyroid gland is difficult to palpate in a patient who is obese or has a very short muscular neck.

3. Palpation may be facilitated by having patient swallow water.
4. The isthmus crosses the trachea at the first or second tracheal ring and the lobes of the thyroid move upward with swallowing.
5. Examiner should note the size, consistency, tenderness, and nodularity of the gland.
6. The normal gland is "gelatinous", pliant. Hyperplastic glands are soft.
7. Carcinomas may be hard and firm, and may have associated adenopathy or be adfixed to adjacent structures.
8. Thyroiditis may be nodular or diffuse, rubbery, and may be accompanied by local pressure symptoms.
9. A palpable lymph node in the midline just above the isthmus is associated with thyroid carcinoma or thyroiditis (**Delphian node**).

E. **Suppressive therapy** — Synthroid® 1.5–2.0 μg/lb PO every day for well–differentiated causes (post–operation). Document decreased TSH levels. Supplemental therapy: Synthroid® 1.0 μg/lb for benign disease.
1. Useful in patients who have an elevated TSH level or have adenomatous goiters (by cytopathologic examination) that are hypofunctioning as opposed to non–functioning.
2. *Not* useful in differentiating thyrotropin–dependent and (presumably) benign nodules from thyroid cancer.
3. Soft nodules in pregnant patients warrant a 3–6 month trial (if cytology indicates benign disease).
4. Nodules which persist after 3 months require excision.

F. **Aspiration cytology** — the single most helpful first procedure to evaluate a thyroid nodule.
1. Technique — identify and immobilize lesion between 2 fingers.
   a. Insert 20 or 22 gauge needle into the lesion using a 10 cc syringe or special aspirating holder.
   b. While suction is applied, move the needle within the lesion to aspirate clumps of epithelial cells (with large lesions, aspirate near periphery for highest diagnostic accuracy).
   c. Release suction prior to removing the needle in order to prevent aspiration of the cell sample into the syringe or aspiration of blood.
   d. Expel cells onto slide and fix, or in special preservation solution.
   e. Need experienced cytologist to interpret thyroid aspirates.
2. Results — 7% rate of non–diagnostic samples. Interpreted as neoplasia (it is difficult to distinguish adenomas from well–differentiated carcinomas), indeterminate, or the appropriate benign diagnosis.
   a. Colloid nodules can be diagnosed as such and contain colloid plus normal follicular cells.

b. Cytology is clearly diagnostic of papillary cancer. Accurate and reliable.

c. "Follicular cytology" can represent a benign follicular nodule, a follicular carcinoma, or a follicular area in a mixed papillary/follicular cancer — the diagnosis cannot be made without a careful examination of the entire nodule and its capsule. Excision is **recommended** due to risk of cancer.

d. Intermediate lesions must be removed because 20–60% will be malignant.

e. Accuracy — highly dependent on the cytopathologist's experience.

1) 2.2% false-negative rate is the best reported (Lowhagen, Sweden).

2) 10–20% false-negative rate in U.S. literature (less at University of Cincinnati), 88–99% sensitivity.

f. The 10-20% false-negative rate severely limits the usefulness of aspiration cytology. If a high clinical suspicion of malignancy exists, an excisional biopsy or lobectomy is indicated.

g. If lesion is cystic — malignancy is unlikely if the cyst disappears completely following aspiration; aspiration repeated at 6–8 week intervals if recurs. Thyroid cysts usually refill. Surgical removal advised on third recurrence.

G. **Ultrasound** — can identify nodules as small as 1 mm.

1. Able to identify if nodule is cystic or solid, but provides no information as to whether nodule is benign or malignant.

2. Solid nodules are more likely to be malignant.

3. Most cystic nodules are benign, but some papillary cancers are cystic.

H. **Thyroid scan** — can classify nodule as cold (non–functional), warm (functional), or hot (hyperfunctional). Most cancers appear to be "cold" as do most of the benign lesions. Therefore, carcinomas are found in 20–25% of cold nodules.

I. Thyroid function tests — not very useful as diagnostic test, as most thyroid cancers are euthyroid. Single hot nodule present with hyperthyroidism is less likely to be malignant (0.5%).

II. THYROID CARCINOMA

A. Overview.

1. Most common endocrine malignancy in U.S.

2. 4 cases per 100,000 population (relatively uncommon).

3. Uncommon cause of death, because the majority of these lesions are well differentiated and relatively non–aggressive. Moreover, death usually follows a long disease course — up to 30 years.

B. **Histologic types of thyroid carcinoma.**

1. **Papillary** carcinoma — 70%.

a. Slow–growing and often multicentric.

    b. Most common tumor following neck irradiation.

    c. Commonly spread to regional lymph nodes (50% have nodal metastasis at time of operation), but even then rarely cause rapid death (> 90% 5–year survival if small and intrathyroidal).

    d. Moderately more aggressive in males over age 40 or females over age 50.

    e. Tumors < 1.5 cm rarely metastasize or recur; if ≥ 1.5 cm, 50% have lymph node metastasis.

    f. Distant metastases, usually to lung, are present in 5–15% of patients.

2. Follicular carcinoma — 15–20%.

    a. Usually unilateral.

    b. Rarely metastasize to regional nodes (< 15%).

    c. Hematogenous dissemination has occurred in 50% of cases at time of diagnosis (bone, lung, brain and liver) — Distant metastases are often first indication of malignancy.

    d. 5–year survival.

        1) 85% in the absence of angioinvasion.

        2) 45–50% if angioinvasion is present.

3. Mixed papillary/follicular carcinoma — behaves like papillary, but usually more aggressive.

4. Medullary carcinoma — 7%.

    a. Arise from C–cells (parafollicular) of the thyroid which secrete calcitonin. C–cells are of neural crest origin and part of the APUD system.

    b. Virulence intermediate between well–differentiated and anaplastic lesions.

    c. Frequently metastasize to regional lymph nodes.

    d. Aggressive initial surgical approach (total complete thyroidectomy) is advocated due to ineffective medical adjuvant treatment.

    e. Sporadic cases — usually unilateral.

    f. Familial cases — often bilateral.

        1) Occurs in 50% of offspring of patients with this hereditary form.

        2) Associated with **MEN–II syndrome** (medullary carcinoma of the thyroid, pheochromocytoma, and either hyperparathyroidism [**MEN–IIa**] or mucosal neuromas [**MEN–IIb**).

        3) Calcitonin levels are useful for screening, and if elevated are **diagnostic**.

5. Anaplastic carcinoma — 3%.

    a. Mean survival is 2–5 months.

    b. Outcome unaffected by surgery.

    c. May develop in a well–differentiated lesion which contained an anaplastic component.

    d. Almost 80% have a history of long–standing goiter.

    e. Some evidence suggests that external irradiation to a well–differentiated lesion could contribute to de–differentiation into an anaplastic lesion.

    f. Make sure small–cell type is studied appropriately to rule out lymphoma which has a much better prognosis.

III. INDICATIONS FOR SURGICAL TREATMENT

A. **Carcinoma** — either diagnosed on aspiration cytology or suspected from work–up in high–risk group.

B. **Hyperthyroidism.**
    1. Very large multinodular goiter with relatively low radioiodine uptake which is therefore poorly treated with ^{131}I.
    2. Pregnancy or patients desiring to become pregnant within 1 year.
    3. Children.

C. Large goiter impairing airway — tracheal deviation, stridor, retrosternal position.

IV. TREATMENT

A. Options.
    1. Excisional biopsy of nodule is **contraindicated**.
    2. Lobectomy with removal of isthmus is the minimal biopsy of any nodule.
    3. Ipsilateral lobectomy with contralateral subtotal or intracapsular lobectomy (decreases risk of damage to parathyroid glands and recurrent laryngeal nerves on contralateral side).
    4. Total thyroidectomy.

B. Areas of agreement on surgical treatment.
    1. Papillary carcinoma < 1.5 cm in diameter — lobectomy and isthmectomy alone. Rare recurrence or nodal metastases.
    2. Preoperatively diagnosed metastatic thyroid carcinoma — total thyroidectomy. This facilitates adjuvant treatment with ^{131}I.
    3. Medullary carcinoma — total thyroidectomy with modified lymph node dissection (preserve internal jugular vein and spinal-accessory nerve) on side of lesion or both sides if bilateral disease is present. In familial cases detected by screening calcitonin levels in a subclinical state, total thyroidectomy without lymph node dissection is probably adequate.

C. Management of other well–differentiated carcinomas.
    1. Factors to consider in deciding extent of resection.
        a. There is a 30% incidence of microscopic disease in clinically uninvolved lobe (50% if previous cervical irradiation).
        b. The incidence of contralateral recurrence in patients who have undergone less than total thyroidectomy varies widely from 4.2 to 24%.

    c. Risks of recurrent laryngeal nerve injury — when nerve injuries occur, they are usually injured in removing larger advanced tumors that are adherent or encasing the nerve as it is approaching the thyroid cartilage. The configuration of the cancer, rather than the intent or skill of the surgeon, is more frequently the cause of nerve injury. Risk of injury is 0.2–3%, while risk of injury with re-operation is approximately 6%.

    d. Hypoparathyroidism — any one functional gland can maintain eucalcemia; thus, this complication is seen exclusively in bilateral dissection. Incidence around 3%.

  2. Lymph node dissection — most authors feel that lymph node dissection is indicated only for clinically apparent disease.

    a. 50% of lymph node dissections done in the absence of clinical disease will show microscopic involvement.

    b. 13% of patients who do not undergo lymph node dissection will develop clinically apparent disease.

    c. The presence or absence of nodal metastases has minimal effect on prognosis, and local control is equal if nodes are not removed until they become clinically apparent.

    d. The disease is removed with neck nodes by a modified "conservative" lymphadenectomy when metastases are present. A major purpose is to prevent subsequent airway compromise as metastases grow.

V. PREOPERATIVE PREPARATION OF THE HYPERTHYROID PATIENT

A. **Propylthiouracil (PTU)** — 150 mg PO q 6–8 h or Tapazole® 30–60 mg per day given BID or TID prevent the formation of thyroid hormone. No effect is usually seen for 2–3 weeks until the gland is depleted of stored sources.

B. **Saturated solution of potassium iodide (SSKI)** — 2–5 drops PO every day given for 10–15 days prior to surgery will decrease the vascularity of the thyroid gland.

VI. POST–THYROIDECTOMY CARE

A. All patients should be treated with Synthroid®.

  1. Replacement in patients undergoing total thyroidectomy.

  2. Suppression of TSH in subtotal resections.

B. Radionuclide imaging after 3–4 weeks of Synthroid® therapy is useful to localize metastatic disease.

C. ^{131}I can be used as adjuvant treatment if metastatic disease is present. Usually following total thyroidectomy.

  1. Papillary or follicular cancer with positive nodes, possible residual disease, suspected metastases, angioinvasive.

  2. Hold thyroid replacement for 6 weeks.

3. ^{131}I scan.
    a. No uptake — no therapy.
    b. Local or metastatic uptake identified — therapeutic ^{131}I.
4. Re–evaluate yearly.

VII. THYROID STORM

A. May be precipitated by surgery, anxiety, excessive palpation of gland, or adrenergic stimulants in an otherwise well–controlled hyper-thyroid patient.

B. Prevention — allow enough time for adequate depletion of thyroid stores of T_4 after treatment with PTU prior to surgery.

C. Symptoms.
    1. Hyperpyrexia, tachycardia, numbness, irritability, vomiting, and diarrhea.
    2. High output cardiac failure is the usual cause of death.

D. Treatment.
    1. Mechanical cooling — oxygen–volume restoration.
    2. To prevent adrenal insufficiency, administer 100 mg hydro-cortisone IV.
    3. Beta blockade — may be substituted for prolonged preoperative prep in severe disease in young patients.
        a. Propranolol 1–2 mg slow IVP followed by constant infusion of 50–100 μg/min to control symptoms.
        b. Propranolol starting at 10 mg PO q6h and increased prn to control symptoms may be given pre- or post-operatively, but this only blocks the effects of hyperthyroidism despite persistently elevated T_4 levels.
    4. Begin long–term suppression with PTU.
    5. Digitalization if persistently severe symptoms.

PARATHYROIDISM

I. PRIMARY HYPERPARATHYROIDISM (HPT)

A. Recent increase in incidence, especially asymptomatic cases due to routine serum calcium screening.
   1. 100–200 per 100,000 in–hospital population.
   2. 25–28 per 100,000 general population.
   3. Highest incidence in post–menopausal women.
   4. 50,000–90,000 new cases per year, 60% asymptomatic.

B. **Clinical presentation** — "stones, bones, abdominal groans, and psychic overtones."
   1. Up to 35% of asymptomatic patients have suspected complications.
   2. Urologic most common manifestation, up to 30% of patients.
      a. Presents as nephrolithiasis or nephrocalcinosis.
      b. Stones are usually calcium phosphate. Calcium oxalate or mixed stones less common.
      c. 5-15% incidence of primary HPT in patients with urolithiasis.
   3. Skeletal syndrome — < 10% of symptomatic patients.
      a. Bone pain, arthralgias (secondary to pseudogout), vague aches.
      b. Osteitis fibrosa cystica, bone cysts, pathological fractures are rare.
   4. **Hypercalcemic syndrome** — may present with acute hypercalcemic crisis.
      a. Presenting symptoms — anorexia, nausea, vomiting, polyuria, polydipsia, abdominal pain, nonspecific GI upset, lethargy, bone pain, muscular weakness.
      b. Serum calcium levels > 15 mg/dl are critical and require urgent treatment (see section F).
      c. If untreated, may progress to dehydration, oliguria, renal failure, delirium in hours to days.
   5. Peptic ulcer, pancreatitis, hypertension all reported with primary HPT. No firm clinical evidence to support causal link.
   6. Familial primary HPT — < 10% of patients have associated MEN I or II (see "Miscellaneous Endocrine Disorders"). Be sure to screen for unrecognized pheochromocytoma — big trouble. Must treat pheochromocytoma *first* !

C. Physical exam — parathyroid gland may only be palpable in 5–40% of patients with a large adenoma.

D. **Laboratory studies.**
   1. Elevated serum calcium (normal 8.5–10.5).
      a. Only 20% of patients with elevated calcium have primary HPT.

    b. Major cause of hypercalcemia is **neoplastic** (skeletal metastasis or myelomas).

    c. Other causes — sarcoidosis, drugs, vitamin D intoxication, milk alkali syndrome, ectopic PTH production by tumors (lung, kidney, pancreas, breast, and bladder).

    d. Serum calcium may be intermittently normal in primary HPT — at least 3 determinations are recommended.

2. Serum phosphorus — usually low in primary HPT.

3. Plasma chloride.

    a. Level is increased in those patients with primary HPT without renal disease or being treated with diuretics.

    b. Levels > 102 are present with HPT; if chloride < 102, hypercalcemia most likely due to cause other than HPT.

    c. Chloride/phosphate ratio > 33 virtually diagnostic of HPT.

4. **Serum parathyroid hormone (PTH).**

    a. Increased PTH with hypercalcemia is diagnostic of primary or tertiary HPT.

    b. Level greater than expected for given serum calcium.

    c. Measurement by immunoassay is more difficult than most other polypeptides.

    d. N–terminal — confers the biological effect of the molecule, short half–life (several minutes).

    e. C–terminal — better for diagnosing primary HPT, longer serum half-life (1–2 hours).

    f. "Ectopic" PTH production characterized by a polypeptide with PTH–like actions, but not detected by PTH assay.

    g. An elevated PTH in a patient with impaired renal function does not necessarily indicate HPT. There is a decrease in excretion of PTH fragments by the kidney as the creatinine increases.

5. Urinary calcium excretion.

    a. Rarely exceeds 500 mg/day in primary HPT.

    b. In familial hypercalcemic hypocalcuria — < 200 mg/day of urinary calcium.

6. Roentgenologic findings.

    a. Magnified hand films on industrial grade film reveal subtle changes of osteitis fibrosa cystica.

       1) Fraying of distal phalangeal tufts.

       2) Subperiosteal resorption of margins of middle and distal phalanges (pathognomonic of chronic HPT).

       3) Cysts of the carpal bones.

    b. Solitary bone cysts (Brown tumors).

    c. "Ground glass" demineralization of skull seen in advanced cases.

    d. Excretory urogram.

       1) Detect radiolucent calcium oxalate stones.

       2) Evaluate nephrocalcinosis.

       3) Rule out hypernephroma (the source of "ectopic" PTH in 30% of cases).

    e. Chest x-ray.

       1) Resorption of distal end of clavicle is pathognomonic of chronic HPT.

       2) Rule out lung tumors (frequent source of "ectopic" HPT).

E. Pathology — 3 distinct lesions.

  1. Parathyroid adenoma — most frequent cause, 85–90% of cases.

    a. Usually solitary (multiple adenomas in up to 5%).

    b. Size varies from 70 mg up to several grams.

    c. Histologically indistinguishable from chief cell hyperplasia, although a rim of normal parathyroid tissue may be visible.

  2. Chief cell hyperplasia — about 10% of cases of primary HPT.

    a. Histology — lack of stromal fat. Normal parathyroid in children or malnourished may have an identical appearance.

    b. All four parathyroid glands involved.

    c. All cases of primary HPT in association with MEN syndromes involve hyperplasia.

  3. Parathyroid carcinoma — < 1% of cases.

    a. Usually involves single gland.

    b. Firm, adherent to adjacent structures.

    c. Metastasizes late to regional lymph nodes.

F. Treatment — acute hypercalcemic crisis.

  1. Medical emergency due to rapid dehydration followed by renal failure.

  2. Treatment — rapid rehydration with normal saline.

  3. When urine output is restored, begin forced diuresis with furosemide (20 mg IV at hourly intervals), administer saline equal to urine output.

  4. If due to bony metastases (particularly from breast), steroids may slow bone release.

  5. Watch for hypokalemia.

  6. Etridonate disodium (7.5 mg/kg IV x 3 days, then 5–20 mg/kg PO qd maintenance) can be effective in lowering calcium levels (works by inhibiting bone metabolism). It should *not* be used in the face of renal failure. Very useful in therapy of malignancy induced hypercalcemia.

  7. Administration of mithramycin (25 μg/kg over 4 hrs) will usually return calcium to normal within 24 hrs and maintain for several days.

    a. Mithramycin — used **only in most desperate circumstances** (hypercalcemia in malignancy).

    b. Daily white counts must be carefully monitored — discontinue drug at slightest decrease in WBC.

    c. If not properly used with caution, this is a *deadly* drug due to the frequency and severity of bone marrow "wipe–out".

G. Surgery for hyperparathyroidism.

  1. Symptomatic or complicated disease.

  2. Serum calcium > 11 mg/dl.

  3. Post–menopausal women with mild symptoms and osteoporosis may benefit from early operative intervention to prevent osteopenia.

  4. Recurrent hypercalcemia occurs in ~ 16% of patients operated on for hyperplasia (1–19 years post–op) and 3% of patients with adenomas (average of 12 years and not earlier than 9 years post–op).

  5. Operative strategy.

    a. Attempt to identify all four glands.

    b. If one or two glands are enlarged and the patient does not have MEN, then these glands are removed.

    c. If 3 or more glands are enlarged or patient has MEN, a 31/2 gland parathyroidectomy is performed or total parathyroidectomy with re–implantation of parathyroid tissue in forearm or sternocleidomastoid.

    d. If MEN–II suspected, it is essential to completely explore thyroid, searching for medullary thyroid carcinoma. Should have a pre–op calcitonin level.

    e. If there is a possibility of devascularization of remaining parathyroid tissue, an autotransplant to the sternocleidomastoid muscle or forearm flexor muscles is done.

    f. If 4 normal glands are found, exploration of the superior mediastinum (via cervical incision), the retropharyngeal and retroesophageal spaces, and bilateral carotid sheaths is done. Supernumerary glands present in up to 10%.

    g. If only 4 normal glands located, they are tagged with clips and pre–op localization studies are performed prior to re-operation.

  6. Postoperative results, complications, and care.

    a. Low morbidity — 3% occurrence of vocal cord dysfunction, with up to 10% of these permanent.

    b. Serum calcium usually returns to normal within 1–2 days.

    c. Symptomatic hypocalcemia may occur due to hypoparathyroidism (high serum phosphorus) or "bone hunger" (low serum phosphorus).

      1) Symptoms — anxiety, hyperventilation, circumoral paresthesias, positive Chvostek's and Trousseau's (carpedal spasm) signs.

      2) Treatment with oral calcium carbonate (600 mg q 6 h) and vitamin D will usually alleviate symptoms.

      3) If symptoms severe, treatment with IV calcium gluconate is indicated.

4) Vitamin D may be stopped when eucalcemia established for several weeks.
5) Calcium supplements stopped when parathyroid function returns.
7. Patients in whom initial exploration was unsuccessful should undergo preoperative localization prior to re-exploration.
   a. Ultrasound — detects glands as small as 3 mm. Useful prior to initial exploration, accuracy about 80%. Does not detect retrosternal adenomas.
   b. CT scan — recommended for suspected retrosternal adenoma (dynamic scan with IV contrast). Accuracy about 50%.
   c. Radionuclide scan — subtraction scan using thallium-201 and technetium 99m. Accuracy 80–85%.
   d. Arteriography — selective studies of superior thyroid, inferior thyroid, or internal mammary arteries may demonstrate a tumor blush. Useful in locating mediastinal tumors. Accuracy about 50%.
   e. Selective venous sampling — accuracy up to 70% when combined with arteriography. Requires highly skilled technique, results delayed, is very expensive.
   f. MRI — promising future, but still too little data to evaluate.

II. SECONDARY HYPERPARATHYROIDISM (HPT)

A. Usually found in patients with chronic renal failure.
   1. Phosphate retention secondary to kidney's inability to excrete increased phosphate load leads to decreased serum ionized calcium.
   2. Decreased gut absorption of calcium due to decreased renal activation of vitamin D.
   3. Decreased renal clearance of PTH as renal failure progresses.
   4. All of the above lead to parathyroid hyperplasia.
B. Symptoms.
   1. Renal osteodystrophy — increased bone resorption leads to bone pain and pathologic fractures.
   2. Soft tissue calcification — lead to tendonitis, tendon rupture, limitation of joint movement, vascular calcification, coronary artery calcification.
   3. Other manifestations — psychiatric disorders, headache, muscle weakness, weight loss, fatigue.
C. Medical treatment — prevention of secondary HPT.
   1. Phosphate binding antacids, low phosphate diet — used to lower serum phosphate to under 5 mg/dl.
   2. Oral calcium supplements and vitamin D administration to increase serum calcium.
   3. Adjust dialysate concentrations of calcium (3.1–3.8 mEq/liter).

D. **Surgical treatment.**
   1. Indications — severe bone disease, severe pruritis, extensive soft tissue or vascular calcification, other uncontrollable manifestations.
   2. Operative strategy — subtotal (3 1/2 gland) parathyroidectomy or total parathyroidectomy with autotransplant of parathyroid tissue into the forearm musculature.

III. TERTIARY HYPERPARATHYROIDISM (HPT)

A. Persistent hypercalcemia and hyperparathyroidism following successful renal transplant.
B. Occurs in up to 30% of patients with pre–transplant HPT.
C. **Pathogenesis** — believed to be secondary to hyperplasia of the parathyroid gland before and during hemodialysis. There is an increased number of parathyroid cells, each producing a non-suppressible minimum obligatory PTH secretion. Thus, there is a continued elevated PTH level which leads to hypercalcemia.
D. **Indications for surgery** — hypercalcemia > 11.5 mg/dl persistent for 6 months post–transplant that is not responsive to therapy with phosphate binding antacids, or other disorders as for secondary HPT. Perform subtotal or total (with autotransplant) parathyroidectomy.

ADRENAL GLAND

The adrenals are 3–6 gm triangular–shaped glands at the superiomedial aspect of each kidney. The cortex, of mesodermal origin, produces steroid hormones. The medulla, of ectodermal (neural crest, or APUD) origin, acts as a giant post–synaptic sympathetic nerve ending, producing norepinephrine and epinephrine.

I. ANATOMY AND PHYSIOLOGY

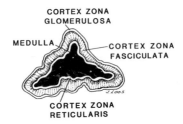

A. **Cortex zona glomerulosa.**
  1. Product – mineralocorticoids (aldosterone).
  2. Stimulus – angiotensin, K+.
  3. Effect – kidney (H_2O and Na+ retention, K+ excretion).
  4. Measure – urine or plasma aldosterone levels.
B. **Cortex zona fasciculata.**
  1. Product – glucocorticoids (cortisol).
  2. Effect – catabolic, gluconeogenic, anti–inflammatory.
  3. Stimulus – stress, ACTH.
  4. Measure – plasma cortisol (diurnal variation), urinary free cortisol, urinary 17–OH–corticosteroids.
C. **Cortex zona reticularis.**
  1. Product – androgens, low levels of other sex steroids.
  2. Measure – urinary 17–ketosteroids, urinary estrogens.
D. **Medulla.**
  1. Product – catecholamines (epinephrine, norepinephrine).
  2. Stimulus – generalized stress response (longer duration than simple sympathetic nerve discharge).
  3. Effect – increased BP, pulse, respirations.
  4. Measure – urinary epinephrine, norepinephrine, VMA (from epinephrine, norepinephrine metabolism), metanephrine (from epinephrine metabolism).

II. PRIMARY HYPERALDOSTERONISM (Conn's Syndrome)

A. High autonomous secretion of aldosterone with low renin levels. If renin is high, increased aldosterone is secondary to decreased renal blood flow (renal artery stenosis, congestive heart failure, cirrhosis, etc.).

B. Clinically–exaggerated physiologic effects – decreased K^+ (weakness, cramps), increased total body Na^+ and H_2O (hypertension, headaches, polyuria, polydipsia, nocturia). More common in women, with mean age at diagnosis 40–50 years. One percent of all hypertension cases are due to primary hyperaldosteronism.

C. 50–80% due to small (< 2–3 cm) cortical adenoma, 15–50% bilateral hyperplasia. Functional carcinoma is extremely rare.

D. **Diagnosis: screening.**
   1. Low K^+ in patient with hypertension on no diuretics – misses 20%.
   2. Plasma aldosterone/renin ratio > 400 reported to be highly accurate.

E. **Diagnosis: confirming** – 24–hr urine for Na^+, K^+, aldosterone.
   1. Serum K^+ < 3.0 with urinary K^+ > 40 is highly suspicious, especially with increased urinary aldosterone.
   2. Renin stimulation test – correct K^+ first to prevent false–negatives. Induce diuresis with Lasix® 80 mg PO, upright posture x 4 hr, then measure plasma renin. Will be low with primary hyperaldosteronism.
   3. Aldosterone suppression – high NaCl diet (9 g/day) for at least 3–4 days. Give Florinef® 0.5 mg/day x 3 days (or 10 mg deoxycortisone IM q 12 hr x 2 doses). Measure plasma aldosterone and 24–hr urine aldosterone. If Conn's, levels will not be suppressed.
   4. Both tests positive – confirms diagnosis.

F. **Diagnosis: adenoma vs. hyperplasia** – draw plasma aldosterone level at 8:00 *am*; upright posture for 4 hr, then redraw level; if aldosterone decreases, it is an adenoma (sensitive to diurnal decrease in ACTH); if level does not change or increases – hyperplasia (sensitive to postural changes in renin–angiotensin system).

G. **Localization.**
   1. CT scan can identify 75–90%, including some adenomas < 1 cm.
   2. Selective venous sampling for aldosterone level is sensitive, but invasive; use if CT scan unsuccessful. Avoid venography due to risk of adrenal hemorrhage.
   3. Adrenal scintigraphy: with NP50 (iodocholesterol) and dexamethasone suppression is nearly as good as CT, but more time–consuming and more radiation exposure, especially to thyroid (radioactive iodine).
   4. 85% unilateral adenoma, < 5% bilateral adenoma, 10% bilateral hyperplasia.

H. **Treatment: adenoma** — unilateral adrenalectomy, 80–90% relief of symptoms; spironolactone for 1–2 wks preoperatively. Posterior (flank) approach has the least morbidity; abdominal approach for very large tumors or suspected carcinoma.

I. **Treatment: hyperplasia** — spironolactone or amiloride, plus anti-hypertensives as necessary; most respond well. Response to surgery (bilateral adrenalectomy) for failed medical management is inter-mediate as patients require life–long adrenal replacement.

III. HYPERADRENOCORTICISM (Cushing's Syndrome and Disease)

A. **Excess glucocorticoid** due to:
  1. Excess pituitary ACTH (Cushing's disease) — 65–70%, most due to microadenoma, some idiopathic (? hypothalamic).
  2. Adrenal tumor — 10–20%, usually adenoma in adult; carcinoma more common in children.
  3. Ectopic ACTH — 5–10%, most commonly from oat–cell carci-noma of lung, but also carcinoids, islet cell tumors, medullary carcinoma of thyroid, thymomas, others.
  4. Non–ACTH–dependent adrenal hyperplasia — rare.

B. **Clinically** — truncal obesity, moon facies, proximal muscle weak-ness, buffalo hump, striae, easy bruising, hirsutism, hypertension, glucose intolerance, personality changes, amenorrhea, osteoporosis, poor wound healing; females > males about 4 : 1.

C. **Diagnosis — screening.**
  1. Plasma cortisol levels often not helpful unless document loss of diurnal variation.
  2. Free urinary cortisol — positive if 24–hr urine with > 100 μg/dl free cortisol; < 5% false–positive, false–negative.
  3. Dexamethasone suppression — 1 mg PO at 11:00 *p.m.*, measure plasma cortisol at 8:00 *a.m.* Normal < 5 μg/dl; > 10 μg/dl is abnormal.

D. **Differentiating cause of excess glucocorticoid.**
  1. Measure ACTH — low to unmeasurable with adrenal source; high with pituitary or ectopic source.
  2. High–dose dexamethasone suppression — 2 mg PO q 6 hr x 48 hr; 24–hr urine on second day sent for 17–OH–corticosteroids, 17–ketosteroids, and free cortisol. Compare to levels on 24–hr urine done prior to dexamethasone. Adrenal tumors, ectopic sources, do not suppress to 40% baseline (however, some say up to 25% of ectopic sources *will* suppress). Pituitary disease will usually suppress to < 40% of baseline urinary cortisol levels. Up to 15% of patients with Cushing's disease (pituitary) may need higher dose of dexamethasone to suppress.
  3. Venous sampling — compare peripheral ACTH level with sample obtained by catheterization of petrosal sinus. Ratio of petrosal to peripheral ACTH >2.0 diagnoses Cushing's disease; ratio < 1.5 suggests ectopic ACTH production.

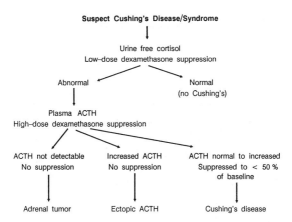

Suspect Cushing's Disease/Syndrome

Urine free cortisol
Low–dose dexamethasone suppression

Abnormal | Normal (no Cushing's)

Plasma ACTH
High–dose dexamethasone suppression

ACTH not detectable — No suppression | Increased ACTH — No suppression | ACTH normal to increased — Suppressed to < 50% of baseline

Adrenal tumor | Ectopic ACTH | Cushing's disease

E. **Localization: pituitary** — CT used most; may miss up to 50%.
F. **Localization: adrenal** — CT identifies > 90%; arteriography is less often necessary with newer generation CT scanners. Venography carries a 5% risk of adrenal hemorrhage and is *not* recommended. Adrenal scintigraphy works, but drawbacks include expense, length of time required to perform test, and exposure of thyroid to ^{131}I.
G. **Localization: ectopic** — CT or x-ray of chest most likely to reveal source; CT of abdomen for pancreatic or gut sources.
H. **Treatment: pituitary** — trans–sphenoidal excision of microadenoma currently the procedure of choice; 80% cure, 95% remission, 6% recurrence, with low morbidity.
   1. Bilateral adrenalectomy has been used for neurosurgical failures and in cases with no demonstrable pituitary lesion (15% later develop adenoma and thus need close follow-up), obviously requires life–long gluco– and mineralocorticoid replacement; these patients may develop **Nelson's syndrome** (hyperpigmentation due to unsuppressed pituitary ACTH/MSH secretion), which can be treated or prevented with pituitary irradiation.
   2. Radiation alone is successful therapy in children up to 80% of time, but results in adults are less impressive (50–60% response with 6–12 month delay).
   3. Chemotherapeutic approaches include cyproheptadin (serotonin antagonist) or bromocriptine (dopamine agonist) to inhibit CRF/ACTH production, metyrapone or aminoglutethimide (inhibitors

of steroid synthesis), and mitotane (causes necrosis of zona fasciculata and reticularis); all are less effective, to some degree toxic, and are used primarily as palliative therapy.

I. **Treatment: adrenal** — unilateral adrenalectomy for adenoma or carcinoma; rare case of non–ACTH–dependent hyperplasia treated with bilateral total adrenalectomy; same criteria for approach (flank vs. abdominal) as with Conn's.

J. **Treatment: ectopic ACTH** — remove primary lesion if possible.

IV. ADRENOCORTICAL INSUFFICIENCY (Addison's Disease)

A. Rare in surgical patient; need high index of suspicion.

B. **Primary causes** — autoimmune (may be associated with other autoimmune endocrine disorders as Schmidt's syndrome), adrenal hemorrhage (secondary to sepsis, coagulopathy), metastatic cancer to adrenals, tuberculosis, prolonged hypotension. Symptoms of aldosterone deficiency (hyperkalemia, hyponatremia, volume depletion) are seen only with primary disease.

C. **Secondary causes** — most commonly adrenal atrophy due to chronic exogenous steroid therapy; rarely due to pituitary insufficiency. Any sick patient on chronic steroids may suffer an acute adrenal crisis.

D. **Clinical picture: chronic** — weakness, fatigue, weight loss, anorexia, GI complaints; diffuse hyperpigmentation of skin; dizziness, dehydration, amenorrhea; can develop acidosis and renal failure picture. May have lymphocytosis and eosinophilia.

E. **Acute (crisis) presentation** — can mimic intra–abdominal catastrophe, septic shock, or MI; classic signs are hypotension, hypoglycemia, hyperkalemia, hyperthermia, abdominal pain.

F. **If suspect** diagnosis, treat immediately with 200 mg hydrocortisone IV and hydration — may be life-saving. Continue with hydrocortisone 50–100 mg IV q 6 hr. Blood may be sent for cortisol, ACTH, but may not be helpful. Look for underlying cause (sepsis, or other) and treat.

G. **ACTH stimulation test** — for diagnosis of a chronic state, measure plasma cortisol before and 15, 30 and 60 min after 250 μg ACTH IV; diagnosis depends on subnormal response (absolute values depend on type of assay used).

H. Thyroid function should also be checked to rule out Schimdt's syndrome or other complicating metabolic abnormalities.

I. **Prevention: perioperative steroids** — any patient currently on steroids, on steroids in the past year, known insufficiency, or pre-op for adrenalectomy (see "Preoperative Preparations" for dosing).

V. ADRENOGENITAL SYNDROME

A. Excess adrenal androgen secretion; one in 15,000 live births.

B. **Etiology.**

   1. One of 6 possible enzyme defects in childhood, most common being C–21 hydroxylation defect.

2. Adrenal carcinoma (child or adult), ovarian carcinoma can rarely cause the syndrome.

C. Diagnosis.

1. 24–hr urine for 17–ketosteroids; plasma testosterone levels.
2. Dexamethasone suppression — 0.5 mg q 6 hr x 7 days, then collect 24–hr urine. Failure to suppress suggest tumor; suppression is consistent with virilizing hyperplasia (enzyme defect).
3. Pelvic exam for ovarian tumors, which also do not suppress with dexamethasone.

D. Treatment.

1. Enzyme defects are treated with glucocorticoid to suppress ACTH; abnormal external genitalia in infants/children may require surgical correction.
2. Surgery for adrenal or ovarian tumors.

VI. PHEOCHROMOCYTOMA

A. Functional adrenal medullary tumor (APUD cell origin), producing excess catecholamines; rare, seen in 0.1–1.0% of hypertensive patients.

B. "10% tumor" — 10% are bilateral, malignant, extra–adrenal, multiple, familial, and in children; 25–30% in children can be extra-adrenal and/or bilateral; 3 x more likely to be malignant in a woman. Malignancy determined by metastases or invasion (histology not helpful).

C. Associated with other neuroectodermal disease — neurofibromatosis, von Hippel–Lindau disease, tuberous sclerosis, others.

D. Associated with Multiple Endocrine Neoplasia (MEN) IIa (Sipple's syndrome) and MEN–IIb (see "Miscellaneous Endocrine Disorders"), both genetic disorders with autosomal dominant transmission. Family members of patients with pheochromocytoma should be screened; 80% of pheochromocytomas associated with MEN–II are bilateral.

E. Clinical — affects all age groups, races, sex; peak incidence in 30's and 40's. About half have paroxysmal hypertension, half with sustained hypertension with exacerbations.

1. Other symptoms related to catechol excess can be acute (headache, palpitations, anxiety, tachycardia, sweating, intermittent neuropsychiatric symptoms) or chronic (cardiovascular, cerebrovascular, or renal effects secondary to prolonged hypertension).
2. Attacks can be precipitated by almost any stress, including exertion, emotion, changes in position or intrathoracic/abdominal pressures, surgery, diagnostic procedures; can occur spontaneously; occasionally are fatal.
3. Suspect pheochromocytoma in any patient with hypertension associated with postural *hypo*tension and tachycardia, any patient with poor blood pressure control on anti–hypertensive medications, or any patient with wide fluctuations in blood pressure.

F. **Differential diagnosis** ("great mimic") — essential hypertension, migraine, supraventricular arrhythmias, thyrotoxicosis, carcinoid, neuroblastoma, hypoglycemia, diabetes, seizure disorder, autonomic hyperreflexia, pre–eclampsia or eclampsia, or simple hypertension of pregnancy.

G. **Diagnosis** — 24–hr urine for free catechols, metanephrine, and vanillylmandelic acid (VMA).
   1. Can get false–positive if on MAO inhibitor, sympathomimetic drugs, or recent angiographic contrast.
   2. Plasma catecholamine levels are only intermittently elevated; therefore, are unreliable for diagnosis.
   3. **Avoid provocative tests.** Extremely dangerous.

H. **Localization** — CT scan (90–95% accurate) and MIBG scintiscan (appears to be very sensitive and specific).
   1. Morbidity and mortality with angiography and venography make these less useful; if required, need α– and β–blockade just as if for surgery.
   2. 10% extra–adrenal, most commonly in paraganglionic tissue at aortic bifurcation (organ of Zuckerkandl), but can be in any paraganglionic tissue (including urinary bladder, renal hilum, mediastinum, neck).

I. **Treatment** — surgical resection for both benign and malignant disease (debulk if resection not possible); most are refractory to radiation or chemotherapy. Most adrenal surgery is best done through a flank approach; however, pheochromocytomas should be approached through the abdomen in order to perform a complete exploration for extra–adrenal, bilateral, or occult multifocal disease, as well as to remove gallbladder if necessary (25–30% have associated gallstones).

J. **Preoperative preparation.**
   1. α–blockade with phenoxybenzamine, 20–40 mg divided bid–tid; increase by 10–20 mg/day until blood pressure and symptoms controlled; start 10–14 days prior to surgery (some increase dose until have postural hypotension).
   2. β–blockade — most would add propranolol 10 mg tid–qid *after* α–blockade achieved, for 3–5 days pre–op to control rate and rhythm, especially if an epinephrine producing tumor. Patients with pheochromocytoma are very sensitive to propranolol.
   3. Steroids (see Addison's Disease) — pre–op glucocorticoids are recommended by some, especially if familial with anticipated bilateral adrenalectomy. If both adrenals are not removed, steroids can be stopped post–op.

K. **Intraoperative management.**
   1. Knowledgeable anesthesiologist — avoid MSO_4, demerol (both cause catechol release) and atropine (tachycardia). Ethrane, droperidol, nitrous, and thiopental all seem to be okay.
   2. Arterial line with CVP or Swan–Ganz catheter monitoring.

3. Drugs available in operating room — phentolamine (α–blocker), propranolol (β–blocker), nitroprusside, Levophed® or phenylephrine, Lidocaine®, and blood.

L. **Abdominal approach** — full exploration. Once all gross tumor is resected, can give 1 mg glucagon to check for occult residual tumor; if get tachycardia and hypertension, look again. Unilateral adrenalectomy for single tumor; bilateral adrenalectomy for bilateral disease, MEN–II, or familial disease. Debulk malignant tumors to help reduce symptoms; metastases most commonly to bone, liver, lung, nodes; right–sided tumors may invade IVC.

M. **Prognosis** — 96% 5–year survival with benign disease (recurrences are usually with familial disease); 44% 5–year survival if malignant (more common in females, bilateral, or extra–adrenal tumors).

N. **Follow–up** — exam every 6 months; urinary catechols every 3 years, then yearly or if new symptoms; CT scan if necessary by clinical picture. All family members should be screened yearly for pheochromocytoma, medullary thyroid cancer, and hyperparathyroidism.

VII. INCIDENTAL ADRENAL MASS

A. Discovered more often with increased use of CT scan — 0.6% of all abdominal scans will show a mass; 92% of adrenal carcinomas > 6 cm in diameter.

B. Benign lesions or metastatic disease much more common than non–functioning carcinoma.

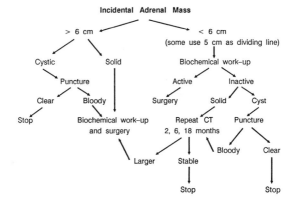

Incidental Adrenal Mass

MISCELLANEOUS ENDOCRINE DISORDERS

I. **APUD CELL (AMINE PRECURSOR UPTAKE AND DECARBOXYLATION) CONCEPT**
A. Concerns a group of cells (of supposed neuroectodermal origin) which possess similar biochemical characteristics.
B. Provides a *theoretical* framework for understanding the normal and pathologic biosynthesis of over 40 polypeptides by cells in the GI (bowel, pancreas) system, thyroid, parathyroid, adrenal medulla, carotid body, and neurologic system.
C. Symptoms arise due to overproduction of these polypeptides in endocrine, paracrine and neurotransmitter activities.
D. Range from benign to malignant disorders.
E. General approach — confirm diagnosis (biochemically and/or histologically), locate tumor and control symptoms (with medication or surgical removal).
F. **Overview** (all tumors can be multihormonal, with predominant symptoms related to the most biochemically potent):

Tumor	Site	Predominant Hormone	Symptoms
Carcinoid	– Appendix, ileum – Other GI sites, bronchial tree – Often multicentric	Bradykinin; serotonin	Flushing, diarrhea, cramping
Gastrinoma	– Pancreas (D-cell), duodenum – Ectopic	Gastrin	Severe peptic ulcer disease, diarrhea, abdominal pain
Insulinoma	– Pancreas (β-cell)	Insulin	Symptoms of hypoglycemia often misdiagnosed as neuro or psych problem
Glucagonoma	– Pancreas (α-cell) (50% in tail)	Glucagon	Migratory necrolytic erythema, mild diabetes, glossitis, thrombosis
VIP–oma	– Pancreas (D-cell) (80% body/tail) – 10-20% extra-pancreatic	Vasoactive intestinal polypeptide (VIP)	Watery diarrhea, hypokalemia, and achlorhydria (WDHA syndrome)
Somato-statinoma	– Pancreas (D cell)	Somato-statin	Mild diabetes, steatorrhea, indigestion, often incidental finding (e.g., at time of cholecystectomy)

II. CARCINOID TUMORS

A. Most common GI APUD–oma, most common tumor of small bowel; all potentially malignant tumors of enterochromaffin cell origin.

B. Can originate from foregut (including bronchial tree, pancreas, gallbladder), midgut (small bowel), or hindgut (large bowel).
   1. Bronchial and metastatic midgut carcinoids most likely to cause **carcinoid syndrome.**
   2. Appendix — most common site (41%) followed by small bowel (20%), rectum (16%) [overall 85–90% in GI tract]; lungs and bronchial tree (10%), larynx, thymus, kidney, ovary, prostate, skin (5%).
   3. Except for appendiceal and rectal carcinoid, lesions tend to be multicentric.
   4. Survival depends on growth rate and presence or absence of metastases.

C. **Hormone production.**
   1. Serotonin predominates; also may produce kallikrein, tachykinin (substance P), and others.
   2. Hindgut tumors are rarely hormonally active.
   3. Some hormones are deactivated by the liver prior to entering systemic circulation.

D. **Symptoms.**
   1. Mechanical obstruction due to tumor or secondary desmoplastic reaction; occasionally rectal bleeding from rectal carcinoid.
   2. **Carcinoid syndrome** requires elaboration of active hormone by tumor *outside* portovenous drainage.
   3. Most common symptoms of the syndrome and probable cause:
      a. Flushing (94%) — kallikrein (bradykinin).
      b. Diarrhea (78%) — serotonin.
      c. Cramping (51%) — serotonin.
      d. Valvular heart lesions (50%) — ? serotonin.
   4. Other symptoms can include telangectasias, wheezing, edema.

E. **Diagnosis.**
   1. Most are found during surgery for intestinal obstruction or appendectomy; pre–operative search unusual, but angiography, endoscopy, barium studies, and CT scan can all be useful; bronchial lesions diagnosed by CXR and/or bronchoscopy.
   2. **5–HIAA** (hydroxyindoleacetic acid) levels > 10 mg in 24–hour urine is diagnostic of hormonally active tumor, if the patient is not on phenothiazines (false negatives) and is not eating serotonin–containing foods (e.g., pineapple, chocolate, bananas, walnuts, avocados).
   3. Bronchial carcinoids may cause elevated **5–HTP** (hydroxytryptophan) levels with normal 5–HIAA values.

F. **Treatment — surgical resection** is the most likely chance for cure. *Always* consider lesions to be **malignant**.
1. Appendiceal carcinoid < 2 cm — simple appendectomy.
2. Appendiceal carcinoid > 2 cm, at base of cecum, serosal invasion, or local nodal disease requires right hemicolectomy.
3. Treatment of small bowel carcinoids — high incidence of other primary tumors.
4. Rectal carcinoids locally excised unless > 2 cm, locally invasive or nodal disease, in which case APR is recommended, or LAR if possible.
5. Often multicentric, thus careful exploration is necessary; all gross disease should be resected to reduce hormone production.
6. Bronchial carcinoids are resected as indicated based on location.
7. If pre–operative diagnosis is made (e.g., carcinoid syndrome), the patient should be prepared for surgery with hydration, serotonin antagonists, and possibly α- and/or β-adrenergic blockers to avoid extreme response to tumor manipulation (see "Adrenal Gland" section VI).

G. **Treatment — medical** (symptomatic treatment).
1. Anti–hormonal measures — serotonin antagonists (methysergide, ciproheptadine, ketanserin); treats only GI symptoms, not flushing.
2. Anti–secretory measures — somatostatin analogue (Sandostatin®) has alleviated both flushing and GI symptoms in clinical trials.
3. Chemotherapy — variable results in small series; most common regimens include streptozotocin and 5–FU; some add doxorubicin; most respond poorly.
4. Some reports of long-term remission with hepatic artery embolization for liver metastates.

H. **Prognosis** (5–year survival).
1. Overall — 65–80%.
2. Localized disease — up to 95%.
3. Regional nodal disease — approximately 65%.
4. Distant metastases — 20%.
5. Appendix best (99%); lungs and bronchi next (96% local disease, 87% all stages).

III. GASTRINOMA (ZOLLINGER–ELLISON SYNDROME)

A. **Delta–cell pancreatic tumor**; 15–20% duodenal or ectopic (splenic hilum, gastric wall, mesentery, liver). More than 50% malignant, over half of those are metastatic at time of diagnosis (to nodes, liver, spleen, peritoneum, mediastinum). Very slow-growing tumors; prolonged survival if ulcers are controlled. Of patients with PUD, 0.1–1.0% have gastrinoma, 25% of gastrinoma patients have MEN–I syndrome (see section VIII below), half of patients with MEN–I have gastrinoma. Duodenal tumors are usually solitary, 75% benign — benign tumors elsewhere tend to be multicentric; head of pancreas most common.

B. Clinical presentation — severe PUD with atypical location of multiple ulcers, often resistant to medical therapy. Associated complications (bleeding, perforation, outlet obstruction) are common.

    1. Diarrhea — secondary to acid secretion, inactivated enzymes, and gastrin–stimulated increased motility.

    2. Abdominal pain — present in > 90% of patients. May become malnourished and dehydrated.

C. Diagnosis — elevated fastin **gastrin** levels (> 500 pg/ml) in a patient with *increased* gastric acid (differential diagnosis: gastrinoma, retained antrum, outlet obstruction, renal failure, short bowel syndrome); if gastric acidity is *decreased*, elevated gastrin is **secondary** (chronic gastritis, gastric carcinoma, pernicious anemia, vagotomy, H2 blockers).

    1. If gastrin above normal (20–150 pg/ml) but < 500, need provocative test (off H2 blockers at least 24–48 hours).

    2. **Secretin stimulation** (positive in ≥ 90% of cases; peak usually at 2–5 minutes) — test of choice.

Measure serum gastrin
↓
Secretin 2 U/kg IV bolus
↓
Serum gastrin at 2, 5, 10, 20, 30 minutes after infusion
↓
Positive test if gastrin increased 200 pg/ml above baseline
(some say 100 pg/ml)

    3. **Calcium stimulation** (may cause arrhythmias, need to monitor) — 80% sensitive, 50% specific.

Monitor patient
↓
Ca^{++} gluconate 5 mg/kg/hr infusion x 3 hours
↓
Serum gastrin every 30 minutes
↓
Positive is 300 pg/ml rise above baseline
(some say 400 pg/ml)

    4. Acid output measurement.

        a. **Basal acid output (BAO)** > 15 mEq/hr or > 100 mmol HCl/ 12 hrs suggests gastrinoma.

        b. **Maximal acid output (MAO)** with pentagastrin stimulation shows minimal increase over BAO with gastrinoma. BAO/ MAO ratio usually > 0.6 with gastrinoma, since parietal cells already maximally stimulated endogenously.

     c. Acid outputs less accurate than secretin stimulation test.
    5. Gastrin levels > 5000 pg/ml, or presence of α-HCG in serum suggests metastatic disease.
    6. Always check serum Ca^{++} to screen for MEN–I.
D. Localization — often not possible pre–op due to small tumors. Duodenal tumors can sometimes be identified endoscopically.
    1. Transhepatic portal venous sampling/mapping — up to 90% success in some hands, but others report much poorer results.
    2. CT scan — 20–80% success; various series, most on lower end of range. Angiography, ultrasound < 25% successful.
    3. Intraoperative ultrasound is very successful, and when combined with thorough palpation of the pancreas, can locate the majority of gastrinomas.
E. **Treatment.**
    1. High–dose H_2 blockade often controls secretory and PUD symptoms, but break-through acid secretion can occur with time; some patients never respond.
    2. Role of **omeprazole** (Losec®) ($H^+ - K^+$ ATPase inhibitor) not yet clear, but may provide better control of acid secretion.
    3. All patients with Zollinger–Ellison syndrome deserve exploration to attempt cure (only possible cure), diagnose metastases, and debulk tumor if necessary (10–20% cure rate).
    4. Some authors report good symptomatic results with parietal cell vagotomy and H_2 blockade when unresectable.
    5. Classic surgical approach in past: total gastrectomy; cures the symptoms, but late deaths still occur due to metastatic disease; variable nutritional consequences following gastrectomy.

* Possible role for parietal cell vagotomy
** Or omeprazole

IV. INSULINOMA

A. Functional β-cell tumor of pancreatic islet; second most common endocrine tumor of pancreas. Another "10% tumor" — 10% malignant, 10% multiple (includes nesidioblastosis), 4–10% associated with MEN–I; multiple lesions associated with MEN–I over half the time. Tumors are small (60–70% < 1.5 cm), equally distributed through pancreas, up to 90% solitary and benign, usually are resectable. Insulin is produced as proinsulin which is cleaved into equimolar amounts of C–peptide and insulin. Both fragments are secreted by the β-cell. C–peptide has a much longer half-life.

B. **Clinical.**

1. Symptoms of **hypoglycemia** (primarily neurologic) with reactive epinephrine release (adrenergic) brought on by fasting or exercise; often occurs in the *a.m.*; patients are often obese due to learned habit of frequent ingestion of sweets to alleviate the symptoms.

2. Can include diplopia, blurred vision, confused behavior, amnesia, weakness, focal or generalized seizures, paralysis, coma. Sweating, hunger, tremor, and palpitations occur with sympathetic response to hypoglycemia.

3. With repeated attacks, permanent neurologic damage can occur; often initially confused with neuropsychiatric problems; average 33 months from onset of symptoms to diagnosis.

C. **Diagnosis .**

1. **Whipple's Triad** strongly suggests diagnosis (diagnosis is 95% accurate with up to 72–hour fast).
   a. Symptoms of hypoglycemia with fasting.
   b. Blood glucose < 50 mg/dl at time of symptoms.
   c. Symptoms relieved by glucose.

2. Some use insulin/glucose (I/G) ratio > 0.30 during fast as diagnostic, or insulin > 6 μU/ml.

3. Measure insulin antibodies, urinary sulfonylureas and **proinsulin/ C–peptide** (both *low* with self–administered human insulin) to search for factitious hyperinsulinemic hypoglycemia.

4. Most useful (although rarely necessary) suppression test may be the euglycemic (administer *both* insulin and glucose to maintain euglycemia) **C–peptide suppression test** (positive if C–peptide does not decrease).

5. Provocative tests (tolbutamide test, calcium gluconate infusion) are less reliable than 72–hr fast; both risk severe side–effects; not recommended by most authors.

6. Malignant tumor is suggested by very high proinsulin level and/ or presence of HCG in serum.

D. **Localization** — generally proceeds with ultrasound → CT scan (or MRI) → percutaneous transhepatic portal vein sampling (**PTPVS**).

1. **Angiography** with subtraction techniques can be up to 90% successful; shows localized, dense tumor blush on capillary phase;

false positives can occur (accessory spleens, inflamed lymph nodes), but test is invasive.

2. **CT scan, ultrasound** in general are less than 50% successful in localizing these small tumors, but if positive, save patient from angiography.

3. **PTPVS** has variable but encouraging results when other methods fail; but is tedious, costly, uncomfortable, requires skilled angiographer; safe and useful in selected cases.

4. **Intraoperative ultrasound** is extremely accurate (and should be available); however, so is intraoperative bimanual pancreatic palpation.

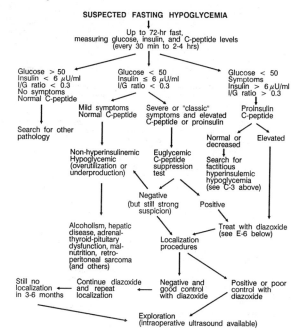

SUSPECTED FASTING HYPOGLYCEMIA

E. **Treatment** — surgical resection is goal, with up to 90% success (cure).

1. Pre–op maintenance of glucose levels with frequent meals and/or glucose infusion; frequent intraoperative glucose measurements.

2. Mobilize and palpate entire gland, even if single tumor localized preoperatively (Kocher maneuver and mobilization of pancreatic tail and spleen).

3. Enucleate small tumors near surface; pancreatic resection for others, including Whipple procedure if necessary for tumor located in head; frozen section to confirm pathology. **Caution** for enucleation in tail or deep in head for possible damage to pancreatic duct.

4. If no tumor is found — intraoperative ultrasound.

    a. Biopsy or resection of pancreatic tail — if frozen section reveals nesidioblastosis (adenomatosis), 75–80% resection is said to provide best control of symptoms with the least morbidity; may require subsequent medical therapy.

    b. Do not blindly resect head of pancreas.

5. Metastatic disease should be treated by debulking as much tumor mass as possible.

6. **Medical treatment** — for patient who cannot tolerate general anesthesia, for control of symptoms preoperatively, or to treat metastatic disease.

    a. **Diazoxide** — inhibits insulin release, decreases peripheral glucose utilization; multiple side–effects may preclude use (edema, hirsutism, nausea, bone marrow depression, hyperuricemia); diuretic may control edema.

    b. **Streptozotocin** with 5–FU to treat malignant insulinoma; 50–66% achieve partial remission, 17–33% with complete remission; up to 95% experience nausea and vomiting, sometimes severe; renal tubular, hepatic toxicity also possible.

V. GLUCAGONOMA

A. Rare α-cell pancreatic islet tumor, < 100 reported cases.

B. Clinical — see chart in section I; mean age 55.

C. **Diagnosis.**

1. Skin lesions best clue — migratory annular erythematous eruptions, superficial necrosis ("**migratory necrolytic erythema**").

2. Mild, easily controlled diabetes.

3. Confirm with elevated plasma glucagon. **Note:** Levels may also be elevated with renal failure, liver failure, and severe stress.

4. Provocative test (arginine infusion: elevates plasma glucagon in patient with glucagonoma) is rarely needed.

D. **Localization** — arteriography, CT scan, selective venous sampling can all localize tumor; MRI appears best for liver metastases; ultrasound is occasionally useful.

1. Most are bulky (> 3 cm) and vascular, therefore easier to find.
2. 50% in tail, 50% malignant, 50% metastatic at time of exploration (to nodes, liver, adrenal, spine).

E. **Treatment** — surgical excision if possible; approximately 30% are completely resectable.
   1. Debulking unresectable primaries and metastases has resulted in prolonged survival.
   2. Chemotherapy for recurrent or unresectable tumors can relieve symptoms; DTIC, or 5–FU/streptozotocin have both been used.
   3. Hepatic artery embolization has been used for liver metastases.
   4. A somatostatin analogue (**Sandostatin®**) has been effective in treating clinical symptoms.
   5. Rash is treated with zinc, high–protein diet, and control of the diabetes.

VI. VIPoma (VERNER–MORRISON SYNDROME, PANCREATIC CHOLERA SYNDROME, WDHA SYNDROME)

A. Rare (< 100 cases) syndrome due to production of vasoactive intestinal polypeptide (VIP: normally a neurotransmitter), pancreatic islet cell tumor (70%), extrapancreatic tumor (10–20%, includes ganglioneuroblastoma, adrenal medulla, pulmonary sites), or possibly islet cell hyperplasia (10–20%). About 50–60% are malignant, most are metastatic at the time of diagnosis; extrapancreatic tumors are *rarely* malignant.

B. **Clinical: WDHA** — 2-10 liters/day of watery diarrhea, resulting in dehydration, hypokalemia, acidosis; associated with achlorhydria (hypochlorohydria more common) due to suppressive action of VIP on gastric acid secretion.
   1. Up to 20% of patients will exhibit spontaneous flushing similar to carcinoid syndrome.
   2. Hyperglycemia and hypercalcemia occur in 50–75% of VIPoma patients for unclear reasons.
   3. Occasionally associated with MEN–I.

C. **Diagnosis** —presence of WDHA syndrome (with associated electrolyte abnormalities) with *low* gastric acid secretion and elevated VIP levels.
   1. VIP is invariably elevated, but assay is difficult and requires a reliable lab.
   2. **Pancreatic polypeptide** (PP) may also be elevated with pancreatic VIPomas.

D. **Localization** — use CT and/or ultrasound first; 80% will be body or tail; if unsuccessful, use angiography; transhepatic venous sampling may prove helpful in difficult cases.

E. **Treatment.**
   1. Vigorous pre–op fluid resuscitation, then surgical resection.

    2. If no tumor is found, some authors feel subtotal pancreatectomy is indicated if tumor markers (VIP, PP) are consistently elevated pre–op.

    3. For unresectable or metastatic disease — debulk; some recommend hepatic artery embolization.

        a. Steroids may provide temporary symptomatic relief in 50%, but relapse is the rule.

        b. > 90% remission rate with streptozotocin, many lasting for years; DTIC and 5–FU have also been used successfully.

        c. Several series have shown symptomatic relief using somatostatin analogue (**Sandostatin®**), with a suggestion of tumor mass regression.

VII. SOMATOSTATINOMA

A. Very rare tumor of pancreatic islet; duodenal tumors also reported.

B. Termed **"inhibitory syndrome"**; classic triad of gallstones, diabetes, and steatorrhea are vague, duodenal tumors are asymptomatic; therefore most tumors discovered late in course with metastases already present.

C. In general, these are malignant, solitary, and virulent.

D. **Symptoms** are due to inhibition of exocrine and endocrine pancreas, gallbladder contraction, and gastric emptying (resulting in bloating, indigestion, nausea and vomiting).

E. **Diagnosis** — usually discovered *incidentally* at cholecystectomy; plasma somatostatin can be measured and is markedly elevated.

F. **Localization** — most discovered incidentally, but CT and angiography are useful.

G. **Treatment** — resection should be attempted if possible; debulking is recommended otherwise.

    1. Duodenal somatostatinomas should be treated like carcinomas.

    2. Tumor is rare; no information on chemotherapy is available.

H. **Prognosis** — in cases described is poor, with most patients surviving several months; early diagnosis and resection might be curative.

VIII. MULTIPLE ENDOCRINE NEOPLASIA (MEN) SYNDROMES

A. All are **autosomal dominant.**

MEN-I	MEN-IIa	MEN-IIb
Pituitary adenoma	Medullary thyroid CA	Medullary thyroid CA
Parathyroid hyperplasia	Pheochromocytoma	Pheochromocytoma
Pancreatic islet cell tumor	Parathyroid hyperplasia	Multiple mucosal neuromas

B. **MEN–I (Wermer's syndrome**, "3 P's" — pituitary, parathyroid, and pancreas).

1. Peak incidence in 20's for women, 30's for men; most commonly present with PUD symptoms/complications; next most common is hypoglycemia (insulinoma); less common is headaches, visual field deficits, amenorrhea (pituitary adenoma).

2. **Pituitary** — 60–70% have adenoma, usually chromophobe with hypofunction; occasionally have functional tumor (e.g., acromegaly).

3. **Parathyroid** — most consistent lesion; > 90% with generalized hyperplasia and hypercalcemia; may have renal stones, peptic ulcer disease (PUD).

4. **Pancreas** — 80% with pancreatic lesion; most common in gastrinoma, followed by insulinoma; *any* islet cell tumor is possible, including simple islet cell hyperplasia; tumors usually multicentric, often malignant, but slow–growing.

5. Diagnosis.
   a. Screen all patients with pancreatic tumor for hyperparathyroidism (Ca^{++}, PTH).
   b. Screen all family members of patients with gastrinoma or any other MEN–I associated lesions (pituitary, parathyroid).
   c. Pancreatic polypeptide may be a good marker; appears to be elevated in nearly *all* cases.

6. **Treatment.**
   a. Hyperparathyroidism — **treat first**, with subtotal parathyroidectomy; if PUD present and persists with normal Ca^{++}, do work–up for gastrinoma.
   b. Since gastrinoma and other pancreatic lesions in MEN–I are often multiple and/or malignant, surgery may not be curative (see above sections for approach to these lesions).
   c. Pituitary lesions — addressed surgically as indicated.

C. **MEN–IIa (Sipple's syndrome) and IIb.**
   1. Both MEN–IIa and IIb are **autosomal dominant**, but sporadic cases have been reported.
   2. **Medullary thyroid carcinoma**, preceded by thyroid C–cell hyperplasia, is present in 100% of these patients; multicentric and bilateral, unlike sporadic cases; **much more aggressive** tumor in IIb syndrome, making early total thyroidectomy critical for successful treatment.
   3. **Pheochromocytoma** — present in 40–50%; 80% bilateral, almost always benign; peak incidence in teen's, 20's.
   4. **Parathyroid hyperplasia** is present in approximately 60% of MEN–IIa patients.
   5. MEN–IIb patients have characteristic physical appearance with multiple **cutaneous neuromas**.
   6. **Diagnosis** — elevated plasma calcitonin level.

    a. Measurement of plasma calcitonin after **pentagastrin stimulation** (0.5 μg/kg IVP, measure calcitonin at 1-3 min, 30 min) detects medullary thyroid carcinoma in clinically normal patients that will have microscopic disease when their thyroid is removed.

    b. Symptoms of pheochromocytoma (see "Adrenal Gland" section VI for work–up).

    c. Blood Ca^{++}, PTH levels for hyperparathyroidism.

7. Treatment.

    a. Look for and treat **pheochromocytoma** first — abdominal, bilateral exploration due to frequency of bilateral lesions.

    b. Total thyroidectomy, with resection of nodes between jugular veins from thyroid cartilage to sternal notch; neck dissection for more extensive lymphatic involvement; follow pentagastrin stimulation test to check for adequacy of resection, recurrence.

    c. Subtotal parathyroidectomy for patients with hyperparathyroidism, or total parathyroidectomy with reimplantation.

8. Prognosis.

    a. Related to the extent of thyroid tumor.

    b. Extremely variable, even in same family. Overall, 10–year survival of patients with medullary thyroid carcinoma is 50%.

NON-INVASIVE VASCULAR LABORATORY STUDIES

The non-invasive vascular laboratory provides the clinician with an objective means of non-invasively and reproducibly assessing the hemodynamic effects of a variety of vascular lesions as well as following these patients after medical or surgical intervention.

I. PERIPHERAL ARTERIAL

A. **Doppler arterial survey.**
   1. The presence of an audible signal in any vessel confirms its patency.
   2. A normal multiphasic signal strongly suggests the absence of a significant proximal lesion.

B. **Segmental limb pressures** — measurement of multilevel, segmental, systolic pressures.
   1. Most generally accepted and widely applied non-invasive technique for diagnosing extremity arterial occlusive disease.
   2. Simple, reproducible, inexpensive, and well-tolerated.
   3. Ankle/brachial index (ABI) [or the ankle pressure index (API)] is a simple ratio of ankle pressure to arm pressure that can establish the severity of the extremity ischemia. This can be performed at the bedside with a blood pressure cuff and a hand-held Doppler instrument.
      a. ABI 0.9 – 1.0 — normal.
      b. ABI 0.75 – 0.9 — mild occlusive disease.
      c. ABI 0.5 – 0.75 — moderate disease.
      d. ABI < 0.5 — severe; symptoms of rest pain usually present.
      e. ABI < 0.2 — symptoms of severe rest pain or gangrene usually present.
   4. **Disadvantages:** localization of specific responsible lesions may be difficult.
      a. Aortoiliac disease in the presence of superficial femoral artery occlusion is particularly difficult to identify.
      b. Segmental limb pressures in patients with calcified vessels which are not compressible (diabetes mellitus or chronic renal failure) are meaningless.
      c. Examiner must remember that distal pressures may represent the combined effects of more than one lesion.

C. **Waveform analysis** — segmental pulse volume waveforms.
   1. Excellent assessment of segmental limb perfusion.
   2. Less technician-dependent.
   3. Not limited by vessel wall calcification.
   4. Rapidly obtained utilizing the same cuffs placed for segmental limb pressures.
   5. Can be analyzed qualitatively with much accuracy.

D. **Stress testing** — allows quantitation of the physiologic impact of arterial lesions and the resulting functional disability.
   1. Useful in studying patients who have exercise-related peripheral arterial complaints.

    2. Treadmill exercise best reproduces the exercise-induced reactive hyperemia in symptomatic patients.

    3. In patients who cannot exercise, temporary, pneumatic cuff occlusion is utilized to produce reactive hyperemia.

E. **Transcutaneous oximetry** (TcPO$_2$).

    1. Relative newcomer to vascular lab that measures skin oxygen tension and reflects adequacy of arterial/capillary perfusion.

    2. Particularly useful in patients with incompressible calcified vessels (e.g., diabetes) in which segmental pressures and PVR are less accurate.

    3. Has been used to classify severity of disease (claudicators *vs.* rest pain *vs.* impending gangrene) to predict the patient's healing potential (ulcers and amputation level) and to predict success of revascularization. In one study, results were ($p < 0.001$):

Normal	Claudication	Rest Pain	Impending Gangrene
64 ± 8	46 ± 10	17 ± 9	5 ± 2

    4. The technique is somewhat complex and is based on diffusion of O$_2$ and its electrochemical reduction by a cathode.

    5. **Disadvantages** include sensitivity of measurements to environmental conditions and unreliability of measurements in extremities with marked edema, hyperkeratosis, cellulitis, and obesity.

F. **Upper extremity evaluation.**

    1. Atherosclerotic arterial occlusion is rare in the upper extremity; however, vasospasm, emboli, and trauma may result in ischemic symptoms, and non-invasive vascular studies may be helpful.

    2. Useful in evaluating the patency of the palmar arch prior to cannulation of the radial or ulnar arteries.

    3. Useful in differentiating between vasospasm and collagen vascular disease of the upper extremity.

    4. Helpful in evaluating the vascular complications of the thoracic outlet syndrome.

G. **Penile blood flow.**

    1. Detect impotence due to vascular insufficiency.

    2. Penile-brachial index (PBI).

       a. PBI < 0.60 is compatible with vasculogenic impotence.

       b. PBI $\geq$ 0.75 is the lower limit of normal.

II. CEREBROVASCULAR

A. A great variety of tests are available. They are "indirect" if they evaluate hemodynamic alterations, and "direct" if they examine the anatomy at the carotid bifurcation.

B. **Ocular plethysmography** (OPG) — indirect measure of cerebrovascular occlusive disease. Two types available: One device detects delay in pulse arrival in the eye (OPG-K). Second device measures ophthalmic systolic pressure (OPG-G); this is most commonly used.

    1. **Advantages.**

    a. Sensitive and specific in recognizing hemodynamically significant lesions.

    b. More objective and less technician–dependent than other forms of indirect testing.

  2. Disadvantages.

    a. Small risk of minor eye irritation.

    b. Sensitive to only the most severe stenoses.

  3. Criteria for significant stenosis (OPG-G).

    a. Right-to-left ophthalmic pressure difference ≥ 5 mmHg.

    b. Right-to-left ophthalmic pressure difference of 1-4 mmHg with an ophthalmic-brachial pressure index < 0.66.

    c. No ophthalmic pressure difference, but ophthalmic-brachial pressure index < 0.60. (Invalid if patient is severely hypertensive.)

    d. Difference of ocular pulse amplitude ≥ 2 mmHg.

C. Carotid imagers.

  1. Real-time B-mode ultrasound allows visualization of the carotid bifurcation.

    a. Unable to penetrate heavily-calcified plaque.

    b. When used alone, unable to identify complete occlusion with reliability.

    c. Sensitivity and specificity in detecting larger than 50% stenoses are limited.

  2. Duplex scanner — combination of real-time B-mode scanner with pulse Doppler real-time frequency analysis of resulting waveform.

    a. Sensitivity and specificity have surpassed those for previous techniques. This is the current gold standard in carotid artery non-invasive testing.

    b. Disadvantages include: highly technician-dependent, significant patient cooperation required, most expensive devices presently used in clinical vascular laboratory.

III. NON-INVASIVE TESTING IN VENOUS DISEASE

A. Venous Doppler survey — inexpensive, simple means of assessing presence of *proximal* venous obstruction.

  1. Portable Doppler velocity meter with insonation of the major deep veins of the leg.

  2. Normal venous signals are phasic with respiratory variability and augment with compression of the extremity distal to the point of investigation.

  3. A continuous signal lacking augmentation reflects proximal venous obstruction with collateral venous flow.

  4. Advantages.

    a. Applicability at the bedside.

    b. Ability to repeat the study frequently without patient discomfort.

    c. Low cost.

5. **Disadvantages.**
   a. Accuracy is very technician-dependent.
   b. Limited to proximal (iliofemoral) venous obstruction.
   c. Accuracy falls with isolated calf clot due to the presence of paired veins and extensive collaterals.
6. Useful screening test in differentiating venous obstruction from other causes of leg swelling (edema secondary to CHF, cellulitis, lymphangitis).

B. ^{125}I–fibrinogen leg scanning. [Not a true "non-invasive" technique used in the vascular laboratory, but rather a less invasive method (as compared to phlebography) of imaging acute thrombi.]
   1. Detects thrombi which are actively accreting fibrin in the calf veins and the distal half of the thigh.
   2. Sensitive and specific for acute calf and lower thigh vein thrombosis.
   3. Fails to detect proximal thrombi in upper thigh and iliac vein in approximately 30% of patients, and therefore should not be used as the only diagnostic test in patients with clinically suspected venous thrombosis.
   4. Valuable diagnostic test when using with IPG in patients with clinically suspected venous thrombosis.
   5. **Disadvantages.**
      a. False-positive results occur if scanning is performed over a hematoma, large wound or area of inflammation.
      b. In some patients with symptomatic acute venous thrombosis, it may take 48 or even 72 hours for enough radioactivity to accumulate in the thrombus to allow a positive diagnosis. Thus, it should not be done in the evaluation of acute DVT.

C. **Plethysmography** — the study of changes in limb volume.
   1. Two principal types.
      a. Occlusive techniques — strain-gauge plethysmography, impedance plethysmography (IPG).
      b. Non-occlusive techniques — phleborheography (PRG).
   2. IPG studies the changing resistance to passage of an electrical current (impedance) through the lower extremity relative to changes in its blood volume.
   3. IPG measures resting limb volume and records the response to temporary venous occlusion and its subsequent relief.
      a. A pneumatic cuff is placed on the thigh, temporarily inflated to 50-60 cm of H_2O pressure, and changes in calf volume (as reflected in decreasing electrical impedance) are measured.
      b. When tracing plateaus, the cuff is released and the decrease in venous volume (as reflected in increased electrical impedance) is measured over 3 seconds.
      c. During cuff inflation, a normal limb will exhibit a rapid increase in calf volume due to unobstructed arterial inflow.

       d. Upon release of the cuff, the veins will empty rapidly and cuff volume will return to baseline within 3 seconds.

       e. The obstructed venous system will frequently demonstrate reduced filling, since the obstruction has already engorged the veins and venous emptying through collateral channels is inefficient and results in a marked slowing of venous outflow.

  4. Numerous studies comparing IPG to venography document a sensitivity of 93% and specificity of 94%.

  5. Disadvantages.

       a. False–positive studies may occur due to other causes of venous outflow obstruction (gravid uterus, tumor, edema, etc.) or hemodynamic impairment (CHF, severe arterial insufficiency, chronic lung disease).

       b. Patient who is cold, anxious, or uncooperative may present difficulties in interpretation due to vasoconstriction or muscular contraction.

  6. False–negative results are rare and seen with non–occlusive thrombi, chronic obstruction with abundant collateralization, and superficial phlebitis.

D. Venous Photoplethysmography (PPG) — used to assess the degree of chronic venous insufficiency.

  1. Measures changes of skin blood content after standard exercise.

  2. Photo-electric cells placed on the skin over the malleolus, and venous refilling time is recorded after repeated dorsiflexion of the foot.

       a. Normal — venous refilling time is often > 25 sec.

       b. In venous valvular incompetency — refilling time is much shortened (< 20 sec) because of constant reflux from incompetent venous valves.

  3. Tourniquet is then applied to thigh, calf and ankle at a pressure of 50 mmHg to occlude the superficial venous system.

       a. Test is then repeated.

       b. Differentiates superficial from deep venous insufficiency.

E. Duplex Venous Imaging.

  1. Duplex scanning as described previously (see I.-E) combines real-time B-mode ultrasound images of blood vessels with spectral analysis of the Doppler velocity signals from within the vessels, providing both anatomic and hemodynamic information.

  2. Normal veins are easily compressible with gentle pressure on the ultrasound probe and exhibit functioning venous valve leaflets and normal biphasic blood flow within their lumens.

  3. Veins containing intraluminal thrombus lose compressibility and exhibit abnormal or absent Doppler flow signals.

       a. Only the actual visualization of intraluminal thrombus permits the definitive diagnosis of DVT.

       b. Loss of compressibility or alteration of Doppler signals provide only indirect evidence subject to interpretative errors.

    c. Duplex scanning may differentiate fresh from chronic thrombus and can even identify new clot superimposed on preexisting chronic disease.

4. With experienced technicians, accuracy of the study approaches 100% and has all but replaced venography in the evaluation of lower extremity DVT.

5. **Disadvantages.**
    a. Accessibility is limited to vessels of the upper and lower extremity and extrathoracic jugular system. Imaging of the iliac veins and intrathoracic veins are less accurate due to interference by intraabdominal and intrathoracic structures.
    b. An expensive, time-consuming, technician-dependent study.

F. **Diagnosis of suspected acute DVT** (see algorithm).
1. Use of any one of the non-invasive venous tests is superior to the clinical diagnosis of DVT.
2. A combination of IPG and duplex scan theoretically takes advantage of the strength of each and minimizes the possibility of missing clinically important thrombosis, but results in a decrease in specificity.
    a. A negative IPG rules out the possibility of proximal venous obstruction.
    b. A scan is able to evaluate calf veins for thrombosis.
3. Visualization of thrombus on a scan is sufficient to warrant institution of therapy, as is an unequivocally positive IPG in a patient without a previous history of ipsilateral DVT.
4. Venography is reserved for confirmation of positive or equivocal Duplex scan when one of the clinical sources of a false-positive study (CHF, arterial insufficiency, etc.) is present.

Suspected Acute DVT

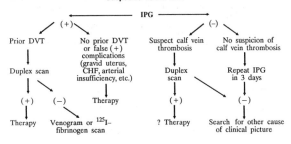

THE DIABETIC FOOT

There are approximately 10 million diabetics in the United States (20% being Type I and 80% being Type II). Lower extremity disease is the most common disorder requiring operation in diabetics. Twenty-five percent of diabetics (1.5 million) develop foot problems. Greater than 50% of all non–traumatic lower extremity amputations are performed on patients with diabetes.

I. **ETIOLOGY**
A. Typical diabetic foot problems are the foot or toe ulcer, the mal perforans ulcer (a plantar ulcer with a long, narrow tract that extends to the joint at the tarsal–metatarsal level), the Charcot foot (a joint deformity that produces "hammer toes" or inversion or eversion at the ankle), and the septic limb.
B. The major causes of foot problems in diabetics are related to atherosclerosis, peripheral neuropathy and infection.
   1. **Atherosclerosis.**
      a. Peripheral vascular disease tends to be bilateral and multi-segmental, involving peripheral arteries.
      b. "Small vessel disease" in diabetics is most likely related to altered basement membrane permeability, and not to obstructive lesions of the microcirculation.
   2. **Peripheral neuropathy.**
      a. Occurs in diabetics with disease of 10 years or more duration.
      b. The cause is unknown, but may be related to sorbital metabolites deposited in nerves.
      c. Affects the motor, sensory and sympathetic nerve supply to the lower limbs.
      d. Peripheral neuropathy and motor weakness lead to deformities such as Charcot's foot, neuropathic (mal perforans) ulcer, hallux valgus, and hammer toes.
   3. **Infection.**
      a. Begins most often from minor foot trauma or a trivial break in the skin.
      b. May present as an innocuous fissure, ulcer, cellulitis, deep abscess or gangrene.
      c. Infections are **polymicrobial**.
         1) *B. fragilis*, anaerobic *Streptococcus*, enterococci, *Proteus*, *Clostridium*.
         2) Gas in tissue is most often produced from gram-negative rods, enterococcus and rarely *Clostridia*.
      d. Impaired PMN activity in the poorly controlled diabetic may contribute to the onset and aggressiveness of diabetic foot infections.

II. TREATMENT

A. Primary treatment of foot ulcers.

1. Assess the extent and severity of ulcer.
2. Determine the degree of neuropathy and vascular insufficiency.
3. Obtain radiograph of foot — rule out soft tissue gas or osteomyelitis.
4. Control blood glucose and metabolic abnormalities.
5. Debride necrotic tissue — be judicious.
6. Obtain aerobic and anaerobic **tissue** cultures.
7. Parenteral antibiotics if infection present.
8. Absolute non–weight bearing of injured foot.
9. Local wound care and dressings.
10. Improve circulation (revascularization if indicated).
11. Treatment after healing should include careful follow-up and podiatric appliances.

B. Treatment of foot abscess or gangrene.

1. These patients require operative intervention to drain the abscess cavity or amputate the nonviable tissue.
2. Tissue cultures.
3. Parenteral antibiotics.
4. Local wound care and dressings.
5. Correct metabolic abnormalities.
6. Revascularization may be indicated once infection has resolved.
7. May require skin graft or local tissue flap for wound closure.
8. Treatment after healing should include careful follow–up and podiatric appliances.

C. The most important treatment is **prevention**, with conscientious diabetic foot care and frequent examinations.

1. Non–constricting footwear.
2. Nail care, treat mycotic nail infections.
3. Keep web spaces clean and dry, inspect daily.
4. Examine plantar surface (with mirror if needed) for injury or foreign bodies. Unknown injuries are common in patients with neuropathy.

ACUTE LIMB ISCHEMIA

I. **ETIOLOGY**
A. **Arterial embolism.**
1. Cardiac source (80% of emboli from heart).
    a. Thrombus (myocardial infarction, ventricular aneurysm, atrial fibrillation, mitral stenosis).
    b. Endocarditis.
    c. Myxoma.
2. Atheroembolism (blue toe syndrome) from an ulcerating atherosclerotic plaque in a large artery.
3. Aneurysmal source, in order of decreasing frequency — aortic, popliteal, femoral.
4. Paradoxical embolus — venous source across an intracardiac shunt (rare).
B. **Arterial thrombosis.**
1. Atherosclerosis — clot on the surface of a plaque, hemorrhage beneath a plaque, stenosis, aneurysm.
2. Congenital anomaly.
    a. Popliteal entrapment.
    b. Adventitial cystic disease.
C. Arterial trauma — iatrogenic *vs.* incidental.
D. Drug–induced vasospasm — with particular attention to illicit drug use and inadvertent arterial injection.
E. Severe venous thrombophlebitis.
F. Aortic dissection.

II. **INITIAL ASSESSMENT**
A. **History.**
1. Pain — onset, location, duration.
2. Previous claudication.
3. Previous cardiac disease — mitral stenosis, atrial fibrillation, cardiomyopathy, M.I., prosthetic valve.
4. Trauma.
5. History of hypertension, chest or back pain.
6. Drugs — ergotamines, dopamine.
7. Low flow states — septic shock, dehydration, hemorrhage, CHF.
B. **Examination.**
1. **5 P's of acute arterial insufficiency** — pain, paralysis, paresthesias, pallor, pulseless. A 6th "P" that is sometimes added is "polar" (cold).
2. Trophic skin and nail changes.

3. **Complete bilateral** pulse examination including auscultation for bruits and portable Doppler exam when unable to appreciate pulses by palpation.
4. Assessment of limb viability.
   a. Muscle turgor (soft = viable).
   b. Neurologic status — paralysis and anesthesia generally indicate a non–viable limb.
5. Cardiac examination — rhythm, murmurs, rub.
6. **CXR** and **KUB** — look for wide mediastinum and vascular calcifications.
7. **EKG** — look for evidence of M.I.

III. SECONDARY ASSESSMENT

A. Duration — **"golden period"** of 6 hours before ischemia and myonecrosis become irreversible.
B. Non–invasive studies can be helpful, but must **not delay** definitive therapy.
C. **Indications for arteriography.**
   1. Determine site of vascular obstruction.
   2. Suspected thrombosis.
   3. Suspected aortic dissection.
   4. Suspected multiple emboli.
D. **Operative risk.**
   1. Most such patients have underlying heart disease and this, in conjunction with the need for emergent surgery, make operative risk **high** in this setting.
   2. Embolectomy under local anesthesia is preferred and is much less dangerous than amputation or attempted revascularization.

IV. MANAGEMENT OF ACUTE ARTERIAL INSUFFICIENCY

A. In all cases, **immediate heparinization** to prevent further propagation of thrombus — bolus with 10,000 units heparin, then start continuous infusion ($\sim$ 1,000 units/hr) to maintain PTT at 1 1/2 to 2 times control.
B. **Arterial embolism.**
   1. Generally lodges at bifurcations of vessels.
      a. Common femoral — approximately 50%.
      b. Aortic bifurcation — approximately 25–30%.
      c. Popliteal trifurcation — approximately 15%.
   2. Mortality higher with more proximal location — aorta (22%) > iliac (18%) > femoral (9%) > popliteal (7%).
   3. After heparinization, emergent **surgical embolectomy** is the treatment of choice.
      a. Local anesthesia.
      b. Isolation of artery (usually common femoral) with proximal and distal control.

    c. Fogarty® balloon–tipped catheter is introduced through an arteriotomy and passed beyond the area of clot. Balloon is inflated and catheter withdrawn, hopefully bringing clot out in front of it. May need to "milk" the lower leg to remove small vessel clots. (Popliteal arteriotomy may be useful in some cases.)

4. Need **completion angiography** after removal of thrombus.
   a. "Back bleeding" and clinical examination are poor indicators of success.
   b. 20% of patients will have a good functional result after embolectomy despite absent distal pulses.

5. Continue heparin post–op; begin Coumadin® on day 3, continue until patient no longer at risk for further emboli. Discontinue heparin when adequately anticoagulated on Coumadin®.

6. **Identify and treat underlying cause** (atrial fibrillation, mitral stenosis, M.I.)

7. Watch for **myonephropathic–metabolic** syndrome.
   a. Ischemic muscle converts to anaerobic metabolism, with paralysis of the cellular Na^+–K^+ pump. The pH falls while concentrations of K^+, lactic acid, muscle enzymes, myoglobin and oxygen free radicals all rise dramatically. Once the threatened muscle is re–perfused, these toxic metabolites circulate throughout the body and can cause renal failure as well as multiorgan system failure.
   b. As far as the renal failure is concerned, myoglobin precipitates in the renal tubules (acidic environment), leading to necrosis with a worsening spiral of oliguria, hyperkalemia, and metabolic acidosis.
   c. Treatment — when myoglobin is present (red urine).
      1) Correct hyperkalemia.
      2) Alkalinize urine with intravenous $NaHCO_3$.
      3) Give osmotic diuretic — Mannitol® (1 g/kg IV).
      4) Fasciotomy to decompress compromised muscle.
      5) Hemodialysis if necessary.
   d. The mortality with this syndrome is as high as 33%.

C. **Atheroembolism (blue toe syndrome).**
   1. Heparinization acutely — long–term anti–coagulation is of no value.
   2. Elective angiography to search for treatable embolic causes.
   3. Thromboendarterectomy or complete arterial replacement with prosthetic graft if the source is identified.

D. **Arterial thrombosis.**
   1. Generally suspected from history and exam.
   2. Previous collateralization will generally prevent development of myonecrosis.
   3. Arteriography is key for identifying optimal surgical approach.

E. **Arterial trauma.**
   1. Generally results from intimal flap with resultant thrombosis.
   2. Penetrating injuries are most common (missile, blast, fracture, severe ligament tears and dislocation at the knee).
   3. Arteriography mandatory — embolectomy and repair of intimal flap as indicated.
F. **Venous thrombosis** (also see "Thromboembolic Prophylaxis and Management of Venous Thromboembolism").
   1. Major venous thrombosis involving the deep venous system of the thigh and pelvis produces characteristic clinical picture of pain, extensive edema, and blanching, termed **phlegmasia alba dolens.**
   2. As impedance of venous return from the extremity progresses further, there is danger of limb loss from cessation of arterial flow leading to congestion, cyanosis and distended veins, termed **phlegmasia cerulea dolens.**
   3. Risk of venous gangrene if pulses absent mandates heparinization and venous embolectomy with protective distal AV fistula.
G. **Drug–induced vasospasm** — treat by discontinuing drug, occasionally use of IV nitroprusside drip (vasodilatation), phentolamine (alpha blockade), or nitropaste topical.
H. **Aortic dissection.**
   1. Identify by history (hypertension, back/chest pain) and exam (absent pulses throughout).
   2. Aortography (including thoracic arch) if suspected.
I. **Thrombolytic therapy** (streptokinase, urokinase).
   1. Role is still being defined.
   2. Generally effective in patients in whom surgical therapy would work as well, more rapidly and at lower cost.
   3. Requires continuous arterial infusion, ICU monitoring, frequent angiography.
   4. High risk of hemorrhagic complications.
      a. **Contraindications** — liver or renal disease, blood dyscrasias, GI bleeding, GI malignancy, intracranial hemorrhage, severe hypertension, recent surgery (within 48 hours).
      b. Recent streptococcal infection or history of scarlet fever in childhood contraindicates streptokinase (increased chance of allergic reaction).

V. PROGNOSIS
A. 15–30% of patients with arterial embolism die, usually of cardiovascular causes.
B. 5–15% of patients with arterial embolism require **amputation.**
C. Amputation is procedure of choice in patients with irreversible ischemia or those unable to tolerate extensive reconstruction.
D. The major factor in mortality is underlying cardiac disease.

ABDOMINAL AORTIC ANEURYSM

I. ETIOLOGY

A. Atherosclerosis most common (90%), secondary to structural, bio-chemical and hydraulic factors.

B. Inflammatory — ? autoimmune phenomenon (~ 5% of all AAA).

C. Mycotic or bacterial etiology — rare. Most commonly associated with SBE. (In past, syphillis and salmonella were implicated.)

D. Traumatic — much more common in thoracic aorta; rare in abdominal aorta.

E. Marfan's syndrome — cystic medial necrosis.

II. PATHOLOGY

A. Location.
  1. Below origin of renal arteries in 95% of cases.
  2. May extend to involve common iliac arteries, rarely beyond.
  3. May be completely limited to abdominal aorta.

B. Size — from 3–15 cm, usually fusiform aortic dilation. Dilation occurs in accordance with *LaPlace's law* (T = P x r, where T = wall tension, P = intraluminal pressure, r = aortic radius).

C. Associated with other manifestations of diffuse atherosclerosis. De-Bakey (*Ann. Surg.* 160:622, 1964) studied 1400 patients with AAA.
  1. Coronary artery disease — 30%.
  2. Hypertension — 40%.
  3. Associated occlusive arterial disease.
    a. Carotids — 7%.
    b. Renals — 2%.
    c. Iliac — 16%.
  4. Associated with other clinically significant aneurysms — thoracic aorta, femoral and popliteal arteries (4%, 3% & 2% respectively).

III. NATURAL HISTORY

A. Estes (*Circulation* 2:258, 1950) — classic study of untreated AAA of all sizes; published prior to availability of effective surgical therapy.
  1. 102 patients with AAA.
  2. 64 died, 63% secondary to rupture.
  3. Of all aneurysm patients, 20% had ruptured within 1 year and 50% within 5 years. Only 18.9% survived 5 years after diagnosis compared with 79.1% expected 5–year survival.

B. Darling (1970) autopsy studies — 25% of aneurysms between 4 and 6 cm had ruptured and 10% of ruptured aneurysms were < 4 cm.

C. Crisler & Bahnson (*Curr. Prob. Surg.* 9:1,1972) summarized risk of rupture of all AAA is 50% (over 10–year period); 5–year survival with aneurysms 6–7 cm in diameter is 5–10% without resection and 50% with resection; 1-year survival (6–7 cm diameter) was 50%.

D. Increased size = increased risk of rupture.

IV. CLINICAL PRESENTATION

A. Most aneurysms are asymptomatic and discovered on routine abdominal exam.

B. Leaking AAA may present with abdominal, back, or flank pain due to tension on retroperitoneum from aneurysm or from leakage of blood. Complaints may be mild; requires a *high index of suspicion*. Often proceeds rapidly to exsanguination.

C. With leakage or free rupture, patients may present in *shock*, occurs in 20% of ruptured AAA.

V. PHYSICAL EXAMINATION

A. Presence of pulsatile mass on deep palpation at level of umbilicus − 5 cm aneurysm is palpable in most patients.

B. Tortuous aorta may mimic AAA, presenting as pulsating, expansile abdominal mass, as distinct from other abdominal masses which merely transmit aortic pulsations (i.e., pseudocyst, pancreatic carcinoma, etc.).

C. In thin individuals aortic pulsations may be unusually prominent; however, careful bimanual palpation should confirm normal diameter.

D. Important to evaluate other peripheral arteries for associated occlusive disease − pulses and bruits.

VI. DIAGNOSTIC STUDIES

A. Plain film of abdomen is often (85%) diagnostic. Calcific rim of aneurysm often visible ("egg shell"); cross-table lateral view is most helpful to see both calcified walls anterior to the vertebral bodies.

B. **Ultrasound** is the simpler, less expensive mode to detect and confirm the presence of an aortic aneurysm. It is also the best way to serially follow small aneurysms.

C. **Abdominal CT scan** is the most accurate but also most expensive means of diagnosing AAA.

D. **Aortography.**
   1. Authorities disagree and debate value.
      a. Poor study for diagnosis or assessment of size, because thrombus within AAA obscures actual aneurysm size.
      b. Can give important information regarding associated vascular lesions, i.e., renal artery stenosis.
   2. Indications for aortography (most authorities agree).
      a. Hypertension − to rule out renal vascular causes.
      b. History compatible with intestinal angina − to rule out SMA or celiac lesions.
      c. Horseshoe kidney.
      d. Thoracoabdominal aneurysm − suspected by CXR findings.
      e. Lower extremity ischemia or diminished pulses (i.e., evidence of occlusive disease).
      f. Angiogram being performed in another vascular bed.
         1) Coronary arteries.

2) Carotid and/or vertebral arteries.
3. If aortogram not planned, should get IVP.

VII. CARDIAC WORK–UP OF ELECTIVE AAA REPAIR

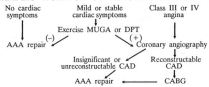

Ref: Hollier LH: Surgical management of abdominal aortic aneurysm in the high-risk patient. *Surg. Clin. North Am.* 66:2:267-279, 1986.

VIII. OPERATIVE INDICATIONS

A. Patients with aneurysms > 4–5 cm are candidates for elective operation unless concomitant medical problems increase operative risk or a second pathological process markedly reduces the patient's life expectancy.
B. Size increase of > 0.4 cm/year.
C. Chronologic age itself is not a contraindication and must be correlated with overall physical condition of patient.
D. When aneurysm becomes *symptomatic*, operation becomes imperative regardless of aneurysm size.

IX. MANAGEMENT OF RUPTURED AAA

A. **Diagnosis.**
   1. Generalized abdominal pain with associated back or flank pain and shock of varying degree (may be very mild).
   2. Abdominal exam — pulsatile mass palpable in 50%; may not be present due to hypotension.
   3. May simulate other intra–abdominal or medical conditions (i.e., renal colic, pancreatitis, myocardial infarction, muscular backache); therefore, need high index of suspicion.
   4. Rupture is frequently contained by retroperitoneal tissue; free intraperitoneal rupture may occur. In the latter case, mortality is usually immediate. Occurs in 20% of ruptured AAA.
   5. Diagnosis based on *clinical* grounds. Hemodynamically unstable patients with clinical evidence of ruptured AAA go *directly to OR*. Stable patients with a question of the presence of AAA may undergo emergent abdominal CT scan.

B. **Therapy.**
   1. There must be rapid replacement of blood loss with crystalloid and blood transfusion. Rapid replacement is maintained to correct hypotension.

2. Midline approach used with rapid isolation of the aorta just below diaphragm for proximal control (approach via the gastrohepatic omentum); clamping for approximately 30 min is possible without significant visceral ischemia.
3. Infrarenal clamp placed after aneurysm incised and surrounding hematoma evacuated, providing better visualization and avoiding damage to renal vasculature.
4. Low porosity woven or PTFE graft should be used with ruptured AAA, as preclotting is next to impossible.
5. Renal insufficiency most common complication postoperatively. May be prevented in part by mannitol (12.5 g) or furosemide (40 mg) infusion prior to anesthesia induction (controversial).
6. Mortality is approximately 50%.

X. ELECTIVE MANAGEMENT OF AAA
A. Preoperative preparation.
1. Optimize cardiovascular function and fluid volume.
2. Mechanical +/- antibiotic bowel preparation. Paregoric pre-op reduces size of small bowel.
3. Establish water diuresis with adquate IV hydration before anesthesia and maintain during surgery. A thermodilution pulmonary artery catheter (Swan–Ganz®) may be helpful during pre–op hydration and perioperative maintenance of adequate filling pressures and cardiac output. Mannitol (50 g) IV prior to cross–clamping aorta helps maintain adequate GFR.
4. Preoperative and intraoperative parenteral antibiotics.
B. Via midline incision, aorta is mobilized and infrarenal clamp is placed for proximal control.
C. Iliac arteries clamped for distal control.
D. IMA ligated from within the aneurysm to avoid injury to collateral vessels to the left colon. (In patients with decreased visceral blood supply and patent IMA, it may be necessary to re–implant artery into graft.)
E. Anterior portion of aneurysm wall is opened and thrombus is removed.
F. Posterior wall is left in place and lumbar vessels suture ligated.
G. Preclotted prosthetic graft sewn in place.
1. Tube graft if iliac arteries normal.
2. Bifurcation graft if iliac arteries are aneurysmal.
H. Non–resective surgical therapy.
1. In high–risk patient, axillo–bifemoral graft with induced aortic aneurysm thrombosis via catheter deposition of thrombogenic material or coil is a rarely used option.
2. High complication rate, including thrombus extension into renal or mesenteric arteries and rupture of aorta, have caused most to abandon this form of therapy.

XI. COMPLICATIONS

(Remember, these patients have diffuse vascular disease.)

A. Myocardial ischemia, arrhythmia and infarction.
   1. Arrhythmias — very common.
   2. Fatal MI in 3% of elective, 10% of symptomatic intact, and 16% of ruptured AAA cases.

B. Stroke — embolic or secondary to hypotension.

C. Renal insufficiency.
   1. Causes.
      a. Preoperative dehydration was formerly most common cause. An actively transporting renal tubule is more resistant to ischemic insult.
      b. Hypotension.
         1) Blood loss — leaking or ruptured aneurysms.
         2) Intraoperatively when aortic cross clamp is removed; prevent by adequate hydration.
      c. Atheromatous debris or thrombus is dislodged and embolizes to the kidneys.
   2. Frank renal failure — < 3% of elective cases, but > 20% of patients with ruptured aneurysms. Mortality rate of patients with renal failure and ruptured AAA is approximately 50%.

D. Colon ischemia.
   1. Normally there are 2 prominent collaterals between the SMA and IMA: (1) marginal artery of Drummond; (2) meandering mesenteric artery (not normally present in absence of SMA or IMA stenosis). These may be occluded or stenosed by the general atherosclerotic process.
   2. Prevent ischemia and assure adequate perfusion by several intraoperative maneuvers.
      a. Palpate the root of the SMA — pulsatile or not?
      b. Examine IMA orifice from within the opened aneurysm sac — open (retrograde bleeding) or not? A large, wide-open IMA should alert you to the need to re–implant artery.
      c. Doppler ultrasound — presence of audible doppler flow over the base of the large bowel mesentery and serosal surface appears to correlate well with colon viability.
      d. Measure IMA stump pressure — if mean pressure < 40 mm Hg, patient appears to be at higher risk of ischemic colitis.
      e. Fluorescein — ultraviolet luminescence.
      f. Experimental methods — bowel surface oximetry, intraluminal pH measurements.
   3. If hematochezia develops postoperatively, **immediate sigmoidoscopy** should be performed.
      a. Mucosal ischemia most common and usually manifested by mucosal sloughing; resolves spontaneously in most cases.
      b. Transmural involvement will require re–exploration and colonic resection with colostomy.

E. Arterial thromboembolic complications of lower extremities — emboli from aneurysmal sac or thrombosis from extended aortic clamp time.

F. **Spinal cord ischemia** (more common with thoracic aneurysm repair).
  1. Syndrome — paraplegia with loss of light touch and pain sensation and loss of sphincter control. Proprioception and temperature reception are spared.
  2. Pathology.
     a. Anterior spinal artery is formed in the neck and supplies the spinal cord.
     b. Several "anterior radicular arteries" feed into the anterior spinal artery.
     c. The lowest (and largest) anterior radicular artery usually arises at the T8–L1 level, but occasionally the origin is lower, leading to obliteration with abdominal aortic surgery (0.5% of cases).

G. Late complications.
  1. **Aortoenteric fistula.**
     a. *De novo* or more commonly from proximal suture line of aortic graft.
     b. Distal portion of duodenum most common location — 82% duodenum, 8% small bowel, 6% large bowel, 5% stomach.
     c. Presentation — GI bleeding with associated abdominal and back pain; may have **"herald bleed"** of more minor degree followed by exsanguinating hemorrhage.
     d. Diagnosis — endoscopy to rule out other source; if no definitive site found, graft–enteric fistula must be assumed.
     e. Treatment — remove graft, oversew aorta, repair enteric defect; drain retroperitoneum (with or without antibiotic irrigation); extra–anatomic bypass (axillo–bifemoral).
  2. Late infection of prosthetic graft material requires extra-anatomic bypass and removal of infected graft material and oversewing the aortic stump.
  3. Sexual dysfunction.
     a. Retrograde ejaculation and/or inability to maintain erection in 30–40% of men due to aorto–iliac surgery.
     b. Caused by injury to sympathetic plexus around the aorta and the left iliac artery.

XII. PROGNOSIS

A. Surgical repair has been shown to double survival time of untreated aneurysm.

B. Operative mortality for elective repair is < 5% (1–2% common).

C. Mortality for emergent repair of **ruptured** AAA ranges from 20% to 80% depending on condition of patient at presentation (persistent shock has high mortality).

CEREBROVASCULAR DISEASE

Unrecognized carotid disease remains a major source of morbidity and mortality. Not every bruit requires intervention. On the other hand, some symptoms require aggressive investigation.

I. GENERAL CONSIDERATIONS
A. Stroke is the 3rd leading cause of death in U.S.
B. 400,000 new strokes occur each year in U.S.; > 300,000 secondary to cerebrovascular disease.
C. Surgical goal is to relieve the symptoms of cerebral dysfunction with prevention of stroke.
D. Internal carotid artery originates at common carotid bifurcation — four distinct anatomic portions:
   1. Cervical — no branches.
   2. Petrous.
   3. Cavernous — ophthalmic artery.
   4. Cerebral — cerebral arteries.
E. External carotid artery branches (caudad — cephalad). In the face of extracranial internal carotid artery occlusive lesions, the external system will provide collateral circulation to the intracranial supply via the ophthalmic artery.
   1. Superior thyroid.
   2. Ascending pharyngeal.
   3. Lingual.
   4. Facial.
   5. Occipital.
   6. Posterior auricular.
   7. Maxillary.
   8. Superficial temporal.

II. CLINICAL MANIFESTATIONS
A. **Transient ischemic attack (TIA).**
   1. Episode of neurologic dysfunction lasting from a few minutes to no more than 24 hours and no residual neurologic deficit.
   2. Commonly affects vision of ipsilateral eye — **amaurosis fugax**, a transient blindness of one eye ("Like a shade closing over my eye").
   3. Ipsilateral hemispheric symptoms — transient paresis and/or paraesthesias of contralateral extremity.
   4. Risk of stroke — 5% per year, highest risk in 1st year of symptoms.
   5. Crescendo TIA — repeated neurologic events without interval neurologic deterioration. An indication for *emergent* cerebral angiography.
B. **Reversible ischemic neurologic deficit (RIND)** — neurologic manifestations lasting from 24–72 hours.

C. Completed stroke — persistent neurologic dysfunction if > 72 hours.
D. Vertebrobasilar system disease causes "posterior" symptoms — headaches, vertigo, equilibrium changes, "drop attacks", bilateral visual disturbances, pharyngeal sensory loss, vasomotor and respiratory center changes.
E. **Subclavian steal syndrome.**
 1. Proximal subclavian artery stenosis (proximal to vertebral artery).
  a. Subclavian artery unable to supply adequate blood flow to the arm during exertion.
  b. The blood flows up the carotid artery, through circle of Willis, and then retrograde down the vertebral artery to supply the subclavian artery distal to the stenosis. Exercise or use of the arm decreases resistance in arm, leading to increased blood flow via the vertebral artery, decreased cerebral flow, and cerebral symptoms.
  c. Cerebral circulation is decreased due to this shunting.
 2. Symptoms — vertigo plus syncopal episodes; very rarely (< 10%) correlated with arm exercise.

III. PATHOLOGY
A. **Etiology.**
 1. In Western countries, atherosclerosis is the primary pathologic event (> 90%).
 2. Non–atherosclerotic causes of carotid stenosis (10%) include inflammatory angiopathies, fibromuscular dysplasia, kinking secondary to arterial elongation, extrinsic compression, traumatic occlusion, spontaneous dissection.
B. Obstruction at the carotid bifurcation with proximal internal carotid involvement is most common location for atherosclerotic disease.
C. **Carotid ulceration.**
 1. Loss of endothelium in the central portion of the lesion exposes loose atheromatous material, resulting in distal embolization of debris.
 2. **Classification of ulcers.**
  a. "A" — minimal discrete cavity within atheromatous plaque.
  b. "B" — large cavity with higher stroke rate.
  c. "C" — multiple cavities or cavernous appearance, causing high stroke and death rate.
D. **Risk factors.**
 1. Age — individuals > 70 years of age have 8 times greater incidence of stroke than those < 50 years of age.
 2. Hypertension, diabetes, smoking, hyperlipidemia.
 3. Associated factors — coronary artery disease, peripheral vascular disease.

IV. DIAGNOSIS — VASCULAR STUDIES
A. **Noninvasive** (also see "Noninvasive Vascular Laboratory Studies").

1. **Doppler ultrasonic periorbital examination.**
   a. Internal carotid stenosis or occlusion is collateralized by flow via the connections between the external carotid and ophthalmic arteries.
   b. Doppler measures the direction and velocity of flow through the superficial temporal artery.
   c. Low equipment cost.
   d. Highly technician–dependent (subjective test results).
   e. No anatomic visualization.
2. **Oculopneumoplethysmography (OPG).**
   a. Determine and compare ophthalmic artery pressure in both eyes.
   b. Ophthalmic artery pressure is unilaterally decreased.
   c. Suggests > 70% stenosis of the ipsilateral internal carotid artery, but does not localize lesion.
   d. Moderate equipment costs.
3. **Duplex scanning** – combines B–mode image plus Doppler spectral analysis.
   a. Provides accurate anatomic and flow information.
   b. High equipment costs. Despite cost, has replaced indirect tests in most labs.
   c. Technician–dependent study.
B. **Cerebral angiography.**
   1. Indications – surgical candidates:
      a. TIA's, RIND's.
      b. Significant carotid artery stenosis indicated by non–invasive testing.
      c. Stroke.
   2. Arteriography.
      a. Visualization of all 4 neck vessels (carotids and vertebrals) and aortic arch.
      b. 75% of patients with strokes have angiographically demonstrable lesions (40% of these are extracranial).
   3. Digital subtraction imaging – contrast may be administered intravenously or intra–arterial. Contrast load is usually reduced. Resolution and visualization of small lesions may be less than conventional arteriography.

V. INDICATIONS FOR OPERATIVE REPAIR

A. History of hemispheric transient ischemia attack plus appropriate carotid stenosis – stroke risk 25–40% within 5 years.
B. **Thromboembolic stroke** with good recovery – 20–35% recurrence within 5 years (1/2 within first year).
C. **Chronic cerebral ischemia** – consider operative repair if mental/intellectual deterioration secondary to carotid disease (*very rare*).

D. In symptomatic patients, **carotid endarterectomy** appears to provide superior stroke prevention for patients with > 70% unilateral stenosis, > 50% bilateral stenosis, internal carotid occlusion in conjunction with 50% contralateral stenosis (Hertzer et al., *Ann. Surg.* 204:154, 1986).
E. **Asymptomatic carotid bruit/stenosis** — controversial.
   1. Evaluate noninvasively initially, confirm with angiography if noninvasive studies suggest significant disease.
   2. Increased risk for neurologic sequelae with > 80% stenosis or > 50% stenosis with contralateral occlusion — controversial.
   3. Preocclusive stenosis or large ulcerated plaques deserve surgical correction; also, severe bilateral stenosis in younger patient.
F. **Concomitant coronary artery disease.**
   1. Patients with coronary artery disease requiring surgical intervention are at risk for stroke if concomitant carotid disease is present (and *vice versa*).
   2. Carotid endarterectomy is followed immediately by coronary revascularization.

VI. CONTRAINDICATIONS TO OPERATIVE REPAIR
A. Overall general condition poor.
B. Stroke in evolution — wait for maximum neurologic recovery (controversial).

VII. COMPLICATIONS OF OPERATIVE INTERVENTION
A. **Wound hematoma** — procedure performed under full heparinization. Potential for airway compromise.
B. **Hypertension/hypotension.**
   1. Interference with baroreceptor mechanisms of the carotid sinus results in BP lability.
   2. Treatment — adequate fluid volume, nitroprusside, dopamine, neosynephrine as needed.
C. **Cranial nerve injury.**
   1. Recurrent laryngeal — vocal cord paralysis, hoarseness, poor cough mechanism.
   2. Hypoglossal — unilateral tongue paralysis.
   3. Marginal mandibular — drooping at corner of mouth.
   4. Superior laryngeal — early voice fatigability, loss of high pitch phonation.
D. Intraoperative neurologic deficit — 2–3%.
E. Postoperative stroke, worsening of neurologic deficits, death.
   1. Embolization of debris secondary to operative manipulations.
   2. Current accepted standards for perioperative mortality < 3%.
F. **Postoperative myocardial infarction** — leading cause of death following surgery.

MESENTERIC ISCHEMIA

Mesenteric ischemia is uncommon. However, successful treatment requires a high index of suspicion and recognition of both the chronic and acute forms.

I. ANATOMY AND PHYSIOLOGY

A. Circulation deficits in GI tract are uncommon, due to abundant collateral circulation between:
   1. Celiac axis.
   2. Superior mesenteric artery (SMA).
   3. Inferior mesenteric artery (IMA).
B. **Collateral vessels.**
   1. Pancreaticoduodenal arcade (celiac and SMA).
   2. Branch of left colic (SMA and IMA).
   3. Marginal artery of Drummond – often small, not continuous, especially at splenic flexure (SMA and IMA).
   4. Arc of Riolan (SMA and IMA).
C. **Physiology.**
   1. Circulation increases with digestion, decreases with exercise.
   2. Mesenteric vessels undergo **vasoconstriction** due to:
      a. Sympathetic stimulation.
      b. Decreased blood flow.
      c. Drugs (e.g., digitalis).

II. ACUTE MESENTERIC ISCHEMIA

A. **Clinical presentation** – hallmark is severe acute mid–abdominal pain *out of proportion* to physical findings.
   1. Early – symptoms of GI emptying are prominent (i.e., nausea, vomiting, diarrhea). Diffuse abdominal tenderness, without peritoneal signs and active bowel sounds, may be present.
   2. Late – symptoms of intestinal infarction. Hypotension, eventually leading to shock. Fever, bloody diarrhea and peritonitis develop late and are previous findings. Mortality at this point 80–85% despite intervention.
   3. Early diagnosis improves survival.
B. **Etiology.**
   1. Embolization of SMA (40%) – 1/3 of patients have antecedent embolic episodes (lower extremity embolus, CVA). Patients with potential sources of emboli (atrial arrythmias, atrial myxoma, mural thrombi) are at risk.
   2. Thrombosis of SMA (40%) – thrombus formation on atherosclerotic plaque. Often preceded by symptoms of chronic mesenteric ischemia (postprandial pain, weight loss, bloating, diarrhea).

3. Non–occlusive ischemia (20%) — vasoconstriction of mesenteric vasculature due to low cardiac output ("low flow state"). Common predisposing conditions are myocardial infarction, CHF, renal or hepatic disease, or trauma or operation leading to hypovolemia or hypotension.

C. **Management** — simultaneous fluid and electrolyte resuscitation and evaluation should be conducted *expeditiously*. Mesenteric angiography (with lateral views of aorta) is the *definitive* diagnostic test.

1. If peritonitis is present, or evidence of intestinal infarction, immediate abdominal exploration should be performed.

2. Embolus — arteriography shows occlusion of SMA, with embolus lodged just beyond inferior pancreaticoduodenal and middle colic arteries ("meniscus sign").

   a. Systemic heparinization should be given.

   b. Angiography catheter may be used to infuse papaverine both pre– and postoperatively.

   c. Following adequate resuscitation, immediate exploration should be performed. Embolectomy is performed via longitudinal arteriotomy in SMA. Arteriotomy may be closed with or without vein patch.

   d. Assess bowel viability by direct inspection and/or fluoroscein examination. Administer sodium fluoroscein (1 g IV) and inspect bowel under UV (Wood's) lamp. Viable bowel has smooth, uniform fluorescence.

   e. Consider "second–look" operation to re–inspect bowel of questionable viability.

3. Thrombosis — arteriogram shows complete occlusion of SMA at origin. Usually very little collateralization.

   a. *Immediate* operation is necessary. Diagnosis is often made late, and extensive bowel necrosis is present. At exploration, bowel is often gray and pulseless.

   b. Revascularization should be attempted with aortomesenteric bypass graft (Dacron® or saphenous vein).

   c. Resect non–viable bowel *after* revascularization. Consider "second–look" operation.

4. Non–occlusive — arteriography shows marked narrowing and "pruning" of distal mesenteric vessels, but not large vessels.

   a. Treatment is primarily non–operative. Patients are often extremely ill and poor surgical risks.

   b. Angiographic catheter should be left in place in SMA and infuse papaverine 20 mg IM initially, then 20 mg/hour (tolazoline; Priscoline® is an alternate choice).

   c. Optimize cardiac output (if possible).

III. CHRONIC MESENTERIC ISCHEMIA
A. Atherosclerotic involvement of 2 of 3 main visceral arteries.
B. **Diagnosis** — symptoms often applicable to multiple etiologies (i.e., gallbladder disease, occult GI cancer, etc.).
   1. Chronic epigastric abdominal pain, colicky occurring 30–60 min after meal. May be relieved by defecation.
   2. Involuntary weight loss ("food fear").
   3. Presence of abdominal bruit.
   4. Angiography — utilized after other disease entities ruled out. Should include lateral view of aorta and take–off of vessels.
C. **Treatment** — surgical revascularization is indicated.
   1. Nutritional repletion.
   2. Bypass grafting.
      a. 2-Vessel aortomesenteric graft (saphenous vein or Dacron®).
      b. Combined infra–renal aortic implant and aortomesenteric graft.
   3. Transaortic endarterectomy — for multiple vessel disease.
D. **Prognosis** — relief of pain in 90%.
   1. Best long–term results with 3–vessel revascularization.
   2. Recurrence 40% with 3–vessel revascularization *vs.* 50% for single–vessel.

RENOVASCULAR HYPERTENSION

I. GENERAL CONSIDERATIONS

A. Renovascular hypertension is hypertension induced by obstructed blood flow to the kidney.

B. The most common of surgically correctable forms of hypertension. Included in this group are coarctation of the aorta, pheochromocytoma, Cushing's syndrome (adrenal hyperplasia, cortical adenoma/carcinoma), primary hyperaldosteronism, and unilateral parenchymal disease. Renal artery stenosis is present in an estimated 5–10% of both adults and children with hypertension.

C. First clearly elucidated by Goldblatt in the 1930's.

D. **Mechanism:** A stenotic renal artery causes a decreased pressure and flow to the kidney. The juxtaglomerular apparatus in response to the low pressure secretes renin. Renin converts angiotensin to angiotensin I, a decapeptide. Angiotensin I is cleaved of 2 amino acids by angiotensin converting enzyme (ACE) to angiotensin II. Angiotensin II acts on the adrenal cortex to cause aldosterone secretion.

  1. Angiotensin II is a powerful vasoconstrictor.
  2. Aldosterone causes increased retention of sodium and water by the kidney.

II. PATHOLOGY OF RENAL ARTERY STENOSIS

A. **Atherosclerosis** causes two–thirds of renal artery stenosis.

  1. Tends to be in men in the 5th, 6th, 7th decades of life.
  2. Tends to occur near the origin of the renal artery.
  3. About one–third have bilateral lesions.
  4. Can decrease kidney function and lead to occlusion.

B. **Fibrous dysplasia** (also called fibromuscular dysplasia) − 4 types: 30% of renal artery stenosis.

  1. Medial fibrodysplasia − 70% of fibrous dysplasia.
    a. Occurs in women in 4th and 5th decades, causing a series of stenosis alternating with true aneurysmal outpouchings.
    b. Histologically, smooth muscle is replaced by fibrous tissue.
    c. Rarely affects renal function.
  2. Perimedial dysplasia.
    a. Predominantly young women.
    b. Focal stenosis of renal artery without aneurysms.
    c. Histologically has excessive elastic tissue at junction of media and adventitia.
  3. Internal fibrodysplasia − rare. Build–up of subendothelial mesenchymal cells.
  4. Medial hyperplasia − very rare. Caused by proliferation of medial smooth muscle.

C. Others — hypoplastic stenosis, AV malformation, renal artery dissection or thrombosis, and emboli to the kidney.

III. CLINICAL MANIFESTATIONS
A. A neurovascular cause of systemic hypertension should be suspected in certain situations:
   1. Onset of hypertension at a young age or over 55 years old.
   2. Acceleration of hypertension after previously good control.
   3. Resistance to triple drug therapy.
   4. Hypertension accompanied by deterioration in renal function.
   5. Presence of a continuous abdominal bruit in the epigastrium or upper quadrants of the abdomen. The presence of a systolic bruit is non-specific.

IV. DIAGNOSTIC METHODS
A. **Rapid sequence IVP** (at 1, 2, and 3 min following injection of dye).
   1. A positive exam will show:
      a. A delay in uptake of concentration of contrast, followed by a paradoxical hyperconcentration of the dye in the collecting systems.
      b. A decreased size of the affected kidney by 1.5 cm or greater when compared to the contralateral kidney.
   2. Sensitivity only 70% with a 10% false–positive rate.
B. **Renal arteriography.**
   1. Establishes the existence of a lesion.
   2. Provides anatomic localization of the lesion(s), along with the delineation of the extra- and intrarenal arterial anatomy and the presence of any collateral circulation.
   3. Does *not* give **functional** significance of a lesion, that is, the mere existence of a lesion in a hypertensive patient is not proof that the patient has renovascular hypertension.
C. **Renal vein renin measurements** — used to determine which stenoses are significant and are actually causing hypertension.
   1. Peripheral measurement of serum renin activity is *not* a useful screen.
   2. Simultaneous renal vein renins are obtained along with an IVC renin.
   3. A ratio of 1.5 or greater from the vein of the suspect kidney compared to the normal side indicates a significant stenosis.
   4. Patients must be off beta blockers and aortic sympathetic drugs prior to the test.
   5. Captopril administration 1/2 hour prior to testing increases the sensitivity of the tests by magnifying the difference in the renal vein renins.
D. **Color flow Dopper ultrasound** — a new technique, not frequently used.
   1. Difficult to see the origins of renal arteries in most people.

    2. A normal test precludes the diagnosis of renal artery stenosis.

**V. TREATMENT OF RENOVASCULAR STENOSIS
CAUSING HYPERTENSION**
A. Medical therapy — anti–hypertensive medications.
B. Percutaneous transluminal angioplasty.
    1. Treatment of choice for fibromuscular dysplasia.
    2. Can be used for the treatment of atherosclerotic stenosis. Approximately 75% have initial success; 25% of these recur at 3 months. Renal artery ostial lesions do not respond to dilation.
C. Endarterectomy.
D. Bypass of the renal artery.
    1. Saphenous veins, Gortex and Dacron are all used. None is superior to the other in terms of long–term patency.
    2. Autogenous internal iliac artery is probably the graft material of choice for children under 15 years old.
    3. Renal artery bypass often accompanies aortic bypass or replacement for occlusive or aneurysmal disease.
    4. Bypass procedure for other special circumstances — splenic artery to left renal artery and gastroduodenal artery to right kidney.
E. Results.
    1. 90% are cured or improved after surgery.
    2. Operative mortality is 2–3%.
    3. One study suggests that a patient with surgically treated hypertension is 2 times more likely to be alive 9 years post–op when matched to a control population treated medically despite comparable blood pressure control.

PEDIATRIC SURGICAL EMERGENCIES

Children, particularly neonates, are not small adults. They have their own patterns of disease and physiological responses. Dosages are different. In general, however, surgical philosophy and approaches are similar.

I. FLUID REQUIREMENTS & RESUSCITATION MEDICATIONS

A. Maintenance fluids.

Weight (kg)	Amount of Fluid (crystalloid) per 24 hours
0 – 10	100 cc/kg
11 – 20	1000 cc + 50 cc/kg over 10 kg
21 – 40	1500 cc + 20 cc/kg over 20 kg
≥ 40	2500 cc/24 hrs (adult requirement)

B. Maintenance electrolytes.

1. Na^+ – 3–4 mEq/kg/24 h.
2. K^+ – 2–3 mEq/kg/24 h.
3. Ca^{++} – 2 mEq/kg/24 h.

C. Blood products (Note: May be infused over shorter times for a patient in shock).

1. Whole blood – 10–20 cc/kg.
2. Plasma – 10–20 cc/kg.
3. 5% albumin – 10–20 cc/kg.
4. Packed RBC – 5–10 cc/kg.
5. 25% albumin – 2–4 cc/kg.

II. CARDIOPULMONARY RESUSCITATION IN CHILDREN

A. Drugs.

Medication	Initial Dose (IV)
$NaHCO_3$ (1 mEq/ml)	1-2 mEq (1-2 ml)/kg
*Epinephrine 1:10,000	10 μg (0.1 ml)/kg
Atropine (1.0 mg/ml)	0.02 mg (0.02 ml)/kg
Calcium chloride 10%	20 mg (0.2 ml)/kg
Lidocaine 2%	1 mg (0.05 ml)/kg
Dopamine 40 mg/ml – 60 mg (1.5 ml)/100 ml D_5W = 500 μg/ml	1 ml/kg · hr = 10 μg · min (Moderate dose – predominant β-adrenergic effects)
Epinephrine 1:1000 – 6 mg (6 ml)/100 ml D_5W = 60 μg/ml	1 ml/kg · hr = 1 μg/kg · min (High dose – α- and β-adrenergic effects)
Isoproterenol 1:5000 – 0.6 mg (3.0 ml)/100 ml D_5W = 6 μg/ml	1 ml/kg · hr = 0.1 μg/kg · min (Low dose)
Lidocaine 4% – 120 mg (3 ml)/100 ml D_5W = 1200 μg/ml	1 ml/kg · hr = 20 μg/kg · min (Moderate dose)

* May be given via endotracheal tube if unable to achieve venous access.

B. Defibrillation – 2 joules/kg.

Ref: Eichelberger MR, Randolph JG. *J. Trauma* 23:91, 1983. Adapted with permission.

III. TRAUMA

A. **Principles of assessment and resuscitation** — same in children as adults:
   1. Establish airway, breathing.
   2. Control external bleeding.
   3. Vascular access/fluid resuscitation.
   4. Abdomen/chest/neurologic/orthopedic exam.
   5. Diagnostic procedures.

B. **Special considerations.**
   1. **Battered child syndrome** (reportable to authorities in some states if suspected).
      a. Suspect if parent gives inappropriate history not corroborated by physical findings.
      b. Characteristics of child abusers.
         1) Parents, relatives, guardians, baby-sitters.
         2) All socioeconomic levels.
         3) Parents with history of abuse during their own childhood.
         4) Often history of alcoholism or divorce.
      c. Characteristics of abused child.
         1) Majority < 3 years old.
         2) History of prolonged interval between injury and seeking medical attention.
         3) No racial or sexual differences.
      d. Types of injuries.
         1) Soft tissue — multiple bruises, abrasions, burns (often stocking distribution of feet and legs).
         2) Skeletal — often multiple fractures in various stages of healing. Rib and skull fractures common.
         3) Nervous system — acute and chronic subdural hematoma.
         4) Visceral — bowel perforation, mesenteric tears, liver/spleen/pancreas/kidney injuries.
         5) Genitalia — sexual abuse common.
      e. **Treatment.**
         1) Admission for observation and protection of child.
         2) Complete exam, including skeletal survey (**Silverman series**).
         3) Consultation for psychological evaluation.

C. **Abdominal trauma** — Principles of initial assessment of blunt and penetrating trauma in adults also pertains to pediatric age group.
   1. Significant differences — management of pediatric abdominal trauma include:
      a. Routine liver enzymes in all patients with blunt abdominal trauma; SGOT > 200, SGPT > 100 IU has high correlation with presence of hepatic injury.
      b. Use of CT scan in patient suspected of having intra-abdominal injury by physical exam or elevated liver enzymes.

    c. CT scan has virtually replaced emergency peritoneal lavage for evaluation of intra-abdominal trauma injury in many pediatric centers.

    d. Non-surgical treatment if significant parenchymal injuries to liver or spleen. Bedrest and supportive therapy will result in resolution of these injuries in the majority of cases.

    e. Criteria for surgical exploration.
        1) Continued hemodynamic instability.
        2) Multiple, large devitalized tissue fragments (liver and spleen) noted on CT.
        3) Persistent hemorrhage (blood requirements > 50% of calculated blood volume – 8% of body weight in kg – over 24 hours.
        4) Splenic injury with known pre-existing splenic disease (e.g., mononucleosis, leukemia, lymphoma).
        5) Intraperitoneal free air.

Ref: Ryckman FC, Noseworthy J. *Surg Clin N Am* 65:1287, 1985.

IV. INTESTINAL OBSTRUCTION

A. Principles of diagnostic assessment similar to that of adults (see "Intestinal Obstruction" chapter). In general, **bilious vomiting** in the neonate warrants urgent diagnosis and therapy.

B. Etiology of obstruction — dependent on **age** of patient and level of obstruction (listed in order of anatomic occurrence).

    1. Newborns (< 30 days old).
        a. Gastric/duodenal obstruction.
            1) Esophageal atresia stenosis.
            2) Gastric volvulus.
            3) Pyloric stenosis.
            4) Duodenal atresia.
            5) Duodenal web.
            6) Annular pancreas.
            7) Malrotation.
        b. Distal intestinal obstruction.
            1) Meconium ileus.
            2) Ileal/jejunal atresia.
            3) Necrotizing enterocolitis.
            4) Functional ileus (sepsis, CNS, drugs).
            5) Omphalitis/omphalomesenteric duct remnant.
            6) Intestinal duplication.
            7) Mesenteric cysts.
            8) Strangulated malrotation.
        c. Colonic obstruction.
            1) Aganglionosis (Hirschsprung's disease).
            2) Cloacal anomalies.

       3) Necrotizing enterocolitis.
       4) Colonic duplications.
       5) Colonic atresia.
       6) Imperforate anus.

2. **Infants (1–24 months).**
   a. Gastric/duodenal obstruction.
      1) Pyloric stenosis.
      2) Malrotation.
      3) Duplication.
   b. Distal intestinal obstruction.
      1) Intussusception.
      2) Inguinal hernia.
      3) Intestinal duplication.
      4) Mesenteric cysts.
      5) Omphalomesenteric duct remnants.
      6) Necrotizing enterocolitis.
      7) Appendicitis.
   c. Colonic obstruction.
      1) Intussusception.
      2) Aganglionosis.
      3) Colonic duplication.
      4) Necrotizing enterocolitis.

3. **Children (> 2 years old).**
   a. Gastric/duodenal obstruction — uncommon.
      1) Trauma (duodenal hematoma).
      2) Duplication.
      3) Granulomatous enterocolitis (Crohn's disease).
   b. Distal intestinal obstruction.
      1) Inguinal hernias.
      2) Appendicitis.
      3) Crohn's disease.
      4) Adhesions (previous surgery or inflammation).
   c. Colonic obstruction.
      1) Ulcerative colitis or Crohn's disease.
      2) Adhesions.

V. FOREIGN BODIES

Common problem in infants; aspiration or ingestion of small objects, or unchewed food.

A. Laryngeal.
   1. **Symptoms** — choking, loss of voice, dyspnea, stridor, retraction.
   2. **Treatment.**
     a. If soft food, may attempt modified Heimlich maneuver or turn child upside down and percuss back.

    b. Laryngoscopy — for more pointed objects.
       1) Never do alone! Have nurse assistant, circulating nurse, anesthesiologist as head holder.
       2) Place IV and use sedation — diazepam (Valium®) 0.1–0.3 mg/kg slow IVP.
       3) Apply a local anesthetic to posterior pharynx (topical Cetacaine® spray).
       4) Insert laryngoscope slowly and remove foreign body with forceps when first seen.

B. Tracheobronchial — majority in right main stem bronchus.
    1. Symptoms — coughing, wheezing, choking, or an unexplained persistent or recurrent pneumonitis.
    2. Diagnosis and treatment.
      a. Chest x-ray — inspiratory and expiratory films.
        1) During expiration, mediastinum will shift away from involved side.
        2) Note atelectasis or hyperinflation distal to foreign body.
      b. Bronchoscopy.
        1) For diagnosis and treatment.
        2) Narrow and inflamed lumen suggests distal foreign body.

C. Esophageal.
    1. Symptoms — pain, drooling, inability to swallow.
    2. Diagnosis and treatment.
      a. PA and lateral chest x-ray (with view of neck) — to locate foreign body and determine its character. If object is radiolucent, have patient swallow barium.
      b. Balloon retrieval — perform *only* with fluoroscopy and patient sedation.
        1) Pass Foley catheter beyond object.
        2) Inflate balloon of catheter and withdraw object.
        3) Grasp object with forceps once in mouth.
        4) Use this technique only in presence of blunt or flat object (*not* sharp).
      c. Esophagoscopy — requires general anesthesia.

D. Gastrointestinal — 95% pass through entire GI tract without difficulty in 24–48 hours.
    1. Round/oval/cuboid objects (marbles, buttons, etc.).
      a. May repeat abdominal x-rays in 4–5 days.
      b. No need for hospitalization.
    2. Sharp/pointed objects (pins, sharp glass, etc.).
      a. Admit and observe with serial abdominal films.
      b. Keep patient on usual diet for age.
      c. Do *not* administer cathartics, enemas, etc.
      d. Indications for laparotomy — failure of sharp object to move, signs of peritonitis, lower GI bleeding.
    3. Elongated/slender objects (pencils, nails, etc.).

    a. Greatest incidence of complications.
    b. Admit and observe with serial abdominal x-rays.
    c. Indications for operation — same as #2 above.
  4. Batteries — if ingested, should be surgically removed if failure
    to progress as noted by serial abdominal x-rays.

VI. CONGENITAL DIAPHRAGMATIC HERNIA (Bochdalek)

A. Anatomy.
  1. Size of defect ranges from 1 cm to absence of entire hemi-
    diaphragm.
  2. 85% occur on left side, usually involves posterolateral portion
    of diaphragm.
  3. Abdominal contents herniate into pleural cavity, compressing
    lung.

B. Associated anomalies.
  1. High incidence of GI anomalies (Meckel's diverticulum, in-
    testinal malrotation, incomplete attachment of colon).
  2. Congenital cardiac defects 10–15%.
  3. Pulmonary hypoplasia 2–20%.
  4. Genitourinary–associated anomalies are rare.

C. Diagnosis.
  1. Respiratory distress (dyspnea, cyanosis, apnea).
  2. Scaphoid abdomen with bulging chest.
  3. Displacement of heart sounds away from side of herniation.
  4. Onset of symptoms may be immediately after birth, but may
    also appear hours to days after birth ("**honeymoon period**").
    Time of development of respiratory distress:
    a. < 12 hours — 61%.
    b. 12–24 hours — 44.4%.
    c. 24–72 hours — 38.4%.
    d. > 72 hours — 4.7%.
  5. Chest x-ray — usually confirms diagnosis by findings of loops
    of gas–filled bowel within chest. If infant very young (< 24
    hrs), little opportunity to swallow air and bowel loops may be
    opacified.
  6. If diagnosis in doubt, may place NG tube and instill small
    amounts of contrast (1–2 cc) into stomach under fluoroscopy.
    Other conditions confused with diaphragmatic hernia include
    congenital pulmonary emphysema, pneumatoceles, etc.

D. Treatment.
  1. Urgent transabdominal repair of diaphragmatic defect.
  2. Preoperative preparation.
    a. Place NG tube (8 French) and connect to intermittent
    suction.
    b. Maintain body temperature in warm isolette.

    c. Avoid positive pressure ventilation via mask — may create further gastric distention and compromise pulmonary function.

    d. Correct metabolic acidosis (see section I).

    e. Place at least two IV's.

    f. Type and cross–match.

  3. **Mortality** — contributing factors:

    a. With associated anomalies: 65%; without associated anomalies: 14%.

    b. Weight.

      1) < 5.5 pounds — 28.6%.

      2) > 5.5 pounds — 14.3%.

  4. May require **ECMO** (extracorporeal membrane oxygenation) support for persistent hypoxia after repair (pulmonary hypoplasia).

VII. ACUTE SCROTUM

Most urgent concern is possible torsion of testicle with subsequent infarction.

A. Presentation.

  1. Testicular torsion.

    a. Acute onset of generalized scrotal pain, edema, discoloration, nausea, vomiting, retracted testicle.

    b. Undescended testicle in inguinal canal simulates incarcerated hernia.

    c. Intra-abdominal testicle simulates acute appendicitis.

  2. Torsion of testicular appendages (appendix testis or appendix epididymis) — scrotal pain localized to small area.

  3. Epididymitis — more gradual onset of scrotal pain, with associated fever, pyuria.

  4. Mumps orchitis — onset after puberty, 3–7 days after onset of parotid swelling.

B. Diagnosis.

  1. Physical exam — mainstay of diagnosis.

  2. Doppler and radioisotope scans helpful.

    a. If Doppler scan indicates absence of testicular artery pulsations, consider testicular torsion.

    b. Radionuclide scan — if flow absent to testicle, consider torsion, tumor; if increased flow is present, consider epididymitis.

  3. Often impossible to differentiate between torsion and infectious etiologies.

C. Treatment.

  1. Emergency scrotal exploration/orchidopexy (with/without contralateral orchidopexy) for suspected testicular torsion or equivocal cases.

    2. Torsion of testicular appendage — excision of appendage.

    3. Epididymitis — antibiotics and scrotal elevation.

VIII. OMPHALOCELE/GASTROSCHISIS

A. Omphalocele.

    1. Considered a hernia of umbilical cord.

    2. Rectus muscle displaced laterally — defect medial to rectus.

    3. Associated anomalies (up to 67%) — incomplete rotation of small bowel, exstrophy of bladder, cardiovascular, etc.

    4. **Preoperative preparation.**

       a. Maintain normal body temperature in warm isolette.

       b. Placement of NG tube.

       c. IV hydration and replacement of GI losses.

       d. Cover exposed sac and/or bowel with plastic sheet or bag to decrease evaporative fluid loss.

       e. Type and cross–match.

       f. Prophylactic systemic antibiotics.

          1) Ampicillin 50–100 mg/kg/day divided q 12 h IM or IV.

          2) Gentamicin 5 mg/kg/day divided q 12 h IM or IV.

    5. **Treatment.**

       a. Silastic "silo" sewn around circumference of larger defects with gradual reduction of abdominal contents over 1-2 weeks.

       b. Primary closure of skin over smaller defects with repair of ventral hernia later.

B. Gastroschisis.

    1. Defect in abdominal wall **lateral** to rectus abdominus muscle.

    2. Fewer associated abnormalities.

    3. **Preoperative preparation** — same as for omphalocele.

    4. **Treatment** — same as for omphalocele. If bowel is edematous, anticipate prolonged ileus and requirements for TPN.

IX. TRACHEO–ESOPHAGEAL FISTULA

A. History.

    1. Usually presents in newborn period or infancy.

    2. Excessive salivation, drooling, or gagging.

    3. Episodes of cyanosis, coughing, labored breathing, choking on feeding, inability to pass NG tube.

B. Diagnosis.

    1. Suspicion of any newborn with above history.

    2. Pass catheter (8-10 French) into esophagus until obstruction is met.

    3. Obtain chest x-ray (upright PA and lateral) and note inability of tube to advance into stomach. Also note **distention of GI tract** or **absence of gas** in abdomen.

    4. If doubt still exists as to diagnosis, 0.5 cc of radiopaque contrast material can be injected into catheter and repeat chest x-rays obtained.

    5. Ultrasound used to verify position of aortic arch (right or left).

C. **Types of tracheo-esophageal fistulas** (Fig. 1).

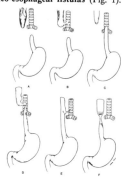

FIGURE 1
Types of Tracheo-esophageal Fistulas

    1. Type A (6-7%) — isolated esophageal atresia; gasless abdomen.

    2. Type B (1%) — esophageal atresia with proximal tracheo-esophageal fistula.

    3. Type C (86.5%) — esophageal atresia with distal tracheo-esophageal fistula — most common.

    4. Type D (1-5%) — proximal and distal tracheo-esophageal fistula with esophageal atresia.

    5. Type E (5%) — tracheo-esophageal fistula without esophageal atresia.

    6. Type F (1%) — esophageal atresia without tracheo-esophageal fistula.

D. **Preoperative preparation.**

    1. Maintain esophageal catheter to intermittent suction.

    2. Maintain NPO.

    3. Place IV's.

    4. Elevate head of bed.

    5. Type and cross–match.

    6. Preoperative antibiotics.

        a. Penicillin 50–100,000 units/kg/day q 12 h.
        b. Gentamicin 7 mg/kg/day divided q 12 h IM or IV.

E. Treatment.
    1. Gastrostomy — usually the initial procedure to prevent further aspiration and allow resolution of pneumonia (7–10 days).
    2. Repair of tracheo-esophageal fistulas.
        a. Extrapleural right thoracotomy preferred (except with right-sided aortic arch) — potential anastomotic leak isolated from pleural space.
        b. If proximal esophagus too short for anastomosis, consider:
            1) Spiral myotomy of upper segment.
            2) Preoperative bougienage.
            3) Colon or small bowel interpositions (but deferred until infant ≥ 1 year of age).

X. GI BLEEDING

A. History — try to obtain information on the following:
    1. Note ingestion of iron, beets, cherry Jello, or sources of red food coloring.
    2. Quantity of blood vomited or passed and how long patient has been bleeding.
    3. Character of blood — coffee-ground, bright red, clots.
    4. History of familial bleeding tendencies or polyposis.
    5. Pain when defecating.
    6. Stool mixed with blood or blood–streaked.
    7. In adolescents — excessive alcohol ingestion, especially first experience.

B. Physical examination.
    1. General — signs of shock or hypovolemia.
    2. Skin.
        a. Hemangiomas/telangiectasia.
        b. Circumoral melanin spots (Peutz–Jeghers syndrome).
        c. Purpura (Henoch–Schonlein syndrome).
        d. Petechiae — generalized bleeding disorders.
    3. Nasopharynx — inspect for evidence of bleeding.
    4. Abdomen.
        a. Hepatomegaly — associated with portal hypertension.
        b. Mass — if mobile, suggests bowel etiology of bleeding.
        c. Caput medusa — associated with portal hypertension.
    5. Anus/rectum — examine for fissures, trauma, hemorrhoids, rectal prolapse, polyps.

C. Diagnosis.
    1. Place NG tube to determine whether source of bleeding is upper or lower GI tract.
        a. CBC initially and follow serially.

    b. Platelet count, bleeding time, partial thromboplastin and pro-thrombin time.

    c. Type and cross–match.

  2. Depending upon initial assessment, further studies may be indicated.

    a. Flexible fiberoptic esophagogastroscopy — may reveal gastric or duodenal ulcer, gastritis, Mallory–Weiss tear, esophageal varices, etc.

    b. Technetium scan (Meckel's scan) — ^{99m}Tc Pertechnetate concentrates in ectopic gastric mucosa cells of the Meckel's diverticulum.

    c. Sigmoidoscopy — may detect juvenile polyps, congenital polyposis, or colitis.

    d. For further work-up, see "GI Bleeding" chapter.

  3. Neonatal GI bleeding — rarely requires operative correction.

    a. Hematemesis/melena may result from swallowed maternal blood during delivery.

    b. Melena produced by as little as 2.6 ml of swallowed blood.

    c. Apt–Downing test — differentiates between fetal and maternal blood.

      1) 1 volume of stool to 5 volumes H_2O; mix, centrifuge, and separate 5 ml of clear, pink supernatant.

      2) Add 1 ml of 1% NaOH and wait 2 minutes.

      3) If supernatant remains pink, blood is fetal in origin; if it turns brown–yellow, blood is of maternal origin.

    d. Etiology.

      1) Hemorrhagic disease of newborn (vitamin K deficiency).

      2) Peptic ulcer — high gastric acidity noted in neonates.

      3) Stress ulcer — associated with CNS injury, sepsis, shock.

      4) Necrotizing enterocolitis.

      5) Anal fissures.

      6) Intestinal volvulus with infarction.

      7) Infectious diarrhea.

      8) Idiopathic — common.

  4. Infants and children — blood pressure deceptive, as substantial blood loss can occur with normal blood pressure before irreversible shock *suddenly* occurs.

D. Common causes of GI hemorrhage in children/adolescents.

  1. Esophagitis, Barrett's ulcer, varices.

  2. Peptic ulcer, gastritis, duodenitis.

  3. Duplications of alimentary tract.

  4. Polyps, hamartomas (Peutz–Jeghers syndrome).

  5. Intestinal trauma.

  6. Liver trauma — hematobilia.

  7. Foreign bodies, bezoars.

8. Meckel's diverticulum.
9. Inflammatory bowel disease.
10. Henoch–Schonlein purpura.
11. Intussusception.
12. Volvulus with infarction.
13. Parasitic infestation.
14. Hemangiomas, arteriovenous malformations, telangiectasis.
15. Acute colitis.
16. Rectal prolapse, fissures, proctitis.
17. Blood dyscrasia with or without any of the preceding conditions.
E. **Management** – same as adult GI bleeding.
  1. Blood replacement guidelines.
    a. Estimation of blood volume.
      1) Premature – 85–100 ml/kg.
      2) Term newborn – 85 ml/kg.
      3) > 1 month – 75 ml/kg.
    b. Infuse blood at volume of 10 cc/kg over several hours and repeat as needed to keep Hct > 30%.
  2. Treatment of etiologic cause.

XI. ACUTE ABDOMEN (Non–Traumatic)
A. Less than 5% of all abdominal pain (pediatric) seen in emergency room will ultimately require surgical intervention.
B. **History.**
  1. Pain – note duration, location, radiation, character (crampy, constant), association with movement, eating, etc.
  2. Vomiting – note character (bilious, bloody), time in relation to food intake and pain.
  3. Change in bowel habits – consistency and color of stool, last bowel movement, constipation.
  4. Urine – dysuria, hematuria, urgency, anuria.
  5. Vaginal discharge, bleeding, menstrual history.
C. **Physical exam** – *thorough* examination is critical, since etiology of abdominal pain may not be found on abdominal exam alone.
  1. General appearance – note facial expression, skin color, turgor.
  2. Chest – signs of intrathoracic inflammatory process (dullness to percussion, decreased breath sounds, wheezing, etc.).
  3. Abdomen.
    a. Appearance – distended, scaphoid, visible loops of bowel, erythema.
    b. Auscultation – note presence or absence of bowel sounds. If present, note character (high pitched, hyperactive).
    c. Palpation – lightly palpate all quadrants and note presence of obvious mass, location of pain, tone of abdominal wall.
      1) Liver/spleen – note pain, size, contour.

2) CVA tenderness.
3) Note palpable loops of bowel or fecal material.
4) Inguinal region – note presence or absence of hernia, undescended testicle, lymphadenopathy, etc.
5) Scrotum – see section VII.
6) Rectal exam – should be done on every patient with abdominal pain; important to detect induration, localize tenderness or mass, and character of stool.
7) Pelvic exam – insure patency of hymen in all female patients.
   a) Exam deferred if patient pre-pubertal and not sexually active, but mandatory in all adolescent females and older, as well as all sexually active patients (regardless of age).
   b) Note vaginal bleeding or discharge, pain with cervical motion, open cervical os, adenexal tenderness/mass, or enlarged uterus.

D. Laboratory studies.

1. CBC with differential – examine peripheral smear for evidence of RBC destruction.
2. Urinalysis.
3. Electrolytes, BUN, creatinine if history of diarrhea or vomiting.
4. Sickle cell prep.
5. Serum pregnancy test if even *a remote* possibility of pregnancy in adolescents (β-HCG).
6. Liver function studies if evidence of hepatobiliary trauma or disease on history or physical exam.
7. Chest x-ray.
8. Flat and upright (or left lateral decubitus) abdominal films.
9. Abdominal ultrasound if mass is palpated, hepatomegaly, or suspected pelvic or biliary pathology.

E. Common conditions requiring surgical exploration.

1. **Acute appendicitis** – most common intra-abdominal indication for surgery in children > 2 years of age.
   a. If diagnosis in question, always admit patient and observe with serial abdominal exams.
   b. Progression of signs and symptoms – pain (initially periumbilical, then localized to RLQ), low-grade fever, anorexia and vomiting, mild leukocytosis.
   c. X-ray of abdomen may reveal appendicolith in RLQ, ileus, mass effect in RLQ.
   d. **Treatment** – urgent appendectomy.
   e. **Preoperative preparation.**
      1) Place IV line.
      2) Prophylactic antibiotics given to prevent wound infection and intra-abdominal abscess in cases of suspected perforation or abscess.

3) Choice of antibiotic should provide coverage for enteric organisms and anaerobes (e.g., ampicillin, gentamicin, clindamycin).
4) High fever must be controlled with salicylates, cooling blanket if necessary. Use rectal thermometer intraoperatively.

2. **Intussusception** — more common in children < 2 years old.
   a. History of sudden onset of pain with drawing up of legs and periods of quiescence.
   b. Associated with passage of "currant jelly" stool, vomiting.
   c. Abdominal mass.
   d. Hydrostatic reduction of intussusception with barium is indicated unless peritonitis or bowel obstruction present.
   e. Surgery indicated if barium enema unsuccessful.

3. **Necrotizing enterocolitis** — most common GI emergency of the neonate.
   a. Frequently affects premature and low–birth–weight infants.
   b. Signs and symptoms — ileus, vomiting, bloody stools, abdominal distention, hypothermia, shock.
   c. X-ray findings — pneumatosis intestinalis is classic; also ascites, intestinal distention, portal venous gas.
   d. **Management.**
      1) Medical.
         a) Place NG or orogastric tube (10 French sump).
         b) Systemic antibiotics.
         c) Parenteral nutrition.
         d) Monitor with serial platelet counts and abdominal x-rays (every 6 hours).
         e) Correct acidosis and restore intravascular volume.
      2) Surgical indications.
         a) Progressive clinical deterioration — uncorrectable acidosis, worsening thrombocytopenia.
         b) Signs of diffuse peritonitis.
         c) Free air on abdominal x-rays.
         d) Palpation of abdominal mass.
         e) Abdominal wall erythema or induration.
         f) Abdominal paracentesis suggestive of non-viable bowel if fluid brown and cloudy, extracellular bacteria on gram stain, large number of WBC's with differential > 80% neutrophils.

4. **Incarcerated hernia.**
   a. History may or may not reveal prior hernias.
   b. Examination reveals immobile, tender mass in groin with mass extending along spermatic cord all the way to internal ring.

    c. Attempt at reduction of hernia indicated except if peritonitis and/or bowel obstruction are present.

    d. Reduction facilitated by firm pressure in the direction of inguinal canal. Sedation, in addition to elevation of legs and torso, may also be helpful.

    e. Hospitalization and close observation indicated following successful reduction; then elective repair of hernia.

    f. Surgery warranted in presence of peritoneal signs or bowel obstruction.

5. Other important causes of abdominal pain.

    a. Chronic non–specific pain of childhood — diagnosis by exclusion.

    b. Constipation — most common etiology of non–surgical abdominal pain in childhood.

    c. Acute gastroenteritis — history of severe diarrhea with vomiting and fever followed by abdominal pain. Consider salmonellosis, shigellosis, etc.

    d. Mesenteric adenitis (commonly mistaken for acute appendicitis) — abdominal pain often preceded by viral upper respiratory symptoms (1–2 weeks).

    e. Crohn's disease — may mimic acute appendicitis.

    f. Meckel's diverticulitis — rectal bleeding more common than pain; may mimic appendicitis.

    g. Primary peritonitis.

        1) Gram–negative organisms are responsible for 70% of infections.

        2) Diffuse peritoneal infection without apparent source.

        3) Vast majority require celiotomy for diagnosis.

    h. Pneumonia — usually in right lower lobe, causing referred abdominal pain.

    i. Acute pyelonephritis.

    j. Pelvic inflammatory disease — pain most frequent during menses.

    k. Mittelschmerz — ovulatory pain midway through menstrual cycle.

    l. Henoch–Schonlein purpura — hemorrhagic rash, usually on lower extremities. May also be associated with arthritis and/or nephritis.

    m. Herpes–Zoster — abdominal pain precedes development of vesicular rash that usually corresponds to dermatome.

    n. Cholecystitis — usually associated with hemolytic disorder.

    o. Cystitis.

    p. Diabetic ketoacidosis (sometimes the presenting episode with juvenile–onset diabetes is manifest by severe abdominal pain).

    q. Intestinal parasites.

NEUROSURGICAL EMERGENCIES

Neurosurgical emergencies represent clinical conditions in which rapid evaluation and appropriate intervention may decrease morbidity and mortality. Early assessment of altered consciousness and prompt initial management will ensure the best possible outcome, particularly in the head trauma patient. This chapter provides the basic principles necessary for the early care of the patient with an acute neurosurgical problem.

I. **APPROACH TO THE UNCONSCIOUS PATIENT**
A. Unconsciousness requires either bilateral cerebral dysfunction or depression of reticular activating system (RAS) function.
B. **Etiology.**
   1. Supratentorial mass causing compression of diencephalon or brainstem. Initial focal change with rostral to caudal deterioration due to uncal herniation. Neurologic signs may aid in anatomically localizing etiology, i.e., motor exam asymmetry.
   2. Infratentorial — unconsciousness by a direct effect on RAS. Initial brainstem signs or sudden onset of coma, often oculovestibular abnormalities, such as gaze palsies. Cranial nerve palsies are often present. Abnormal respiratory patterns may be seen, often with vomiting.
   3. Metabolic and diffuse — confusion and stupor precede coma; motor signs are absent or symmetric; pupillary reflexes are intact. Often accompanied by acid/base disturbances. Seizures are common, often with asterixis, tremor and myoclonus.
   4. Psychiatric causes — objective findings are **absent**. Active lid closing, normal pupillary response, physiologic reflexes; normal motor tone, normal EEG.
C. **History** — important features include an abrupt *vs.* gradual onset, presence of a lucid interval, and recent neurologic complaints. A medication history is essential, especially psychotropics, sedatives, and opiates.
D. **Physical examination.**
   1. General — vital signs, respiratory pattern, evidence of trauma or IV drug abuse.
   2. **Level of consciousness.**
      a. Awake and alert — responsive to verbal stimuli.
      b. Lethargic — sleeps, but arousable to full waking state.
      c. Obtunded — sleeps unless continually stimulated, but can be fully aroused.
      d. Stupor — responds to physical stimuli, but cannot be aroused to full waking.
      e. Coma — unarousable.
   3. **Glasgow Coma Scale (GCS)** — range of 3–15:

Eye Opening	Verbal	Motor	Points
–	–	Obeys	6
–	Oriented	Localizes	5
Spontaneous	Confused	Withdraws	4
To speech	Inappropriate	Decorticate	3
To pain	Incomprehensible	Decerebrate	2
None	None	None	1

4. Evaluation of central reflexes and responses.
   a. Pupillary responses (CN II, III).
   b. Corneal reflexes (CN V, VII).
   c. Extraocular movements; conjugate or dysconjugate gaze (CN III, IV, VI).
   d. Oculocephalic reflex (doll's eyes) — only if C–spine clear (CN VIII).
   e. Oculovestibular reflex — tested with iced water lavage into ears; normal response is tonic deviation of eyes toward stimulus with rapid component nystagmus away (CN VIII).
   f. Gag response (CN IV, X).
   g. Response to central stimulation (pain) using sternal or supra-orbital pressure — use if not following commands.
5. Motor system — tone, strength.
6. Sensory system — pin prick, light touch.
7. Evaluation of superficial reflexes, deep tendon reflexes (DTR's), presence or absence of pathologic reflexes and sphincter tone.

E. **Initial management of coma.**
   1. Airway/breathing — O_2.
   2. Circulation — brain injury rostral to low brainstem is rarely a primary cause of systemic hypotension.
   3. Laboratory — CBC, renal profile, Ca^{++}, Mg^{++}, osmolarity, toxicology screen; type and crossmatch; hold bloods for LFT's, coags, endocrine, cultures, alcohol level.
   4. Glucose — 25 grams (50 ml of 50% dextrose) IV push (often administered by EMT's in the field).
   5. Decrease intra-cranial pressure (ICP).
      a. Elevate head of bed and maintain head in neutral position if general condition allows.
      b. Hyperventilate to $PaCO_2$ 25–30 torr in adults, 20–25 torr in children.
      c. Consider mannitol 1 gm/kg IV bolus.
      d. Consider steroids — useful for cerebral edema due to CNS tumors, metastatic tumors, +/– in sub- and epidural hematomas; equivocal response with contusions, lacerations, intra-cerebral hemorrhage, infarction and anoxic insults.
   6. Control seizures.
      a. Lorazepam 1.5 mg or valium 5–10 mg IV push first; simultaneous use of longer acting anticonvulsant (Phenytoin).
      b. See management of status epilepticus.
   7. Pan–culture if febrile.

      a. Consider lumbar puncture (see Table 1).
      b. Consider treatment of infections.
  8. Normalize pH.
  9. Normalize temperature.
10. Administer thiamine 100 mg IV push.
11. Antidotes — i.e., nalaxone.
12. Protect eyes.
13. Sedation as needed for agitation.

TABLE 1

CSF Findings in Various Pathologic Conditions (Adult Values)

Condition	Opening Pressure (cm H_2O)	Appearance	Cells (per mm^3)	Protein (mg%)	Glucose (% serum)	Miscellaneous
Normal	7-18	Clear, colorless	0 PMN, 0 RBC, 0 mono	15-45	50	
Acute purulent meningitis	Frequently increased	Turbid	Few-20 K (WBC's mostly PMN's)	100-1000	< 20	Few cells early or if treated
Viral meningitis and encephalitis	Normal	Normal	Few-350 (WBC's mostly monos)	40-100	Normal	PMN's early
Guillain-Barr	Normal	Normal	Normal	50-1000	Normal	Protein ↑, frequently IgG
Polio	Normal	Normal	50-250 (monos)	40-100	Normal	
TB meningitis	Frequently increased	Opal, yellow, fibrin clot	50-500 (monos)	60-700	< 20	PMN early, (+) AFB culture, (+) Ziel-Neelson stain
Fungal meningitis	Frequently increased	Opal-escent	30-300 (monos)	100-700	< 30	(+) India ink for cryptococcus
Traumatic (bloody) tap	Normal	Bloody, super-natant colorless	RBC:WBC as in peripheral;	Slight ↑	Normal	Blood ↓ in succeeding tubes, xanthochromia takes hours
Sub-arachnoid hemorrhage	Increased	Bloody Super-natant xantho-chromic	Early ↑ RBC's Late ↑ WBC's	50-400 100-800	Normal	RBC's disappear in 2 weeks, xanthochromia may persist for weeks
Multiple sclerosis	Normal	Normal	5-50 (monos)	Normal-800	Normal	Usually ↑ gamma globulins (oligoclonal)

II. HEAD TRAUMA (Figure 1)

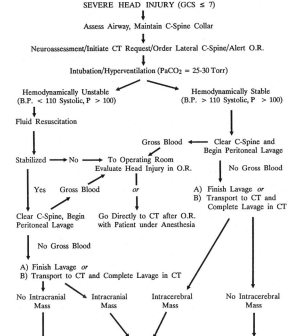

FIGURE 1
Severe Head Injury Protocol

A. **General categories of head trauma.**
  1. **Mild** — GCS = 15; often asymptomatic, may have headache, dizziness, with or without scalp lacerations or contusions. Requires short–term observation for neurologic change.
  2. **Moderate** — GCS 9–14; altered level of consciousness; amnestic of event; basilar skull fracture; severe facial injuries; multiple traumatic injuries. Consider obtaining head CT scan, especially if patient is going to the O.R. for other reasons.
  3. **High–risk** — GCS ≤ 7; depressed level of consciousness; focal neurologic deficit; depressed skull fracture; penetrating head injury; 50–60% will have multisystem trauma, 5% spinal injury.
B. **Indications for mannitol therapy in the E.R.**
  1. Clinical evidence of mass effect or herniation.
  2. Sudden neurological deterioration prior to CT scan.
  3. After CT if:
     a. A lesion associated with increased ICP is found.
     b. Neurosurgical lesion on CT requiring O.R. intervention.
  4. Mannitol is contraindicated if hypotension is present.
C. **Indications for burr holes in the E.R.**
  1. A patient dying from brain compression who has had witnessed transtentorial herniation en route to, or in the ER.
  2. Should be performed by the most qualified available physician.
D. **Increased intracranial pressure (ICP).**
  1. Clinical manifestations.
     a. Classical signs of headache, oculomotor palsies, Cushing's triad (hypertension, bradycardia, respiratory irregularities), papilledema are often not seen in trauma patients.
     b. Suspect elevated ICP if there is a deterioration in neurologic exam, drop in GCS or progression of focal neurologic deficits.
     c. Upper limits of normal = 10–15 cm H_2O; treatment is indicated if ICP ≥ 16 cm H_2O for 10 minutes; sustained ICP at 25–30 cm H_2O increases mortality.
  2. Indications for ICP monitoring (intraventricular catheter or subarachnoid bolt).
     a. GCS ≤ 7 if not improved after 6 hours of empiric therapy.
     b. Multisystem trauma where other therapies may have an adverse effect on ICP or on ability to follow neurologic examination (e.g., paralytics, heavy sedation).
     c. Relative contraindication in coagulopathies — if absolutely needed, use sub-arachnoid bolt (not intraventricular catheter) after correction of coagulation profile with FFP, vitamin K or platelets.
  3. Management of elevated ICP.
     a. Postural — elevate head of bed 30–45°, maintain neck in neutral position to facilitate venous return and avoid kinking of the jugular veins.

b. Hyperventilation — hyperventilate to $PaCO_2$ of 25–30 torr; works by arteriolar constriction to rapidly lower ICP. Duration of effectiveness is controversial, probably not effective after 48–72 hours. However, a rapid rise in $PaCO_2$ even after that time will elevate ICP, so hyperventilation should be slowly weaned.

c. Dehydration.
   1) Mannitol — use lowest possible effective dose, usually 0.25 g/kg IVPB q 6 h or 25 g IVPB q 6 h; in emergent situations may bolus with up to 1 g/kg.
   2) Lasix — 20–40 mg IVP q 6 h on alternating schedule with mannitol; an effective adjunct to mannitol therapy.
   3) Follow renal profile and measured serum osmolarity q6h and hold diuretics for serum osmolarity ≥ 310.

d. Hypertension control.

e. Control agitation — sedation as needed; boluses of short acting agents preferred (fentanyl 50 μg IVP q 30–60 min or nembutal 2–5 mg/kg IVP q 4 h).

f. IV fluids — goal is euvolemia or mild fluid restriction. Preferably use isotonic fluids. In multisystem trauma, other injuries may dictate fluid management. In severe head injuries, vasopressors are often preferable to fluid boluses for mild hypotension during dehydration therapy.

g. Steroids — controversial, presently not used at our institution in cases of traumatic closed head injury. (When used, and even when not, head injured patients require aggressive stress ulcer prophylaxis with antacids and H_2 blockers.)

h. CSF drainage — via intraventricular catheter.

i. Pentobarbital coma — patients with good neurologic function who deteriorate secondary to increased ICP may be candidates for this.

j. Surgical techniques — used in the most extreme cases; involves resection of "silent" areas of the brain (right anterior temporal, right frontal), areas of contusion, or decompressive removal of skull and dura.

III. SPINE AND SPINAL CORD INJURIES

A. **General considerations** — These injuries are usually due to severe cervical spine fractures and dislocations. They may or may not be associated with paralysis. More than half of patients with spinal injuries have a normal motor, sensory and reflex exam. Any patient sustaining injury above the clavicle or a head injury resulting in an unconscious state should be suspected of having an associated cervical spinal column injury.

B. **Assessment.**
   1. General assessment.

    a. Examination must be carried out with patient in neutral position on back–board and with C–spine immobilized.

    b. Other associated injuries must be ruled out.

    c. Paralyzed patient can often identify pain at the injury site.

2. Cervical vertebral assessment.

    a. Pain, tenderness, posterior "step–off" deformity.

    b. Pain radiation, prominence of spinous process, local tenderness.

3. Neurological assessment.

    a. Complete *vs.* incomplete spinal cord lesions.

        1) Pin–prick and deep pain discrimination indicates an incomplete lesion.

        2) Light touch is often the last sensory modality preserved.

        3) Assess for sacral sparing in anal, perianal and scrotal areas.

    b. Sensory/motor function.

        1) Determine the level of injury by assessing sensorimotor function level.

        2) See motor chart (Table 2) and sensory dermatomal diagram (Fig. 2).

        3) Injuries at C4 or higher will have impairment of ventilation.

TABLE 2
Motor Level Assessment

Segment	Muscle	Action to Test	Reflex
C1-3	Neck muscles		
C4	Diaphragm, trapezius	Inspiration	
C5	Deltoid		
C5-6	Biceps	Elbow flex	Biceps
C6	Extensor carpi radialis	Wrist extension	Supinator
C7	Triceps, extensor digitorum	Elbow extension	Triceps
C8	Flexor digitorum	Hand grasp	
T1	Hand intrinsics		
T2-T12	Intercostals		
T7-L1	Abdominals		Abdominal cutaneous
L2	Iliopsoas, adductors	Hip adduction	
L3-4	Quadriceps	Knee extension	Quadriceps
L4-5	Medial hamstrings, tibialis anterior	Ankle dorsiflex	Medial hamstrings
L5	Lateral hams, posterior tibialis, peroneals	Knee flexion	
L5-S1	Extensor digitorum, EHL	Great toe extension	
S1-2	Gastrocnemius, soleus	Ankle plantarflex	Ankle jerk
S2	Flexor digitorum, flexor hallucis		
S2-4	Bladder, lower bowel		Anal wink and bulbocavernosus

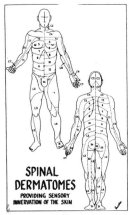

FIGURE 2

Ref: *The Harriet Lane Handbook*, 10th Ed. (C.H. Cole, ed.). Chicago: Year Book Medical Publishers, 1984, p. 365. Reproduced by permission.

4. Spinal shock — may occur immediately after spinal cord injury.
   a. Hemodynamics — unchanged pulse, decreased blood pressure to systolic about 80 mmHg (due to blood pooling in dilated vessels).
   b. Neurological findings — flaccid paralysis, flaccid sphincters, absent pathological and normal reflexes.
   c. Treatment — shock usually responds to crystalloid resuscitation; vasopressors (neosynephrine) occasionally needed.
5. X-rays.
   a. Cervical spine.
      1) Lateral C–spine — all 7 cervical vertebrae and C7–T1 interface must be seen; best obtained while pulling down on shoulders; swimmer's view often necessary.
      2) AP cervical and odontoid views — completes series to fully clear C–spine; should only be obtained once patient has been stabilized.
      3) Tomograms, lateral flexion and extension, CT and MRI — often needed to complete workup of specific injuries.
   b. Thoracolumbar.
      1) AP and lateral views.
      2) Must be cleared prior to removing back–board.

C. Treatment — neurosurgical consultation is *mandatory*.
1. Immobilization.
   a. Semi–rigid cervical (Philadelphia) collar and spine board — standard for pre–hospital care and during ER evaluation.
   b. Cervical fractures/dislocations require definitive stabilization with cervical traction (halo or tongs) and/or internal fixation.
   c. Thoracolumbar injuries may require corset or spica cast and internal fixation.
2. IV fluids — limit to maintenance fluids unless more are needed for shock management.
3. Medications — steroids (controversial).
4. Airway — intubation or tracheostomy often required for high C–spine injuries.
5. Effective nursing care (skin care, bowel and bladder programs).

IV. NEUROSURGICAL EMERGENCIES
A. Epidural hematoma.
1. Seen in about 1% of head trauma patients.
2. Classic presentation is brief loss of consciousness followed by lucid interval, then progressive obtundation, ipsilateral pupillary dilatation and contralateral hemiparesis (seen in 60%). Other presentations include headache, nausea, vomiting, seizure, unilateral hyperreflexia and positive Babinski sign.
3. Usually arterial etiology (85%), often in area of a temporal/parietal skull fracture.
4. On CT, one usually sees a biconvex mass with high attenuation.
5. Optimally treated epidural hematoma has a 5–10% mortality.

B. Subdural hematoma.
1. Twice as common as epidural hematomas.
2. Source of bleeding is usually venous; two types are described:
   a. Tear of bridging vessels from acceleration/deceleration; often presenting with a lucid interval followed by later deterioration secondary to mass effect.
   b. Subdural hematoma associated with parenchymal laceration; usually presents with coma, localizing signs and severe, underlying brain injury.
3. On CT scan a cresent–shaped mass is seen, usually over the convexities and with high attenuation (but less dense than epidural hematoma due to dilution of blood in CSF).
4. Classified as hyperdense from 0–48 hours, subacute at 1–3 weeks, and chronic at 3 weeks to 4 months.
5. If evacuated in O.R. in less than 4 hours — 30% mortality; if > 4 hours elapses — 90% mortality. Also, much worse outcome if postoperative ICP > 20.

C. Status epilepticus.

1. Defined as recurrent seizures occurring too frequently for consciousness to be regained between events.
2. Management involves control of seizures as follows.
   a. Valium 10 mg IVP (at IVP rate of < 2 mg/min) q 20 min x 3 if needed, or Ativan 1.5 mg IVP over 2 min q 3 min x 3 if needed.
   b. Simultaneous Dilantin loading.
      1) If patient not on Dilantin — load with 18 mg/kg (1200 mg/70 kg) at a rate not exceeding 50 mg/min.
      2) If on Dilantin — bolus with 500 mg at ≤ 50 mg/min.
   c. If seizure activity persists:
      1) Dilantin 8 mg/kg at < 50 mg/min.
      2) Then:
         a) Phenobarbital infusion at < 100 mg/min, up to 20 mg/kg (1400 mg/70 kg) *or* (but not both):
         b) Valium infusion of 100 mg in 500 ml D5W at 40 ml/min.
   d. If still seizing — notify anesthesiologist, then begin either:
      1) Paraldehyde 5 ml in 500 ml D5W at 50 cc/hr and titrate to stop seizures, *or*:
      2) Lidocaine 2–3 mg/kg IVP at 50 mg/min, then infusion at 1–2 mg/min.
D. **Brain death.**
   1. Criteria determined by Cincinnati Society of Neurologists and Neurosurgeons. These may vary in different locations.
      a. Absence of brainstem function.
         1) Pupillary light reflex absent.
         2) Corneal reflex absent.
         3) Oculocephalic reflex ("doll's eyes") absent.
         4) Oculovestibular reflex (cold–water calorics) absent.
            a) 60–100 cc ice water flushed into each ear with eyes held open.
            b) Intact response is nystagmus toward opposite ear.
         5) Oropharyngeal (gag) reflex absent.
      b. No response to central pain stimulation (supraorbital notch pressure).
      c. No spontaneous respirations for 3 min in normocarbic patient.
   2. Exceptions.
      a. Hypothermia must be ruled out as cause of coma.
      b. Remediable endogenous or exogenous intoxication must be ruled out, especially barbiturates, paralytics, benzodiazepines.
      c. Shock.
      d. Immediately post–resuscitation.
   3. Two examinations 6 hours apart meeting criteria of 1 and 2 confirm brain death.
   4. No laboratory diagnostic tests (including EEG) are necessary.

UROLOGIC PROBLEMS IN SURGICAL PRACTICE

I. UROLOGIC INFECTIONS
A. Cystitis.
1. Female cystitis is typically an ascending bacterial infection associated with sexual activity, pregnancy, and the post–partum period.
2. Male cystitis is usually associated with urologic pathology such as obstruction (BPH, cancer, stricture), urine stasis (neurogenic bladder), foreign body (calculus, indwelling catheter) and inadequate treatment of persistent urinary pathogens (chronic bacterial prostatitis).
3. Etiology – gram–negative organisms predominate (*E. coli, Proteus, Enterobacter, Klebsiella, Pseudomonas*); occasionally *Streptococcus faecalis* and *Staphylococcus* species are cultured.
4. Clinical presentation – dysuria, frequency, urgency, incontinence, hematuria, supra–pubic pain.
5. Laboratory findings – a catheterized urine specimen from the female and a clean–catch midstream voided specimen from the male are equivalent. Urinalysis shows 5–10 WBC's per high power field, often with hematuria and bacteruria. Urine culture typically grows greater than 100,000 CFU/ml.
6. Treatment – in males investigation into and correction of the underlying disorder is essential. Treatment consists of empirical use of broad–spectrum oral antibiotics with gram–negative organism coverage.
   a. Nitrofurantoin macrocrystals 50 mg PO QID for 7–10 days.
   b. Cephalexin 500 mg PO QID for 7–10 days.
   c. Trimethaprim 160 mg/sulfamethoxazole 800 mg PO BID for 7–10 days.
7. If symptoms and cultures clear on antibiotics in females, no further work–up is necessary. Males require further urologic evaluation.
8. Patients with chronic indwelling Foley catheters or those on intermittent self–catheterization have urine colonized with bacteria. If these patients are asymptomatic, treatment is not necessary and only rarely successful in clearing the bacteria. Adequate hydration and good bladder emptying are essential in preventing the progression of colonization to infection.

B. Acute bacterial prostatitis.
1. Clinical findings – typically an acute febrile illness, urgency, frequency, dysuria, chills, low back pain, perineal or rectal pain. Rectal examination reveals an exquisitely tender soft prostate.

Vigorous rectal exam or massage should be *avoided* due to the risk of causing bacteremia.

2. Laboratory findings — leukocytosis with differential left shift. UA shows pyuria, microscopic hematuria, and bacteriuria.
3. Urethral instrumentation should be avoided.
4. Complications — acute urinary retention, prostatic abscess, pyelonephritis, epididymo–orchitis, or septic shock.
5. Treatment — broad–spectrum antibiotics against gram–negative bacilli. In the stable patient, oral antibiotics can be utilized (trimethaprim/sulfamethoxazole attain adequate prostate tissue levels as well as the newer quinolones — ciprofloxacin, norfloxacin). In the unstable patient showing signs of sepsis, combination therapy including an aminoglycoside and ampicillin is indicated.

C. **Acute epididymo–orchitis.**
   1. Etiology — two major groups.
      a. Sexually transmitted organisms — associated with younger men; usually *Chlamydia trachomatis* and *Neisseria gonorrhea.*
      b. Infection associated with concomitant urinary tract infections (UTI) or prostatitis. Associated with urinary tract obstruction in older men. Usually *E. coli*, *Proteus*, *Klebsiella*, *Enterobacter*, *Pseudomonas.*
   2. Clinical findings — symptoms may follow an acute lifting or straining type activity. Typically a painful, swollen, tender epididymis and testicle is found. Overlying scrotal skin may be red, swollen, and warm. A tense reactive hydrocoele may be present which makes testicular palpation difficult. The spermatic cord is often thickened.
   3. Laboratory findings — leukocytosis with left shift often present. UA shows pyuria and bacteriuria. UC may grow gram–negative bacilli listed above. Special techniques are usually required for isolation of *Chlamydia* and *Neisseriae* (often unsuccessful).
   4. Treatment.
      a. Bedrest during the acute phase.
      b. Scrotal elevation — athletic supporter, ice pack to scrotum.
      c. Analgesia and antipyretics.
      d. Avoidance of sexual activity and physical activity.
      e. Antibiotics.
         1) Sexually transmitted organisms — doxycycline 100 mg PO BID for 21 days or tetracycline 500 mg PO QID for 21 days. Both patient and partner should be treated. Use of condom protection in sexual activity is encouraged.
         2) Non–sexually transmitted organisms — antibiotics are determined by UC and sensitivity results. Usually those listed for prostatitis are appropriate empirically.

D. Acute pyelonephritis.
1. An acute bacterial inflammation of the renal parenchyma initiated by ascending bacteria (reflux), hematogenous and lymphatogenous routes of infection.
2. Organisms — *E. coli, Proteus, Enterobacter, Klebsiella.*
3. Clinical findings — fever, chills, severe costovertebral angle pain and tenderness, frequency, urgency, dysuria, nausea and vomiting.
4. Laboratory findings — significant leukocytosis with left shift. UA is significant for pyuria, bacteriuria, occasional hematuria, and occasional leukocyte or granular casts. UC typically positive for greater than 100,000 CFU/ml.
5. Differential diagnosis — includes pancreatitis, basal pneumonia, appendicitis, cholecystitis, diverticulitis, pelvic inflammatory disease, and renal or perirenal abscess.
6. Treatment — minimally symptomatic patients who are tolerating their diet can be treated expectantly with oral broad-spectrum antibiotics against gram-negative bacilli. In the severely ill patient, prompt treatment is essential to prevent sepsis, renal scarring, and loss of renal function. Initial empiric treatment should consist of an aminoglycoside and ampicillin. Antibiotics should be guided by UC results. Parenteral therapy is continued until patient is afebrile for 24 hours. Conversion to appropriate oral antibiotics can then be initiated.

II. UROLOGIC EMERGENCIES
A. Trauma.
   1. Renal trauma.
   a. Etiology.
      1) Blunt renal trauma — usually MVA's. Accounts for 70–90% of renal trauma; 80% will have injuries to other organ systems. Any patient sustaining injury to the flank, abdomen, or lower chest should be suspected of having renal trauma.
      2) Penetrating renal trauma — usually knife or gun-shot wounds; 80% will involve other organ systems.
   b. Classification.
      1) Minor injuries — 85% of cases.
         a) Renal contusion — contusion of renal parenchyma.
         b) Cortical laceration — superficial laceration of parenchyma not associated with collecting system.
      2) Major injuries — 10–15% of cases.
         a) Deep laceration — renal parenchymal laceration extending into collecting system. Includes renal rupture where multiple lacerations separate portions of parenchyma.
         b) Renal pedicle injury — involves renal veins and/or artery.

c. Diagnosis.
   1) Intravenous pyelography yields definitive diagnosis in 90% of renal injuries. Failure to visualize a kidney suggests a pedicle injury. Prompt function without extravasation of contrast material suggests a minor injury such as renal contusion or cortical laceration. Extravasation of contrast indicates a laceration involving the collecting system.
   2) Computed tomography – can show all of the above plus evidence of retroperitoneal hematoma, and define the vascular perfusion.
   3) Angiography – essential when renal pedicle injury is suspected.
d. Treatment.
   1) Penetrating renal trauma almost always requires immediate exploration.
   2) Blunt renal trauma.
      a) 85% of cases can be managed non–surgically, i.e., renal contusion, cortical laceration, and some deep lacerations.
      b) Renal pedicle injuries always require exploration and repair or nephrectomy.
      c) Intermediate injuries may involve surgical or non–surgical treatment dependent on the patient's overall condition and severity of injury.

2. **Ureteral trauma.**
   a. Ureters are rarely injured due to external violence. Most injuries are iatrogenic from pelvic surgery with transection or ligation of the ureter.
   b. Treatment is dependent upon the injury. Excretory urograms, retrograde pyelograms, and CT scans often define the injury.
      1) Simple ureteral ligation – prompt recognition may be treated by release of ligature. Late recognition may require partial ureterectomy and ureteral re–implantation into the bladder. Prevention is the best treatment.
      2) Simple surgical transection – requires immediate uretero–ureterostomy and stent placement.
      3) Gun–shot wounds – require exploration and wide debridement of injured segment. An ureteroureterostomy or transureteroureterostomy may be required dependent on severity of injury.

3. **Bladder trauma.**
   a. Etiology – external blunt trauma (blow to lower abdomen), pelvic fracture, penetrating injury, iatrogenic (gynecologic or pelvic surgery).
   b. Presentation – bony pelvis generally protects the bladder from external violence. Nevertheless, 15% of patients with

pelvic fracture will have a bladder or urethral injury. Bladder rupture may present as an acute abdomen with extravasation of urine into the peritoneal cavity (intraperitoneal rupture). Alternatively, bony spicules from a fractured pelvis may penetrate the bladder with pelvic extravasation of urine (extraperitoneal rupture).

c. Diagnostic evaluation.
   1) History of lower abdominal trauma (steering–wheel blow in MVA) or pelvic fracture.
   2) Patients may be unable to urinate or may have lower abdominal pain, gross hematuria or pelvic hematoma.
   3) X-ray examination.
      a) Abdominal/pelvic plain film — examine for pelvic fractures, soft tissue masses, deviated bowel gas pattern suggesting pelvic hematoma or urinoma.
      b) Excretory urogram — documents function of kidneys and may show bladder extravasation, but is often inadequate.
      c) Cystogram — urethral injury in males must be **ruled out** by **retrograde urethrogram** (see "Urethral Trauma" below) prior to inserting urethral catheter. Cystography is performed after catheterization of the bladder. Fill the bladder with 50–75 cc of contrast material and examine x-ray film for gross extravasation. If no extravasation is seen, follow with an additional 200–300 cc contrast. Repeat x-ray, again examine for extravasation, bone spicules, etc. Finally, completely drain bladder and repeat pelvic x-ray. Final film is essential for identifying subtle extravasation and rupture. Helpful to obtain AP as well as oblique films when evaluating pelvis and bladder. Cystogram should *always* precede excretory urogram.

d. Treatment.
   1) Penetrating injuries — usually require prompt exploration, debridement and repair. Most patients with penetrating injuries are at high risk for concomitant rectal injury.
   2) Blunt injuries.
      a) Extraperitoneal bladder ruptures with sterile urine and no intra–abdominal injuries can be managed with catheter drainage. If free bony spicules are seen on work–up, the injury will require exploration and removal of the penetrating foreign bodies.
      b) Intraperitoneal bladder ruptures require immediate exploration, repair and drainage.

4. **Urethral trauma.**

a. Anatomy — the urethra in the male is divided into anterior and posterior divisions. The anterior urethra consists of the urethra distal to the urogenital diaphragm. The posterior urethra extends from the inferior edge of the urogenital diaphragm to the proximal bladder neck. Anterior injuries are often associated with straddle–type trauma to the perineum or urethral instrumentation. Posterior urethral injuries most often occur with pelvic fractures. Female urethral injuries are unusual.

b. Anterior urethral injuries may extravasate blood along fascial planes. An injury to the urethra limited by Buck's fascia (i.e., urethral instrumentation injury) will result in blood extravasation along the penis. An injury through Buck's fascia will demonstrate extravasation of blood along the fascial planes of the abdomen (Scarpa's fascia) and scrotum, penis, and perineum (Colle's fascia).

c. Posterior urethral injuries almost always occur with pelvic fractures, and are usually associated with pelvic hematoma. Blood at the urethral meatus, inability to void, and high-riding prostate gland on rectal exam is highly suggestive of a posterior injury.

d. Diagnostic procedures — **all suspected urethral injuries in males must be evaluated by a retrograde urethrogram prior to insertion of a bladder catheter.** Urethral catheterization can easily convert a partial tear into a complete urethral transection and must be avoided. Retrograde urethrogram is simply performed by injecting 10–15 cc of contrast material into the urethra with a syringe and taking oblique pelvic x-ray films. If no extravasation is seen with complete filling of the urethra into the bladder, a catheter can be passed gently. If any obstruction or difficulty in passing the catheter is encountered, the procedure should be terminated, and immediate urology consult obtained.

e. Treatment.
   1) Minor anterior urethral lacerations can be managed with bladder catheter drainage alone. Penetrating injuries require exploration, debridement, and repair.
   2) More severe anterior urethral injuries, usually straddle–type injuries, may require exploration.
   3) Management of posterior urethral injuries is controversial. Two options exist: immediate exploration with primary urethral reanstomosis, or supra–pubic catheter placement for urinary diversion. In general, due to the severity of other life–threatening injuries with pelvic fracture, the conservative approach of supra–pubic urinary catheter diversion is preferred.

5. **Acute scrotum.**
   a. Etiology — the acute scrotum refers to the swollen, tender scrotum associated with a testicular, epididymal or spermatic

    cord abnormality. Differential diagnosis includes testicular torsion, torsion of testicular appendages, acute epididymo–orchitis, or acute incarcerated inguinal hernia. Correct diagnosis and expeditious treatment is essential to prevent organ loss.

b. Testicular torsion is the spontaneous twisting of the testicular pedicle, causing acute testicular ischemia. Most commonly presents as an acute onset of testicular or unilateral scrotal pain, swelling and tenderness in the 10–18 year old age group. Pain is severe and UA is normal. Many patients complain of a similar event within the past year which spontaneously resolved. The testicle is usually elevated in the scrotum, and is exquisitely tender. If the diagnosis is in doubt, a radionuclide testicular scan can be obtained; however, delay in treatment may result in further organ damage. Surgical treatment consists of exploration, de-torsion, and suturing the testicle to the scrotal wall to prevent recurrence. The contralateral testicle is sutured in place as well to prevent torsion. Orchiectomy is performed if a non–viable testicle is found.

c. Acute epididymo–orchitis occurs in the sexually active pubertal male on up into the elderly male age groups. The onset of pain is gradual and may be accompanied by irritative voiding complaints. UA may show pyuria. Scrotal elevation may decrease the pain, and the opposite testis is normal. Treatment consists of symptomatic relief and appropriate antibiotics (see section I).

d. Torsion of testicular or epididymal appendages — vestigial remnants of the müllerian ductal system persist as small pedunculated appendages from the testis and epididymis. Occasionally, these appendages can spontaneously twist on their pedicles causing acute ischemia and a painful scrotum. Patients are usually pre-pubertal and voiding complaints are absent. UA is normal. Examination reveals an exquisitely tender, pea–sized mass near the head of the epididymis. The testicle is usually not tender. A "blue dot" sign is described on scrotal transillumination; however, it may be obscured by localized scrotal edema and redness. Treatment is conservative: bedrest, ice packs, and analgesics. If the diagnosis is in doubt, surgical exploration may be necessary to rule out testicular torsion, and excise the appendage.

e. Incarcerated inguinal hernia — usually only confused with testicular torsion in young male patients. May be acute onset, severe pain with scrotal swelling and hyperemia. Nausea and vomiting may be present. UA is normal. Often the hernia can be manually reduced with immediate resolution of symptoms; however, surgical exploration and repair may be required.

III. URINARY RETENTION

A. **Etiology** — bladder emptying requires a coordinated bladder contraction in the absence of bladder outlet obstruction.

   1. Factors which inhibit a coordinated bladder contraction:

      a. Neurogenic dysfunction — results from a neurologic process that gives a hyporeflexic ("flaccid") neurogenic bladder such as injury to the sacral spinal cord, cauda equina, or the pelvic nerves. Also present during the initial stages of any level of spinal cord injury (spinal shock).

      b. Decompensated bladder — overdistention of the bladder can overstretch the detrusor muscle and inhibit its ability to contract.

   2. Factors which cause bladder outlet obstruction:

      a. Male — BPH, prostate cancer, urethral stricture, bladder neck contracture, bladder calculi.

      b. Female (very uncommon causes of urinary retention) — urethral stenosis, urethral trauma, urethral diverticulum, cystourethroceles.

B. **Presentation and diagnosis.**

   1. Acute symptoms — urgency and supra–pubic pain.

   2. Chronic symptoms — progressive obstructive voiding symptoms leading eventually to anuria or **overflow incontinence**.

   3. Asymptomatic and present with an abdominal mass, renal insufficiency, or bilateral hydronephrosis.

   4. Diagnosis usually confirmed by placement of a foley catheter with return of a large quantity of urine.

C. **Treatment.**

   1. Attempt is made to pass an 18 Fr foley catheter.

      a. Common causes for inability to pass a foley catheter:

         1) Inadequate lubrication (lubrication can be injected up the urethra with a small syringe).

         2) Young male patient who overtightens external sphincter (will fatigue after about 30 sec).

         3) Urethral strictures (scar tissue occluding urethral lumen).

         4) Enlarged median lobe of the prostate or defect from a previous TURP (transurethral resection of the prostate) can create an acute angulation in the prostatic urethra. A **coude' catheter** may be successful because of its angulated tip.

      b. If initial attempts at passing an 18 Fr foley or coude' tip catheter are unsuccessful, a urologist should be consulted. Use of filiforms and followers, percutaneous cystotomy, or formal cystoscopy may be required.

2. Definitive treatment of urinary retention varies with the causative factors:
   a. BPH — usually managed with TURP or open prostatectomy (removal of only the inner adenoma of the prostate through a surgical incision).
   b. Prostate cancer — prostate cancer which has progressed to urinary obstruction often has metastasized to bone or lymph nodes; is therefore usually treated hormonally (orchiectomy, DES, LHRH agonist). Prostate cancer can also cause urinary retention by spinal cord compression from vertebral metastasis (neurogenic hyporeflexic bladder).
   c. Bladder neck contracture — caused by scarring at the bladder neck, usually following TURP. Managed by transurethral incision of the bladder neck.
   d. Urethral stricture — managed by transuretheral incision or urethroplasty.
   e. Hyporeflexic neurogenic bladder — usually managed with ISC (intermittent straight catheterization).
   f. Decompensated bladder — also managed by ISC.
3. Post–obstructive diuresis — following relief of urinary retention there may be a significant diuresis.
   a. Post-obstructive diuresis is primarily due to excess water and solute retained during period of urinary retention (physiologic diuresis).
   b. Rarely a diuresis will occur due to a tubular defect with loss of the kidney's ability to concentrate urine. A hypovolemic state can result from this pathologic diuresis. The patient's vital signs should be closely monitored for orthostatic changes in the event IV fluid replacement is needed (D5$\frac{1}{2}$ NS).

IV. UROLITHIASIS

A. Etiology.

1. **Calcium oxalate** or mixed calcium oxalate/calcium phosphate stones.
   a. Account for 70% of urolithiasis.
   b. Usually they are "idiopathic" and due to either excessive absorption (in GI tract) or excretion (by kidney) of calcium, causing hypercalcuria.
   c. Approximately 5% have hyperparathyroidism with hypercalcemia.
   d. Less than 1% of calcium stones are caused by other metabolic diseases such as Type 1 renal tubular acidosis (distal RTA) or primary hyperoxaluria.
   e. Calcium stones are radiopaque.

2. **Struvite** or infection stones.
    a. Contain magnesium ammonium phosphate.
    b. Account for 15% of urolithiasis.
    c. Must be infected with urease–producing bacteria (usually *Proteus* but also *Klebsiella*, *Pseudomonas*, and *Staphylococcus*) which produces an alkaline urine.
    d. Struvite stones are less radiopaque than calcium–containing stones.
3. **Uric acid stones.**
    a. Account for about 8% of stones.
    b. May be associated with hyperuricemia or gout, or may result from the hyperuricuria during the acute stages of chemotherapy for myeloproliferative diseases.
    c. Most are idiopathic and associated with normal serum and urine uric acid levels.
    d. Often the urine pH is persistently low, which will precipitate uric acid stones.
    e. Uric acid stones are radiolucent.
4. **Cystine stones.**
    a. Accounts for less than 3% of stones.
    b. Result from an inherited defect of the renal tubule causing loss of cystine, ornithine, arginine and lysine in the urine.
    c. UA will show characteristic hexagonal–shaped microscopic crystals.
    d. Cystine stones are faintly radiopaque.
B. **Presentation.**
1. Stones may be asymptomatic or may cause symptoms from obstruction at the ureteropelvic junction, at the neck of a calyx, or along the course of the ureter.
2. Renal colic is caused by distention of the urinary tract and is related to the rapidity of development, not to the degree of distention.
3. Pain may be referred to the flank, the abdomen, the testicle, or into the scrotum or labia.
4. Distal ureteral stones often cause irritative bladder symptoms of urinary urgency and frequency.
5. Many general surgical intra–abdominal emergencies can be confused with renal colic including appendicitis, small bowel obstruction, diverticulitis, ovarian torsion, and ectopic pregnancy.
6. Bladder stones cause irritative symptoms of urgency, frequency and dysuria, and occasionally bladder outlet obstruction. Usually caused by bladder outlet obstruction with urinary stasis.
7. Occasionally obstructing calculi are associated with infected urine causing pyohydronephrosis. Can produce life–threatening sepsis and is a **surgical emergency.**

C. **Diagnosis.**
1. UA shows microscopic hematuria usually, and occasionally py-uria. Struvite stones are associated with alkaline urine and uric acid stones are associated with acidic urine.
2. IVP (intravenous pyelogram) — best method to diagnose uro-lithiasis and should demonstrate the size and location of the stone as well as the degree of obstruction.
3. Retrograde pyelograms (done through cystoscope) — sometimes necessary in patients who cannot tolerate an IVP (patients with renal insufficency or allergy to contrast).
4. Serum calcium, uric acid, and phosphorous levels should be obtained. BUN and creatinine are important to evaluate renal function.
5. Strain urine to obtain any passed calculi for stone analysis.

D. **Treatment.**
1. Usually patients with small, uncomplicated ureteral or renal calculi can be managed with oral analgesics and followed as outpatients.
2. Patients with an obstructing calculus associated with a solitary kidney, persistent vomiting, fever, suspected UTI, or pain un-controlled with oral analgesics should be admitted.
3. Patients with pyohydronephrosis (obstructing calculus with UTI) who are septic should have emergent placement of a ureteral stent by cystoscopy or placement of percutaneous nephrostomy.
4. Current urologic management of ureteral stones usually involves transurethral endoscopic manipulation, either fragmenting and extracting the stone, or pushing it up into the kidney for ESWL (extracorporeal shock–wave lithotripsy).
5. Most renal stones are now managed with ESWL, using shock waves to fragment the stone. Larger renal calculi are sometimes managed with percutaneous nephroscopy (endoscopic manipula-tion through a percutaneous flank approach) or open surgical removal (pyelolithotomy, nephrolithotomy, partial nephrectomy or nephrectomy).
6. Bladder calculi are usually removed transurethrally with simul-taneous correction of the underlying bladder outlet obstruction.

Recommended References:

1. Gillenwater JY, Grayhack JT, Howards SS, Duckett JW. *Adult and Pediatric Urology* (Chicago: Year Book, 1987). General urology text with in–depth discussions of common urologic diseases.
2. Hauno PM, Wein AJ. *A Clinical Manual of Urology* (Norwalk, CT: Appleton-Century-Crofts, 1987). A condensed handbook of urology.
3. Smith DR. *General Urology* (Los Altos: Lange, 1981).

THE HAND

Hand injuries and infections should never be underestimated because a seemingly "minor" problem can result in prolonged recovery, loss of employment, and permanent disability. One must have thorough knowledge of the complex anatomy and biomechanics of the hand prior to treating any of its injuries or infections. One should also be able to recognize when the services of a hand specialist are required.

I. PERTINENT HISTORY
A. Age, past medical history, **tetanus** status, allergies, last meal.
B. Details of injury (cut, crush, bite, etc.), degree of **contamination**.
C. Hand **dominance**, condition of hand prior to injury or infection.
D. Time **elapsed** since onset of injury or infection.
E. Previous treatment.

II. HAND INJURIES
A. Introduction.
1. Aim of treatment is restoration of function and anatomical continuity.
2. Initial management may determine final outcome.
   a. **Beware** of nerve and tendon lacerations, fractures in open wounds, compartment syndromes and skeletal injuries in closed wounds.
   b. Refer complicated cases to a specialist.
3. Prevent infection.
   a. Irrigate all open wounds thoroughly.
   b. Give antibiotics and tetanus prophylaxis where indicated.
4. Dressings and splints should be comfortable, conforming and not circumferential.
5. **Elevate** every injured hand above the heart.
6. Major injuries involving tendons, nerves, arteries or massive contamination should be explored in the OR.
B. Vascular injuries.
1. Temporarily control bleeding with local pressure and elevation. Do not use a tourniquet around the base of a finger; if needed, apply blood pressure cuff to arm and inflate to 250 mm Hg.
2. Check radial and ulnar pulses. May perform Allen's test to assess collateral blood supply. Assess skin temperature and capillary refill.
3. **Never blindly clamp** bleeding vessels because further damage to the vessel and/or accompanying nerve may result.
4. Injuries with significant bleeding often require operative exploration.

C. Nerve injuries.
1. Sensory assessment.
   a. Assess each nerve by its distribution (Fig. 1).
   b. Use pinprick and 2–point discrimination along longitudinal axis (6 mm distinction at fingertip).
   c. **Never** administer anesthetic before completing sensory exam.

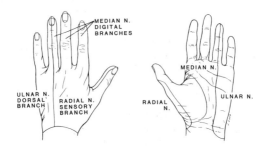

Figure 1
Sensory Areas of the Left Hand

2. Motor assessment.
   a. <u>Median</u> nerve.
      1) Assess innervated muscles (Fig. 2a).
      2) Thenar muscles (abductor pollicis brevis, flexor pollicis brevis, opponens pollicis) can be tested by *opposition* of thumb to ring or little finger (Fig. 2b).
   b. <u>Ulnar</u> nerve.
      1) Assess innervated muscles (Fig. 3a).
      2) Test flexion of ring and little finger, ability to cross index and long fingers or ability to spread fingers apart (finger abduction) (Fig. 3b).
   c. <u>Radial</u> nerve.
      1) Assess innervated muscles (Fig. 4).
      2) *No* intrinsic muscles of hand are innervated.
      3) Test wrist and MCP extension, also thumb abduction and extension.

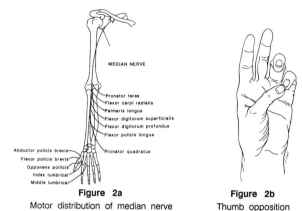

Figure 2a

Motor distribution of median nerve

Figure 2b

Thumb opposition

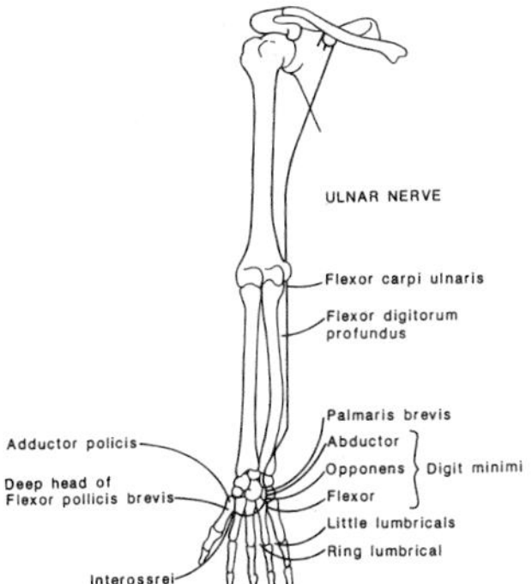

Figure 3a

Motor distribution of ulnar nerve

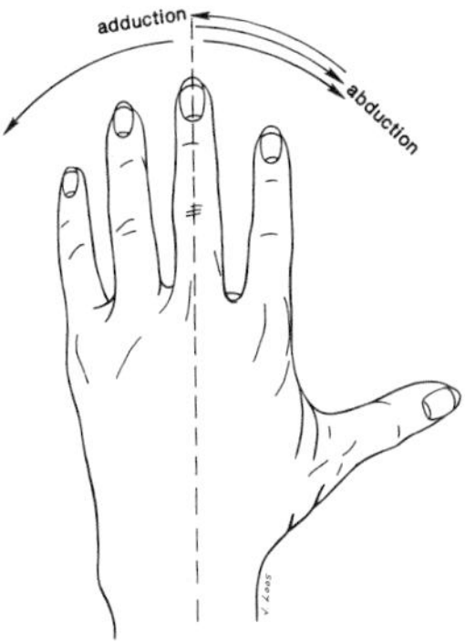

Figure 3b

Finger abduction

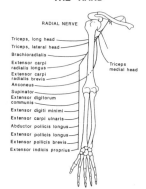

Figure 4

Motor distribution of radial nerve

D. Tendon injuries.
  1. Flexors.
     a. Flexor digitorum profundus (FDP) – stabilize proximal interphalangeal (PIP) joint and have patient flex distal joint (Fig. 5).
     b. Flexor digitorum superficialis – block FDP by placing all but finger being tested in extension and have patient flex individual finger at PIP joint (Fig. 6).

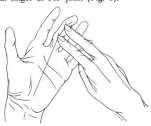

Figure 5

Examination of flexor digitorum profundus

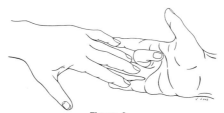

Figure 6

Examination of flexor digitorum superficialis

    c. Flexor tendon injuries in *"no man's land"* (between the distal palmar crease and the middle of the middle phalanyx) should only be repaired by hand specialist.

  2. Extensors.

    a. Extensor tendons can be tested by having patient extend each finger independently.

    b. Extensor proprius tendons can be tested by having the patient make a fist and extending index and little finger independently.

E. Bone and joint injuries.

  1. If there is *any* question about a foreign body, dislocation or fracture, obtain an x-ray.

  2. A fracture is highly suspected if **hematoma, deformity** or **persistent local tenderness** follows any closed injury.

  3. Obtain x-ray in **three planes** to avoid missing small fractures.

F. Soft tissue injuries — principles of wound management. In general, nonabsorbable monofilament sutures should be used for skin closure. Exception is in infants/children where chromic may be used to avoid suture removal. Absorbable sutures should be used for re-approximation of deeper tissues.

  1. Tidy wounds.

    a. Irrigate thoroughly with saline, remove any clots, close with fine sutures or steri-strips.

    b. Tetanus prophylaxis, splint, elevate.

  2. Untidy wounds.

    a. Excise devitalized tissue.

    b. Irrigate with saline, remove clots, leave wound open or close loosely with minimum number of sutures.

    c. May need formal repair in OR.

  3. Puncture wounds.

    a. Check for foreign body by x-ray and exploration (if indicated).

    b. Ellipse skin around wound to check for damage to deep structures.

    c. Leave open for drainage.

4. Flap wounds.

    a. If base of flap is proximal, it usually has good blood supply and will survive.

    b. If base of flap is distal, the tip is less likely to survive.

    c. A flap sutured under tension is likely to become ischemic.

    d. A long flap has a greater chance of survival if the subcutaneous fat is trimmed away and the skin then used as a full-thickness skin graft (FTSG).

5. Avulsed flap.

    a. May be sutured in place after defatting as a FTSG.

    b. Usually does better with a formal split-thickness skin graft (STSG).

    c. **Fingertip avulsion** (based on severity) may be managed by allowing wound to granulate and close, closing primarily, replacing avulsed tip as FTSG after defatting, V–Y advancement flap or more advanced finger flap techniques.

6. Skin defects.

    a. Most defects > 1 cm in diameter will need a STSG.

    b. Larger, complicated defects may require a flap graft.

7. Bite wounds.

    a. Human or animal bites are prone to severe infection despite appearing innocuous on initial presentation.

    b. Usually located on dorsal surface of phalanges (over MCP joints) when due to punching mouth with clenched fist.

    c. Require thorough wound excision and irrigation.

    d. Leave wound open with wet dressing, splint and elevate.

    e. For human bites, admit patient to hospital and provide systemic antibiotics and hand soaks.

    f. Most common pathogen in human bites is *Eikenella corrodens* and in animal bites is *Pasteurella multocida*. Both are sensitive to penicillin.

8. Nailbed injury.

    a. Drain subungual hematoma with heated tip of paper clip.

    b. For a fractured nail or visible extension of laceration into matrix, remove loose nail and repair matrix with fine chromic suture, replace nail (with holes for drainage) as splint or pack edges of epo- and paronychium with non-adherent dressing to avoid adhesions to matrix.

III. HAND INFECTIONS (Table 1)

A. Obtain complete history.

B. Do complete examination to assess extent of infection.

C. Elevate all hand infections.

D. Antibiotics are indicated for cellulitis and sometimes for suppuration.
E. Do not wait for fluctuation before incising for suspected pus.
F. Flexor tendon sheath infections are characterized by **Kanavel's four cardinal signs:**
 1. Finger held in slight flexion.
 2. Finger is uniformly swollen and red.
 3. Intense pain on attempted extension.
 4. Tenderness along line of sheath.

IV. TECHNIQUES FOR NERVE BLOCKS
 (see "Anesthesia" section X).

V. TREATMENT OF PATIENT AND AMPUTATED PART FOR POSSIBLE REIMPLANTATION
A. With refinements in microsurgical technique and post-operative rehabilitative and reconstructive techniques, reimplantation is a treatment option which needs to be considered immediately in the evaluation of a severely injured patient. However, because this often requires referral to other centers or physicians, the initial examining surgeon should be aware of the contraindications to reimplantation.
 1. **Strong contraindications.**
  a. Significant associated injuries which make the patient too unstable for the prolonged initial reimplantation procedure and multiple subsequent procedures which are often necessary.
  b. Multilevel, crush or degloving injury to the amputated part which precludes functional recovery.
  c. Severe chronic illness.
 2. **Relative contraindications.**
  a. Single digit amputation, especially proximal to FDS insertion.
  b. Avulsion injuries, as evidenced by:
   1) Nerves and tendons dangling from the part.
   2) "Red streaks" — bruising over the digital neurovascular bundles indicating vessel disruption.
  c. Previous injury or surgery to the part.
  d. Extreme contamination.
  e. Lengthy warm ischemia time (applicable to macroreimplantation in which the part contains significant muscle mass).
  f. Age — advanced or very young.
B. Handling of an amputated part.
 1. Cleanse off gross debris with saline.
 2. Wrap in a moist saline sponge — do *not* place in a container of saline as dessication and excessive softening of tissues will occur. Place in plastic bag.

3. Place on top of crushed ice with several layers of gauze between part and ice. Do *not* immerse part in ice or ice-cold saline; freezing and thawing of cells can occur.

C. Care of the patient.

1. Examine carefully for life-threatening associated injuries which can be overlooked, particularly in the macro-reimplantation candidate.

2. Use direct pressure, not tourniquets, to control bleeding.

3. Transport after the patient's stability has been carefully assessed.

TABLE 1
Differential Diagnosis in Hand Infections

Type of infection	History	Examination	Finger movement	Investigations*	Differential diagnosis	Organism	Treatment†	Complications
Cellulitis (it can be the 1st stage of any of the following infections)	Acute pain (14-48 hr) Malaise	Signs of inflammation: fever, lymphangitis	Restricted due to pain and swelling	Urinalysis X-ray for foreign body Blood sugar Full blood count	Exclude any deep infection	Streptococci	Antibiotics (penicillin or erythromycin). Incision is required only if deep pus is suspected	Suppuration
Acute paronychia	Pain for 2-5 days	Tender swelling around the nail fold. Often an abscess. Pulp normal	Usually no restriction of movement	Swab discharge for organisms	Lateral pulp infection	Mixed organisms. Staphylococci predominate	Antibiotics (cloxacillin for cellulitis). Drain the abscess by lifting the nail fold or removing the nail	Local spread
Distal pulp space	Increasing throbbing pain for 3-5 days. Sleepless night(s)	Tender and tense pulp. Rest of finger normal	Restricted at DIP joint because of pain	X-ray for osteomyelitis and foreign body	Extensive paronychia Haematoma	Staphylococci	Do not wait for fluctuation – incise and drain early	Osteomyelitis of distal phalanx
Boil or carbuncle	Pain for 2-3 days (history of older boils or diabetes). Usually some discharge	Dorsal cellulitis with a central core. Slight fever	Restricted by pain and swelling	Swab for culture and sensitivity; blood sugar. X-ray for osteomyelitis and foreign body	Space infection Web infection	Staphylococci	Control diabetes. Antibiotics (cloxacillin). Remove core if it does not separate	Local necrosis
Bites	Painful knuckle wound usually after a fight	Infected wound of MCP or IP joint. Extensor tendon laceration	Restricted because of tendon and joint involvement	Swab discharge. X-ray for osteomyelitis, arthritis and foreign body	Infected laceration with or without foreign body	Mixed organisms	Antibiotics (tetracycline). Wound toilet. Cover for tetanus	Septic arthritis and tenosynovitis
Teno-synovitis	Increasing pain after a puncture wound of a digital crease	Severe pain on passive joint extension (touching only the finger nail). Tender over tendon sheath. Swelling of finger.	Marked restriction of both active and passive movements	X-ray for foreign body	Cellulitis Space infection Septic arthritis	Mixed organisms. Streptococci or gram-negative organisms predominate	Antibiotics (tetracycline). Cover for tetanus. Incise tendon sheath if no response to conservative treatment within 24 hr	Spread to other tendon sheaths. Necrosis of tendon with stiff finger(s). Spread to deep palmar spaces.
Osteomyelitis Septic arthritis	Appear 3-4 weeks after a deep infection, a neglected bite, or a penetrating wound	Signs of inflammation are modified by antibiotics and previous surgery. There is usually tenderness.	Restricted movement because of bone and joint involvement	X-ray for extent of bone and joint damage. Swab discharge	Deep infection (e.g. tendon sheath)	Staphylococci (or mixed organisms)	Antibiotics. Surgical toilet including sequestrectomy	Permanent loss of function which may necessitate amputation. Metastatic infection.

* All patients with hand infections should have the following investigations:
swab discharge for culture and sensitivity, urinalysis, x-ray, blood sugar, blood count.

† In every infection, distinguish between the stage of cellulitis (treat by splintage in correct posture, elevation, and antibiotics) and the stage of suppuration (treat by incision and drainage).

PERIOPERATIVE MANAGEMENT OF
THE CARDIAC SURGERY PATIENT

I. **PREOPERATIVE EVALUATION**
A. **History and physical examination** — important factors.
  1. Control of anginal symptoms, recent myocardial infarction.
  2. Signs or symptoms of congestive heart failure.
  3. Arrhythmias, presence of pacemaker.
  4. History of congenital heart defects, rheumatic fever.
  5. Presence of neurologic symptoms, carotid bruit, claudication and evidence of peripheral vascular disease or aortic aneurysms.
B. **Preoperative testing.**
  1. Baseline EKG — presence of arrhythmia or ischemia.
  2. Review of cardiac catheterization and echocardiogram results.
    a. Significance of coronary disease.
    b. Evaluation of myocardial function by wall motion and ejection fraction.
    c. Presence of valvular disease.
  3. Laboratory tests — as per usual pre-op, include bleeding time and type & cross-match for blood.
  4. PA and lateral chest X-ray.
C. **Medications.**
  1. Digoxin — continue up to surgery.
  2. Beta-blockers, calcium channel antagonists, and long-acting nitrates — continue up to surgery.
  3. Antiarrhythmics — these should be continued *unless* the patient will be undergoing arrhythmia ablational surgery, at which time the attending surgeon may have them discontinued.
  4. Aspirin — continue up to surgery; coumadin should be discontinued prior to surgery, PT corrected to < 15 sec.
  5. Bronchodilators — continued to surgery.
  6. Anticonvulsants — continued, often require loading dose post-op due to dilutional changes after cardiopulmonary bypass.
  7. MAO inhibitors and TCA's — stop at least one week prior to surgery.
  8. Insulin — one-half usual *a.m.* dose given subcutaneously prior to surgery; oral agents should not be administered.
  9. Steroids — recent use requires perioperative coverage (see "Preoperative Preparation" section VII).
D. **Pre-op orders.**
  1. Accurate height and weight recorded in chart.
  2. Hibiclens® shower the night before; enema or suppository.
  3. NPO after midnight.
  4. Sleeping pill — usually Halcion® 0.125–0.25 mg.

5. Antibiotics on call — cefazolin or cefuroxime 1 g PO qhs IVPB.

II. OPERATIVE PROCEDURES

A. Coronary artery bypass grafting.
1. Current mortality rates 0.5–3.5%.
2. Prolonged periods of hypo-/hypertension must be avoided postop.
   a. **Hypotension** — determine cause, treat accordingly (see following section on postoperative complications).
   b. **Hypertension** — increases afterload and myocardial oxygen consumption, aggravates bleeding aorto-coronary suture lines. Make certain of adequate pain relief prior to beginning vasodilator treatment.
3. Internal mammary artery grafts — now the procedure of choice due to superior patency rates (*in situ* and segmental grafts).

B. Valve repair/replacement.
1. Control of hypertension is most important in these patients, especially aortic valve replacements.
2. Cerebral embolism — risk of either air or embolic debris from manipulation of calcified heart valves entering the cerebral circulation is high in these patients.
3. Anticoagulation — mechanical prosthetic valves require permanent anticoagulation to prevent thromboembolic complications, and therapy is usually deferred until drainage tubes and pacing wires have been removed.
4. Severe congestive heart failure often seen in patients with valvular heart disease may persist postoperatively, requiring prolonged inotropic support and afterload reduction.

C. Arrhythmia ablation.
1. Refractory ventricular tachycardia and pre-excitation syndromes (i.e., Wolf–Parkinson–White syndrome) are the most common arrhythmias treated surgically.
2. Temporary pacing wires are used to obtain ventricular and atrial EKG's postop to confirm ablation. These should not be removed prior to formal postop electrophysiologic studies.
3. Amiodarone is frequently used as an antiarrhythmic in these patients. This medication should be stopped **6–8 weeks** prior to surgery, as it can result in severe myocardial depression and pulmonary complications following cardiac surgery.

D. Thoracic aortic aneurysms.
1. Multiple etiologies — atherosclerosis, dissection (i.e., Marfan's syndrome), trauma.
2. Preoperative control of hypertension to prevent rupture — require intra-arterial pressure monitoring, blood pressure control with nitroprusside or labetalol drips.
3. Dissection may advance proximally to disrupt coronary blood flow or induce aortic valve incompetence.

    4. Postoperative — renal failure, GI or spinal cord ischemia are common complications.

    5. Traumatic aortic tear — thorough examination postoperatively for associated injuries that may have been missed in the course of emergency surgery.

E. **Congenital cardiac surgery** — a formal description of the multiple procedures for repair of congenital anomalies is beyond the scope of this chapter.

III. POSTOPERATIVE COMPLICATIONS

A. Arrhythmias.

    1. Ventricular ectopy — most common.

        a. For frequent (> 6–10/min) or multifocal PVC's, treat with lidocaine bolus of 1 mg/kg, followed by drip at 2–4 mg/min.

        b. Cardioversion needed if progresses to ventricular tachycardia.

    2. Nodal or junctional rhythm.

        a. Many times no treatment necessary (assure no hypotension).

        b. Rule out digoxin toxicity, make certain serum $K+ > 4.5$.

        c. May require A-V sequential pacing if loss of atrial kick has significant hemodynamic sequelae.

    3. Supraventricular tachycardia (SVT) — includes atrial fibrillation and flutter.

        a. Onset may be heralded by multiple PAC's.

        b. Atrial EKG using atrial pacing leads often helpful in distinguishing fibrillation from flutter during rapid rates.

        c. Atrial fibrillation — digitalization.

        d. Atrial flutter.

            1) Rapid atrial pacing > 400 bpm.

            2) Digitalization followed by IV propranolol.

            3) IV verapamil followed by digitalization.

        e. In both instances, if any significant drop in blood pressure or cardiac output, the arrhythmia should be treated with DC cardioversion 25–50 joules. This should be done prior to digitalization, however, to prevent onset of ventricular arrhythmias.

B. Bleeding.

    1. Etiology — include medications, clotting deficits, reoperation, prolonged operation, technical factors, hypothermia, and transfusion reactions.

    2. Treatment.

        a. Assure normothermia.

        b. Transfusion reaction protocol if suspected.

        c. Measurement of clotting factors — PT, PTT, platelet count, activated clotting time.

        d. Correction.

       1) FFP, cryoprecipitate, platelets.

       2) Protamine for continued heparinization.

  3. Reoperation — indications: mediastinal tube output of > 300 cc/hr; technical factors found as the etiology > 50% of time.

C. **Renal failure** — incidence is 1–30%.

  1. Diagnosis — renal *vs.* pre-renal (see other chapters).

  2. Management.

    a. Optimize volume status and cardiac output.

    b. Discontinue nephrotoxic drugs.

    c. Maintain urine output > 40 cc/hr (low-dose dopamine, furosemide, ethacrynic acid as indicated).

    d. Dialysis — either peritoneal or hemodialysis may be used.

    e. Outcome — mortality rates 0.3–23% depending upon the degree of azotemia; if dialysis is required, up to 80%.

D. **Respiratory failure.**

  1. Mechanical — mucous plugging, malpositioned endotracheal tube, pneumothorax.

  2. Intrinsic — volume overload, non-cardiogenic pulmonary edema, pulmonary embolus, atelectasis, pneumonia.

E. **Low cardiac output syndrome** — cardiac index < 2.0 $L/min/m^2$.

  1. Signs — decreased urine output, acidosis, hypothermia, altered sensorium.

  2. Assessment — heart rate and rhythm (EKG: possible acute MI), pre-load and afterload states (Swan–Ganz readings), measurement of cardiac output.

  3. Treatment.

    a. Stabilize rate and rhythm.

    b. Optimize volume status, systemic vascular resistance.

    c. Correct acidosis, hypoxemia if present (CXR for pneumothorax).

    d. Inotropic agents if necessary.

    e. Persistent low cardiac output despite inotropic support may require intra-aortic balloon pump.

F. **Cardiac tamponade.**

  1. Onset — suggested by increasing filling pressures with decreased cardiac output, decreasing urine output and hypotension, eventual equalization of right and left–sided atrial pressures.

  2. High degree of suspicion when coincides with excessive postoperative bleeding.

  3. Treatment — transfusion to optimize volume status and inotropic support; avoid increased PEEP; emergent re-exploration may be needed at bedside for sudden hemodynamic decompensation.

G. **Perioperative myocardial infarction** — incidence 5–20%.

  1. Diagnosis — new onset Q waves post-op; serial isoenzymes, increased MB fractions; bedside dipyridamole scan.

2. Treatment — vasodilation (IV nitroglycerine preferred to nitroprusside). Continued hemodynamic alterations should be treated with immediate intra-aortic balloon counterpulsation. This "unloads" the ventricle, and may preserve non-ischemic adjacent myocardium.
3. Outcome — associated with increased morbidity and mortality, as well as poorer long–term results.

H. **Postoperative fever.**

1. Very common in the first 24 hours postoperatively; etiology unknown, may be associated with pyrogens introduced during cardiopulmonary bypass. Treat pyrexia with acetaminophen and cooling blankets, as associated hypermetabolism and vasodilation can be detrimental.
2. Fevers post-op for valve patients should be cultured. CABG patients should have work-up on 5th post-op day.
3. Perioperative antibiotics should be continued until all invasive monitors and drainage tubes have been removed.
4. Sternal wound — daily inspection for drainage and stability. Sternal infections may be disastrous in the cardiac patient.
5. Post-pericardiotomy syndrome — characterized by low-grade fever, leukocytosis, chest pain, malaise, and pericardial rub on auscultation. Usually occurs 2–3 weeks following surgery, and is treated with NSAID's. Steroids are necessary for some cases.

I. **CNS complications.**

1. Etiologies — pre-existing cerebrovascular disease, prolonged cardiopulmonary bypass, intraoperative hypotension, emboli (either air or particulate matter).
2. Transient neurologic deficit — occurs in up to 25% of patients. Improvement usually occurs within several days.
3. Permanent deficit — suspect in patients with delayed awakening postoperatively; may have pathologic reflexes present.
4. Post-cardiotomy psychosis syndrome — incidence 10–24%. Starts around postoperative day 2 with anxiety and confusion; may progress to disorientation and hallucinations. Treat with rest and quiet environment, antipsychotics as necessary.
5. CT scan early for suspected localized lesions; EEG in patients with extensive dysfunction.
6. Treatment — optimize cerebral blood flow, avoid hypercapnia.
   a. Postoperative seizures treated with lorazepam and loading with diphenylhydantoin.
   b. Mannitol may be needed in presence of increased intracranial pressure, depending on hemodynamic status.

LUNG CARCINOMA

I. GENERAL CONSIDERATIONS
A. **Solitary pulmonary nodules (SPN)** should be *considered malignant until proven otherwise.*
B. **Metastatic lesions** are most often multiple and/or subpleurally based. The incidence of a metastatic solitary nodule from an asymptomatic primary malignancy is exceedingly low. Therefore, an extensive meta-static work–up is unnecessary for a SPN.
C. Granulomatous disease and bronchogenic carcinoma account for 80% of SPN.
D. **Indicators of malignancy.**
   1. Incidence of malignancy increases with age.
      a. 35–44 years − 15%.
      b. 60–69 years − 50%.
      c. > 80 years − > 90%.
   2. 4 : 1 ratio of malignancy vs. benign when > 4 cm in diameter.
   3. Smoking history > 20 pack–years.
   4. X-ray patterns showing lobulated or spiculated contours.
E. **Indicators of benign nodule.**
   1. Calcium in nodule − only 0.5% are malignant.
   2. Laminated or "popcorn" lesions associated with hamartomas. Smooth contours are more commonly associated with benign lesions.
   3. Complete lack of growth in over 2 years − the doubling time of lung carcinomas is between 37 and 465 days.

II. DIAGNOSIS
A. **Thorough history,** including smoking and environmental/occupa-tional exposures. **Physical exam**: extensive search for adenopathy.
B. **Sputum cytology.**
   1. Low cost and risk, with 40–80% yield. Requires at least three morning specimens.
   2. Highest yield for squamous cell (usually more centrally located lesions).
   3. Does not contribute to the diagnosis of a benign lesion.
C. **Pleural fluid cytology** (if effusion present on chest x-ray).
   1. Yield is 40–75%.
   2. Highest yield for adenocarcinoma.
D. **Bronchoscopy.**
   1. Yield is 55–80%.
   2. Best for large or central nodules.
   3. Provides staging information in the event of carcinoma, and may be performed at the time of thoracotomy.

E. **Percutaneous needle biopsy.**
  1. *Often unnecessary*, as a negative yield does not rule out carcinoma, and a positive biopsy would require thoracotomy for treatment.
  2. **Indications.**
    a. Suspected small cell carcinoma, when surgery is most likely *not* in the treatment plan.
    b. Poor risk patients who cannot tolerate thoracotomy.
  3. **Contraindications.**
    a. Bleeding diathesis.
    b. Bullous disease near the lesion.
  4. Yield is 96% with 2 attempts.
  5. **Complications.**
    a. Pneumothorax has 24% incidence, but only 10% of patients require chest tube placement.
    b. Minor hemoptysis — 6% incidence.

III. CARCINOMA OF THE LUNG
A. **General considerations.**
  1. 144,000 newly diagnosed cases per year.
  2. Responsible for 126,000 cancer deaths per year. The leading cause of cancer deaths in men and women. In 1986, overtook breast cancer as the leading cause of cancer death in women.
  3. 5-Year survival of all patients after diagnosis is 13%.
B. **Histology: 99%** of lung cancers are epithelial in origin.
  1. Squamous cell (epidermoid) carcinoma — 30–35% incidence, which is decreasing; usually centrally located.
  2. Adenocarcinoma — 30–35% incidence, which is increasing; usually peripherally located; most common carcinoma in *non-smokers.*
  3. Adenosquamous carcinoma.
  4. Small cell (oat cell) carcinoma — 25% incidence; a distinct clinicopathologic entity marked by rapid growth and poor prognosis. Three cell types: lymphocyte–like, spindle cell, and polysomal cell.
  5. Undifferentiated (large cell) carcinoma — 10% incidence. Two types: giant cell and clear cell.
  6. Mucous gland carcinoma — includes adenoid cystic carcinoma and mucoepidermoid carcinoma.
  7. Carcinoid tumor — typical, spindle cell, atypical.
  8. Pancoast tumor — carcinoma of superior sulcus, Horner's syndrome.

IV. STAGING CLASSIFICATION
A. TNM nomenclature of lung cancer.

T_x - Positive cytology only

T_0 - No evidence of tumor

T_{is} - Carcinoma *in situ*

T_1 - < 3 cm in diameter; no bronchial invasion

T_2 - > 3 cm or invades pleura, hilum or bronchus

T_3 - Any invasion of parietal pleura, chest wall, diaphragm, mediastinum

N_x - Unable to assess

N_0 - No nodes

N_1 - Ipsilateral nodes (peribronchial or hilar)

N_2 - Ipsilateral mediastinal nodes

N_3 - Contralateral mediastinal nodes

M_x - Unable to assess

M_0 - No metastasis

M_1 - Distant metastasis

B. Stages of lung cancer according to TNM classification.

Occult carcinoma — $T_xN_0M_0$.
Stage I — $T_{is}N_0M_0$, $T_1N_0M_0$, $T_2N_0M_0$.
Stage II — $T_1N_1M_0$, $T_2N_1M_0$.
Stage IIIa — $T_3N_0M_0$, $T_3N_1M_0$, $T_3N_2M_0$, $T_1N_2M_0$, $T_2N_2M_0$.
Stage IIIb — Any TN_3.
Stage IV — M_1.

V. STAGING PROCEDURES
A. Physical exam, chest x-ray, bronchoscopy, chest CT scan.
B. Mediastinal staging by chest CT.
1. False–positive 20%, false–negative < 10%.
2. Assess liver and adrenal glands for metastatic disease by a small caudad extension of the scan.
C. Cervical mediastinoscopy — false–negative 3–5%; mortality 0.8%; morbidity 1.6%; aortopulmonary window nodes inaccessible.
D. Anterior mediastinotomy (Chamberlain procedure) — biopsy access to aortopulmonary window, left hilum, and internal mammary nodes (morbidity 10%).
E. Scalene node biopsy — 90% yield, indicated for palpable supra-clavicular nodes.

VI. TREATMENT OF NON–SMALL CELL CARCINOMA: SURGICAL
A. Assessment of pulmonary reserve.
1. **Pulmonary function test criteria** (see also "Respiratory Care"):

	Pneumonectomy	Lobectomy	Wedge/Segmental Resection
MVV	> 55%	> 40%	> 35%
FEV_1	> 2.0 L/min	> 1.0 L/min	> 0.6 L/min

    2. Clinical assessment of function — step climbing at a normal
rate without significant increase in pulse or respiratory rate.
      a. One flight — tolerate thoracotomy.
      b. Two flights — tolerate lobectomy.
      c. Three flights — tolerate pneumonectomy.
B. Thoracotomy (if adequate pulmonary reserve and no evidence of
metastasis).
    1. Wedge resection or segmentectomy.
      a. Some series report no difference *vs.* lobectomy while others
report a high recurrence rate.
      b. Indications — marginal pulmonary reserve or metachronous
or synchronous tumors.
    2. Lobectomy.
      a. Procedure of choice in most resectable lung cancers. Pre-
serves pulmonary function and quality of life.
      b. Includes entire first level lobar lymphatics.
      c. Mortality rate of 0–5%.
    3. Pneumonectomy.
      a. Hilar involvement or tumor extension across the fissure.
      b. Mortality rate of 5–10%.
      c. Can result in poor pulmonary reserve with *significant* change
in lifestyle.
    4. Mediastinal lymph node sampling is usually carried out during
thoracotomy. A positive frozen section should be treated with
a lymphadenectomy of the nodal area.

VII. TREATMENT OF NON–SMALL CELL CARCINOMA: NON–SURGICAL

A. Radiation.
    1. Palliation — may relieve superior vena cava obstruction, hemop-
tysis, pain, and dyspnea.
    2. Preoperative — no difference in outcome, with increased post-
op complication rate. The exception occurs in superior sulcus
(Pancoast) tumors, which show improved survival (45% *vs.* 30%)
after pre–op radiation and *en bloc* resection.
    3. Postoperative — improves local control with squamous cell
carcinomas, but no change in survival rates.
B. Chemotherapy — used mainly to treat disseminated disease, but
remains controversial. Patients with low tumor burdens appear to
do best.
C. Immunotherapy — currently no useful regimens have been found
for the treatment of lung cancer.
D. Laser therapy — may be useful in relief of endobronchial obstruction in unresectable tumors.

E. **Combination therapy.**
   1. Early studies have shown postoperative chemotherapy and radiation in complete and incomplete resections to have improved survival over postoperative radiation alone.
   2. Small studies using preoperative chemotherapy/radiation regimens have shown increased survival.
F. **Five–year survival rates.**
   1. Stage I.
      a. $T_1N_0M_0$ — 80%.
      b. $T_2N_0M_0$ — 62%.
   2. Stage II — 20–25%.
   3. Stage III — 0%.
   4. Stage IIIa — 8–30%.
   5. Stage IIIb — 0–57%.

VIII. TREATMENT OF SMALL CELL CARCINOMA

A. **Chemotherapy/radiation mainstay of treatment.**
   1. **Tumor response** seen in 75–95% of patients.
      a. Complete response seen in 50% with limited disease (confined to one hemithorax), and 20% with widespread disease.
      b. Partial response will occur in 45%.
   2. **Limited disease** — 0–10% cured; median survival > 18 months.
   3. **Extensive disease** — 5% cured; median survival ~ 12 months.
B. **Surgical treatment** — may be useful to increase survival in stage I disease, but this is a very limited group of patients.

PART III

PROCEDURES

VASCULAR ACCESS TECHNIQUES

I. PERIPHERAL VENOUS ACCESS
A. Sites.
1. The veins of the hands and arms are most often used for intra-venous catheter placement. Simple blood drawing is most easily done in the antecubital fossa, while IV catheters function best in the veins on the dorsum of the hand, forearm, and upper arm. Choices in order of preference:
   a. Cephalic vein ("intern's vein").
   b. Basilic vein.
   c. Median vein.
   d. Greater saphenous vein.
2. IV access or phlebotomy may be gained in the saphenous veins under certain circumstances such as major trauma, cardiac arrest, etc., but generally should be avoided due to the risks of phlebitis, DVT and infection (especially in patients with diabetes and patients with peripheral vascular disease). The saphenous vein may be found ~ 1 cm anterior and superior to the medial malleolus.

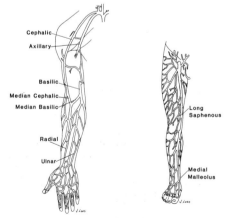

FIGURE 1
Anatomy of Veins of Upper and Lower Extremities

B. **Technique of peripheral venous cannulation.**
1. In patients who need rapid volume expansion, use the largest gauge catheter available (14 gauge or 16 gauge). When giving blood, use at least an 18 gauge catheter.
2. The more distal veins of the hand should be used first. In circulatory collapse the antecubital veins are the largest veins of the arm and are used for rapid access.
3. Apply tourniquet proximally.
4. Locate vein and cleanse the overlying skin with alcohol or betadine.
5. Local anesthesia may be considered in the awake patient if a large–bore catheter is to be placed.
6. Hold the vein in place by applying pressure on the vein distal to the planned point of entry.
7. Puncture the skin with the needle bevel upward; enter the vein from either side or from above.
8. When blood return is noted, advance approximately 1 mm further, stabilize the needle and slide the catheter into place.
9. Remove the tourniquet and needle, attach the IV tubing and cover with a sterile dressing.

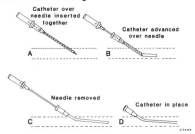

FIGURE 2
Insertion of the Over–Needle Catheter

In *A*, needle and catheter have been inserted through the skin. In *B*, the needle tip has been inserted into the vein. Blood returns, but the catheter is not yet in the vein. The tip of the needle must be raised to avoid impaling the back wall, and the needle must be advanced further to carry the catheter into the vein as in *C*. In *D*, the catheter is threaded into the vein, over the needle.

II. CENTRAL VENOUS ACCESS

Access to central venous system may be required for many reasons.

A. **Indications.**
1. Inadequate peripheral venous access.
2. Total parenteral nutrition.
3. Central venous pressure monitoring.
4. Placement of pulmonary artery catheter.

B. **Anatomy for central venous catheter placement.**
1. **External jugular vein** — formed at the angle of mandible by the posterior facial veins and the posterior auricular vein, passes caudally over the sternocleidomastoid (SCM) to enter the subclavian vein lateral to the anterior scalene muscle.

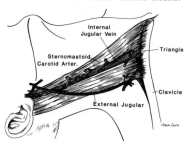

FIGURE 3
Anatomy of External Jugular Vein

2. **Internal jugular vein** — arises from base of skull in the carotid sheath *posterior* to internal carotid artery and terminates in subclavian vein anterior and lateral to common carotid artery. Runs medial to SCM in its upper part, posterior in triangle between two heads of SCM and behind clavicular head in its lower part.
3. **Subclavian vein** — continuation of axillary vein at lateral border of first rib, passes over first rib anterior to anterior scalene muscle, continues *behind medial third* of clavicle where it is fixed to the rib and clavicle. Joins the IJ to form innominate vein behind sterno–costoclavicular joint. Subclavian artery and apical pleura lie behind vein at medial third of the clavicle.
4. **Femoral vein** — used as a last resort because of the increased frequency of thrombosis, embolism, and infection. The vein is located *medial* to the femoral artery in the femoral sheath below the inguinal ligament. The artery may be found at the midpoint of a line connecting the anterior superior iliac spine and the pubic symphysis; the vein is one fingerbreadth medial.

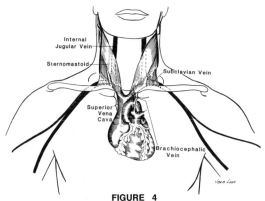

FIGURE 4
Venous Anatomy of Thoracic Inlet

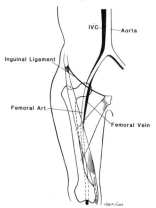

FIGURE 5
Anatomy of Femoral Vein

C. Central line placement techniques.

    1. External jugular vein — not a preferred site due to positional functioning and difficulty maintaining a dressing.

        a. Patient is prepped, draped, and placed in Trendelenburg position. Turn patient's head to opposite side.

        b. Compress the vein at the base of the neck to distend it.

        c. Insert 18 gauge needle, directed caudally, into vein.

        d. Thread .089 cm diameter, 35 cm long J–tipped flexible guide wire into vein to negotiate junction of external and internal jugular veins.

        e. Insert 14–16 gauge catheter over wire, remove wire, suture in place.

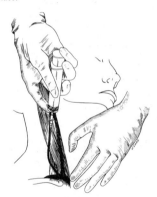

FIGURE 6
Cannulation of External Jugular Vein

    2. General principles of internal jugular and subclavian vein catheterization.

        a. Check PT, PTT and platelet count before puncture attempts, to rule out coagulopathy.

        b. Equipment needed:

            1) Povidone–iodine or Hibiclens® prep solution.

            2) 4 x 4 gauze sponges.

            3) Sterile towels.

            4) Local anesthesia (1% lidocaine/carbocaine) and 20, 25 gauge needles.

    5) 2–0 silk suture.

    6) #11 scalpel blade.

    7) 3 cc, 5 cc, or 10 cc syringe, non–Leur lock tip.

    8) 18 gauge thin–walled needle at least 6 cm long with Seldinger wire.

    9) Single or multilumen catheter (15–20 cm long).

    10) Rolled towel or sheet.

    11) 75 mg lidocaine if Swan–Ganz planned.

  c. Place a rolled towel vertically between shoulder blades, put in Trendelenburg position with neck extended.

  d. Wear gown, mask and gloves, then prep and drape patient.

  e. Infiltrate local anesthesia at puncture site with 25 gauge needle, then 20 gauge needle; infiltrate tract toward vein, aspirating prior to instilling anesthetic. This is especially important for subclavian venipuncture as the clavicle edge should be anesthetized.

  f. Flush catheter with sterile fluid, estimate length to sterno-manubrial junction to place in superior vena cava.

  g. Mount 18 gauge thin–walled needle on syringe (smaller needle if internal jugular).

  h. Insert slowly, while aspirating, until blood returns, advance a few millimeters farther until blood return increases. Bright red blood usually means arterial puncture; remove needle and apply pressure for 10 min.

  i. If no blood returns, withdraw needle *slowly* under negative pressure; blood may still return into syringe. If still no blood return, re-attempt.

  j. After blood returns, stabilize needle, carefully unscrew syringe and prevent air embolism by occluding needle with finger.

  k. Place guide-wire through needle gently; it should advance *easily*. Withdraw needle, holding the wire in position.

  l. Nick skin with #11 blade, slide dilator over wire to enlarge skin site and tract, remove dilator, then advance catheter over wire into desired position.

  m. Remove wire, check blood return, attach IV tubing.

  n. Suture at skin, place sterile occlusive dressing.

3. Internal jugular — central approach.

  a. Locate the triangle formed by the 2 heads of SCM and the clavicle.

  b. Insert 22 gauge localizing needle at apex of triangle formed by two heads of SCM.

  c. Aim needle parallel to clavicular head toward ipsilateral nipple at 45–60° angle until vein is entered.

  d. If needle is inserted 3 cm without blood return, attempt new puncture in slightly more lateral position.

  e. Do *not* proceed medially, as carotid artery will be punctured.

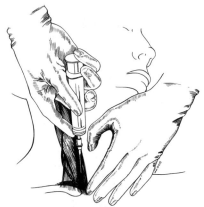

FIGURE 7
Central Approach for Internal Jugular Venipuncture

4. **Internal jugular — posterior approach.**
   a. Insert needle under SCM at junction of middle and lower thirds of posterior border, aiming anteriorly to suprasternal notch at 45° angle to sagittal and horizontal planes.
   b. Vein should be entered within 5–7 cm of needle penetration.

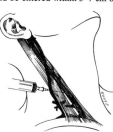

FIGURE 8
Posterior Approach for Internal Jugular Venipuncture

5. **Internal jugular — anterior approach.**
   a. Retract carotid artery medially from anterior border of SCM.
   b. Introduce needle at mid-point of anterior border of SCM at point 5 cm below mandible and 5 cm above clavicle.
   c. Aim needle at 30–45° toward ipsilateral nipple.

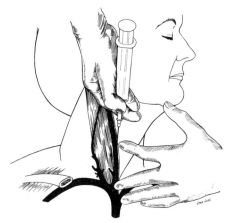

FIGURE 9
Anterior Approach for Internal Jugular Venipuncture

6. **Subclavian vein catheterization (infraclavicular).**
   a. Insert needle 1–2 cm below junction of medial and middle third of clavicle.
   b. Advance needle parallel to frontal plane until clavicle located.
   c. March the needle down the clavicle until it just passes below it, aiming at the suprasternal notch.
   d. When the vein is entered, carefully rotate the needle 90° to aim the bevel caudally so the wire will pass into the bracheocephalic vein.
   e. Vein can also be entered via supraclavicular approach, but higher incidence of arterial puncture.

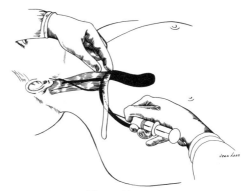

Figure 10
Infraclavicular Subclavian Venipuncture

7. **Contraindications** to central venous catheterization.
   a. Thrombosis of central veins.
   b. Coagulopathy — this is a relative contraindication. Many coagulopathies can be temporarily overcome with transfusion of fresh frozen plasma, cryoprecipitate or platelets, followed by immediate venipuncture. It is preferable to place deep lines in areas that are compressible in the event of bleeding (i.e., femoral, brachial, internal jugular). Also consider cutdown of antecubital veins.
   c. Bullous emphysema — avoid subclavian approach.
8. **Complications.**
   a. Catheter misplacement — poor blood return, cardiac irritability, pain in neck or ear. Corrective options include:
      1) Reposition under fluoroscopy.
      2) Re-attempt entire procedure.
   b. Arterial puncture (subclavian, carotid, femoral).
   c. Hemorrhage — venous/arterial.
   d. Pneumothorax — always check chest x-ray prior to re-attempting central venipuncture on contralateral side.
   e. Thoracic duct injury with or without chylothorax.
   f. Extravasation of fluid, hyperalimentation, etc.
   g. Neural injury (brachial plexus).
   h. Air embolism.
   i. Catheter or wire embolization.

    j. Hydrothorax.
       1) Primary — placement of catheter into pleural or mediastinal spaces.
       2) Secondary — erosion of catheter through SVC after successful placement.
    k. Infection.
       1) Cellulitis at puncture site.
       2) Bacteremia from catheter colonization (catheter sepsis).
       3) Increased incidence with use of multilumen catheters.
    l. Thrombosis (central venous) — clinical signs include unilateral upper extremity edema, upper extremity and neck venous distention and neck pain. **Treatment:** Similar to iliofemoral DVT. Remove catheter, heparinization followed by coumadinization.

III. ARTERIAL ACCESS
A. Indications.
    1. Continuous blood pressure measurement.
      a. Shock from hypovolemia, hemorrhage, burns, trauma.
      b. Use of IV vasopressors or vasodilators.
      c. Major operations in which major fluid losses can be expected.
      d. Severe cardiac disease or respiratory disease.
      e. Patients in whom changes in blood pressure could be deleterious — cardiovascular, cerebrovascular disease.
    2. Need for frequent blood sampling.
      a. Blood gases for ventilator management.
      b. Serial electrolytes, blood counts in ICU setting.
      c. Avoids discomfort, difficulty, and complications of frequent arterial and venous puncture.
B. Sites of cannulation (in order of preference).
    1. Radial.
    2. Femoral.
    3. Axillary.
    4. Ulnar.
    5. Dorsalis pedis.
    6 Brachial — not routinely used because of high risk of embolic and ischemic hand complications.
C. Radial artery cannulation.
    1. Begin with an assessment of collateral circulation — modified **Allen's test.**
      a. Compress radial and ulnar arteries.
      b. Patient clenches fist to exsanguinate palmar skin.
      c. Release pressure over ulnar artery.

d. Return of skin color in ≤ 6 seconds indicates patency of ulnar artery and superificial palmar arch; therefore, it is okay to cannulate radial artery.

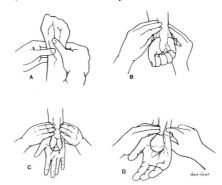

FIGURE 11
Allen's Test

2. Several studies have shown that the Allen's test is *not* a predictor of ischemia post cannulation; thus, after an abnormal Allen's test, the radial artery may still be used if no peripheral vascular disease is present.
3. **Technique.**
   a. Apply armboard to hand and forearm dorsally.
   b. Place roll of gauze behind wrist to dorsiflex hand 60°.
   c. Prep wrist and palm.
   d. Wear mask, sterile gloves.
   e. Drape area with sterile towels.
   f. Infiltrate local anesthetic into proposed insertion site.
   g. Use 20 gauge 11/4–2 inch long, Teflon™ coated angiocath.
   h. Insert catheter/needle at 30–45° angle to skin and advance slowly until blood returns to needle hub.
   i. Tilt needle and catheter down slightly and, while holding needle in place, slide catheter over needle into artery.
   j. Remove needle, attach T–piece extension and pressure tubing, flush catheter, and make certain good waveform is present.

    k. Suture catheter securely with 2–0 or 3–0 silk.
    l. Apply sterile dressing.

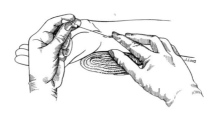

FIGURE 12
Cannulation of Radial Artery

D. Femoral artery cannulation.
    1. Has the same rate of complications as radial cannulation.
    2. Is safer than a difficult radial cannulation.
    3. Has longer average catheter duration than radial (about 2 days more).
    4. Has twice the rate of complications of radial cannulation in patients with peripheral vascular disease (17% vs. 8%).
    5. Should be performed in hemodynamically unstable patients for speed and facility of procedure.
    6. Technique.
        a. Shave groin.
        b. Use 19–20 gauge, 16 cm long catheter.
        c. Insert needle/catheter 2 cm below inguinal ligament at 45°.
        d. Secure catheter to skin with 2–0 silk.
E. Axillary artery cannulation.
    1. Shave axilla, hyperabduct and externally rotate arm.
    2. Palpate pulse just below biceps muscle.
    3. Use 20 gauge, 5 cm long needle with guide wire, 16 cm long catheter.
    4. Insert needle as high as possible within axilla, 35° angle to skin.
    5. Insert guide-wire, remove needle.
    6. Place catheter and secure to skin.

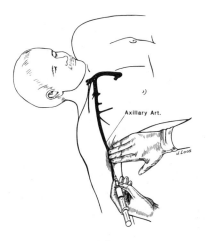

FIGURE 13
Cannulation of Axillary Artery

F. **Dorsalis pedis artery cannulation.**
   1. Best utilized in younger patients. Not to be used in patients with diabetes or peripheral vascular disease.
   2. Same technique as radial artery.
G. **Disparities between A–line and cuff pressure measurements.**
   1. Variance of 5–20 mmHg is within expected range. Peak central pressures slightly lower than peak peripheral pressures due to inertia of entrainment of a column of blood meeting resistance.
   2. Cuff pressure > 20 mmHg over A–line pressure.
      a. Improper cuff size (usually cuff too small) or placement.
      b. Severe peripheral vascular disease with catheter in a distal artery.
      c. Improperly calibrated sphygmomanometer or transducer.
      d. Dampened waveform – look for tubing problems.
         1) Air bubbles or blood in line.
         2) Clotting at catheter tip.
         3) Loose connections.
         4) Line occlusion.
         5) Kinked catheter from dressing position.

    3. A–line pressure > 20 mmHg higher over cuff pressure.
      a. Severe vasoconstriction – use cuff pressure.
      b. Catheter in small vessel in high–flow state.
      c. Resonance of catheter system – use larger, more compliant tubing with length ≤ 36".

H. Complications – overall incidence of A–line-related complications is about 7% for radial and femoral lines. In the presence of peripheral vascular disease, however, this doubles to 17%. The incidence of complications is also increased with different percutaneous or cutdown techniques. Catheter size and material appear to have little or no effect on complication rates.

    1. **Ischemia/thrombosis** – most common complication.
      a. Radial artery is occluded in 25% of all cannulations, yet almost no ischemic damage to hand occurs.
      b. Increased incidence with peripheral vascular disease, use of vasopressors.
      c. Not predicted by Allen's test.
      d. Use continuous line flush with heparin at 2–4 U/ml.
    2. **Infection** – catheter–related sepsis. Change catheter when erythema develops at insertion site or positive blood cultures are drawn through the catheter.
    3. **Embolism.**
      a. From clots in catheter tip or air in tubing.
      b. Increased incidence with intermittent line flush.
    4. **Hemorrhage.**
      a. Rapid blood loss/exsanguination may follow any disconnection in system between patient and transducer.
      b. Decreased incidence with ≥ 5–10 minutes of direct pressure post decannulation.
    5. **Pseudoaneurysm.**
      a. May occur when periarterial hematoma develops.
      b. If present – resect and repair artery.

IV. PULMONARY ARTERY CATHETERIZATION

The Swan–Ganz pulmonary artery catheter was designed to provide a clinical means for frequent and reliable assessment of left ventricular preload. In the absence of severe cardiopulmonary dysfunction, the pulmonary capillary wedge pressure provides an index of the left atrial pressure and, hence, the left ventricular end–diastolic pressure (preload). Starling's law describes the relationship of preload to cardiac function.

A. Swan–Ganz catheters:
    1. Allow measurment of right atrial, right ventricular, pulmonary artery and pulmonary capillary wedge pressure.
    2. Allow calculation of cardiac output and other hemodynamic parameters by thermodilution.

3. Allow sampling of pulmonary arterial (mixed venous) and right atrial blood.

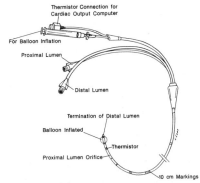

FIGURE 14
Triple–Port, 4–Lumen, Swan–Ganz® Catheter

B. Indications — see "Cardiopulmonary Monitoring".
C. Equipment needed for insertion.
   1. Swan–Ganz catheter.
   2. Pressure monitoring lines.
   3. Two 3–way stopcocks to connect to proximal and distal ports.
   4. 3 cc syringe for balloon inflation (comes with Swan–Ganz).
   5. Equipment for central venous cannulation, catheter sheath (Cordis® introducer), and optional Swan–Ganz plastic sheath that allows catheter adjustment under sterile conditions.
   6. Transducers, pressure monitors.
   7. Sterile gowns, gloves, mask, drapes.
   8. An assistant, preferably an experienced SICU nurse !
D. Preparing for catheter insertion.
   1. Peripheral IV line must be in place for fluids and emergency medications.
   2. Lidocaine, atropine, and defibrillator must be available.
   3. Continuous ECG monitoring.
   4. Set up transducer and connecting tubing.
   5. Zero and calibrate transducer.
   6. Prep area with antiseptic solution and drape widely.

E. Insertion sites.
  1. Subclavian vein (left is preferred over right).
  2. Internal jugular vein (right preferred over left).
  3. Femoral vein.
  4. Brachial vein via antecubital cutdown — only as last resort; highest risk of complications.
F. Testing catheter before insertion.
  1. Flush the proximal, distal lumens with sterile saline containing 2–4 units heparin/cc to eliminate air bubbles and test system.
  2. Test balloon with 1.5 cc air to rule out leaks.
  3. Connect thermistor to cardiac output computer, note increase in temperature after warming the thermistor between fingertips.
  4. Shake the catheter tip to confirm pressure wave changes on the monitor.
G. Insertion of catheter.
  1. Use meticulous aseptic technique.
  2. Cannulate central vein, introduce catheter sheath (Cordis®) and suture in place after blood return is confirmed.
  3. Attach IV tubing to Cordis® line. After this, catheter is brought into the sterile field, set up and tested (see section F, above).
  4. A clear plastic collapsible sheath may be placed over the catheter at this time that allows sterile manipulation of catheter after insertion.
  5. Insert catheter through Cordis® slowly until CVP tracing is seen (15 cm), then ask assistant to inflate balloon ("balloon up").
  6. Slowly advance catheter into right atrium, then right ventricle; when right ventricle waveform is identified, advance catheter smoothly and quickly into pulmonary artery. While advancing, hold catheter firmly and close to Cordis® to avoid kinking.
  7. Slowly advance to wedged position in pulmonary artery and deflate balloon ("balloon down").
     a. If PA waveform returns — good position.
     b. If wedge waveform persists — withdraw slightly and re-check.
  8. *Always* deflate balloon before withdrawing catheter.
  9. Confirming wedge position.
     a. Catheter flushes easily before inflating balloon (excludes catheter obstruction).
     b. Loss of PA tracing with balloon inflation; returns with deflation.
     c. PCWP ≤ PAD pressure (normal 6–12 mmHg).
  10. To determine wedge, inflate balloon slowly while monitoring waveform. To prevent pulmonary artery rupture, stop inflation when wedged waveform is achieved. Always disconnect inflation syringe and unlock port prior to reconnecting and inflating the balloon. This avoids inadvertent overdistention or rupture of balloon and pulmonary artery.

11. Conditions of low cardiac output, tricuspid regurgitation or pulmonary hypertension may require multiple attempts or fluoroscopy to pass the catheter. Mitral regurgitation may cause poor changes in waveform, also making catheter placement difficult. Changes in patient position (Trendelenburg's or left or right decubitus) are sometimes helpful.
12. If IJ or SC vein used, PA should be within 50 cm of catheter insertion; 70 cm for femoral or antecubital sites.
13. Document location of catheter tip and rule out pneumothorax with CXR, preferably upright.
14. Monitor the waveform continuously to recognize inadvertent wedging ("over-wedging") which can cause pulmonary infarction. If catheter is noted to be over-wedged, adjust immediately.

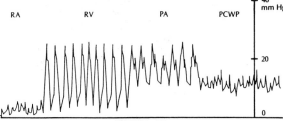

FIGURE 15
Characteristic Waveform Changes

Ref: Shuck JM, Nearman HS. Technical skills in patient care. In *Clinical Surgery* (Davis JH, ed). St. Louis: CV Mosby, 1987, with permission.

H. **Waveforms seen during passage of Swan–Ganz catheter.**
   1. Vena cava — dampened waveform, gentle sinusoidal motion with breathing. Abrupt increase with cough.
   2. Right atrium — similar to vena cava, but less dampened.
   3. Right ventricle — an abrupt increase in systolic pressure, which rapidly falls toward zero. Diastolic waveform has appearance of square root sign.
   4. Pulmonary artery.
      a. Systolic pressure same as RV.
      b. Dicrotic notch present (best distinguishing factor).
      c. Diastolic pressure rises (tracing does not fall to zero as in RV).
   5. Wedge (PAO, PCWP).
      a. Small A, V waves; fluctuates with ventilation.

      b. Mean pressure ≤ PAD.

      c. Read mean number at end–expiration, preferably off the ventilator.

I. **Complications of Swan–Ganz catheter placement.**

    1. **Catheter kinks/knots** — if a knot is suspected, confirm with CXR and call invasive angiographer to untie knot via femoral vein deflecting wire.

    2. Pulmonary infarction from prolonged balloon occlusion of pulmonary artery.

    3. Pulmonary artery rupture.

      a. Incidence — .06%.

      b. Risk factors — pulmonary hypertension, anticoagulation, hypothermia.

      c. Caused by tip if catheter advanced too far, eccentric balloon inflation or balloon overinflation which ruptures PA.

      d. Symptoms — hemoptysis, hypotension.

      e. Treatment.

        1) < 30 cc hemoptysis — observe.

        2) > 30 cc hemoptysis — consider wedge angiogram performed through catheter to show extravasation.

        3) If massive, bronchoscopy with/without a double–lumen endotracheal tube may be indicated.

    4. Sepsis — site cellulitis/positive blood cultures.

      a. Infection rate related to duration of catheter being in place:

        1) If ≤ 3 days — 5%.

        2) If 4 days — 10%.

        3) If 5 days — 15%.

      b. Recommend removing or changing catheter every 72 hours.

    5. **Dysrhythmia.**

      a. Related to passage of catheter through right ventricle.

      b. Transient PVC's develop in majority of patients (75%).

      c. Persistent PVC's in 3–13%.

      d. Risk factors for ectopy — acidosis, hypokalemia, hypothermia, hypoxia, prolonged time to pass catheter.

      e. Advanced ventricular arrhythmias 3–12%; however, prophylactic lidocaine rarely indicated.

      f. Treatment.

        1) Intravenous lidocaine with/without cardioversion.

        2) Withdraw catheter if unable to suppress (sometimes a large loop in the RV may be the cause).

    6. Balloon rupture — replace catheter.

    7. **Transient RBBB** — patients with pre-existing LBBB are therefore at risk for developing complete heart block. Would consider placement of transvenous pacemaker prior to PA catheter insertion or use of a pacing Swan–Ganz catheter (less reliable).

    8. Endocarditis — from sepsis; more common in burn patients.

AIRWAYS

I. ENDOTRACHEAL INTUBATION

A. Definition — placement of a tube (polyvinylchloride) with a balloon cuff via oral or nasal route into the trachea to facilitate ventilation.

B. **Indications.**
   1. Protection of airway from aspiration.
   2. Relief of upper airway obstruction.
   3. Facilitate tracheobronchial suctioning.
   4. Ventilatory support.

C. **Methods.**
   1. **Orotracheal intubation.**
      a. Primarily for unconscious or anesthetized patients.
      b. Passed orally using direct laryngoscopy.
      c. Advantages — rapid introduction, able to use larger sized endotracheal tube.
      d. Disadvantage — patient discomfort.
   2. **Nasotracheal intubation.**
      a. Passed via nasal route blindly or with laryngoscopy. Requires more skill for placement.
      b. Method of choice in trauma patients with possible cervical spine injury.

D. **Technique.**
   1. Preparation.
      a. Obtain permission if patient's condition allows.
      b. Equipment — ambu bag, laryngoscope, endotracheal tubes (a variety of sizes), suction device, lubricant, tube stylet, Cetacaine® spray.
      c. Select tube size (rule of thumb) — in adults, approximate diameter of fifth digit is an appropriate tube size.
   2. **Orotracheal intubation.**
      a. Preoxygenate patient with mask ventilation, 100% O_2.
      b. Place in sniffing position (neck flexed, head extended) — *contraindicated* in patients with possible cervical spine injury.
      c. Anesthetize posterior pharynx with Cetacaine® spray.
      d. Open mouth widely using crossed finger technique with the right hand (thumb on lower incisors, index finger on upper incisors).
      e. Insert laryngoscope using left hand in right–hand corner of mouth and advance, sweeping the tongue to the left.
      f. When the epiglottis is visualized, the tip of the laryngoscope is placed above (for curved laryngoscope blades) or below (for straight blades) the epiglottis (Fig. 1). Handle of the laryngoscope is then lifted, **not tilted**, to visualize cords.

    Pharynx may require suctioning for adequate visualization of cords (Figs. 2 & 3).

 g. Insert tracheal tube **under direct vision** *through* the vocal cords. Time insertion with patient's inhalation.

 h. If unsuccessful, after 15 seconds remove laryngoscope and return to step (a), and re-oxygenate the patient.

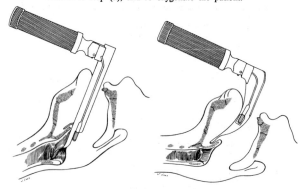

FIGURE 1

Straight vs. Curved Blade Laryngoscopy Positioning

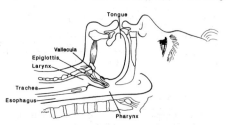

ANATOMY DURING DIRECT LARYNGOSCOPY

FIGURE 2

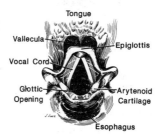

Anterior

Tongue

Vallecula — Epiglottis

Vocal Cord

Glottic — Arytenoid
Opening — Cartilage

Esophagus

Posterior

ANATOMY DURING DIRECT LARYNGOSCOPY

FIGURE 3

3. Post–intubation.
   a. Check for adequate and **symmetric** ventilation by inspection and auscultation of the chest.
   b. Inflate cuff with minimal amount of air that will prevent leakage around cuff during ventilation.
   c. Secure tube with adhesive or trach–tape to prevent dislodgement.
   d. Check tube position by CXR.
   e. After 10–20 minutes, obtain arterial blood gas and adjust ventilator accordingly.
4. **Nasotracheal intubation.**
   a. Prepare and position patient as for orotracheal intubation.
   b. Anesthetize nasal mucosa with cocaine or lidocaine and small dose of phenylephrine. This will provide both anesthesia and vasoconstriction to avoid epistaxis.
   c. Preoxygenate patient.
   d. Gently advance tube through well–lubricated nares, going up from nostril (to avoid the large inferior turbinate) and then posterior and down into the nasopharynx. Rotate tube to facilitate passage. The curve of the tube should be aligned to facilitate passage along this course.
   e. Listen for patient breath sounds *through* the nasotracheal tube. Advance tube into trachea blindly by advancing during inspiration.

    f. If unable to pass tube into trachea blindly, use laryngoscope and Magill forceps to introduce nasotracheal tube into the larynx under direct vision.

    g. Follow same post–intubation procedures as for orotracheal tube insertion.

E. Complications of intubation.

    1. Aspiration during attempted intubation.

    2. Malposition — esophageal intubation, extubation, endobronchial intubation. (Most common **lethal** error is esophageal placement; most common malposition is inserting tube too far into right mainstem bronchus, obstructing the left mainstem bronchus.)

    3. Tube obstruction — kinking, compression, foreign body, secretions.

    4. Traumatic intubation and tracheal erosion due to long–term intubation.

    5. Tracheoesophageal fistula — results from tracheal ischemia due to excessive pressure from tube and cuff.

    6. Spinal cord injuries resulting from hyperextension of neck in patients with unstable cervical spine injuries.

    7. If any question about tube placement, tube patency, or tube obstruction, remove tube and re–intubate.

II. CRICOTHYROTOMY

A. Definition — surgical transtracheal intubation through cricothyroid membrane.

B. Indications — **emergent** need for artificial airway in a patient who cannot be intubated via the oral or nasal routes.

C. Technique.

    1. Palpate thyroid and cricoid cartilage to define anatomy and identify cricothyroid membrane (Fig. 4).

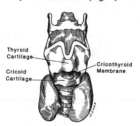

Thyroid Cartilage

Cricoid Cartilage

Cricothyroid Membrane

FIGURE 4
Anatomy of Cricothyroid Membrane

2. Make midline incision through the skin overlying cricothyroid membrane and expose membrane. If no scalpel is available, a 14 gauge IV catheter attached to oxygen source may provide temporary oxygenation. (**Caution:** Prolonged ventilation via the small catheter will result in hypercarbia due to inadequate exhalation of CO_2.)

3. Incise cricothyroid membrane with scalpel (horizontal incision) and enlarge ostomy by turning scalpel handle 90°.

4. Insert appropriate size (usually 6 or 7 mm) tracheostomy or endotracheal tube through ostomy (Fig. 5).

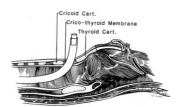

FIGURE 5
Insertion of Cricothyroid Airway

5. Check position of tube by auscultation and obtain CXR to confirm position.

6. Consider converting cricothyroidotomy to formal tracheostomy or endotracheal intubation when patient's condition allows.

D. **Complications.**
   1. Early — hemorrhage, creation of false passage, subcutaneous emphysema, perforation of esophagus, and mediastinal emphysema.
   2. Late — tracheal stenosis, especially in pediatric age group. Consider converting to formal tracheostomy early in children.

III. TRACHEOSTOMY

A. Definition — operative placement of an artificial airway through the anterior portion of the 2nd or 3rd tracheal ring.

B. **Indications.**
   1. Where surgery in upper airway may cause airway compromise, tracheostomy is done electively (head & neck surgical patients).
   2. Prolonged intubation.

       a. With the introduction of high–volume, low–pressure cuffed endotracheal tubes and minimal seal technique, prolonged intubation appears to be without significant complications as compared with tracheostomy where the respiratory support period is measured in days.

       b. Tracheostomy provides better patient comfort and may facilitate the weaning process if prolonged intubation is anticipated.

   3. Upper airway obstruction.

       a. Emergency airway control is more quickly accomplished by cricothyroidotomy.

       b. Anticipate problems or an inability to perform elective intubation when there is a large goiter, neck mass causing tracheal compression, laryngeal tumor, previous head and neck irradiation, etc.

C. Complications.

   1. Hemorrhage — bleeding occurs early due to inadequate hemostasis and can usually be managed with direct pressure, but occasionally requires reoperation. Late hemorrhage results from erosion into major vessel, usually innominate artery. Temporary control of bleeding should be obtained by placing a finger anterior to the trachea down into the mediastinum through the tracheostomy incision and compress innominate artery against sternum while patient is returned to O.R. for emergent ligation through a median sternotomy.

   2. Pneumothorax, pneumomediastinum, pneumoperitoneum — obtain CXR after tracheostomy tube placement and for any respiratory deterioration.

   3. Accidental extubation — in the early postoperative period, it may be very difficult to replace the tracheostomy tube since a mature tract has not yet developed. Replacement may be facilitated by passing a small red rubber catheter through the skin incision and into the trachea. Tracheostomy tube can then be passed over the catheter into proper position. (Remember, you can use any clamp or tool to hold soft tissues apart to allow air exchange.) It is preferable to place oral endotracheal tube until the situation is stabilized.

   4. Tube malposition — insertion of tracheostomy tube into bronchi or mediastinum may occur. Tube position should be confirmed postoperatively with CXR.

   5. Obstruction — foreign bodies, blood, inspissated secretion, and floppy cuffs may cause obstruction, requiring replacement of the tracheostomy tube.

   6. Swallowing dysfunction — the tracheostomy tube may cause difficulty swallowing, which resolves with removal of the tube or deflation of the cuff.

7. Tracheoesophageal fistula — reported incidence as high as 0.5% results from tracheal ischemia due to pressure from tracheostomy tube and cuff.
8. In the obese patient, a standard tracheostomy tube may not be long enough. If used, it easily becomes displaced into the pretracheal soft tissues. For overweight patients, a spiral–wound flexible endotracheal tube (Anode®) may be required.

TUBE THORACOSTOMY

I. DRAINAGE APPARATUS
A. **The 3–bottle system** (Fig. 1) — trap, underwater seal and suction regulation.

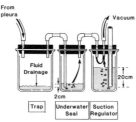

FIGURE 1

1. **Bottle 1 — the trap.** Fluid drained from pleural cavity remains in bottle.
2. **Bottle 2 — underwater seal.** Air is forced out from the pleural space during inspiration, when intrapleural pressure is negative.
3. **Bottle 3 — suction control.** Suction of –20 cm H_2O is achieved by placing tip of the tube 20 cm below H_2O surface of bottle 3, and increasing suction until air bubbles gently through the water.

B. **Compartmental plastic chest drainage units** (Fig. 2) — analogous to the bottles of the 3–bottle system.

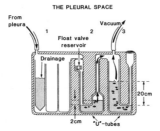

FIGURE 2

II. CHEST TUBE INSERTION

A. **Indications** — drainage of intrapleural air (pneumothorax) or fluid collections (pleural effusion, hemothorax, empyema).

1. Blood, pus, and pleural effusions are drained with a large (32-36 Fr.) tube placed through the 5th intercostal space in the midaxillary line, and directed posteriorly.

2. A simple pneumothorax is evacuated with a smaller (24-28 Fr.) tube in either the same position, or less commonly in the 2nd or 3rd intercostal space in the midclavicular line.

B. **Placement of chest tube** (5th intercostal space, midaxillary line).

1. Position the patient in a slightly oblique manner using a folded towel beneath the scapula. The arm is moved from the field by placing the hand behind the head.

2. Wear a mask, sterile gown and gloves. Prepare a wide field with bactericidal solution (i.e., povidone–iodine) and drape with sterile towels.

3. Infiltrate a wide area of skin and subcutaneous tissue over the 6th rib in the midaxillary line with local anesthetic agent (i.e., 1% lidocaine). [**Never place a chest tube very far inferior to the nipple line.**] Advance the needle down to the rib and inject the periosteum.

4. Advance the needle through the intercostal space superior to the 6th rib (this avoids the intercostal neurovascular bundle which lies inferior to the rib) until the pleural space is entered. Usually a small "pop" is felt during this, and aspiration of the syringe yields air or fluid.

5. The needle is then slowly withdrawn while aspirating until nothing further is returned. At that point a large bolus of local anesthetic (10 cc) is injected, which provides pleural anesthesia.

6. Using a # 10 scalpel blade, a skin incision is made down to the 6th rib. The incision should be large enough to admit the index finger.

7. Tunnel above the 6th rib into the 5th intercostal space using a Kelly clamp (Fig. 3). The intercostal muscles are split by spreading the clamp *gently*.

8. Once the pleura is reached, close clamp, grip the shaft of the clamp firmly, and carefully push the tip through the pleura (Fig. 4). There will usually be a rush of air, blood, or fluid when the pleural cavity is entered.

9. Spread the jaws of the clamp to create a hole large enough to admit an index finger, which is then placed into the pleural cavity to check for the presence of adhesions. The lung should be palpable during inspiration, insuring entrance into the pleural cavity.

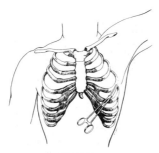

FIGURE 3

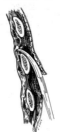

FIGURE 4

10. Grasp the chest tube at the tip (fenestrated end) with a Kelly clamp and guide the tube into the pleural space (Fig. 5). Ideal placement for most chest tubes is posterior to the lung and directed toward the apex. **Be sure the most proximal hole on the chest tube is intrapleural !!!**
11. Secure the tube to the skin with an 0 silk suture and connect the tube to a drainage apparatus (see Part I). Check for movement of fluid in the tubing during respiration. This is a good indicator of adequate intrapleural placement of the tube.
12. Apply an occlusive dressing using petroleum gauze, dry sterile gauze, benzoin, and cloth tape. Secure all connections with cloth tape.

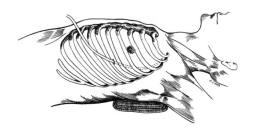

FIGURE 5

13. Obtain a STAT portable chest x-ray to document proper positioning of the tube, evacuation of air or fluid collections, and inflation of the lung.
14. REMEMBER: The procedure is NOT complete until the chest x-ray has been checked and a procedure note written.

C. **Maintenance.**
   1. Obtain daily portable chest x-rays until the tube is removed.
   2. Change dressing periodically to inspect the site, making sure the suture remains intact. Redress tube as described earlier.
   3. Never clamp a chest tube (risks a tension hydro/pneumothorax); only leave on water seal.

III. CHEST TUBE REMOVAL

A. Iatrogenic pneumothorax is the common complication.
B. Patient cooperation is essential.
C. **Procedure** (Figs. 6-8).
   1. Remove all dressings and cut the anchoring suture.
   2. Cleanse the skin with alcohol.
   3. Prepare a small dressing sponge by applying a generous amount of Betadine® ointment.
   4. With sterile gloved hand, pinch skin together around chest tube.
   5. Rapidly remove the chest tube while pinching skin together to avoid introduction of air.
   6. Apply generous amount of Betadine® ointment to thoracostomy site to afford a barrier to air.
   7. Release skin and apply dressing sponge to site.
   8. Cover dressing in an air-tight fashion with adhesive tape.
   9. Dressing should remain in place for 24–48 hrs.

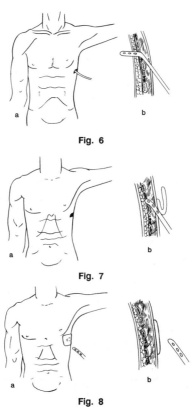

Fig. 6

Fig. 7

Fig. 8
Chest Tube Removal
(a = frontal view, b = sagittal view)

THORACENTESIS

I. INDICATIONS
A. Diagnostic evaluation of pleural effusion.
B. Therapeutic aspiration of fluid or air to return lung volume.

II. MATERIALS
A. Thoracentesis kit — become familiar with the set available. Most are based on a catheter–over–needle design.
B. Without a kit:
  1. Local anesthetic, sterile drapes, prep kit, gloves.
  2. 25 gauge needle, 22 gauge 1½" needle, 5 cc syringe.
  3. 16–18 gauge angiocath, 20–60 cc syringe.
  4. Three–way stopcock.
  5. IV tubing, collection container, hemostat.
C. 500–1000 cc evacuated bottle.

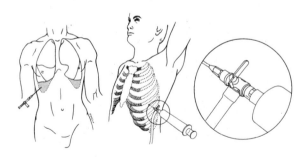

FIGURE 1
Thoracentesis

III. PROCEDURE

A. Review CXR to localize fluid. Blunting of the costophrenic angle on PA view indicates > 250 cc is present. **Ultrasound guidance** is useful to localize loculated effusions.

B. Obtain informed consent.

C. The patient should be sitting comfortably, leaning forward with arms resting on a bedside table.

D. Generally performed along the **posterior axillary line** from the back. The fluid level is confirmed by percussion of dullness and counting ribs on CXR. The correct site is 1–2 interspaces *below* the level of the effusion, but *NOT* below the 8th intercostal space.

E. Using sterile technique, the area is prepped and draped. Local anesthetic is infiltrated intradermally over the superior margin of the rib below the chosen interspace. This is continued with the 1½" needle through the subcutaneous tissue to infiltrate the periosteum and intercostal muscles. Care is taken to aspirate with each move. When the pleura is entered and fluid returned, note depth with a clamp and withdraw the syringe 0.5 cm and inject to anesthetize the pleura. Then remove needle.

F. Insert a 16–18 gauge angiocath through the anesthetized area to the previous depth while **continuously aspirating**. Care must be taken to avoid the neurovascular bundle (by advancing *over* the superior portion of the rib). The pleura has been entered when fluid returns. Advance the angiocath over the needle and withdraw the needle. Occlude the catheter lumen with a finger to prevent a pneumothorax. Interspace a 3–way stopcock between the angiocath and large syringe. The third lumen is directed to the collecting chamber.

G. Confirm position by aspirating into syringe with the stopcock "off" to the collection chamber. If good return is noted, turn the stopcock "off" to the patient and expel the contents of the syringe into the collection chamber. Repeat this procedure until the desired amount of fluid is removed or no further fluid is obtained. When an evacuated bottle is used, after confirming position of the catheter, turn the stopcock "off" to the syringe and allow free aspiration.

H. Remove the angiocath and apply a sterile dressing.

I. Recommended **pleural fluid studies** — specific gravity; pH; cell count and differential; LDH; amylase; glucose; protein; gram stain; bacterial, fungal, and AFB cultures. Cytology should be obtained if malignancy is suspected (requires increased volume of fluid into a heparinized bottle). Specific protein subsets if collagen vascular, or rheumatoid disease suspected.

J. Obtain a CXR to confirm the efficacy of the aspiration and to rule out a pneumothorax.

IV. INTERPRETATION OF THE RESULTS

Labs	Transudate	Exudate
Protein	< 3 g/dl	> 3 g/dl
Specific gravity	< 1.016	> 1.016
LDH	Low	High
LDH ratio (effusion:serum)	< .5	> .6
Glucose	2/3 serum glucose	Low
Amylase		500 Units/ml
RBC	< 10 k/mm^3	> 100k/mm^3
WBC	< 1000/mm^3	> 1000/mm^3

V. DIFFERENTIAL DIAGNOSIS
A. Transudate — cirrhosis, nephrotic syndrome, CHF, lobar atelectasis, viral infection.
B. Exudate — bacterial or viral infection, neoplasm, intra–abdominal infection, pancreatitis, TB, trauma, pulmonary infarction, chylous effusion.
C. Grossly bloody — iatrogenic injury, pulmonary infarction, trauma, tumor, hepatic or splenic puncture.
D. Extremely low glucose consistent with rheumatoid process.

VI. COMPLICATIONS
A. Pneumothorax.
B. Hemothorax.
C. Hepatic or splenic puncture.
D. Parenchymal tear.
E. Infection (may lead to empyema).

BLADDER CATHETERIZATION

I. URETHRAL CATHETERIZATION

A. **Continuous catheterization** – indications:
   1. Monitor urine output (indication of perfusion in trauma, shock, and perioperative fluid management).
   2. Relieve urinary retention secondary to obstruction or loss of bladder tone.
   3. Urinary incontinence.
   4. Perineal wounds (burns, operative, traumatic) to prevent soilage.

B. **Intermittent catheterization** – indications:
   1. Determine post–void residuals secondary to obstruction or neurogenic bladder.
   2. Sterile diagnostic urinalysis and cultures.
   3. Management of neurogenic bladder and chronic urinary retention.

C. **Contraindications:**
   1. Urethral disruption – of concern in males with pelvic trauma or deceleration accidents (see "Urologic Problems" section II).
   2. Prostatic or urethral infection (relative).
   3. Recent urethral or bladder neck surgery or repair of urethral or vesical fistula.

D. **Materials** – 16–20 Fr. foley catheter with 5 cc balloon (18 Fr. most common). Pediatric feeding tube in infants (no balloon).
   1. Sterile catheterization kit with water soluble lubricant, gloves, prep solution, cotton balls, drapes, and water for balloon inflation.
   2. Closed drainage system.
   3. Normal saline irrigation and a catheter syringe.

E. **Technique – males.**
   1. Position patient in the supine position. Lay out equipment in a convenient array with both hands sterilely gloved. Confirm integrity of foley balloon. Drape field with opening in drape over the penis.
   2. Grasp the penis with non–dominant hand and hold erect with modest tension (this hand is now contaminated and must remain in place). Prep the glans, foreskin and meatus. Be sure that the foreskin is retracted in an uncircumsized male to allow for an adequate prep.
   3. Insert the well–lubricated catheter into the meatus while maintaining tension on the penis. There will be some resistance as the catheter passes the prostate and sphincter. The catheter should be inserted a sufficient distance so as to ensure the balloon will not lie within the urethra (to the hub of the catheter), and urine should return confirming the catheter tip is within the bladder. If no urine is obtained, irrigate with

20–30 cc of normal saline to clear the ports. If there is free return of irrigation, it is unlikely that the catheter resides in the urethra.

4. When confident that the balloon lies within the bladder, inflate the balloon with 5 cc of sterile water and withdraw catheter to seat balloon against the prostate or bladder neck. Connect the catheter to closed–drainage system.

5. Advance foreskin to **prevent paraphimosis**. Secure catheter to patient's thigh or abdomen to prevent accidental dislodgement.

F. **Technique – females.**

1. Position patient supine with knees flexed and legs fully abducted ("frog–leg" position). Arrange equipment in a convenient array with both hands sterilely gloved. Drape patient.

2. Spread labia with fingers of non–dominant hand to expose the urethral meatus (this hand is now contaminated and must remain in position). Prep introitus from anterior to posterior.

3. Sterilely insert well–lubricated catheter into urethral meatus to approximately 15 cm. The return of urine confirms position in the bladder. If no urine returns, irrigate the catheter with 20–30 cc of sterile saline. Free return of urine makes it unlikely that the catheter remains within the urethra.

4. Inflate balloon with 5 cc of sterile water. Withdraw catheter gently to seat against the bladder neck. Attach closed–drainage system to catheter and secure to the patient's thigh or abdomen to prevent accidental dislodgement.

G. **Difficult urethral catheterizations.**

1. Causes – meatal stricture, urethral stricture, prostatic hypertrophy, urethral disruption.

2. Possible solutions.

   a. Assure that catheter is well lubricated, and repeat attempt.

   b. Attempt intubation with larger or smaller catheters.

   c. Inject 5–10 cc sterile lubricant into urethral meatus.

   d. If pain limits procedure, xylocaine jelly can be used as lubrication.

   e. Meatal strictures can be dilated with a hemostat.

   f. Filiform and followers may be necessary to obtain access to the bladder if a catheter will not pass. This should be done by a urologist.

   g. If still unable to pass a catheter by these methods:

      1) Consider the possibility of urethral disruption and obtain a retrograde cystourethrogram.

      2) Consider urologic placement of a catheter with endoscopic aid or placement of a suprapubic catheter for bladder drainage.

H. **Care of urethral catheters.**

1. Aseptic technique during insertion.

2. Remove catheter as soon as feasible.

GI INTUBATION

I. **STOMACH**

A. **Nasogastric (NG) tubes** —used primarily for gastric decompression. Pass the largest size tolerable to the patient. Feeding is best accomplished by nasoduodenal tubes.

1. **Levin tube** — a straight tube with a single lumen. It must be connected to intermittent suction to prevent the gastric mucosa from occluding the tube. Relatively soft, fairly well tolerated.

2. **Salem sump tube** — more popular.

   a. This stiffer tube permits easier placement at the cost of increased patient discomfort.

   b. The main lumen should be placed on low continuous suction. A sideport (blue) vents the tube to allow continuous sump suction.

   c. The vent must be kept open while on suction or the gastric mucosa will occlude the tube.

   d. The vent should be flushed with 30 cc of air and the main lumen with 30 cc of saline every 3–4 hrs to ensure patency. The vent is patent when it "whistles" continuously.

3. **Method of insertion.**

   a. Elevate the head of the patient at least 30°.

   b. Inspect nostrils for patency.

   c. Lubricate the tube with water soluble lubricant or lidocaine jelly.

   d. Insert the tube into a nostril and pass it into the nasopharynx. The patient should swallow when the tube is felt in the back of the throat. Sips of water will facilitate passage of the tube into the esophagus in an awake patient.

   e. Advance into the esophagus and stomach.

   f. A guide to the length of tube inserted (Salem sumps) is a series of four black marks on the main lumen. The proximal mark, at the nares, indicates insertion to the distal esophagus, the middle two marks to the body of the stomach, and the distal mark to the pylorus/duodenum.

   g. Inadvertent naso–tracheal intubation is confirmed by the patient gasping for air, coughing, or an inability to speak. These signs may be absent. You must confirm intragastric position of tube prior to using the tube.

   h. Confirm tube position by instilling 20–30 cc of air while listening over the stomach with a stethoscope and by aspiration of gastric contents. Aspiration of gastric contents is a more reliable method.

   i. Use of viscous lidocaine and Cetacaine® spray minimizes patient discomfort.

    j. Secure the tube with tape. Tubes taped tightly to the nostril or nasal septum may lead to pressure necrosis.
    k. Patients with a Zenker's diverticulum may need endoscopic guidance for safe insertion.

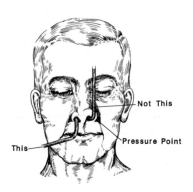

FIGURE 1

B. Orogastric tubes.
    1. Preferred if NG intubation is contraindicated (anterior basilar skull fracture, nasopharyngeal trauma).
    2. **Ewald tube** — especially suited for lavage of the stomach and emergency evacuation of blood, toxic agents, medications, or other substances. Evacuation of blood cannot be accomplished through a Levin or Salem sump tube.
      a. Large (18–36 Fr) double–lumen tube.
      b. The 36 Fr lumen is connected to continuous suction, the 18 Fr lumen is used for irrigation.
      c. **Method of insertion** — in patients with loss of consciousness or loss of the gag reflex, insertion of a cuffed endotracheal tube prior to orogastric tube insertion is preferred.
        1) Lubricate the tube.
        2) Insert the tube into the mouth and down the esophagus into the stomach. If the patient is conscious, have the patient sip water.
        3) Verify the position of the tube by aspiration of gastric contents and by auscultation.

4) Connect to suction; begin irrigation when the stomach is empty. The amount of irrigant used should be monitored. The large bore of this tube may allow rapid overdistention of the stomach with the resultant risk of aspiration.

II. DUODENAL / SMALL BOWEL TUBES
A. Nasoduodenal feeding tubes.
1. Tubes are smaller, soft, and flexible; better tolerated than NG tubes.
2. **Prior to institution of tube feedings, the tube position must be verified by x-ray.**
3. Types of tubes.
   a. **Corpak®** — unweighted, has a bullet at the tip to prevent passage of tube into regions of the tracheobronchial tree that lack cartilaginous support; a wire stylet may be used to pass tube into duodenum under fluoroscopic guidance.
   b. **Frederick–Miller** — has a stylet with flexible and stiff ends. Must only be placed under fluoroscopic guidance to prevent inadvertent tracheobronchial placement. This tube is much easier to pass into the duodenum.
   c. Dobbhoff®, Entriflex®, and Flexiflow® tubes are associated with accidental tracheobronchial placement, and are less popular.
   d. Passage of the tube past the ligament of Treitz eliminates most of the potential for aspiration.
   e. Nasoduodenal tubes allow for early institution of enteric feedings, prior to full resolution of ileus.
B. Nasointestinal tubes for decompression of the small bowel.
1. **Cantor tube** — single–lumen tube with a mercury–filled balloon at the distal end.
   a. To prepare the balloon tip, inject 5 cc of mercury into the middle of the balloon tangentially with 21 gauge needle, then withdraw all air from the balloon.
   b. Lubricate the tube.
   c. While the patient is sitting upright, use a cotton–tipped applicator to help guide the balloon into the nasopharynx. When the tube falls into the back of the throat, have the patient swallow and the tube will travel by gravity into the stomach.
   d. Once the tube is in the stomach, aspirate stomach contents, then place to gravity.
   e. Tape the tube to side of face with 4–6" loop. This permits the tube to advance by peristalsis.
   f. Place the patient on their right side and advance the tube to the "P" position as marked on the outside of the tube. Have the patient remain in this position until the "D" mark is at external nares, indicating passage into the duodenum.

    g. Confirm duodenal position by x-ray. The tube may be positioned at the pylorus under fluoroscopic guidance.

    h. Place the patient on their left side until the tube has advanced several inches. Allow the patient to resume activity and the tube to be drawn downward by peristalsis. Leave a 4" loop free. Pass the tube 3" every 4 hours. Irrigate with 15 cc saline before advancing the tube.

    i. When the tube will no longer advance by peristalsis, place on low intermittent suction.

    j. To remove the tube, slow gentle withdrawal is necessary. The tube should be withdrawn approximately 1 foot per hour to prevent intussusception.

  2. Miller–Abbott tube — dual lumen with 1 lumen for intermittent suction and the other to a balloon which can be filled with mercury or water once the tube enters the stomach.

C. Tubes for intraoperative intestinal decompression.

  1. Types.

    a. Baker tube — dual lumen.

      1) Balloon.

      2) Suction port.

      3) 16 French soft pliable plastic.

    b. Dennis — triple lumen.

      1) Balloon.

      2) Suction port.

      3) Sump port — made of same plastic as a Salem sump.

    c. Leonard — dual lumen.

      1) Balloon.

      2) Stylet.

      3) Firm–coiled spring in the distal 7 feet to facilitate passage and allow removal of the stylet.

  2. Placement.

    a. Introduce tube into stomach via oral or nasogastric route.

    b. Inflate the balloon and pass manually through the duodenum into the small bowel.

    c. May be placed through an enterotomy at the risk of intra–abdominal enteric spillage.

III. SENGSTAKEN–BLAKEMORE TUBE

A. Designed for balloon tamponade of bleeding esophageal or gastric varices.

B. Insertion — prior to insertion, an accurate endoscopic diagnosis is preferable to rule out alternative bleeding sites and document the source of bleeding. In an unstable patient with a high clinical suspicion of varices, it is often necessary to use empirically.

  1. Check the balloons under water to assure that no leaks are present and to verify patency of all 3 lumens of the tube.

2. Measures to prevent aspiration.
   a. Endotracheal intubation in virtually all patients.
   b. Gastric lavage to empty stomach.
   c. Have wall suction available.
   d. Pharynx is *not* anesthetized so as to maintain the gag reflex if the patient is not intubated.
3. Lubricate the tube and pass it into the stomach via the mouth.
4. The tube is advanced fully and air is injected into the suction lumen while auscultating over the stomach region.
5. Confirm the intragastric location of the gastric balloon by instilling small amount of water soluble contrast into the balloon and obtaining an x-ray *before* inflating balloon fully.
6. Inflate the gastric balloon slowly with 200–300 cc of air and double clamp with rubber–shod surgical clamps. Stop air inflation *immediately* if the patient complains of epigastric pain or if insufflation of air is not audible over the epigastric region.
7. Apply gentle traction on the tube until resistance indicates that the balloon is at the esophagogastric junction.
8. Tape the tube to the facemask of a football helmet or attach to 1–2 pounds of traction to maintain gentle traction of tube.
9. Aspirate the gastric tube (suction tube) or lavage with saline. If there is no evidence of continued bleeding, there is no need to inflate the esophageal balloon.
10. A second nasoesophageal tube is passed into the proximal esophagus to monitor continued bleeding above the gastric and/or esophageal balloons and to aspirate salivary secretions. The Minnesota tube is a modification which has an esophageal port to obviate the need for this extra tube.
11. If bleeding continues, the esophageal balloon is slowly inflated to 40 mm Hg; a standard sphygmomanometer can be attached to monitor pressure. Use the lowest pressure that stops bleeding. Double clamp balloon inlet with rubber–shod surgical clamps. **Do not** inflate the esophageal balloon > 40 mm Hg.
12. Gastric and esophageal lumens are connected to intermittent suction.
13. Tape scissors to the head of the bed in plain view if urgent transection and removal of the tube is required.
14. Irrigate the gastric lumen tube frequently and record the appearance of the return fluid.
15. Both balloons are inflated for 24 hrs after which the esophageal balloon is slowly deflated and the patient is observed for signs of rebleeding. If rebleeding occurs, the esophageal balloon is reinflated.
16. If no rebleeding, the gastric balloon is deflated after 24 hrs and the patient is observed.

17. If no further bleeding occurs 24 hrs after the gastric balloon is deflated, mineral oil should be given prior to removal. The tube is completely transected with scissors and removed. This ensures that balloons are deflated completely and that the tube is not re-used.
18. The esophageal balloon is always deflated first to prevent the risk of migration then asphyxiation.
19. Constant nursing supervision is essential. Complications are frequent and include aspiration, mucosal bleeding, and perforation.

PARACENTESIS

I. INDICATIONS
A. Diagnostic.
   1. Peritoneal fluid for diagnostic studies.
   2. Determine presence of intraabdominal hemorrhage.
B. Therapeutic.
   1. Removal of ascitic fluid to decrease intraabdominal pressure and relieve respiratory compromise.
   2. Control of ascites refractory to medical management.

II. ETIOLOGY OF ASCITES
A. Transudate.
   1. Cirrhosis — most common etiology.
   2. Congestive heart failure, particularly right sided with hepatic congestion.
   3. Nephrotic syndrome.
B. Exudate.
   1. Malignancy — most common etiology.
   2. Peritonitis.
   3. Pancreatitis.
   4. Tuberculosis.
   5. Chylous ascites.
C. Composition characteristics:

	Transudate	Exudate
Total protein	< 3 g/dl	> 3 g/dl
Specific gravity	< 1.016	> 1.016
LDH	< 200 IU	> 200 IU
Fibrinogen	No	Yes
WBC	< 1000/mm^3	> 1000/mm^3
RBC	< 100/mm^3	> 100/mm^3

III. TECHNIQUE
A. Empty urinary bladder.
B. Identify anatomic landmarks (Fig. 1).
   1. Site most commonly used is the left iliac fossa.
   2. Right iliac fossa may be used if splenomegaly is suspected.
   3. Avoid epigastric vessels and previous surgical scars.
C. The patient is rolled slightly toward the operator.
D. Check for shifting dullness to percussion.
E. Prep and drape, use local anesthetic for skin wheal. Small ascitic collections (< 500 cc) may require ultrasound guidance.
F. Insert an 18–20 gauge angiocath with a 1½" needle while aspirating until the free flow of fluid is obtained; the catheter is advanced

and the needle is withdrawn. The angiocath should be connected by extention IV tubing to a 3-way stopcock to decrease the risk of accidental dislodgement.

G. Removal of large amounts of fluid is facilitated by the use of an evacuated IV bottle connected to non-collapsible tubing.

H. **Diagnostic.**
1. 50–100 cc of fluid is sufficient for evaluation.
2. Fluid is sent for the laboratory studies outlined in the table above — amylase, cytology, gram stain, and bacterial, fungal, and TB culture when appropriate.

I. **Therapeutic.**
1. Up to 5 liters of ascitic fluid can be removed safely at one 30–90 min setting; reaccumulation of ascites with hypovolemia usually results and subsequent volume replacement should be undertaken if peripheral edema is not present.
2. Must be coupled with sodium and fluid restriction, as well as diuretic therapy for long–term ascites control.
3. If repeated paracentesis is required to control ascites, then a peritoneovenous shunt should be considered.

IV. COMPLICATIONS

A. Persistent ascites leakage — 3–5% incidence.
B. Bleeding — 1–2% incidence.
C. Infection — < 1% incidence.
D. Perforated viscus.
E. Hemodynamic instability.
F. Renal failure.
G. Protein depletion.
H. Electrolyte abnormalities.

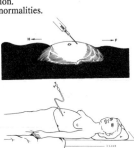

FIGURE 1
Anatomic landmarks for paracentesis

DIAGNOSTIC PERITONEAL LAVAGE (DPL)

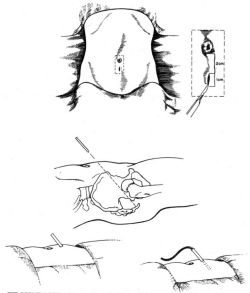

I. TECHNIQUE (Semi-Open) (Favored Technique at Our Institution)

A. Insert NG tube and Foley catheter — stomach and bladder must be decompressed to avoid injury.

B. Restrain patient.

C. Sedate patient if necessary.

D. Shave periumbilical region — above and below umbilicus.

E. Prep region widely with betadine.

F. Drape with sterile towels.

G. Decide on supra- or infra–umbilical incision.

H. Infiltrate proposed site (skin and subcutaneous tissue) with 1% xylocaine with epinephrine — enhances local hemostasis, use even in comatose or anesthetized patient.

I.   Incise skin (1–5 cm vertical incision needed depending on body habitus) and subcutaneous tissue down to midline fascia.

J.   Using #11 scalpel blade, make a 2–3 mm stab incision in fascia.

K.   Place towel clips on both sides of this fascial incision for traction.

L.   With strong upward traction on the towel clips by the assistant, the operator places the trochar–catheter apparatus through the fascial opening and then pushes it through the peritoneum (+/– posterior fascia). This initial push should be done perpendicular to the skin and must stop after one feels the "pop" of the peritoneum. At this point, the trochar–catheter apparatus is tilted down, the catheter alone is advanced toward the pelvis and the trochar removed.

M. Attach the aspirating device and aspirate using a 12 cc syringe.

N. If aspirate is negative, instill 1 liter (10 cc/kg in children) Ringer's lactate or normal saline hung from a pressure bag. Shake the patient's abdomen periodically.

O. When only a small level of fluid remains in the bag, drop the near–empty bag to the floor to drain the fluid. The fluid drains by siphon action, hence if all the fluid is allowed to run in along with some air, the siphon is lost and must be re–started by applying suction via a needle and syringe to a port in the tubing. Tubing used must *not* have a one–way filter device.

P. While the fluid is draining, one must keep a sponge packed into the wound for hemostasis and constantly hold the catheter in place.

Q. After the fluid has returned (at least 300 cc), clamp the tubing and withdraw catheter (avoids siphoning blood from wound into bag).

R. Wound closure — an optional heavy suture may be placed to close the fascial defect, skin closure with skin staples (hold ends of wound taut with towel clips).

II. TECHNICAL VARIATIONS

A. Open technique — midline fascia is incised over 3–4 cm, posterior fascia/peritoneum is held with hemostats and opened under direct vision, catheter without trochar is advanced into peritoneal cavity. Fascial closure required at completion.

B. Closed technique — #11 scalpel blade is used to incise a tract of skin, subcutaneous tissue and midline fascia, catheter–trochar is pushed through as in semi–open technique. *Not* recommended due to greater potential for intra–abdominal injury.

C. Closed, Seldinger technique — uses needle/trochar, guide wire and advancing catheter.

III. TROUBLE–SHOOTING

A. Slow fluid return — adjust catheter position, twist catheter, place patient in reverse Trendelenburg position, apply manual pressure to abdomen, instill an additional 500 cc fluid.

B. Siphon lost (air in tubing) — check all connections, make certain catheter is advanced far enough to avoid exposed side holes, re–establish siphon as described above.

PRINCIPLES OF ABSCESS DRAINAGE

I. **DEEP ABSCESSES**
A. Intra–abdominal, intramuscular, and deep breast abscesses require drainage in the O.R. for adequate analgesia, exposure, and equipment.
B. CT scan or ultrasound–guided drainage catheter placement can be considered in specific cases.

II. **SUPERFICIAL ABSCESSES**
A. Usually subcutaneous and should be easily accessible if E.R. or bedside drainage is considered.
B. **Technique.**
   1. IV sedation with narcotic (e.g., sublimaze, morphine, meperidine) and sedative (e.g., diazepam, midazolam).
   2. IM less well controlled, but an alternative.
   3. Narcan® should be available.
   4. Sterile prep and drape.
   5. Local anesthesia (see "Anesthesia") with field block. Relative acid environment of infected tissue diminishes efficacy of local infiltration anesthetics.
   6. Aspirate fluctuant area with 18–gauge needle to collect good sample of purulent material for anaerobic and aerobic culture.
   7. If in the head and neck region, observe pus for "sulfur granules" characteristic of *Actinomyces israelii*. If present, send sample to mycology for KOH prep and culture, then treat with penicillin or tetracycline.
   8. Adequate incision over fluctuant area.
   9. Swab for culture.
   10. Break down loculations with finger or instrument.
   11. Irrigate liberally with NS; antibiotic–containing solution is of little benefit.
   12. Pack cavity with thin–strip gauze.
   13. Remove pack at 48 hrs and treat as indicated based on status at that time.
C. Use of systemic antibiotics (PO or IV) will depend on degree of surrounding cellulitis and condition of patient. Broad–spectrum coverage at first, then specific therapy, if still indicated, based on culture results.
D. Superficial abscesses or furunculosis are sometimes early harbingers of diabetes. Check 2–hour post–prandial blood sugar.
E. Superficial abscesses in a known diabetic require careful follow–up. It is usually necessary to administer systemic antibiotics and adjust insulin.

F. **Hidradenitis suppurativa** — chronic infection of the cutaneous apocrine glands, subcutaneous tissue, and fascia; confined to areas in which these glands are found (e.g., axilla, areola of the nipple, groin, perineum, and circumanal and periumbilical regions).
  1. Culture yields a variety of saprophytic and pathogenic bacteria (preponderance of *Staphylococci* and *Streptococci*).
  2. Mild cases respond to high dosages of tetracycline.
  3. If suppurative, incision and drainage is necessary.
  4. Treatment of chronic cases involves excision of the involved area (may require skin graft for coverage).
G. **Sebaceous cyst** — plugged ducts of the ceruminous skin glands cause accumulation of sebum and formation of a cyst. These glands are most numerous on the face and the midline of the trunk. They are usually painless and non–tender, but may become secondarily infected.
  1. If infection is present, incision and drainage should be performed followed by planned excision at a second stage once the infection has totally resolved.
  2. If non–infected, surgical excision of the entire cyst is indicated.

GRAM STAIN TECHNIQUE

I. Smear thin layer of material to be stained on slide using a wire loop which has been previously flame sterilized and cooled.

II. Allow material to air dry. Three quick passes through flame may accelerate this, but heat may destroy organisms due to protein denaturing.

III. Apply in order:

	Normal prep	Quick prep
Gentian violet	1 minute	15 seconds
Iodine	1 minute	15 seconds
Alcohol	few seconds	few seconds
Wash in water	few seconds	few seconds (distilled preferred)
Safranin	1 minute	15–20 seconds

The alcohol should be applied in amount and length of time sufficient only to decolorize.

IV. Under oil immersion:

Gram-positive organisms retain the Gentian violet and appear dark blue/purple.

Gram-negative are decolorized, re-stain with Safranin, and appear red.

PART IV

FORMULARY

CATEGORIES

GENERIC DRUGS

AMMONIA DETOXIFIERS, AIDS IN HEPATIC ENCEPHALOPATHY

DRUG	SUPPLIED	DOSE/ROUTE	REMARKS
Lactulose (Cephulac, Chronulac)	Solution: 3.33 g/5 ml	**Portal-systemic encephalopathy:** <u>PO</u>: 30-45 ml 3-4 times daily initially, then adjust dose to produce 2-3 soft stools per day or stool pH of 5. Usual dose is 90-150 ml/day. <u>PR</u>: 300 ml diluted with 700 ml water or 0.9% sodium chloride administered rectally and retained for 30-60 min during 4-6 h as necessary. **Constipation:** <u>PO</u>: 15-30 ml daily.	Indicated in portal-systemic encephalopathy, constipation. *Contraindicated* in low-galactose diet. Results are comparable to those achieved with neomycin. Decreases blood ammonia concentration by 25-50% as a result of acidification of colon contents and formation of ammonium ion. May be used in renal failure or partial deafness. Less than 3% is absorbed from the small intestine following oral administration. Can be given concomitantly with oral neomycin.
Neomycin sulfate (Mycifradin)	Tabs: 0.5 g Solution: 125 mg/5 ml	**Hepatic coma:** <u>PO</u>: 4-12 g/day in 4 divided doses. <u>PR</u>: 1% solution as a retention enema as necessary. **Bowel preps:** a. Condon-Nichols: 1 g neomycin and 1 g erythromycin base po at 1 pm, 2 pm, 11 pm day before surgery. b. Hunter: 1 g neomycin po q 1 h for 4 h, then q 4 h for 36 h. Erythromycin base 1 g po q 6 h for 36 h.	*Contraindicated* in intestinal obstruction and neomycin sensitivity; 97% unabsorbed. *Caution* with concurrent use of other nephrotoxic and ototoxic drugs.

ANTI-ARRHYTHMICS

DRUG	SUPPLIED	DOSE/ROUTE	REMARKS
Bretylium (Bretylol)	Vial: 50 mg/ml	**Acute ventricular arrhythmias:** 5 mg/kg undiluted IVP over 1 min; may repeat with 10 mg/kg if no response as necessary. **Maintenance therapy:** 5-10 mg/kg IM/IV q 6-8 hrs or 1-2 mg/min via continuous infusion.	Useful in ventricular fibrillation and ventricular tachycardia, but no better than lidocaine. Second drug of choice following lidocaine for treatment of ventricular fibrillation. Frequent hypotension may develop within first hour of therapy.
Procainamide HCl (Pronestyl)	Vial: 100 mg/ml, 500 mg/ml	100 mg IV over 1 min; repeat 100 mg every 5 min until arrythmia is controlled or to a total of 1 g. <u>Infusion</u>: 0.02-0.08 mg/kg/min.	Secondary drug for ventricular arrhythmias that are not digitalis induced. Therapeutic plasma concentration is 4-8 μg/ml.

ANTI–ARRHYTHMICS (continued)

DRUG	SUPPLIED	DOSE/ROUTE	REMARKS
Propranolol HCl (Inderal)	Tabs: 10,20,40,60, 80,90 mg. Amp: 1 mg/ml. Extended release caps: 80,120, 160 mg	Parenteral: 1-3 mg IV slowly (< 1 mg/min), may repeat initial dose after 2 min; then wait at least 4 h before additional doses. Oral: Hypertension: 40 mg po bid initially, then gradual increments up to 640 mg/day. Usual maintenance dose: 120-240 mg/day. Angina pectoris: 10-20 mg po tid or qid initially, then gradual increments q 3-7 days up to 320 mg/day until optimal response. Usual maintenance dose: 160-240 mg/day.	Contraindicated in sinus bradycardia, cardiogenic shock, heart block greater than first degree, bronchial asthma. Non-selective β-adrenergic blocking agent. Cardiac arrhythmias: 10-30 mg tid or qid. Migraine prophylaxis: 80 mg/day in divided doses initially, then up to 240 mg/day by gradual increments. Pheochromocytoma (as adjunct to α-adrenergic blocking agents): 60 mg/day in divided doses for 3 days prior to surgery, or 30 mg/day in divided doses for inoperable tumors. Myocardial infarction: 180-240 mg daily, bid, tid or qid beginning 5-21 days after infarction.
Quinidine gluconate (Quinaglute, Duraquin)	Extended release tabs: 324,330 mg Vial: 80 mg/ml	IM: 600 mg, then up to 400 mg q 2 h adjusting dose by the effect of the previous dose. IV: 800 mg diluted with 40 ml D5W and administered at a rate of 16 mg/min.	Can decrease myocardial contractility. Comparable activity to procainamide in the treatment of atrial or ventricular arrhythmias. With IV administration, monitor blood pressure during infusion.
Quinidine polygalacturonate (Cardioquin)	Tabs: 275 mg	PO: 275-325 mg initially, followed by 2nd dose in 3-4 h if necessary; usual daily dose 275 mg 2-3x/day.	
Quinidine sulfate (Quinidex, Cin-Quin)	Caps: 200,300 mg Tabs: 100,200,300 mg Extended release tabs: 300 mg Vial: 200 mg/ml	PO: 200-400 mg q 2-4 h until normal sinus rhythm returns or toxic effects occur; usual daily dose is 200-400 mg 3-4 times daily.	

ANTI-ARRHYTHMICS (continued)

DRUG	SUPPLIED	DOSE/ROUTE	REMARKS
Tocainide (Tonocard)	Tabs: 400,600 mg	PO: initially 400 mg q 8 h; usual maintenance dose is 1.2-1.8 g daily in 3 divided doses.	Electrophysiologically and hemodynamically similar to lidocaine. Therapeutic plasma concentration is usually 4-10 µg/ml. Appears as effective as disopyramide, procainamide or quinidine in preventing and/or suppressing PVC's and/or ventricular tachycardia.
Verapamil (Calan, Isoptin)	Amps: 2.5 mg/ml Tabs: 80,120 mg SR tabs: 240 mg	IVP: 5-10 mg slow IV bolus over 2-3 min; dose may be repeated after 30 min if unsatisfactory initial response. IV infusion: 2.5-5.0 µg/kg/min to maintain rate.	Contraindicated in severe CHF and shock. Metabolized in liver; renal excretion. Onset of action is within 1-2 min with peak effect occurring in 10-15 min. Used in rapid conversion to sinus rhythm of paroxysmal reentrant SVT's that incorporate the AV node as part or all of the reentrant circuit. Also used for temporary control of rapid ventricular rate in atrial flutter or atrial fibrillation. Can cause bradycardia, high-degree AV block and asystole, and transient ventricular ectopy.
Xylocaine (Lidocaine)	Vial: 100 mg/ml and others	IV loading dose: 1 mg/kg; additional 0.5 mg/kg bolus infusions q 10 min as needed to a total of 3 mg/kg. Infusion: 2-4 mg/min.	Drug of choice for ventricular tachycardia, fibrillation, and premature beats. Elevates fibrillation threshold. Therapeutic plasma concentration is 1-5 µg/ml.

MISCELLANEOUS ANTIBIOTICS

DRUG	SUPPLIED	DOSE/ROUTE	REMARKS
Bacitracin	Parenteral: 10,000 units, 50,000 units	IM: 10,000 - 25,000 U q 6 h. PO: 500 mg (non-absorbed). Most commonly used as a topical ointment.	Not administered intravenously. Covers gram-positives, especially Staphylococcus, Clostridium difficile. May increase or prolong skeletal muscle relaxation produced by neuromuscular blocking agents or anesthetics. Can cause nephrotoxicity and albuminuria. Total adult daily dose should not exceed 100,000 units. Has been replaced by the penicillinase-resistant penicillins or cephalosporins.

MISCELLANEOUS ANTIBIOTICS (continued)

DRUG	SUPPLIED	DOSE/ROUTE	REMARKS
Chloramphenicol (Chloromycetin)	Caps: 250 mg Susp: 150 mg/5 ml Parenteral: 1 g	PO/IV: 50 mg/kg/day in divided doses q 6 h.	Adverse effects: non-dose-related irreversible bone marrow depression leading to aplastic anemia; dose-related reversible bone marrow depression (plasma concentrations of greater than 25 µg/ml); gray syndrome; GI disturbances. Due to toxicity, should not be used for trivial infections, prophylaxis, or when other less toxic antibiotics can be used.
Clindamycin (Cleocin)	Caps: 75, 150 mg Solution: 75 mg/5 ml Parenteral: 150 mg/ml	IV/IM: 600 mg q 6 h or 900 mg q 8 h. PO: 150-450 mg q 6 h.	Adverse side-effects: diarrhea (7%); pseudo-membranous colitis with toxic megacolon, rare with 1:7500 due to C. difficile toxin; rash; neutropenia; eosinophilia; occasional elevated SGOT and alk. phos. Covers gram-positives (not Neisseria or enterococci), C. diphtheriae, Actinomyces, anaerobes, 5% B. fragilis resistant. Clostridia variable sensitivity; C. difficile resistant.
Colistin (Coly-Mycon) **Colistimethate** (Coly-Mycin)	Solution (oral): 25 mg/ 5 ml Parenteral: 150 mg	PO: 5-15 mg/kg/day in 3 divided doses. IM/IV: 2.5-5 mg/kg/day in 2-4 divided doses. Maximum daily dose is 5 mg/kg.	Covers gram-negatives, especially Pseudomonas, not Proteus. Can cause neurotoxicity, fever, nephrotoxicity, neuromuscular blockage (apnea). Not recommended due to availability of more effective and less toxic agents.
Metronidazole (Flagyl)	Tabs: 250, 500 mg Vials: 5 mg/ml (100 ml) for IV infusion.	PO (Adults): **Trichomoniasis:** 250 mg tid for 7 days or 2 g in a single dose. **Amoebic dysentery:** 750 mg tid for 5-10 days. IV (Adults): 15 mg/kg followed by 7.5 mg/kg q 6 h.	For oral use in the treatment of Trichomonas vaginalis and asymptomatic consorts, as well as amebiasis. For IV use in the treatment of intra-abdominal abscess, peritonitis, septicemia, CNS infections and lower respiratory tract infections. Effective against obligate anaerobes. Should not be used with alcohol, in pregnancy, with known hypersensitivity, or liver dysfunction. Potentiates coumarin effects on anticoagulation.

MISCELLANEOUS ANTIBIOTICS (continued)

DRUG	SUPPLIED	DOSE/ROUTE	REMARKS
Pentamidine (Pentam 300)	Parenteral: 300 mg	**Pneumocystis carinii:** IM: 4 mg/kg once daily for 14 days. IV: 4 mg/kg once daily for 14 days (infused over at least one hour).	For use in patients with Pneumocystis carinii who are unresponsive to trimethoprim/sulfamethoxazole, trypanosomiasis, and visceral leishmaniasis. Nephrotoxicity (25%), hypotension, hypoglycemia (5-10%), leukopenia, and thrombocytopenia can occur.
Polymyxin B (Aerosporin)	1 mg = 10,000 units Parenteral: 500,000 units Urogenital irrigant: 200,000 units of polymyxin B per ml with neomycin sulfate 57 mg/ml.	IM/IV: 1.5-2.5 mg/kg daily in 2 divided doses.	Covers gram-negatives, especially *Pseudomonas*, not *Proteus*. Can cause local pain on injection, neurotoxicity, nephrotoxicity, neuromuscular blockade (apnea). *Not* recommended due to availability of more effective and less toxic agents.
Spectinomycin (Trobicin)	Parenteral: 2.4 g	IV: 2 g as a single dose	Drug of choice for treatment of infections caused by non-penicillinase-producing *N. gonorrheae* in patients who are allergic or do not respond to penicillins, cephalosporins or tetracyclines. Should be reserved for use in penicillinase-producing strains of *N. gonorrhea*.
Trimethoprim/ sulfamethoxazole (Bactrim, Septra)	Tabs: 80 mg trimethoprim, 400 mg sulfamethoxazole (available as D.S.) Susp: 40 mg trimethoprim/5 ml, 200 mg sulfamethoxazole/5 ml. Parenteral: 80 mg trimethoprim (16 mg/ml), sulfamethoxazole (80 mg/ml)	PO (Adults): 1 double strength or 2 regular strength tabs q 12 h. IV: For *Pneumocystis carinii*: 15-20 mg/kg/day in 3 or 4 divided doses. For urinary tract infections or *Shigella* enteritis: 8-10 mg/kg/day in 2-4 divided doses.	For use in urinary tract infections, acute otitis media, adult chronic bronchitis, Pneumocystis carinii pneumonia. *Contraindications:* hypersensitivity to trimethoprim or sulfa drugs, megaloblastic anemia secondary to folate deficiency, and pregnancy at term and nursing mothers. Excretion is renal. Trimethoprim inhibits production of tetrahydrofolic acid from dihydrofolic acid. Sulfamethoxazole inhibits production of dihydrofolic acid.

MISCELLANEOUS ANTIBIOTICS (continued)

DRUG	SUPPLIED	DOSE/ROUTE	REMARKS
Vancomycin (Vancocin)	Solution: 1,10 g Parenteral: 500 mg	IV: 500 mg q 6 h or 1 g q 12 h. PO: 500 mg q 6 h or 1 g q 12 h.	Can cause hypotension if given IV push in 10 min or less ("red-neck syndrome"). Should be given over 1 h IV. Desire serum peak level 35-45 μg/ml, trough 5-10 μg/ml. Can cause phlebitis, fever, rash, nausea, nephrotoxicity, neutropenia, eosinophilia, flushing over upper chest, anaphylaxis, ototoxicity. Increased incidence of nephrotoxicity when administered concomitantly with aminoglycosides. Not appreciably absorbed from GI tract; therefore, oral therapy should not be used for infections other than C. difficile colitis.

AMINOGLYCOSIDES

DRUG	SUPPLIED	DOSE/ROUTE	REMARKS
Amikacin (Amikin)	Parenteral: 50,250 mg/ml	IV/IM: 15 mg/kg/day divided q 8 h or 12 h.	All aminoglycosides may cause or increase neuromuscular blockade. Use with caution in patients with myasthenia gravis, Parkinsonism, botulism, with neuromuscular blocking drugs or with massive transfusion of citrated blood. Avoid concurrent use with ethacrynic acid, furosemide or methoxyflurane. Do not give in "heparin lock" without first flushing the lock. Can cause nephrotoxicity; ototoxicity usually with high frequency loss, especially with larger total dose over 10 g. Toxicity is associated with greater than 10 days of therapy, prior aminoglycosides, peak serum level > 32 μg/ml, trough level > 10 μg/ml. Rare eosinophilia, arthralgia; fever, skin rash.
Gentamicin (Garamycin)	Parenteral: multiple strengths	IM/IV: 3.0-5.0 mg/kg/day divided q 8 h	Can cause nephrotoxicity, ototoxicity, fever, skin rash, neuromuscular blockade. Serum peak levels: 5-10 μg/ml; serum trough levels < 2.0 μg/ml.
Netilmicin	Parenteral: 25,100 mg/ml	IM/IV: 4-7 mg/kg/day in divided doses (8-12 h).	No significant advantage over gentamicin or tobramycin.

AMINOGLYCOSIDES (continued)

DRUG	SUPPLIED	DOSE/ROUTE	REMARKS
Kanamycin (Kantrex)	Caps: 500 mg Injection: 37.5,250,333 mg/ml	IV/IM: 15 mg/kg/day divided q 8 or 12 h. Total daily dose not to exceed 1.5 g. PO: 8-12 g daily in divided doses as an adjunct in the treatment of hepatic encephalopathy.	Adjust dose in renal insufficiency. Can cause ototoxicity, nephrotoxicity, neuromuscular blockade, skin rash, fever. Serum peak levels: 15-25 μg/ml.
Neomycin sulfate (Mycifradin, Neobiotic)	Tabs: 500 mg Liquid: 125 mg/5 ml	Hepatic coma: PO 4-12 g/day in divided doses. Enteropathogenic E. coli: PO 50 mg/kg/day in divided doses.	Can cause nausea, vomiting, diarrhea; interferes with absorption of digoxin; about 3% of an oral dose is absorbed and if a sufficient amount is absorbed, ototoxicity, nephrotoxicity, and neuromuscular blockade can result.
Streptomycin	Injection: 400,500 mg, 1,5 g	IM/IV: Tuberculosis: 15 mg/kg/day. Endocarditis: 1 g bid for 1 week followed by 500 mg bid for 1 week.	Other aminoglycosides are more effective against gram-negatives. Major indications are treatment of TB and, with penicillin, treatment of endocarditis caused by S. viridans. Can cause vestibular damage, rash, peripheral neuritis, anaphylaxis, renal damage, rarely blood dyscrasias, neuromuscular blockade. IM injection should be deep to avoid pain and sterile abscesses.
Tobramycin (Nebcin)	Injection: 1.2,10,40 mg	IV/IM: 3-5 mg/kg/day in divided doses	Serum peak levels: 5-10 μg/ml; serum trough levels < 2.0 μg/ml.

CARBAPENEMS (THIENAMYCINS)

DRUG	SUPPLIED	DOSE/ROUTE	REMARKS
Imipenem and Cilastatin (Primaxin)	Parenteral: 250,500 mg	0.5-1.0 g IV over 30 min q 6 h.	Highly stable against beta lactamases. Can be associated with risk of suprainfection, emergence of resistant P. aeruginosa, pseudomembranous colitis, phlebitis, hypersensitivity, rash, Coombs positive, elevated SGOT, SGPT, alk. phos., confusion, seizures, nausea, vomiting.

CEPHALOSPORINS

DRUG	SUPPLIED	DOSE/ROUTE	REMARKS
Oral:			
Cefaclor (Ceclor) (2nd generation)	Caps: 250,500 mg Susp: 125,250 mg/5 ml	PO: 0.25 - 0.5 g q 8 h.	Can cause serum sickness-like reactions (1-2%), joint aches, erythema, multiforme, rash, purpura. Effective against ampicillin-resistant strains of *Haemophilus influenzae.*
Cefadroxil (Duricef) (1st generation)	Caps: 500 mg Susp: 125,250, 500 mg/ 5 ml Tabs: 1 g	PO: 1-2 g qd for cystitis; 1 g q 12 h for other indications.	Can cause GI distress, rash. Can be administered once or twice a day because of a prolonged half-life (1-2 hours).
Cephalexin (Keflex) (1st generation)	Caps: 250,500 mg Susp: 125,250 mg/5 ml; 100 mg/1 ml Tabs: 1 g	PO: 0.25 - 0.5 g q 6 h.	Can cause GI distress, skin rash, eosinophilia, leukopenia, Coombs + and elevated SGOT. Comparable spectrum of activity & duration of action to that of cephradine at a significantly lower cost.
Cephradine (Velosef, Anspor) (1st generation)	Caps: 250,500 mg Susp: 125,250 mg/5 ml Injection: 250,500 mg, 1,2,4 g	PO: 0.25 - 0.5 g q 6 h. IM: 1-2 g q 6 h.	Delayed absorption when given with food. Comparable spectrum of activity & duration of action to that of cephalexin at a significantly higher cost.
Parenteral:			
Cefamandole (Mandol) (2nd generation)	Injection: multiple strengths	IM/IV: 0.5-1.0 g q 4-8 h	Can cause pain on IM injection, phlebitis, vasodilation, hypersensitivity, rash, urticaria, eosinophilia, fever, weakly + Coombs, neutropenia, thrombocytopenia, mild elevation of BUN/Cr, SGOT, SGPT, alk. phos. Rare disulfiram-like reactions after alcohol. Effective against ampicillin-resistant species of *Haemophilus influenzae.*
Cefoxitin (Mefoxin) (2nd generation)	Injection: 1,2 g	IM/IV: 1-2 g q 6-8 h	Adequate activity against anaerobic organisms.

CEPHALOSPORINS (continued)
Parenteral (continued):

DRUG	SUPPLIED	DOSE/ROUTE	REMARKS
Cefazolin (Ancef, Kefzol) (1st generation)	Injection: multiple strengths	IM/IV: 0.5-1.0 g q 8 h	Adverse side-effects: rash, elevated SGOT and alk. phos.; phlebitis, Coombs +; abnormal coagulation tests in uremia. Can be administered q 8 h because of an extended half-life. Similar spectrum of activity to cephalothin & cephapirin.
Cefonicid (Monocid) (2nd generation)	Injection: 500 mg, 1 g	IM/IV: 1-2 g q 24 h	Can be administered once a day due to an extended half-life (4-8 h). Minimal activity against anaerobic organisms.
Ceforanide (Precef) (2nd generation)	Injection: 500 mg, 1 g	IM/IV: 0.5-1.0 g q 12 h.	Most strains of *B. fragilis* and *C. difficile* are resistant. Can be administered q 12 h due to an extended half-life (2-3 h).
Cefotaxime (Claforan) (3rd generation)	Injection: 1,2 g	IM/IV: 1-2 g q 6-8 h	Can be administered q 8 h in mild infections. Active metabolite has antibacterial activity similar to a 1st-generation cephalosporin.
Cefotetan (Cefotan) (2nd generation)	Injection: 1,2 g	IM/IV: 1-2 g q 12 h	Comparable spectrum of activity to that of cefoxitin.
Cefuroxime (Zinacef) (2nd generation)	Injection: 750 mg, 1.5 g	IM/IV: 0.75-1.5 g q 8 h	Minimal anaerobic activity.
Ceftriaxone (Rocephin) (3rd generation)	Injection: multiple strengths	IM/IV: 1-2 g once or twice a day	Extended half-life (5-10 h) allows for BID or qd dosing.
Ceftazidime (Fortaz) (3rd generation)	Injection: multiple strengths	IM/IV: 1-2 g q 8 h.	Best activity of all 3rd-generation cephalosporins against *P. aeruginosa*.

CEPHALOSPORINS (continued)
Parenteral (continued):

DRUG	SUPPLIED	DOSE/ROUTE	REMARKS
Cefoperazone (Cefobid) (3rd generation)	Injection: 1,2 g	IM/IV: 2-4 g q 8-12 h	In severe infections should be administered q 8 h. Very high biliary concentrations can be obtained in unobstructed biliary disease. Can cause hypoprothrombinemia. Minimal anaerobic activity.
Cephalothin (Keflin) (1st generation)	Injection: multiple strengths	IM/IV: 0.5-1.0 g q 4-6 h	Can cause phlebitis, rash, fever, eosinophilia, elevated SGOT, neutropenia, anaphylactoid reaction convulsions when given in high doses in renal failure, Coombs +, thrombocytopenia, nephrotoxicity, false + "clinitest", pain on IM injection. At 300 mg/kg/day, it may cause defect in platelet function and coagulation with delayed fibrinogen-fibrin polymerization. Similar spectrum of activity to cefazolin, but must be administered q 6 h. Similar spectrum of activity and duration of action to that of cephapirin at a significantly higher cost.
Cephapirin (Cefadyl) (1st generation)	Injection: multiple strengths	IM/IV: 0.5-1.0 g q 4-6 h	Can cause phlebitis, rash, eosinophilia, fever, pain on IM injection, elevated SGOT, neutropenia, anemia, Coombs +, elevated BUN in patients > 50. Similar spectrum of activity and duration of action to that of cephalothin at a significantly lower cost. Similar spectrum of activity to that of cefazolin, but must be administered q 6 h.
Moxalactam (Moxam) (3rd generation)	Injection: multiple strengths	IM/IV: 2-4 g q 8-12 h	Bleeding can occur in patients treated over 4 days with doses > 4 g/day. Platelet dysfunction. If ≥ 4 g/day for < 3 days, need to monitor bleeding times. Hypoprothrombinemia. Rare immune thrombocytopenia. Watch for supra-infection with enterococci.

CEPHALOSPORINS (continued)

Parenteral (continued):

DRUG	SUPPLIED	DOSE/ROUTE	REMARKS
Ceftizoxime (Cefizox) (3rd generation)	Injection: 1,2 g	IM/IV: 1-2 g q 8-12 h	Similar in spectrum of activity to cefotaxime.

ERYTHROMYCINS

DRUG	SUPPLIED	DOSE/ROUTE	REMARKS
Erythromycin base (E-mycin, Ilotycin)	Caps: 125,250 mg Tabs: 250,333,500 mg	PO: 250 mg q6h or 333 mg q8h. **Prophylaxis of streptococcal infections: Bacterial endocarditis** (prior to dental procedure): 1 g 1 h before the procedure and 500 mg 6 h later. **Rheumatic heart disease:** 250 mg bid. **Syphilis:** 500 mg qid for 15 days. **Gonorrhea:** 500 mg qid for 7 days. **Chlamydia/mycoplasma:** 500 mg qid for 7 days.	Administer on an empty stomach.
Erythromycin estolate (Ilosone)	Caps: 125,250 mg Susp: 125 mg/5 ml, 250 mg/5 ml Tabs: 500 mg Chewable tabs: 125,250 mg	PO: 250 mg q 6 h.	May cause reversible cholestatic hepatitis, and is *contraindicated* in patients with hepatic dysfunction or pre-existing liver disease.
Erythromycin ethylsuccinate (EES)	Susp: 100 mg/2.5 ml, 200 mg/5 ml, 400 mg/5 ml Tabs: 400 mg Chewable tabs: 200 mg	PO: 400 mg q 6 h.	Erythromycin ethylsuccinate (400 mg) is equivalent to erythromycin base, stearate, or estolate (250 mg).
Erythromycin stearate (Wyomycin)	Tabs: 250,500 mg	PO: 250 mg q 6 h.	

ERYTHROMYCINS (continued)

DRUG	SUPPLIED	DOSE/ROUTE	REMARKS
Erythromycin gluceptate (Ilotycin)	Parenteral: 250,500, 1000 mg	IV: 15-20 mg kg daily in 4 divided doses. Legionnaires' disease: 1-4 g in divided doses, alone or in conjunction with rifampin.	Not administered IVP due to local irritative properties.
Erythromycin lactobionate (Erythrocin, Lactobionate-IV)	Parenteral: 500, 1000 mg	IV: 15-20 mg/kg daily in 4 divided doses	

MONOBACTAMS

DRUG	SUPPLIED	DOSE/ROUTE	REMARKS
Aztreonam (Azactam)		IV: 1.0 - 2.0 g q 8 h.	Highly stable against beta lactamases. Covers gram-negatives. Highly active against *Neisseria, H. influenzae, Enterobacteriaceae;* moderate against *P. aeruginosa.* Not active against acinetobacter, *P. maltophilia, P. capacia, Staph., Strep.,* anaerobes. Can cause phlebitis, hypersensitivity, rash, mild elevation of SGOT in 1/3 of patients. Should not be used for surgical prophylaxis or treatment of suspected or documented gram-positive infections.

PENICILLINS

Natural Penicillins:

DRUG	SUPPLIED	DOSE/ROUTE	REMARKS
Penicillin G procaine (Wycillin)	Parenteral: 300,000 units/ml, 500,000 units/ml, 600,000 units/ml	**Staphylococcal and Streptococcal infections:** IM: 600,000 units - 1.2 mu qd for 10 days. **Uncomplicated gonorrhea:** IM: 2.4 mu in each buttock as a single dose with 1 g of oral probenecid.	IM administration only. Serum concentrations are more prolonged but lower than those achieved with an equivalent IM dose of penicillin G potassium or sodium.

PENICILLINS (continued)
Natural Penicillins (continued):

DRUG	SUPPLIED	DOSE/ROUTE	REMARKS
Penicillin G benzathine (Bicillin, Bicillin L-A)	Tab: 200,000 units <u>Parenteral:</u> 300,000 units/ml, 600,000 units/ml	**Staphylococcal and Streptococcal infections:** IM: 1.2 mu as a single dose. **Early syphilis (primary and secondary):** IM: 2.4 mu as a single dose. **Syphilis (> 1 year's duration):** IM: 2.4 mu once a week for 3 consecutive weeks. **Neurosyphilis:** IM: 2.4 mu once a week for 3 consecutive weeks. **Rheumatic fever prophylaxis:** IM: 1.2 mu once every 4 weeks, *or* 600,000 units once every 2 weeks, *or* 200,000 units *orally* BID.	IM administration only. IM penicillin G benzathine results in serum concentrations of penicillin G that are more prolonged but lower than those achieved with an equivalent IM dose of penicillin G procaine or penicillin G potassium or sodium. Used *only* in mild to moderate infections caused by organisms susceptible to *low* concentrations of penicillin G, for prophylaxis of infections, or as follow-up therapy to penicillin G potassium or sodium. Penicillin G potassium or sodium should be used when high concentrations of penicillin G are required. Oral penicillin G benzathine is poorly absorbed and should *not* be used for the *initial* treatment of severe infections.
Penicillin G potassium,	<u>Solution:</u> 200,000 U/5 ml 250,000 U/5 ml 400,000 U/5 ml	**Staphylococcal and Streptococcal infections:** PO: 200,000–500,000 U q 6-8 h for 10 days. IV: 1-2 mu q 4 h.	Susceptible to acid hydrolysis and only 15-30% of an oral dose is absorbed. Food will decrease the rate and extent of oral absorption. Should *not* be used for initial treatment of severe infections.
Penicillin G sodium	<u>Tabs:</u> 200,000 U 250,000 U 400,000 U 500,000 U 800,000 U <u>Parenteral:</u> multiple strengths	**Neisseria meningitidis infections:** IV: 1-2 mu q 2 h or 20-30 mu daily as a continuous infusion. **Clostridium infections:** IV: 20 mu daily in divided doses. **Neurosyphilis:** IV: 2-4 mu q 4 h for 10 days, followed by benzathine penicillin 2.4 mu IM once weekly for 3 weeks. **Bacterial endocarditis prophylaxis:** IV/IM: 2 mu 30 min prior to the procedure, followed by 1-2 mu IM or IV 6-8 h later.	Achieves rapid and high concentrations of penicillin G in the treatment of severe infections caused by organisms susceptible to penicillin G following IM or IV administration. Dosage modification in renal failure is necessary.

Gentamicin should also be administered 30 min prior to the procedure and again 6-8 h later in patients with prosthetic heart valves or a history of endocarditis.

PENICILLINS (continued)

Natural Penicillins (continued):

DRUG	SUPPLIED	DOSE/ROUTE	REMARKS
Penicillin V, Penicillin V potassium	Susp: 125,250 mg/5 ml Tabs: 125 mg (PEN VK), 250, 500 mg Film-coated tabs: 250, 500 mg (PEN VK)	**Staphylococcal and Streptococcal infections:** PO: 125-250 mg q 6-8 h for 10 days or 500 mg q 12 h for 10 days. **Prophylaxis of recurrent rheumatic fever:** PO: 125-250 mg twice daily. **Prophylaxis of bacterial endocarditis:** **Dental procedures:** 2 g 1 h prior to procedure and 1 g 6 h later. **Prophylaxis of Pneumococcal infections:** PO: 125 mg twice daily (age < 5 years); 250 mg twice daily (age > 5 years).	Penicillin V is more resistant to acid-catalyzed inactivation than penicillin G. Administer 1 h before or 2 h after meals. 250 mg of penicillin V is equivalent to 400,000 units of the drug.

Penicillinase-Resistant Penicillins:

DRUG	SUPPLIED	DOSE/ROUTE	REMARKS
Cloxacillin	Caps: 250,500 mg Solution: 125 mg/5 ml	PO: 250-500 mg q 6 h.	Administered 1 h before or 2 h after meals.
Dicloxacillin	Caps: 125,250,500 mg Susp: 62.5 mg/5 ml	PO: 125-500 mg q 6 h.	Administered 1 h before or 2 h after meals.
Methicillin	Injection: multiple strengths	IM/IV: 1 g q 4-6 h	Acute interstitial nephritis is reported more frequently than with any other penicillinase-resistant penicillin. Dosage reduction in renal failure is recommended.
Nafcillin	Caps: 250 mg Solution: 250 mg/5 ml Tabs: 500 mg Injection: multiple strengths	PO: 250-500 mg q 4-6 h. IM: 500 mg q 4-6 h. IV: 500 mg - 1 g q 4 h. **Endocarditis/osteomyelitis:** 1-2 g IV q 4 h.	Orally at least 1 h before or 2 h after meals.
Oxacillin	Caps: 250,500 mg Solution: 250 mg/5 ml Injection: multiple strengths	PO: 500 mg - 1 g q 4-6 h. IM/IV: 250-500 mg q 4-6 h. **Severe infection:** 1 g q 4-6 h.	Adverse hepatic effects are reported more frequently than with any other penicillinase-resistant penicillin. Orally at least 1 h before or 2 h after meals.

PENICILLINS (continued)

Aminopenicillins:

DRUG	SUPPLIED	DOSE/ROUTE	REMARKS
Amoxicillin (Amoxil, Larotid)	Caps: 250,500 mg Susp: 50,125,250 mg/5 ml Chewable tabs: 125,250 mg	PO: 250-500 mg q 8 h.	May be given with meals. Single doses of 3 g have been effective for initial treatment of acute, uncomplicated UTI's in non-pregnant women.
Amoxicillin and clavulanic acid (Augmentin)	Susp: 125,250 mg/5 ml Chewable tabs: 125,250 mg Tabs: 250,500 mg	PO: 250-500 mg q 8 h.	May be given with meals. Clavulanic acid has very weak antibacterial activity when used alone. Use should be reserved for infections caused by beta-lactamase-producing bacteria. Two 250 mg tabs has twice the clavulanic acid of one 500 mg tab.
Ampicillin (Amcil, Omnipen)	Caps: 250,500 mg Susp: 100,125,250, 500 mg/5 ml Parenteral: multiple strengths	PO: 250-500 mg q 6 h.	May be administered with meals, but maximum absorption is obtained if given 1 h before or 2 h after meals.
Bacampicillin (Spectrobid)	Tabs: 400 mg Susp: 125 mg/5 ml	PO: 400-800 mg q 12 h.	Hydrolyzed *in vivo* to ampicillin. Tablets may be administered with meals; suspension should be given 1 h before or 2 h after meals. Each mg of bacampicillin is equivalent to 700 µg of ampicillin.
Cyclacillin (Cyclapen)	Tabs: 250,500 mg Susp: 125,250 mg/5 ml	PO: 250-500 mg q 6 h.	Less active *in vitro* on a weight basis than other aminopenicillins. May be given with meals.
Hetacillin (Versapen)	Caps: 225 mg Susp: 112.5 mg/5 ml	PO: 225-450 mg q 6 h.	Administered 1 h before or 2 h after meals. Hydrolyzed *in vivo* to ampicillin.

Extended-Spectrum Penicillins:

DRUG	SUPPLIED	DOSE/ROUTE	REMARKS
Azlocillin (Azlin)	Parenteral: multiple strengths	IV: 3-4 g q 4-6 h.	May cause hypokalemia and functional thrombocytopenia with large doses in patients with severe renal impairment. One gram of azlocillin has 2.17 mEq of sodium. Dosage adjustment in renal failure is necessary.

PENICILLINS (continued)
Extended–Spectrum Penicillins (continued):

DRUG	SUPPLIED	DOSE/ROUTE	REMARKS
Carbenicillin disodium (Geopen)	Parenteral: multiple strengths	IV/IM: 5 g q 4 h.	May cause hypokalemia and functional thrombo-cytopenia with large doses in patients with severe renal impairment. One gram of carbenicillin has 4.7–6.5 mEq of sodium. Dosage adjustment in renal failure is necessary.
Carbenicillin indanyl-sodium (Geocillin)	Tabs: 382 mg	PO: 382–764 mg 4 times daily.	Used only for the treatment of acute or chronic infections of upper and lower urinary tract.
Mezlocillin (Mezlin)	Parenteral: multiple strengths	IV/IM: 3–4 g q 4–6 h.	May cause hypokalemia and functional thrombo-cytopenia with large doses in patients with severe renal impairment. One gram of mezlocillin has 1.75–1.85 mEq of sodium. Dosage adjustment in renal failure is necessary.
Piperacillin (Pipracil)	Parenteral: multiple strengths	IV/IM: 3–4 g q 4–6 h.	May cause hypokalemia and functional thrombo-cytopenia with large doses in patients with severe renal impairment. One gram of piperacillin has 1.85 mEq of sodium. Dosage adjustment in renal failure is necessary.
Ticarcillin (Ticar)	Parenteral: multiple strengths	IV/IM: 3 g q 4 h.	May cause hypokalemia and functional thrombo-cytopenia with large doses in patients with severe renal impairment. One gram of ticarcillin has 5.2–6.5 mEq of sodium. Dosage adjustment in renal failure is necessary.
Ticarcillin and clavulanic acid (Timentin)	Parenteral: 3 g ticarcillin, 100 g clavulanic acid	IV: 3 g q 4 h.	Dosage adjustment in renal failure is necessary. One gram of Timentin has 4.75 mEq of sodium.

TETRACYCLINES

DRUG	SUPPLIED	DOSE/ROUTE	REMARKS
Demeclocycline (Declomycin)	Caps: 150 mg Tabs: 150,300 mg	PO: 600 mg in 2 or 4 divided doses. SIADH: 600 mg in 3-4 divided doses.	Administer 1 h before or 2 h after meals. Adverse reactions: GI distress, skin rash, deposition in teeth, hepatotoxicity, phototoxicity (17-35%), benign elevated CSF pressure, onycholysis, anaphylaxis, vasopressin-resistant diabetes insipidus (almost 100% at doses of 1200 mg/day). May be useful in "inappropriate" ADH secretion. Covers gram-positives and gram-negatives, *Mycoplasma pneumoniae* and *Chlamydia*. Tetracycline of choice in patients with impaired renal function.
Doxycycline (Vibramycin, Doxycaps, Vivox, Doxy-100 or Doxy-200	Susp: 50 mg/5 ml Caps: 50,100 mg Tabs: 50,100 mg Parenteral: 100,200 mg	PO/IV: 0.1 g q 12 h on 1st day, then 0.1-0.2 g/day.	Covers gram-positives and gram-negatives, *Mycoplasma pneumoniae, Chlamydia, Bacteroides* and *Rickettsiae*. As with other tetracyclines, avoid administration with antacids and other drugs containing aluminum, calcium, iron and Mg.
Methacycline (Rondomycin)	Caps: 150,300 mg	PO: 0.15 g q 6 h.	Covers gram-positives and gram-negatives, *Chlamydia*. Should be administered 1 h before or 2 h after meals.
Minocycline (Minocin)	Caps: 50,100 mg Susp: 50 mg Tabs: 50,100 mg Parenteral: 100 mg	PO/IV: 200 mg initially, followed by 100 mg q 12 h.	Covers gram-positives and gram-negatives, some acinetobacter, *Chlamydia*. Vestibular symptoms occur more often than with other tetracyclines (30-90%).
Oxytetracycline (Terramycin, Oxymycin)	Tabs: 250 mg Caps: 250 mg Injection: 50,125,250, 500 mg	PO: 0.25-0.5 g q 6 h. IV: 0.5-1.0 g q 12 h. IM: 250 mg as a single dose daily	Outdated drug can cause Fanconi syndrome. Administered 1 h before or 2 h after meals.

ANTICOAGULANTS AND THROMBOLYTICS, COAGULANTS, ANTIPLATELET AND ANTIFIBRINOLYTIC AGENTS

Dipyridamole (Persantine)	Tabs: 25 mg	25 to 75 mg po tid.	

ANTICOAGULANTS AND THROMBOLYTICS, COAGULANTS, ANTIPLATELET AND ANTIFIBRINOLYTIC AGENTS (continued)

DRUG	SUPPLIED	DOSE/ROUTE	REMARKS
Aminocaproic acid (Amicar)	Tabs: 500 mg Syrup: 250 mg/ml Vials: 250 mg/ml	Adult: initially 5 g po or slow IVP, then after 1 h give 1 to 1.25 g/h for 8 h or until bleeding is controlled, up to 30 g/24 h.	Antifibrinolytic. For treatment of excessive bleeding caused by systemic hyperfibrinolysis. Reduces fibrinolysis by inhibiting plasminogen activator substance. *Contraindicated* with evidence of active intravascular clotting process. Rapid IV infusion may induce hypotension, bradycardia, or arrhythmias. Give initial IV dose of 4-5 g in 250 ml NS, LR or D₅W over 1 h. Subsequent hourly doses of 1 g in 50 ml diluent over 1 h. In **primary hyperfibrinolysis**, platelet count is normal, precipitation does not occur when protamine is added to citrated blood, and the time required for lysis of a euglobin clot is less than normal, while in **DIC** the platelet count is usually decreased, precipitation occurs in the protamine test, and euglobin test is normal. Amicar can be given to patients with DIC only if heparin is given concomitantly.
Dextran 40 (LMD, Gentran 40, Rheomacrodex)	10% solution of dextran 40 in NS or D₅W	Initially 10 ml/kg continuous infusion over several hours, then 10 ml/kg qod, or 5 ml/kg qd.	Plasma expander, retards rouleau formation and RBC sludging. Can cause severe allergic reactions; carefully monitor renal and cardiac function.
Heparin calcium (Calciparine)	**Parenteral:** Available in a number of dosage strengths and dosage forms.	For venous thrombosis, atrial fibrillation, pulmonary embolism, DIC (controversial), prevention of cerebral thrombosis in evolving stroke, adjunctive treatment in coronary occlusion with acute MI, and in peripheral arterial embolism: 1. Continuous IV infusion: 5000 to 10,000 units IVP bolus, followed by 1000-2000 units/h continuous infusion. 2. Intermittent IV injection: 10,000 units IV bolus, then 5000-10,000 units IV bolus q4-6h. 3. Intermittent SC injection: 5000 units IV bolus, then 8000-10,000 units SC q 8 h. For prevention of post-op DVT and PE: 5000 units SC 2 h before surgery, followed by 5000 units SC q 8-12 h for 7 days or until patient is fully ambulatory, whichever is longer.	Regulate dosage by frequent testing of PTT. Aim for PTT 1½ to 2 times the control value. *Contraindications:* see Heparin sodium

ANTICOAGULANTS AND THROMBOLYTICS, COAGULANTS, ANTIPLATELET AND ANTIFIBRINOLYTIC AGENTS (continued)

DRUG	SUPPLIED	DOSE/ROUTE	REMARKS
Heparin sodium (Panheparin)	**Parenteral:** Available in a number of dosage strengths and dosage forms. *Be certain to check concentrations before administration!*	see Heparin calcium **Treatment of overdosage:** give 1.0-1.5 mg of 1% protamine sulfate by slow IV infusion for every 100 units of heparin given in previous 4 h to be neutralized. Maximum dose 50 mg in any 10 min period.	Use with caution in SBE, arterial sclerosis, dissecting aneurysm, severe hypertension, hemophilia, thrombocytopenia, diverticulitis, ulcerative colitis, recent surgery, PUD, severe hepatic or renal disease. Low-dose prophylaxis is usually ineffective in reducing the incidence of thrombosis after orthopedic surgery.
Protamine sulfate	Amp: 10 mg/ml	**Heparin antidote:** 1-1.5 mg of 1% protamine sulfate solution for every 100 units heparin given in previous 4 h by IV infusion. Maximum dose 50 mg over 10 min period	IV rate not to exceed 5 mg/min. *Monitor blood pressure continuously during administration.*
Streptokinase (Streptase)	Vials: 250,000, 600,000 and 750,000 IU/vial.	**Pulmonary embolism, deep vein thrombosis, arterial thrombosis or embolism:** initially 250,000 IU IV infusion over 30 min, followed by 100,000 IU/h IV continuous infusion for 24-72 h.	**Contraindications:** recent (within past 2 months) CVA or intracranial or intraspinal surgery, active internal bleeding, intra-neoplasm. Pretreatment monitoring: TT, APTT, PT, Hct, platelet count; TT and APTT should be twice normal control values before starting streptokinase. Concomitant use of heparin or oral anticoagulants with IV streptokinase is not generally recommended. To prevent recurrent thrombosis post-streptokinase treatment, administer heparin by IV infusion and follow with oral anticoagulant therapy. *Special caution* with: (1) recent surgical or obstetrical procedure (past 10 days), biopsies, (2) recent trauma or CPR; (3) severe hypertension; (4) suspected left heart thrombus; (5) SBE; (6) hepatic or renal failure related coagulopathies; (7) pregnancy; (8) cerebrovascular disease; (9) diabetes retinopathy; (10) allergic reaction to streptokinase; (11) septic thrombophlebitis.

ANTICOAGULANTS AND THROMBOLYTICS, COAGULANTS, ANTIPLATELET AND ANTIFIBRINOLYTIC AGENTS
(continued)

DRUG	SUPPLIED	DOSE/ROUTE	REMARKS
Urokinase (Abbokinase)	Vials: 250,000 IU/vial for IV only	**Pulmonary embolism:** 4400 IU/kg by IV infusion over 10 min initially, then 4400 IU/kg/h for 12 h.	*Contraindications:* 1. Recent (within past 2 months) CVA or intracranial or intraspinal surgery. 2. Active internal bleeding. 3. Intracranial neoplasm (see Streptokinase for cautions).
Warfarin, sodium (Coumadin, Panwarfin)	Tabs: 2, 2.5, 4, 7.5, 10 mg	Initially 10 mg po qd for 1-3 days, then 2-10 mg po qd or qod. **Control of overcoumadinization:** 1. Discontinuation of coumadin (slow control, days); 2. Vitamin K, po, sc or slow IV (control over 4-8 h); 3. 250-500 ml FFP (immediate effect).	Individualize dosage to maintain PT 1.5 to 2.5 times control value. PT should be monitored daily during initiation of therapy, then every 1-4 weeks thereafter. **Drug interactions:** *Decrease PT:* antacids, adrenocorticoteroids, steroids, antihistamines, barbiturates, carbamazepine, chlordiazepoxide, cholestogramine, ethcholorvynol, estrogens, glutethidimide, griseofulvin, haloperidol, noreprobamate, oral contraceptives, paraldehyde, phenytoin, primidone, rifampin, vitamins C and K. *Increase PT:* allopurinol, aminosalicylic acid, anabolic steroids, antibiotics, bromelaine, chloramphenicol, chymotryprin, cimetidine, cinchophen, clofibrate, dextran, dextrothyroxine, diazoxide, disulfiram, ethacrynic acid, glucagon, indomethacin, MAO inhibitors, methyldopa, metronidazole, narcotics, phenytoin, prophylthrocracil, quinidine, salicylates, sulfas, trimethoprim-sulfamethoxazole. *Increased anticonvulsant blood levels:* phenobarbital, phenytoin. *Increased hypoglycemic effect:* chlorpropamide, tolbutamide.

ANTI-CONVULSANTS

DRUG	SUPPLIED	DOSE/ROUTE	REMARKS
Carbamazepine (Tegretol)	Tabs: 200 mg Chewable tabs: 100 mg	**ADULTS:** Oral: **Trigeminal neuralgia:** 100 mg po bid; increase dose by 100 mg q 12 h (maximum: 1.2 g/24 h); once control of pain is achieved, dose may be reduced to 400-800 mg/day. **Seizures:** 200 mg po bid; increase dose by 200 mg/day (maximum 2.4 g per 24 h); for high doses, administer in 3-4 divided doses to reduce side-effects. **CHILDREN:** Oral: [< 6 years old]: 5 mg/kg/day; increase dose by 10 mg/kg/day and 20 mg/kg/day every 5-7 days; [6-12 years old]: 100 mg po bid; increase dose by 100 mg/day (maximum 1 g/24 h); [13-15 years old]: same as adult except maximum dose 1 g/day; [> 15 years old]: same as adult except maximum dose 1.2 g/day.	Use in partial seizures with complex symptomatology (psychomotor or temporal lobe seizures), generalized tonic-clonic (grand mal) seizures, mixed seizure patterns, trigeminal neuralgia, and for control of pain and/or seizures in a variety of conditions. Adverse reactions include cardiovascular effects, GU and GI tract disturbances, and CNS disturbances. Administer with caution in patients with cardiovascular problems and patients with liver or renal problems. Carbamazepine may increase intraocular pressure. *Contraindications* include history of previous bone marrow depression and/or hypersensitivity to carbamazepine or tricyclic antidepressant agents. Carbamazepine may alter the metabolism of many drugs. Gradual tapering of the drug is necessary to avoid seizures. Therapeutic concentration: 3-14 μg/ml.
Clonazepam (Clonopin)	Tabs: 0.5,1,2 mg	**ADULTS:** Oral: 1.5 mg/day (3 divided doses); increase dose 0.5-1 mg q 3 days (maximum 20 mg per 24 h). **CHILDREN:** Oral: 0.05 mg/kg/day (2-3 divided doses); increase dose 0.5 mg q 3 days (maximum 0.2 mg/kg/24 h).	Use in Lennox-Gastant syndrome and other types of absence (petit mal) seizures. *Contraindications* include hypersensitivity to benzodiazepines, patients with liver disease and acute angle-closure glaucoma. Adverse reactions include CNS depression and behavioral disturbances in children. Doses should be tapered slowly to avoid seizures or withdrawal reactions. Therapeutic concentration: 20-80 ng/ml.

ANTI-CONVULSANTS (continued)

DRUG	SUPPLIED	DOSE/ROUTE	REMARKS
Ethosuximide (Zarontin)	Caps: 250 mg Oral solution: 250 mg/5 ml	ADULTS AND CHILDREN: Oral: 3-6 years old: 250 mg po qd; > 6 years old: 500 mg po daily (2 divided doses); increase dose 250 mg q 4-7 days. Usual dose 20 mg/kg/day. Maximum dose: 1.5 g/24 h; higher given under close supervision.	Use in absence (petit mal) seizures. Adverse reactions include GI tract disturbances and CNS disturbances. *Contraindications* include hypersensitivity to succinimides. Doses should be tapered slowly to avoid seizures. Use with caution in renal or hepatic disease. **Therapeutic concentration:** 40-100 μg/ml.
Phenobarbital sodium	Caps: 16 mg Extended release caps: 65 mg Elixir: 15,20 mg/5 ml Tabs: 8,15,16,30,32, 60, 65,100 mg Amps: 130 mg/ml Vials: 65,130 mg/ml Tubex: 30,60 mg/ml	ADULTS: Oral and Parenteral: Sedation: 30-120 mg po/iv/sc/im daily (2-3 divided doses). Hypnosis: 100-320 mg po/iv/sc/im daily (2-3 divided doses); not recommended for more than 2 weeks. Epilepsy: 100-300 mg po daily at bedtime. Status epilepticus: 200-600 mg iv (maximum 20 mg/kg/24 h). CHILDREN: Oral and Parenteral: Sedation: 6 mg/kg/day po (in 3 divided doses). Epilepsy: 3-5 mg/kg/day po at bedtime. Status epilepticus: 100-400 mg iv.	IV administration may cause respiratory depression if given too rapidly. *Contraindications* include hypersensitivity to barbiturates, patients with bronchopneumonia or other severe pulmonary deficit and porphyria. Administer with caution in patients with renal disease. Reduce dose in liver disease. May cause psychic and physical dependency. Gradual tapering of the drug is necessary to avoid withdrawal reactions. Phenobarbital can alter the metabolism of many drugs including oral anticonvulsants. Adverse reactions include CNS depression and other CNS disturbances, hypersensitivity reactions in children and older patients, GI tract disturbances, and many types of hypersensitivity reactions. Maximum rate of IV administration should not exceed 60 mg/min to avoid respiratory depression. Decrease rate of administration in patients with pulmonary or cardiovascular disease. **Therapeutic concentration:** 15-40 μg/ml.

ANTI-CONVULSANTS (continued)

DRUG	SUPPLIED	DOSE/ROUTE	REMARKS
Phenytoin sodium (Dilantin)	Caps: 30,100 mg Oral susp: 30,125 mg per 5 ml Chewable tabs: 50 mg Amps: 50 mg/ml	**ADULTS:** Oral: 300-600 mg po per day (in 2-3 divided doses), or 6-7 mg/kg/day; do not increase dose more than 100 mg q 2-4 weeks. **Parenteral:** **Status epilepticus:** loading dose 15-18 mg/kg iv at a rate of 25-50 mg/min. **Antiarrhythmic:** 100 mg IV q 5 min, repeat until arrhythmia is stopped or a total dose of 1 g, then 100 mg po 2-4 times a day. **CHILDREN:** Oral: 4-8 mg/kg/day in 2-3 divided doses (maximum 300 mg per 24 h). **Parenteral:** **Status epilepticus:** loading dose 15-18 mg/kg at a rate of 25-50 mg/min.	*Contraindications* include hypersensitivity to phenytoin or other hydantoins. Adverse reactions associated with parenteral therapy include phlebitis, hypotension, cardiac arrhythmias, and cardiovascular collapse. In patients with a compromised cardiovascular system or on sympathomimetic amines, do not exceed a rate of 25 mg/min. Flush the line with normal saline or lactated Ringer's only. *Avoid* extravasation. Additional adverse reactions include GI tract disturbances, CNS changes, gingival hyperplasia, lymphadenopathy, hematologic toxicity, hepatotoxicity, osteomalacia, and dermatologic reactions. GI tract disturbances are associated with oral administration. May interfere with some of the thyroid function tests. Patients in renal failure may require lower doses. Saturation of metabolism may occur with high doses. **Therapeutic concentrations:** 10-20 μg/ml.
Primidone (Mysoline)	Tabs: 50,250 mg Oral susp: 250 mg/ 5 ml	**ADULTS:** Oral: 100-125 mg po qd, increase dose 100-125 mg every several days until 250 mg po tid or qid (maximum 2 g per 24 h). **CHILDREN** (< 8 years old): Oral: 50 mg po qhs, increase dose 50 mg every several days until 125-150 mg tid; usual dose 10-25 mg/kg/ day.	Use in partial (psychomotor) seizures, other partial seizures, akinetic seizures, and tonic-clonic (grand mal) seizures. Adverse reactions include CNS depression and GI tract disturbances. May cause psychic or physical dependency. Can cause hyperexcitability in children. *Contraindications* include hypersensitivity to primidone and barbiturates, and patients with porphyria. Reduce dose in liver or renal disease. **Therapeutic concentration:** 5-12 μg/ml (15-25% of the drug is metabolized to phenobarbital).

ANTI-CONVULSANTS (continued)

DRUG	SUPPLIED	DOSE/ROUTE	REMARKS
Valproate sodium (valproic acid, divalproex sodium, Depakote, Depakene)	Caps: 250 mg Tabs (enteric-coated): 125,250,500 mg Oral solution: 250 mg per 5 ml	**ADULTS AND CHILDREN:** Oral: 15 mg/kg/day (2-3 divided doses); increase dose by 5-10 mg/kg per day every 7 days (maximum 60 mg/kg/24 h). Rectal: Status epilepticus (refractory): 400-600 mg per enema q 6 h; consult reference.	Use in simple and complex absence (petit mal) seizures, status epilepticus and other types of epilepsy. Adverse reactions include GI tract disturbances, CNS depression and other CBS disturbances, hepatotoxicity, acute pancreatitis, alterations in coagulation and cell counts. *Contraindications* include hypersensitivity to valproic acid. Administer with food to reduce GI tract disturbances. Enteric-coated tablets (Depakote) may decrease GI tract disturbances. Valproic acid may alter the metabolism of some drugs. **Therapeutic concentration:** 50-100 μg/ml.

ANTI-DIARRHEALS

DRUG	SUPPLIED	DOSE/ROUTE	REMARKS
Belladonna tincture	Liquid: 30 mg/100 ml	Adult: 0.6-1.0 ml tid or qid	Activity is due to the atropine content. Limited efficacy in the treatment of irritable bowel syndrome, enterocolitis, and neurogenic bowel disturbances.
Camphorated opium tincture (Paregoric)	Liquid: 0.04% morphine (2 mg/5 ml)	Adult: 5-10 ml po q 6 h prn	Contains 25 times less the amount of morphine in tincture of opium.
Diphenoxylate-atropine sulfate (Lomotil)	Tabs: diphenoxylate 2.5 mg; atropine sulfate: 0.025 mg. Elixir: diphenoxylate: 2.5 mg/5 ml; atropine sulfate: 0.025 mg/5 ml	Adult: initially 2 tabs or 10 ml po q 6 h, then 1 tab or 5 ml po q 12 h prn.	*Contraindicated* in diphenoxylate hypersensitivity, jaundice, pseudomembranous enterocolitis, children less than 2 years, acute ulcerative colitis, and use with MAO inhibitors. Diphenoxylate 2.5 mg is equivalent in antidiarrheal efficacy to 5 ml of paregoric.
Kaolin and pectin (Kaopectate)	Liquid: Kaolin 20%, pectin 1%	60-120 ml after each loose bowel movement	Act as absorbants and protectants. *Contraindicated* in intestinal obstruction and undiagnosed abdominal pain.

ANTI-DIARRHEALS (continued)

DRUG	SUPPLIED	DOSE/ROUTE	REMARKS
Lactobacillus acidophilus (Bacid, Lactinex)	Caps: 100 mg Granules: 1 g packet	2 capsules or 4 tablets or 1 packet of granules 3-4 times daily.	A lactic acid-producing bacterium that inhibits the overgrowth of potentially pathogenic fungi and bacteria. Used for uncomplicated diarrhea caused by disruption of the intestinal flora by antibiotics.
Loperamide (Imodium)	Caps: 2 mg Solution: 0.2 mg/ml	Acute diarrhea: Initially 4 mg, followed by 2 mg after each unformed stool. Maximum dose is 16 mg daily. Chronic diarrhea: 4-8 mg daily as a single dose or in divided doses.	Longer acting and 2-3 times more potent on a weight basis than diphenoxylate. As effective as diphenoxylate for control of acute diarrhea.
Opium tincture (Laudanum)	Liquid: 1% morphine (50 mg/5 ml)	0.3-1 ml po q 6 h prn (15 drops/ml)	Contains 25 times the amount of morphine in paregoric. Use with caution in hepatic disease, prostratism, asthma, narcotic dependency. Not for use in children. Contraindicated in diarrhea due to poisoning.

ANTI-EMETICS

DRUG	SUPPLIED	DOSE/ROUTE	REMARKS
Benzquinamide (Emete-Con)	Vial: 50 mg	IM: 50 mg q 3-4 h prn.	Comparable antiemetic effects to those of perphenazine, prochlorperazine or thiethylperazine. May be more effective than trimethobenzamide. IV administration may result in sudden increases in blood pressure and transient cardiac arrhythmias.
Buclizine (Bucladin-S Softab)	Tabs: 50 mg	Motion sickness: PO: 50 mg 30 min before exposure to motion and q 4-6 h prn. Vertigo: PO: 50 mg 1-3 times daily; usual maintenance dose is 50 mg bid.	Used in the prevention and treatment of motion sickness and vertigo associated with diseases of the vestibular system. Less effective than the phenothiazines in controlling nausea and vomiting unrelated to vestibular stimulation.

ANTI-EMETICS (continued)

DRUG	SUPPLIED	DOSE/ROUTE	REMARKS
Cyclizine (Marezine)	Vial: 50 mg/ml Tabs: 50 mg	PO: 50 mg 30 min before exposure to motion and q 4-6 h prn. IM: 50 mg q 4-6 h prn.	Beneficial in prevention and treatment of motion sickness. Comparable activity to meclizine. Less effective than the phenothiazines in controlling nausea and vomiting unrelated to vestibular stimulation.
Prochlorperazine (Compazine)	Tabs: 5,10,25 mg Syrup: 5 mg/5 ml Supp: 2.5,5,25 mg Spans: 10,15,30 mg Amps: 5 mg/ml	PO: 5-10 mg tid/qid; PR: 25 mg bid; IM: 5-10 mg every 3-4 h prn.	*Contraindicated* in phenothiazine hypersensitivity, CNS depression, bone marrow depression. Not effective in preventing vertigo or motion sickness.
Promethazine (Phenergan, Provigan)	Tabs: 12.5,25,50 mg Amps: 25,50 mg/ml Syrup: 25 mg/ml Supp: 12.5,25,50 mg	PO: 25-50 mg 3-4 times daily; PR: 25-50 mg 3-4 times daily; IM: 25-50 mg 3-4 times daily.	*Contraindicated* in promethazin sensitivity.
Thiethylperazine (Torecan)	Tabs: 10 mg Supp: 10 mg Vial: 5 mg/ml	PO: 10 mg 1-3 times daily; PR: 10 mg 1-3 times daily; IM: 10 mg 1-3 times daily.	Similar to other phenothiazines.
Trimetho- benzamide hydrochloride (Tigan)	Caps: 100,250 mg Amps: 100 mg/ml Supp: 100,200 mg	PO: 250 mg 3-4 times daily; PR: 200 mg 3-4 times daily; IM: 200 mg 3-4 times daily.	Less effective as an antiemetic than pheno-thiazines.

ANTI-FUNGAL AGENTS

DRUG	SUPPLIED	DOSE/ROUTE	REMARKS
Clotrimazole (Lotrimin, Mycelex)	Troches: 10 mg Vaginal tabs:100,500 mg Cream: 1% Vaginal cream: 1% Lotion: 1% Solution: 1%	PO: Troche held in mouth 5 times daily. Vaginal: 1 tab per vagina q HS for 7 days.	Indications: *Candida* prophylaxis, skin infection with pathogenic dermatophytes, trichomoniasis in pregnancy. Systemic use is not recommended secondary to hallucinations and disorientation. Adverse reactions include cutaneous erythema, edema, GI disturbance.

ANTI-FUNGAL AGENTS (continued)

DRUG	SUPPLIED	DOSE/ROUTE	REMARKS
Amphotericin B (Fungizone)	**Parenteral:** 50 mg **Topical:** Cream 3%, Lotion 3%, Ointment 3%.	**IV Test dose:** Day 1: 5 mg in 500 ml D5W over 6-8 h Day 2: 10 mg " Day 3: 15 mg " Day 4: 20 mg " Day 5: 25 mg " Day 6: 30 mg " Increase dose by 5 mg increments to 50 mg/day, but do not exceed 1 mg/kg/day. Total dose up to 30 mg/kg. **Bladder irrigation:** 25-50 mg in 500-100 ml sterile H2O or D5W. **Intrathecal:** Mix 0.25-0.5 mg amphotericin B in 5 ml D5W and 25 mg hydrocortisone. First inject 25 mg hydrocortisone into IP site, then inject the hyperbaric amphotericin solution. Place the patient in Trendelenburg position for 45 min.	**Indications:** Candidiasis, cryptococcal infection, blastomycosis, coccidiomycosis, histoplasmosis, mucormycosis, sporotrichosis, aspergillosis. Precipitate in saline solutions. Monitor serum renal profile, CBC, and platelet counts closely. *Acute* adverse reactions: fever, nausea, vomiting, anorexia, headache, thrombophlebitis. Premedication with aspirin or tylenol, compazine, and benedryl. 25 mg hydrocortisone may be added to infusion if needed. Chronic adverse reactions: anemia, hypokalemia, renal failure, hypomagnesemia. Use test doses for serious anaphylactic shock, arrhythmias. No dosage adjustment is necessary in patients with existing renal dysfunction. However, if renal function deteriorates, therapy should be withheld.
Nystatin (Mycostatin, Nilstat)	**Susp:** 100,000 units/ml **Tabs:** 500,000 units **Vaginal tabs:** 100,000 units/tab **Cream/ointment:** 100,000 units/g **Powder:** multiple strength	PO: 500,000 - 1,000,000 units (tab); 500,000 units oral, swish and swallow.	For treatment and prophylaxis of candidiasis. Adverse reactions are mild and rare, but can include nausea, vomiting, diarrhea. Irritation may occur with topical application.
Tolnaftate (Tinactin)	**Topical aerosol:** 1% **Aerosol powder:** 1% **Cream:** 1% **Powder:** 1% **Solution:** 1%	Topically: twice daily	

ANTI-FUNGAL AGENTS (continued)

DRUG	SUPPLIED	DOSE/ROUTE	REMARKS
Griseofulvin [*Microsize*] (Grisactin, Grifulvin, Fulvicin)	Caps: 125,250 Susp: 125 mg/5 ml Tabs: 250,500 mg	PO: 500 mg - 1 g daily as a single dose	Active against species of *Trichophyton*, *Microsporum*, and *Epidermophyton*. Absorption is variable (25-70%). Headache may be severe, but often disappears with continued therapy.
Griseofulvin [*Ultramicrosize*]	Tabs: 125,165,250, 330 mg	PO: 330-660 mg daily as a single dose	Absorption is almost complete.
Miconazole (Monistat)	Parenteral: 10 mg/ml (vehicle is polyethioxylated castor oil). Supp: 100,200 mg Cream: 2% Lotion: 2% Powder: 2%	IV: 200 mg to 3.6 g qd in 2-3 divided doses in 200 ml NS or D5W. Infuse over 60 min. Bladder irrigation: 200 mg in 250 ml NS and instilled 2-4 times daily or by continuous irrigation. Intrathecal: 20 mg indiluted every 1-2 days.	Used as an alternative to amphotericin B and may be used to treat trichomonas infections. Rotate infusion site every 48-72 hours. Hyponatremia secondary to SIADH and anemia may occur. Hepatic metabolism not affected by renal failure.
Ketoconazole (Nizoral)	Tabs: 200 mg	PO: 200 mg qd, usually for 10 days, up to 2 months for cutaneous infection; 400 mg qd for histoplasmosis and coccidiomycosis. Disseminated infections may require 800-1600 mg qd.	For mucocutaneous candidiasis, histoplasmosis, paracoccidiomycosis, pulmonary coccidiomycosis as alternative to amphotericin B. Adverse reactions include nausea and vomiting. Drug absorption is reduced when administered with meals. Reversible hepatitis which is not dose-related has been seen. Adrenal suppression and gynecomastia have also been seen. Antacids and H2 blockers can decrease absorption. In patients with achlorhydria, each tablet should be dissolved in 4 ml of 0.2 N HCl and administered through a straw.
Econazole (Spectazole)	Cream: 1%	Topically: twice daily	Topical treatment of dermatophytoses, superficial mycoses, and cutaneous candidiasis.

ANTI-FUNGAL AGENTS (continued)

DRUG	SUPPLIED	DOSE/ROUTE					REMARKS
Flucytosine (Ancobon)	Caps: 250,500 mg	Dosage schedule depends on renal function:					Variable susceptibility of *Candida* or *Cryptococcus* strains. Adverse reactions: nausea, vomiting, diarrhea. Agranulocytosis and aplastic anemia may be dose-related. Hepatotoxicity is rare.
		CrCl (ml/min)	Individual dose (mg/kg)	Interval (hrs)	Daily dose clearance (mg/kg)		
		> 40	25-50	6	100-200		
		40-20	25-50	12	50-100		
		20-10	25-50	24	25-50		
		< 10	50	> 24 +	—		

ANTI-LIPEMICS

DRUG	SUPPLIED	DOSE/ROUTE	REMARKS
Clofibrate (Atromid-S)	Caps: 500 mg	PO: 500 mg qid.	For hypercholesterolemia and hypertriglyceridemia. May potentiate oral anticoagulants. *Contraindicated* in primary biliary cirrhosis, pregnancy, lactation, hepatic and renal failure. May cause an increased release of ADH.
Cholestyramine resin (Questran, Cuemid)	Powder: 9 g packet	PO: 4 g tid before meals; mixed with 60-180 ml of water, milk, or fruit juice.	Anion-exchange resin produces an increased fecal bile acid excretion. May cause constipation (20%), vomiting, vitamin A, D, E, and K deficiencies. Give other oral meds 1 h before or 4-6 h after cholestyramine dose. Prolonged use may lead to hyperchloremic acidosis. May help as an adjunct to diet in type IIa and type IIb hypercholesterolemia. Also used in treatment of pruritis associated with partial cholestasis.
Colestipol (Colestid)	Susp: 5 g packet	PO: 15-30 g daily in 2-4 divided doses; mixed with 90 ml of a liquid. Do *not* give in dry form.	Anion-exchange resin that binds bile acids in the intestine which is then excreted in feces. May cause constipation (10%), vitamin A, D, E and K deficiencies. Give other oral meds 1 h before or 4-6 h after cholestyramine dose

ANTI-LIPEMICS (continued)

DRUG	SUPPLIED	DOSE/ROUTE	REMARKS
Gemfibrozil (Lopid)	Caps: 300 mg	PO: 300 mg bid, 30 min before meals.	May increase cholesterol excretion in bile and cause cholelithiasis.
Niacin	Tabs: 100,250,500 mg Solution: 50 mg/5 ml	PO: 1.5-6 g daily in 2-4 divided doses with meals	Mechanism of action in the decrease of elevated serum cholesterol is independent of the drug's role as a vitamin. GI upset, facial flushing and skin burning are common. Pre-treatment with a prostaglandin inhibitor (e.g., aspirin) may reduce flushing.
Probucol (Lorelco)	Tabs: 250 mg	PO: 500 mg bid with meals.	Diarrhea can occur in about 10% of patients.

ANTI-VIRALS

DRUG	SUPPLIED	DOSE/ROUTE	REMARKS
Acyclovir (Zovirax)	Ointment: 5% Parenteral: 500 mg Caps: 200 mg	PO: 200 mg q 4 h while awake for 10 days. IV: 5 mg/kg q q 8 h in patients with creatinine clearance > 50 ml/min.	Anti-viral activity against herpes simplex virus types 1 and 2 (HSV-1, HSV-2), varicella-zoster virus, Epstein-Barr virus, herpes virus simiae (B virus), and cytomegalovirus. Impaired renal function occurs in 10% of patients who receive acyclovir by rapid IV injection and 5% of patients who receive it by slow IV infusion (over 1 h), a result of precipitation of drug in the renal tubules.
Amantadine (Symmetrel)	Caps: 100 mg Solution: 50 mg/5 ml	PO: 100-200 mg daily as a single dose or in 2 divided doses.	Used for the prophylaxis and symptomatic treatment of respiratory infections caused by influenza A virus strains. CNS disturbances (nervousness, psychosis, inability to concentrate), livedo reticularis, and seizures are common.

ANTI-VIRALS (continued)

DRUG	SUPPLIED	DOSE/ROUTE	REMARKS
Vidarabine (Vira-A)	Parenteral: 200 mg/ml	**Herpes simplex encephalitis:** IV: 15 mg/kg daily for 10 days. **Herpes zoster:** IV: 10 mg/kg daily for 5 days.	Not to be administered IM or SQ. Administered over 12-24 h using an in-line membrane filter with a pore size of 0.45 µm or smaller. Appears to be less effective than acyclovir in the treatment of herpes simplex encephalitis. Nausea, vomiting, diarrhea, malaise, muscle weakness, and psychosis occur infrequently.

BENZODIAZEPINES

| Diazepam (Valium, Valrelease) | Caps (extended release): 15 mg Tabs: 2,5,10 mg Amps: 5 mg/ml Vials: 5 mg/ml | **ADULTS:** **Oral and Parenteral:** **Anxiety, muscle spasm, prophylaxis of epileptic seizure:** 2-10 mg po/iv tid or qid. Pre-op: 10 mg IM 1-2 h prior to surgery. **Alcohol withdrawal:** 10 mg po tid or qid x 24 h, then 5 mg po tid or qid, or 10 mg iv; repeat every 20-30 min. **Status epilepticus:** 5-10 mg iv; repeat in 10-15 min. **CHILDREN:** Oral: 0.12-0.8 mg/kg/day divided in 3-4 doses. Parenteral: 0.04-0.6 mg/kg per dose q 2-8 h. | Rate of administration for IV use should not exceed 2.5 mg/min for adults and 5 mg over 3 min in children. Geriatric or debilitated patients require lower doses. May cause psychic and physical dependency. Adverse reactions include: CNS depression and other disturbances; paradoxical CNS stimulation; GI tract disturbances; GU disturbances; visual disturbances. Respiratory depression, hypotension, bradycardia and cardiac arrest have been associated with rapid IV administration. May increase LFT's. Use with caution in hepatic or renal disease. *Contraindications* include patients with acute alcohol intoxication with depressed vital signs and patients with hypersensitivity to the drugs. Absorption is slow and erratic with IM administration. Dilution of diazepam in IV solution is not recommended, but diazepam infusion (5 mg/h) has been used in treatment of status epilepticus. Cimetidine may increase the half-life of diazepam. In chronic therapy, discontinue drug gradually to avoid withdrawal reactions. |

BENZODIAZEPINES (continued)

DRUG	SUPPLIED	DOSE/ROUTE	REMARKS
Halazepam (Paxipam)	Tabs: 20,40 mg	**ADULTS** (Oral): **Sedation:** 20-40 mg po tid or qid; increase dose gradually up to 160 mg daily.	See diazepam.
Lorazepam (Ativan)	Tabs: 0.5,1,2 mg Vials: 2,4 mg/ml Tubex: 2,4 mg/ml	**ADULTS** (Oral and Parenteral): **Sedation:** 1-2 mg po/iv/im bid or tid; increase dose gradually up to 10 mg daily. **Hypnosis:** 2-4 mg po at bedtime. **Pre-op:** 0.05 mg/kg deep IM 2 h prior to surgery (up to 4 mg). **Status epilepticus:** 2-15 mg IVP; may repeat dose or 2 mg/min IV infusion.	Lorazepam and oxazepam are recommended in liver disease (little or no change in dosage is necessary). Lorazepam is absorbed more predictably from IM administration than are diazepam and chlordiazepoxide. Lorazepam has been used in the treatment of alcohol withdrawal. See diazepam for additional comments.
Oxazepam (Serax)	Caps: 10,15,30 mg Tabs: 15 mg	**ADULTS** (Oral): **Sedation:** 10-30 mg po tid or qid.	See diazepam and lorazepam.
Prazepam (Centrax)	Caps: 5,10,20 mg Tabs: 10 mg	**ADULTS** (Oral): **Sedation:** 30 mg po daily (one or two divided doses); increase dose gradually up to 60 mg daily.	See diazepam.
Temazepam (Restoril)	Caps: 15,30 mg	**ADULTS** (Oral): **Hypnotic:** 15-30 mg po at bedtime.	See diazepam.
Alprazolam (Xanax)	Tabs: 0.25,0.5,1 mg	**ADULTS** (Oral): **Sedation:** 0.25-0.5 mg po tid; increase dose gradually up to 4 mg daily.	See diazepam.
Clorazepate dipotassium (Tranxene)	Caps: 3.75,7.5,15 mg Tabs: 3.75,7.5,11.25, 15,22.5 mg	**ADULTS** (Oral): **Sedation:** 15 mg po bid; increase dose gradually up to 60 mg daily.	See diazepam.

BENZODIAZEPINES (continued)

DRUG	SUPPLIED	DOSE/ROUTE	REMARKS
Flurazepam hydrochloride (Dalmane)	**Caps:** 15,30 mg	**ADULTS (Oral):** **Hypnotic:** 15-30 mg po at bedtime.	See diazepam.
Chlordiazepoxide (Librium, Libritabs)	**Caps:** 5,10,25 mg **Tabs:** 5,10,25 mg **Amps:** 100 mg powder injection (supplied with 2 ml amp of IM diluent)	**ADULTS (Oral and Parenteral):** **Sedation:** 5-25 mg po/iv tid or qid. **Alcohol withdrawal:** 50-100 mg po/iv; repeat as necessary (600-800 mg daily is not uncommon); reduce dose gradually.	Rate of administration for IV use should not exceed 12.5 mg/min. IM administration is reserved for cases where oral or IV administration is not possible. Special IM diluent provided. Keep refrigerated. See diazepam for additional comments.
Midazolam hydrochloride (Versed)	**Vials:** 5 mg/ml **Disposable syringe:** 5 mg/ml	**ADULTS (Parenteral):** **Pre-op:** 0.07-0.08 mg/kg IM. **Endoscopic or cardiovascular procedures:** 0.1-0.2 mg/kg IV. **Induction of anesthesia:** 0.3-0.35 mg/kg IV.	Short-acting water-soluble benzodiazepine. See diazepam for additional comments.
Triazolam (Halcion)	**Tabs:** 0.125,0.25, 0.5 mg	**ADULTS (Oral):** **Hypnotic:** 0.25-0.5 mg po at bedtime.	Short-acting benzodiazepine. See diazepam for additional comments.

DIURETICS

DRUG	SUPPLIED	DOSE/ROUTE	REMARKS
Bumetanide (Bumex)	**Tabs:** 0.5, 1 mg **Amps:** 0.5 mg/2 ml	**Oral:** 0.5-2 mg/day given in a single dose; if necessary, give 1 or 2 more doses qd but not more than 10 mg/day with a 4-5 h interval between doses. **Parenteral:** 0.5-1 mg slow IV push initially, then 1 or 2 more doses up to 10 mg/day with a 2-3 h interval between doses.	Use with caution in hepatic coma, anuria, or severe electrolyte depletion. *Contraindicated* in patients with a history of hypersensitivity to the drug. Onset of diuresis after IV administration is 5-10 minutes with a duration of 2-4 hours. After oral administration, diuresis occurs within 30 to 60 minutes with a duration of 6-8 hours. One mg of bumetanide has a diuretic potency equivalent to about 40 mg of furosemide.

DIURETICS (continued)

DRUG	SUPPLIED	DOSE/ROUTE	REMARKS
Ethacrynic acid (Edecrin)	Tabs: 25,50 mg Parenteral: 50 mg/vial	Oral: Usual initial dose is 50 mg given as a single dose after a meal. Doses as high as 200 mg per day, given in divided doses after meal, may be required in some patients. Parenteral: 0.5 to 1 mg/kg as an initial dose. Single doses generally should not exceed 100 mg.	Use with caution in hepatic coma, anuria, and severe electrolyte depletion.
Furosemide (Lasix)	Tabs: 20,40,80 mg Oral solution: 10 mg/ml Amps: 10 mg/ml	Edema (oral): 20-80 mg po initially, then increments of 20-40 mg po q 6-8 h up to 600 mg/day. Edema (parenteral): 20-40 mg slow IV push initially, then increments of 20 mg q 2 h until adequate diuresis ensues. Hypotension: 40 mg po bid; adjust dosage to patient response. Acute pulmonary edema: 40-100 mg slow IV push.	Use with caution in hepatic coma, anuria, or severe electrolyte depletion. Contraindicated in patients with a history of hypersensitivity to the drug. Onset of diuresis after IV administration is 5-10 minutes with a duration of action of 2-4 hours. After oral administration, diuresis begins within 30 to 60 minutes with a duration of 6-8 hours.
Hydrochloro-thiazide (Esidrix, Hydroduril)	Tabs: 25,50,100 mg Oral solution: 50 mg/5 ml, 100 mg/ml	25-200 mg/day po.	Use with caution in patients with severe renal disease. Electrolyte disturbances may occur during thiazide therapy. Contraindicated in patients allergic to any thiazides or other sulfonamide derivatives.
Mannitol	Parenteral: 5%, 10%, 15%, 20% and 25% injection	Reduction of elevated ICP: 1-2 g/kg as a 20% solution over 30-60 min. Repeat dose q 4-6 h prn. Prevention of oliguria or acute renal failure: 50-100 g.	Patients with questionable renal function should receive 12.5 g infused over a 3-5 min period as a test dose. A response is considered adequate if at least 30-50 ml of urine per hour is excreted over the next 2-3 hours. If an adequate response is not attained, a second test dose may be given. Fluid and electrolyte imbalances may occur.

DIURETICS (continued)

DRUG	SUPPLIED	DOSE/ROUTE	REMARKS
Metolazone (Diulo, Zaroxolyn)	Tabs: 2.5, 5, 10 mg	Edema: 5-10 mg daily as a single dose. Up to 20 mg per day may be required for edema associated with renal disease.	May be used concomitantly with furosemide to induce diuresis in patients who did not respond to either diuretic alone. Electrolyte disturbances may occur. Severe volume and electrolyte depletion may occur when used concurrently with furosemide. *Contraindicated* in patients allergic to any thiazides or other sulfonamide derivative.
Spironolactone (Aldactone)	Tabs: 25,50,100 mg	25-200 mg/day in divided doses.	May be used for the treatment of diuretic-induced hypokalemia when oral potassium supplements are considered inappropriate. Severe hyperkalemia may occur in patients receiving potassium supplements concomitantly and in patients with renal insufficiency.

GASTROINTESTINAL

Histamine H_2-Receptor Antagonists:

DRUG	SUPPLIED	DOSE/ROUTE	REMARKS
Cimetidine (Tagamet)	Tabs: 200,300,400 mg Vial: 150 mg/ml Syrup: 300 mg/5 ml	Adult: 300 mg po/IV qid or 400 mg po q HS	Histamine H_2-receptor antagonist at the parietal cell level. Antacids can be given concomitantly with PO cimetidine. However, antacids may interfere with absorption of cimetidine. Mental confusion may occur especially in elderly patients with renal insufficiency. In the prophylaxis of stress ulceration, doses greater than 300 mg qid may be necessary to maintain adequate NG pH.
Ranitidine hydrochloride (Zantac)	Tabs: 150 mg Vial: 25 mg/ml	PO: 150 mg po bid or 300 mg po HS IV: 50 mg IV q 8 h.	May need doses up to 6 g/day in divided doses in pathologic hypersecretory conditions such as Zollinger-Ellison syndrome and systemic mastocytosis. Antacids can be given concomitantly. Adjust dosing with renal insufficiency. For patients with creatinine clearance < 50 ml/min, give 150 mg po qd.

GASTROINTESTINAL (continued)

Histamine H$_2$-Receptor Antagonists (continued):

DRUG	SUPPLIED	DOSE/ROUTE	REMARKS
Famotidine (Pepcid)	Tabs: 20, 40 mg Vial: 20 mg	PO: 40 mg po HS for treatment of active ulcer; 20 mg po HS for maintenance therapy.	Comparable to cimetidine or ranitidine in healing duodenal ulcers and preventing their recurrence. No antiandrogenic activity (which can occur with cimetidine). Does not interfere with hepatic metabolism. Experience still insufficient to compare its toxic effects to cimetidine or ranitidine.

Promotility:

Metoclopramide hydrochloride (Reglan)	Tabs: 10 mg Syrup: 5 mg/5 ml Amps: 5 mg/ml	**Intubation of small intestine:** 10 mg IVP. **Gastroesophageal reflux:** PO/IV/IM. **Gastric stasis:** PO/IV/IM 10 mg qid, 30 min before meals and ns. **Chemotherapy-induced emesis:** 2 mg/kg IVPB 30 min before chemotherapy and repeated twice at 2 h intervals following initial dose.	Useful in gastric stasis, gastroesophageal reflux, and prevention of cancer chemotherapy-induced emesis. Contraindicated in GI bleeding, bowel obstruction, epilepsy, pheochromocytoma, hypersensitivity to metoclopramide, and drugs with extra-pyramidal reaction side-effects.

Miscellaneous:

Omeprazole (Losec)	Caps (sustained release): 20 mg	**ADULTS:** **Severe erosive esophagitis or poorly responsive gastroesophageal reflux (GER):** 20 mg PO daily for 4–8 weeks. **Hypersecretory conditions:** Initial adult dose 60 mg PO qd. Individualize dosage. Doses of 120 mg tid have been used. Dosages in excess of 80 mg should be given in divided doses.	Benzimidazole compound suppresses gastric acid secretion inhibition of H$^+$/K$^+$ ATPase system ("acid proton pump"). Causes increase in serum gastrin levels. Effective in treatment of severe GER in terms of healing and symptom control. Use in hypersecretory condition (i.e., Zollinger-Ellison syndrome). Inhibits gastric acid secretion and controls symptoms of diarrhea, pain and anorexia. Well tolerated in Z-E patients with up to 5 years of therapy. Potential interactions with drugs metabolized by cytochrome P-450 system. No dosage adjustment necessary for patients with renal or hepatic dysfunction or in the elderly.

GASTROINTESTINAL (continued)

Miscellaneous (continued):

DRUG	SUPPLIED	DOSE/ROUTE	REMARKS
Misoprostol (Cytotec)	Tabs: 200 µg	NSAIA-induced ulcer prevention: PO: 200 µg qid Benign gastric ulcer: PO: 100-200 µg qid Active duodenal ulcer: PO: 100-200 µg qid or 400 µg bid	Synthetic analog of prostaglandin E₁. Gastric anti-secretory agent; protective effects in gastro-duodenal mucosa. Diarrhea is common side-effect, dose-related. *Contraindicated* in pregnant women.
Octreotide acetate (Sandostatin)	Injectable: 0.05 mg, 0.1 mg, 0.5 mg	**Initial dosage:** 50 µg sc 1-2 times/day Carcinoid tumors: 100-600 µg/day in 2-4 doses during first 2 weeks. Median daily dosage is 450 µg/day for maintenance therapy. VIPomas: 200-300 µg/day in 2-4 doses during first 2 weeks to control symptoms.	Mimics action of natural hormone somatostatin. Suppresses secretion of serotonin, gastrin, vasoactive intestinal peptide, insulin, glucagon, secretin, motilin, pancreatic polypeptide. Use in management of GI fistulas under investigation. Therapy may be associated with cholelithiasis. Initial therapy occasionally associated with hypo- or hyperglycemia. Nausea, diarrhea, abdominal pain, loose stools, pain at injection site may occur.
Sucralfate (Carafate)	Tabs: 1 g	1 g/h before each meal and at bedtime	Does not affect gastric acid output or concentration. Binds to gastroduodenal mucosa and acts as a barrier to gastric acid. *Avoid* co-administration of antacids and sucralfate, as an acidic medium is required for dissolution of sucralfate.
HYPOGLYCEMICS			
Chlorpropamide (Diabenese)	Tabs: 100,200 mg (scored)	**Adults:** Oral: 250 mg po QAM with breakfast; increase dose by 50-125 mg/day every 3-5 days. Geriatric patients: 100-125 mg po QAM initial dose. Doses may be divided in two (Maximum 750 mg in 24 h). Monitor urine sugar/acetone and/or blood sugar.	First generation oral hypoglycemic agent. Adverse reactions include hypersensitivity and idiosyncratic reactions. Disulfiram-like reactions in patients ingesting alcohol may occur. Can cause SIADH secretion, primarily in elderly patients. See acetohexamide for additional comments.

HYPOGLYCEMICS (continued)

DRUG	SUPPLIED	DOSE/ROUTE	REMARKS
Acetohexamide (Dymelor)	Tabs: 250, 500 mg	**Adults:** Oral: 250 mg po QAM with breakfast, increase dose by 250-500 mg/day every 5-7 days. Doses may be divided in two (Maximum: 1.5 g in 24 h). Monitor urine sugar/acetone and/or blood sugar.	First generation sulfonylurea. Elderly patients and severely compromised patients may have exaggerated hypoglycemic response (Monitor carefully during first 24 h). Adverse reactions include GI tract disturbances, cholestatic and mixed hepatic jaundice and hematologic toxicities. *Contraindications* include type I DM, uncontrolled DM, DM secondary to renal dysfunction, patients with major surgery, severe infection and severe trauma. Use with caution in patients with porphyria and in patients with cardiovascular disease. Not recommended in patients with renal or hepatic disease. Monitor for many potential drug interactions. Tolerance may develop.
Glipizide (Glucotrol)	Tabs: 5, 10 mg (scored)	**Adults:** Oral: 5 mg po QAM 30 min before breakfast; increase dose by 2.5-5 mg/day every 3-7 days. **Geriatric patients and hepatic disease:** 2.5 mg po QAM initial dose. Doses may be divided in 2-3 (Maximum: 40 mg in 24 h). Monitor urine sugar/acetone and/or blood sugar.	Second generation sulfonylurea. See acetohexamide for additional comments.
Glyburide (Diabeta, Micronase)	Tabs: 1.25, 2.5, 5 mg (scored)	**Adults:** Oral: 2.5-5 mg po QAM 30 min before breakfast; increase dose by 2.5 mg/day every 7 days. **Geriatric patients:** 1.25 mg po QAM initial dose. Doses may be divided in 2 (Maximum: 20 mg in 24 h). Monitor urine sugar/acetone and/or blood sugar.	Second generation sulfonylurea. See acetohexamide for additional comments.

HYPOGLYCEMICS (continued)

DRUG	SUPPLIED	DOSE/ROUTE	REMARKS
Tolazamide (Tolinase)	Tabs: 100,250,500 mg (scored)	**Adults:** Oral: 100-250 mg po QAM with breakfast; increase dose by 100-250 mg/day every 7 days. **Geriatric patients:** 50-125 mg po QAM initial dose. Maximum: 1 g in 24 h. Monitor urine sugar/acetone and/or blood sugar.	First generation sulfonylurea. See acetohexamide for additional comments.
Tolbutamide (Orinase)	Tabs: 250,500 mg (scored)	**Adults:** Oral: 250 mg po QAM with breakfast; increase dose by 250 mg/day every several days. **Geriatric patients:** may require lower doses. Maximum: 3 g in 24 h. Monitor urine sugar/acetone and/or blood sugar.	First generation sulfonylurea. See acetohexamide for additional comments.
Glucagon hydrochloride	Vials: 1 unit plus 1 ml diluent; 10 units plus 10 ml diluent.	**ADULTS: Parenteral:** Hypoglycemia: 0.5-1 unit sc/im/iv; may repeat dose in 5-20 min. GI tract radiographic exam: 0.25-2 units iv or 1-2 units im. **CHILDREN: Parenteral:** Hypoglycemia: 0.025 mg/kg; may repeat dose.	Adverse reactions include nausea and vomiting. Use with caution in patients with insulinoma and pheochromocytoma. Supplemental carbohydrate source should be administered to patients with hypoglycemia. Short duration of action. Glucagon 1 unit = 1 mg.
INOTROPES			
Amrinone (Inocor)	Vial: 5 mg/ml	**Loading dose:** 0.75 mg/kg IVP over 2-3 min.	Activity is secondary to inotropic and/or vasodilatory properties. Reversible thrombocytopenia may occur in < 5% of patients. Comparable inotropic activity to that of dobutamine.
Dobutamine (Dobutrex)	Vial: 200 mg/5 ml	**Initial dose:** 2.5-15 μg/kg/min.	More potent inotropic agent than dopamine. Not a mesenteric or renal vasodilator; little peripheral vasoconstriction. Predominant β-adrenergic effects (β_1 and β_2).

INOTROPES (continued)

DRUG	SUPPLIED	DOSE/ROUTE	REMARKS
Epinephrine (Adrenalin)	Amp: 1 mg/ml Vial: 30 mg/30 ml Mix 1 mg in 100-250 cc D5W	IV infusions: 1. β-effects: 0.5-1.5 mg/min 2. α- and β-effects: > 1.5 μg/min Intracardiac: 0.5 mg SC or IM: 0.2-0.5 mg q 10 min prn. Prolongation of action of local anesthetics: 0.1-0.2 mg added to local anesthetic solution to a final concentration of 1:100,000 to 1:20,000	α and β (β_1 and β_2) agonist. Action impaired in acidosis. Useful in profound hypotension to maintain organ perfusion. Can support myocardial contractility and heart rate. Stimulates respiration and is potent bronchodilator in low doses. Useful in subcutaneous administration in asthma. Used to treat anaphylactic reactions. High doses may elevate myocardial oxygen consumption. Contraindicated in narrow-angle glaucoma, coronary insufficiency, labor, cyclopropane and halogenated hydrocarbons, local anesthesia of fingers and toes.
Dopamine (Intropin)	Amps: 200 mg/5 ml Vials: 200,400,800 mg/5 ml	Predominant dopaminergic effects: 1. Predominant dopaminergic effects: 1-2 μg/kg/min. 2. Predominant β-adrenergic effects: 2-10 μg/kg/min. 3. Predominant α-adrenergic effects: > 10 μg/kg/min. Initial dose: 2-5 μg/kg/min; then titrate to desired response.	Stimulates α- and β-receptors (β_1 and β_2) and dopaminergic receptors. Supports circulation in a variety of low-output states. In low doses, augments renal blood flow and promotes diuresis. At infusions over 20 μg/kg/min, α-activity predominates and antagonizes dopaminergic effects and increases ventricular afterload; therefore, avoid this agent at this dosage in myocardial ischemia. Contraindicated in pheochromocytoma. May induce tachycardia, requiring a reduction in or discontinuation of dose.
Isoproterenol (Isuprel)	Vial: 0.2 mg/ml, 1 mg/5 ml	Initial dose: 2-10 μg/min IV infusion. Rates greater than 30 μg/min may be used in advanced stages of shock.	β-adrenergic (β_1 and β_2) agonist with chronotopic & inotropic properties. Used for inotropic support, especially when myocardial O_2 supply is not compromised. Can serve as a temporary acceleration of heart rate in heart block. Contraindicated with development of tachyarrhythmia and ventricular irritability. Muscle bed vasodilation can unmask relative hypovolemia and produce hypotension. Avoid in myocardial ischemia.

INOTROPES (continued)

DRUG	SUPPLIED	DOSE/ROUTE	REMARKS
Digoxin (Lanoxin, Lanoxicaps)	Tabs: 125,250,500 μg Caps: 50,100,200 μg Elixir: 50 μg/ml. Amps: 100,250 μg/ml.	**Digitalizing dose (Adults): PO:** 10-15 μg/kg, with 50% of dose given as first dose, then 25% of dose given at 6-8 hr intervals until adequate response is achieved or total digitalizing dose is administered. **IV:** 8-12 μg/kg, with 50% of dose given as first dose, then 25% of dose given at 4-8 hr intervals until adequate response is achieved or total digitalizing dose is administered. Maintenance dose should be adjusted by creatinine clearance.	Usual range (adult) 0.8-2.0 ng/ml. Higher levels may be needed in control of ventricular rate in atrial flutter or fibrillation. Only 60-85% of tablet or elixir dose is absorbed. Capsules are 90-100% absorbed. Doses should be modified when changing from one route of administration to another.

INSULIN

DRUG	SUPPLIED	DOSE/ROUTE	REMARKS
Insulin (*regular* insulin, crystalline zinc insulin)	Vials: Single peak (pork) 100 U/ml Single peak (beef and pork) 100 U/ml Purified (beef) 100 U/ml Purified (pork) 100,500 U/ml Combination purified (pork) 30 U/ml plus Isophane 70 U/ml	**ADULTS: Parenteral:** 5-10 U sc 15-30 min before meals and at bedtime. Doses should be individualized according to urine & blood sucrose. **Diabetic ketoacidosis: Low dose:** initial dose 2.4-7.2 U, then 2.4-7.2 U/hour as an infusion. **CHILDREN: Parenteral:** 2-4 U sc 15-30 min before meals and at bedtime. Individualized dosing is essential. **Diabetic ketoacidosis:** Initial dose 1-2 U/kg in two divided doses (one IV, one sc), then 0.5-1 U/kg q 1-2 h.	Regular insulin can be given sc, IV, IM, or IV infusion. Short-acting insulin. Adverse reactions include hypoglycemic reactions, atrophy or hypertrophy, mental status changes, insulin resistance and allergy. Rotate injection sites to avoid atrophy or hypertrophy. Decrease dose by 20% when converting from single peak insulin to purified insulin. Any changes in insulin preparation or dosage regimen should be made carefully. Purified insulin may be less immunogenic than single peak insulin. Pure pork insulin may be less immunogenic than mixed or beef insulin.
Insulin human (Humulin, Novolin), recombinant DNA and semisynthetic	Vials: Regular 100 U/ml Zinc 100 U/ml Isophane 100 U/ml	**ADULTS AND CHILDREN: Parenteral:** doses should be individualized according to urine and blood glucose.	Regular human insulin can be given sc, IV, IM, or IV. Zinc and Isophane human insulin must *not* be given IV. Human insulin may be less immunogenic than purified insulin. See Insulin (Regular) for additional comments.

INSULIN (continued)

DRUG	SUPPLIED	DOSE/ROUTE	REMARKS
Insulin, Isophane (Neutral Protamine Hagedorin, NPH Insulin)	Vials: Single peak (beef) 100 U/ml Single peak (beef and pork) 40,100 U/ml Purified (beef) 100 U/ml Purified (pork) 100 U/ml Purified combination (pork) 70 U/ml + regular 30 U/ml	ADULTS: Parenteral: 7-26 U sc QAM 30-60 min before breakfast. Some patients may require a smaller dose with supper or at bedtime. Increase dose by 2-10 U/day every few days. Doses should be individualized according to urine and blood glucose.	Isophane insulin must be given by sc only. Intermediate-acting insulin. Equivalent doses can be used when changing from zinc to isophane insulins. See Insulin (Regular) for additional comments.
Insulin, Protamine zinc (PZI)	Vials: Single peak (beef and pork) 100 U/ml Purified (beef) 100 U/ml Purified (pork) 100 U/ml	ADULTS: Parenteral: 7-26 U sc QAM 30-60 min before breakfast. Doses should be individualized according to urine and blood glucose.	Protamine zinc insulin must be given by sc only. Long-acting insulin. Decrease dose by 1/3 when changing form regular insulin to PZI. See Insulin (Regular) for additional comments.
Insulin zinc (Lente)	Vials: Single peak (beef) 100 U/ml Single peak (beef and pork) 40,100 U/ml Purified (beef) 100 U/ml Purified (pork) 100 U/ml	ADULTS: Parenteral: 7-26 U sc QAM 30-60 min before breakfast. Some patients may require a smaller dose with supper or at bedtime. Increase dose by 2-10 U/day every few days. Doses should be individualized according to urine and blood glucose.	Zinc insulin must be given by sc only. Intermediate-acting insulin. Equivalent doses can be used when changing from isophane to zinc insulin. See Insulin (Regular) for additional comments.
Insulin zinc, extended (UltraLente)	Vials: Single peak (beef) 100 U/ml Single peak (beef and pork) 40,100 U/ml Purified (beef) 100 U/ml	ADULTS: Parenteral: 7-26 U sc QAM 30-60 min before breakfast. Doses should be individualized according to urine and blood glucose.	Extended zinc insulin must be given by sc only. Long-acting insulin. Decrease dose by 1/3 when changing from regular insulin to extended zinc insulin. See Insulin (Regular) for additional comments.

INSULIN (continued)

DRUG	SUPPLIED	DOSE/ROUTE	REMARKS
Insulin zinc, prompt (SemiLente)	Vials: Single peak (beef) 100 U/ml Single peak (beef and pork) 40,100 U/ml Purified (pork) 100 U/ml	ADULTS: Parenteral: 10-20 U sc QAM 30 min before breakfast and 2-3 more times/day usually before meals. Doses should be individualized according to urine and blood glucose.	Prompt zinc insulin must be given by sc only. Short-acting insulin. See Insulin (Regular) for additional comments.

NARCOTIC ANALGESICS

DRUG	SUPPLIED	DOSE/ROUTE	REMARKS
Morphine sulfate	Oral solution: 10,20 mg per 5 ml, 20 mg per 10 ml, 20 mg/ml Tabs: extended-release 30 mg.	ADULTS: Oral solution: 10-30 mg po q 4 h prn or as directed. Extended-release tabs: 30 mg po q 8-12 h prn. Parenteral: 5-20 mg sc/im/iv q 3-4 h prn. IV infusion: start at 1-10 mg/h, titrate to 20-150 mg/h (for severe chronic pain associated with cancer). Epidural infusion: 0.6-0.8 mg/kg/day (up to 30 mg as continuous infusion). Rectal: 10-20 mg pr q 4 h prn. CHILDREN: Parenteral: 0.1-0.2 mg/kg up to 15 mg sc/im q 3-4 h prn. IV infusion: 0.025-2.6 mg/kg/h iv; 0.025-1.79 mg/kg/h sc.	For use as a preoperative medication or in severe pain. *Contraindicated* with known hypersensitivity. May cause psychic or physical dependence. Adverse reactions include nausea, vomiting, biliary tract spasm, urinary retention, hypotension, respiratory depression, apnea, cardiac arrest. Administer naloxone (adult 0.4 mg, child 0.01 mg/kg iv) for respiratory depression and overdoses.
Fentanyl citrate (Sublimaze) and combination product (Innovar)	Amps: 0.05 mg/ml (50 mg/ml) Combination product: fentanyl 0.05 mg/ml + droperidol 2.5 mg/ml	ADULTS: Parenteral: 0.002-0.1 mg/kg iv/im; may repeat in 1-2 h; pre-op 0.05-0.1 mg/kg im 30-60 min before surgery. CHILDREN (2-12 years old): Parenteral: 0.02-0.03 mg/kg/20-25 lbs (10 kg).	Less emetic effect, less sedation, and less histamine release than other narcotic analgesics. *Contraindications* include hypersensitivity and monoamine oxidase therapy. Adverse reactions include respiratory depression, muscular rigidity, bradycardia. Administer naloxone (see morphine sulfate) for respiratory depression and overdoses.

NARCOTIC ANALGESICS (continued)

DRUG	SUPPLIED	DOSE/ROUTE	REMARKS
Hydromorphone hydrochloride (Dilaudid) and combination product	Tabs: 1,2,3,4 mg Amps: 1,2,3,4,10 mg/ml Vials: 2 mg/ml Tubex: 1,2,3,4 mg/ml Supp: 3 mg Combination product syrup: hydromorphone 1 mg/ml + guaifenesin 100 mg/5 ml	Analgesic – ADULTS: Oral: 2 mg po q 4-6 h prn. For severe pain 4 mg po q 4-6 h prn. Parenteral: 2 mg sc/im q 4-6 h prn (IV administration over 2-3 min). Rectal: 3 mg pr q 6-8 h prn. Antitussive: Oral: adults and children older than 12 years: 1 mg po q 3-4 h prn; children 6-12 years: 0.5 mg po q 3-4 h prn.	Contraindications include hypersensitivity and in patients with increased intracranial pressure. May cause psychic or physical dependence. Adverse reactions include CNS depression, nausea, vomiting, hypotension, and respiratory depression. Administer naloxone (see morphine sulfate) for respiratory depression and overdoses.
Meperidine hydrochloride (Demerol)	Tabs: 50,100 mg Syrup: 50 mg/5 ml Amps: 25,50,75,100 mg/ml Vials: 25,50,75, 100 mg/ml Disposable syringe: 25,50,75,100 ml	ADULTS: Oral: 50-150 mg po q 3-4 h prn. Parenteral: 50-150 mg sc/im q 3-4 h prn (or slow iv administration). IV infusion: 15-35 mg/h. CHILDREN: Oral: 1.1-1.8 mg/kg po q 3-4 h prn. Parenteral: 1.1-1.8 mg/kg im/sc q 3-4 h prn; pre-op 1-2.2 mg/kg im/sc.	Drug is least effective when given orally. IM route is preferred over SC route when repeated doses are needed. Contraindications include hypersensitivity, monoamine oxidase inhibition therapy, and lactation. May cause psychic or physical dependence. Adverse reactions include CNS alterations, nausea, vomiting, constipation, respiratory depression, cardiac arrhythmias and hypotension. Patient with renal dysfunction may accumulate normeperidine (metabolite) causing seizures. Administer naloxone (see morphine sulfate) for respiratory depression and overdoses.
Sufentanil citrate (Sufenta)	Amps: 50 µg/ml	ADULTS: Parenteral: Analgesia: 1-8 µg/kg iv/im inter-mittent. Anesthesia: 8-30 µg/kg iv infusion. CHILDREN (< 12 years old): Parenteral: Anesthesia: 10-25 µg/kg iv infusion.	Respiratory depression & skeletal muscle rigidity are most common adverse reactions associated with sufentanil. Other side-effects include cardio-vascular changes, nausea, vomiting. Patients on β-blocker therapy require lower doses. Admin-ister with caution in patients with liver and renal disease. Administer naloxone (see morphine sulfate) for respiratory depression and overdoses.

NARCOTIC ANALGESICS (continued)

DRUG	SUPPLIED	DOSE/ROUTE	REMARKS
Codeine sulfate or phosphate and combination products (Tylenol with Codeine #1,2,3,4)	Tabs: 15,30,60 mg Vials: 30,60 mg/ml Disposable syringe: 30,60 mg/ml Combination products: Tabs: 300 mg acetaminophen + 7,5, 15, 30, 60 mg codeine; Oral liquid: 120 mg acetaminophen + 12 mg codeine/5 ml	**ADULTS: Antitussive:** Oral: 10-20 mg po q 4-6 h (maximum 120 mg in 24 h). **Analgesic:** Oral and parenteral: 15-60 mg po, im, sc, iv q 4-6 h. **CHILDREN: Antitussive:** Oral [2-6 years]: 2.5-5 mg po q 4-6 h (maximum 30 mg in 24 h). [6-12 years]: 5-10 mg po q 4-6 h (maximum 60 mg in 24 h). **Analgesic** [> 1 year]: Oral and parenteral: 0.5 mg/kg (15 mg/m^2) po, im, sc q 4-6 h.	*Contraindications* include hypersensitivity to codeine. May cause psychic and physical dependency. Adverse reactions include sedation, dizziness, nausea, vomiting, and respiratory depression. Administer naloxone (see morphine sulfate) for respiratory depression and overdoses.
Pentazocine lactate or hydrochloride (Talwin, Talwin NX) **and combination products**	Tabs: 50 mg pentazocine + 0.5 mg naloxone. Amps: 30 mg/ml Vials: 30 mg/ml Combination products: Tabs: pentazocine 12.5 mg + aspirin 325 mg; Caplets: pentazocine 25 mg + acetaminophen 650 mg	**ADULTS:** Oral: 50-100 mg po q 3-4 h prn (maximum 600 mg in 24 h). Parenteral: 30-60 mg im,sc,iv q 3-4 h prn (maximum 360 mg in 24 h). Combination products: 1 caplet or 2 tablets po q 3-4 h prn.	Narcotic agonist/antagonist. May precipitate withdrawal reactions in patients with narcotic addiction. May cause psychic or physical dependency. *Contraindications* include hypersensitivity to pentazocine. Adverse reactions include nausea, vomiting, dizziness, sedation, cardiovascular changes and respiratory depression. *Not* recommended in patients with increased intracranial pressure. May increase biliary tract pressure. May cause skin and soft tissue changes. Rotate injection sites. IM route is preferred over SC route. *Not* recommended in children under 12 years of age. Administer naloxone (see morphine sulfate) for respiratory depression and overdoses.
Fiorinal® (aspirin, butalbital and caffeine)	Caps: aspirin 325 mg, butalbital 50 mg, caffeine 40 mg. Tabs: same	**ADULTS:** Oral: 1-2 caps or tabs po q 3-6 h.	*Contraindicated* in porphyria, hypersensitivity to aspirin, caffeine or barbiturate. Can cause psychic or physical dependence. Can raise PT. May be beneficial in vascular headaches. Other combination products available.

NARCOTIC ANALGESICS (continued)

DRUG	SUPPLIED	DOSE/ROUTE	REMARKS
Oxycodone hydrochloride and combination products (Percocet-5, Tylox, Percodan)	Tabs: 5 mg Oral solution: 5 mg/5 ml Combination products: Tabs: 5 mg oxycodone HCl + 325 mg acetaminophen (Percocet-5); 4.5 mg oxycodone HCl + 0.38 mg oxycodone terephthalate + 500 mg acetaminophen (Tylox); 4.5 mg oxycodone HCl + 0.38 mg oxycodone terephthalate + 3.25 mg aspirin (Percodan)	ADULTS: Oral: 1-2 tabs po q 4-6 h prn.	*Contraindications* include hypersensitivity to oxycodone, acetaminophen or aspirin (depending on the product). May cause psychic or physical dependency. Adverse reactions include light-headedness, sedation, nausea, and vomiting. Administer naloxone (see morphine sulfate) for respiratory depression or over- doses (in addition to appropriate therapy for aspirin or acetaminophen overdose if combination product).
Propoxyphene hydrochloride (Darvon) or napsylate (Darvon-N) or combination product (Darvocet-N)	Caps: 32,65 mg propoxyphene (Darvon). Tabs: 100 mg propoxyphene napsylate (Darvon-N). Susp: 10 mg/ml propoxyphene napsylate (Darvon-N). Combination product: Tabs: 50,100 mg propoxyphene napsylate + 325,650 mg acetaminophen (Darvocet-N).	ADULTS: Oral: 65 mg propoxyphene HCl po q 4 h prn (maximum 320 mg in 24 h). 100 mg propoxyphene napsylate po q 4 h prn (maximum 600 mg in 24 h).	*Contraindications* include hypersensitivity to propoxyphene, acetaminophen or aspirin (depending on the product). May cause psychic and/or physical dependency. Adverse reactions include dizziness, sedation, nausea, and vomiting. Administer naloxone (see morphine sulfate) for respiratory depression and overdoses (may require repeated doses of naloxone because of the long half-life).
Methadone hydrochloride (Dolophine)	Oral solution: 5,10 mg/ 5 ml x 10 mg/ml (concentrated). Tabs: 5,10 mg Vials: 10 mg/ml	ADULTS: Analgesic: Oral and parenteral: 2.5-10 mg po,sc,im q 6 h prn. (In severe chronic pain in cancer patients, 5-20 mg po,sc,im q 6 h.) Detoxification and maintenance of narcotic addicts: Oral: various dose ranges may be necessary depending on the patient.	Used in severe pain and in detoxification and maintenance of narcotic addicts. *Contra-indications* include hypersensitivity to methadone. May cause psychic and/or physical dependency. Side-effects include nausea, vomiting, biliary tract spasm, urinary retention, respiratory depression, cardiovascular changes, constipation, and sweating. Administer naloxone (see morphine sulfate) for respiratory depression and overdoses (may require repeated doses of naloxone because of the long half-life).

NARCOTIC AGONIST / ANTAGONIST ANALGESICS

DRUG	SUPPLIED	DOSE/ROUTE	REMARKS
Butorphanol tartrate (Stadol)	Amps: 1 mg/ml Vials: 1.2 mg/ml Disposable syringe: 2 mg/ml	ADULTS: Parenteral: 1-4 mg im or 0.5-2 mg iv q 3-4 h prn.	Narcotic agonist/antagonist. May precipitate withdrawal reaction in patients with narcotic addiction. *Contraindications* include hypersensitivity to butorphanol. Adverse reactions include sedation, nausea, vomiting, respiratory depression and blood pressure changes. *Not* recommended in patients with increased intracranial pressure. Low psychic and physical dependence liability. Reduce dose in hepatic disease. *Not* recommended in children < 18 years old. Administer naloxone (see morphine sulfate) for respiratory depression and overdoses. Causes less respiratory depression than morphine sulfate.
Nalbuphine (Nubain)	Amps: 10,20 mg/ml Vials: 10 mg/ml	ADULTS: Parenteral: 10-20 mg sc, im/iv q 3-6 h prn (maximum 160 mg per 24 h).	Narcotic agonist/antagonist (less antagonist action than butorphanol). May precipitate withdrawal symptoms in patients with narcotic addiction. *Contraindications* include hypersensitivity to nalbuphine. Adverse reactions include sedation, nausea, vomiting, respiratory depression, cardiovascular changes, and mental status changes. Low psychic and physical dependence liability. *Not* recommended in patients with increased intracranial pressure. May cause biliary tract spasm. Patients on therapy should receive 25% of the dose. Reduce dose in hepatic or renal disease. *Not* recommended in children < 18 years old. Administer naloxone (see morphine sulfate) for respiratory depression and overdoses. Respiratory depression is equal to morphine, but nalbuphine exhibits a ceiling effect.

NARCOTIC AGONIST / ANTAGONIST ANALGESICS (continued)

DRUG	SUPPLIED	DOSE/ROUTE	REMARKS
Buprenorphine hydrochloride (Buprenex)	Amps: 0.3 mg/ml	Adults and children > 13 years: Parenteral: 0.3-0.6 mg im or slow iv q 6 h prn.	Narcotic agonist/antagonist. May precipitate withdrawal reactions in patients with narcotic addiction. Low physical dependence liability. May cause psychic dependency. *Contraindications* include hypersensitivity to buprenorphine. Side-effects include sedation, nausea, vertigo, dizziness, vomiting, hypotension, and respiratory depression. *Not* recommended in patients with increased intracranial pressure. High doses of naloxone may be required to reverse respiratory depression.

NARCOTIC ANTAGONISTS

Naloxone (Narcan and Narcan Neonatal)	Amps: 0.4,1 mg/ml; Neonatal 0.02 mg/ml	ADULTS: Parenteral: post-op 0.1-0.2 mg iv,sc,im q 3-2 min until response, additional doses q 1-2 h; opiate overdose 0.4-2 mg iv,sc,im q 2-3 min up to 10 mg. Infusion: 0.4 mg/h. CHILDREN: Parenteral: post-op 0.005-0.01 mg q 2-3 min until response, additional doses q 1-2 h; opiate overdoses 0.01 mg/kg iv,sc,im. Infusion: 0.0037 mg/kg/h.	Adverse reactions include nausea, vomiting, sweating, tachycardia. *Contraindications* include hypersensitivity to naloxone. Use with *caution* in patients with preexisting cardiovascular disease. IV administration is preferred in acute situations. In some narcotic overdoses, repeated doses or IV infusion may be necessary (some narcotics may have longer duration of action than naloxone). Naloxone is currently under investigation for many other purposes besides reversal of narcotic actions.

NON–NARCOTIC ANALGESICS

Acetaminophen (Tylenol, Panadol, Datril, and others)	Caps: 325,500 mg Tabs: 325,500,650 mg Chewable tabs: 80 mg Elixir: 120,160,325 mg per 5 ml Oral solution: 100 mg/ ml, 120 mg per 2.5 ml Supp: 120,125,325,650 mg	ADULTS: Oral and rectal: 325 mg po/pr q 4-6 h prn (maximum: short-term 4-6 h, long-term 2.6 g per 24 h). CHILDREN: Oral or rectal: 10 mg/kg/dose (maximum: 5 doses per 24 h).	*Contraindications* include hypersensitivity to acetaminophen; overdosage presents early as nausea, vomiting and malaise, and presents late as clinical and laboratory evidence of hepatotoxicity. Do not use charcoal to treat overdoses. Acetylcysteine (Muco-Myst) may be administered depending on the time after ingestion and the acetaminophen blood levels present.

NON-STEROIDAL ANTI-INFLAMMATORY AGENTS

DRUG	SUPPLIED	DOSE/ROUTE	REMARKS
Ibuprofen (Motrin, Advil, Nuprin, Rufen)	Tabs: 200,300,400, 800 mg	**ADULTS (Oral): Anti-inflammatory:** 400-800 mg po tid or qid with meals or milk. (Maximum 3.2 g in 24 h) **Antipyretic, analgesia and dysmenorrhea:** 200-400 mg po q 4-6 h. **CHILDREN (Oral): Anti-inflammatory:** < 20 kg: 400 mg/day; 20-30 kg: 600 mg/day; 30-40 kg: 800 mg/day; > 40 kg: as an adult.	Non-steroidal anti-inflammatory agent (NSAIA). Adverse reactions include GI tract disturbances (including ulcers and bleeding), CNS changes, hepatotoxicity, hematologic toxicity, renal toxicity and edema. Use with *caution* in patients with PUD, bleeding abnormalities, renal dysfunction, hypertension and cardiac dysfunction. *Contraindications* include hypersensitivity to ibuprofen and in patients in whom asthma, rhinitis or urticaria is precipitated by aspirin or other NSAIA's. May inhibit platelet aggregation. May increase PT in patients receiving oral anti-coagulants.
Diflunisol (Dolobid)	Tabs: 250,500 mg	**ADULTS (Oral): Anti-inflammatory:** 500-1000 mg po q 12 h with meals or milk. **Analgesia:** 500-1000 mg po, then 250-500 mg po q 12 h with meals or milk. Maximum: 1.5 g in 24 h.	Non-steroidal anti-inflammatory agent. See ibuprofen for additional comments.
Naproxen (Naprosyn, Anaprox)	Tabs: 250,375,500 mg	**ADULTS (Oral): Anti-inflammatory:** 250-375 mg po bid with meals or milk; increase dose depending on patient response. Maximum: 1 g in 24 h. **Analgesia and dysmenorrhea:** 500 mg po, then 250 mg po q 6-8 h with meals or milk. Maximum: 1.25 g in 24 h.	Non-steroidal anti-inflammatory agent. See ibuprofen for additional comments.
Sulindac (Clinoril)	Tabs: 150,200 mg (scored)	**ADULTS (Oral): Anti-inflammatory:** 150 mg po bid with meals or milk; increase dose depending on patient response. Maximum: 400 mg in 24 h.	Non-steroidal anti-inflammatory agent. See ibuprofen for additional comments.

NON-STEROIDAL ANTI-INFLAMMATORY AGENTS (continued)

DRUG	SUPPLIED	DOSE/ROUTE	REMARKS
Indomethacin (Indocin, Indocin SR, Indocin-IV)	Caps: 25, 50 mg; Caps, extended release: 75 mg; Oral susp: 25 mg/5 ml; Supp: 50 mg; Vial: 1 mg.	**ADULTS** (Oral or rectal): **Anti-inflammatory:** 25 mg po/pr bid or tid; increase dose 25-50 mg/day every 7 days. Extended-release cap: 75 mg po QAM or QPM; increase dose to 75 mg po bid with meals or milk. Maximum: 200 mg in 24 h. **NEONATES** (premature): **Patent Ductus Arteriosus:** 0.2 mg/kg iv initially, then: < 48 h of age: 0.1 mg/kg q 12-24 h x 2 doses; 2-7 days of age: 0.2 mg/kg q 12-24 h x 2 doses; > 7 days of age: 0.25 mg/kg q 12-24 h x 2 doses; Second and third doses may *not* be given in anuria.	Non-steroidal anti-inflammatory agent. Ocular and otic reactions may occur. *Not* recommended in children younger than 14 years old except for neonates for the treatment of Patent Ductus Arteriorus. GI bleeding, intraventricular hemorrhage and renal insufficiency have been associated with indomethacin therapy in neonates. See ibuprofen for additional comments.
Fenoprofen (Nalfon)	Caps: 200, 300 mg Tabs: 600 mg (scored)	**ADULTS** (Oral): **Anti-inflammatory:** 300-600 mg po tid or qid with meals or milk; increase dose depending on patient response. Maximum: 3.2 g in 24 h. **Analgesia:** 200-400 mg po q 4-6 h with meals or milk.	Non-steroidal anti-inflammatory agent. See ibuprofen for additional comments.
Tolmentin sodium (Tolectin, Tolectin DS)	Caps: 400 mg Tabs: 200 mg	**ADULTS** (Oral): **Anti-inflammatory:** 400 mg po tid with meals or milk; increase dose depending on patient response. Maximum: 2 g in 24 h. **CHILDREN** (Oral): (< 2 years old): **Anti-inflammatory** (< 2 years old): 20 mg/kg/day in 3-4 divided doses with meals or milk; increase dose depending on patient response. Maximum: 30 mg/kg in 24 h.	Non-steroidal anti-inflammatory agent. See ibuprofen for additional comments.

NON-STEROIDAL ANTI-INFLAMMATORY AGENTS (continued)

DRUG	SUPPLIED	DOSE/ROUTE	REMARKS
Phenylbutazone, oxyphenbutazone	Caps: 100 mg Tabs: 100 mg	ADULTS (Oral): Anti-inflammatory: 300-600 mg po daily in 3-4 divided doses with meals or milk.	Non-steroidal anti-inflammatory agent. Use with caution in patients > 40 years of age. Ocular and otic reactions may occur. Hematologic toxicity could be severe (including aplastic anemia). Long-term therapy is *not* recommended. *Contraindications* include: patients with incipient cardiac failure; blood dyscrasias; pancreatitis; parotitis stomatitis; polymyalgia rheumatica; temporal arteritis; senility; drug allergy; severe renal, cardiac, or hepatic disease; history of PUD and known reactions to either drug. See ibuprofen for additional comments.
Piroxicam (Feldene)	Caps: 10,20 mg	ADULTS (Oral): Anti-inflammatory: 20 mg po QD with meal or milk. Maximum: 40 mg in 24 h.	Non-steroidal anti-inflammatory agent. Pediatric dosage recommendations not established. See ibuprofen for additional comments.
Aspirin (ASA, acetyl-salicylic acid)	Caps: 325 mg Tabs: 325,500,650 mg Caps (enteric coated particles): 325,500 mg Tabs (enteric coated): 325,500,650,975 mg Tabs (chewable): 65,81 mg Tabs (extended-release): 650,800 mg Tabs (film coated): 325,500 mg Supp: 60,65,120,125, 130,195,200,300,325, 600,650,1200 mg. Aspirin with buffers also available.	ADULTS (Oral or Rectal): Pain and fever: 325-650 mg po/pr q 4 h prn. Maximum 4 g in 24 h. Inflammatory diseases: Initial: 2.4-3.6 g per day; Maintenance: 3.6-5.4 g per day. Thrombosis: TIA's and stroke: 1.3 g/day in 2-4 divided doses. Myocardial infarction: 300-325 mg once daily. CHILDREN (Oral or Rectal): Pain and fever: 2-11 years old: 65 mg/kg/day po/pr in 4-6 divided doses. ≥ 11 years old: 325-650 mg po/pr q 4 h prn. Maximum: 4 g per 24 h. Inflammatory diseases: Juvenile rheumatoid arthritis: ≤ 25 kg: 60-90 mg/kg/day. ≥ 25 kg: 2.4-3.6 g per day in 4-6 divided doses.	*Caution* in PUD, platelet disorders, anticoagulant therapy (coumadin), hypoprothrombinemia, and asthma. *Contraindications* include hypersensitivity to salicylates and in patients with bleeding disorders. Adverse reactions include GI disturbances, GI bleeding, tinnitus and hearing loss, hepatotoxicity, renal dysfunction.

NON-STEROIDAL ANTI-INFLAMMATORY AGENTS (continued)

DRUG	SUPPLIED	DOSE/ROUTE	REMARKS
Mefenamic acid (Ponstel)	Caps: 250 mg	ADULTS (and CHILDREN > 14): Analgesia or dysmenorrhea: 500 mg po, then 250 mg po q 6 h with meals.	Non-steroidal anti-inflammatory agent. See ibuprofen for additional comments.
Meclofenamate sodium (Meclomen)	Caps: 50,100 mg	ADULTS (Oral): Anti-inflammatory: 200-300 mg po daily in 3-4 divided doses with meals or milk. Maximum: 400 mg in 24 h.	Non-steroidal anti-inflammatory agent. See ibuprofen for additional comments.

PULMONARY

DRUG	SUPPLIED	DOSE/ROUTE	REMARKS
Acetazolamide (Diamox)	Vial: 500 mg Tabs: 125,250 mg Caps (sustained release): 500 mg	125-250 mg IV q 6 h prn, or 125-250 mg po q 6 h prn.	Used when arterial pH exceeds 7.45, serum bicarbonate exceeds 29 mEq/dl, and serum K + is normal.
Albuterol (Proventil, Ventolin)	Oral solution: 2 mg/5 ml Tabs: 2, 4 mg Metered dose inhalers: 90 μg/spray	2-4 mg po tid or 2 inhalations q 4-6 h	β_2 agonist. Use with caution in cardiac disease because it can cause systemic vasodilation and tachycardia.
Isoetharine (Bronkosol, Bronkometer)	Solutions for nebulization: 0.062%-1% Metered dose inhaler: 340 μg/spray	1 or 2 inhalations by a metered dose inhaler q 4 h or 0.25-1 ml of a 1% solution in 2.5 ml NS q 2-4 h via hand-held nebulizer.	β_2 agonist. Use with caution in cardiac disease because it can cause systemic vasodilation and tachycardia.
Metaproterenol (Alupent, Metaprel)	Oral solution: 10 mg/5 ml Metered dose inhaler: 0.65 mg/spray Solution for nebulization: 0.6%, 5%	20 mg po q 6 or 8 h; or 2-3 inhalations by metered dose inhaler, 2.5 ml of the 0.6% solution or 0.2-0.3 ml of the 5% solution in 2.5 ml NS by hand-held nebulizer q 4-6 h.	β_2 agonist. Use with caution in cardiac disease because it can cause systemic vasodilation and tachycardia.

PULMONARY (continued)

DRUG	SUPPLIED	DOSE/ROUTE	REMARKS
Terbutaline (Brethine, Bricanyl)	Tabs: 2.5, 5.0 mg Vial: 1 mg/ml Metered dose inhaler: 200 μg/spray	2.5 to 5 mg po tid, or 0.25 mg sc q 4-6 h, or 2 inhalations q 4-6 h.	β_2 agonist. Use with caution in cardiac disease because it can cause systemic vasodilation and tachycardia.
Theophyllines:			

1. Theophylline	**Short action** (q6h doses):
	1. Elixophyllin:
	  Liquid: 27 mg/5 ml
	2. Slo-Phyllin:
	  Liquid: 27 mg/5 ml
	  Tabs: 100,200 mg
	3. Theolair:
	  Liquid: 27 mg/5 ml
	  Tabs: 125,250 mg
	Sustained release
	(q 8-12 h doses):
	1. Theodur:
	  Tabs: 100,200,300 mg
	2. Uniphyl:
	  Tabs: 200,400 mg
	Parenteral:
	0.4 to 4 mg/ml in 5% dextrose
		<u>IV:</u> Loading dose of 2.5-5 mg/kg of theophylline over 20 mg, then maintenance infusion of 0.08 to 0.39 mg/kg/h.
		<u>PO:</u> Maintenance dose of 400-900 mg/day in divided doses.
			Maintenance dose is adjusted to maintain serum theophylline levels between 10-20 μg/ml. Lower maintenance dose should be used in patients with congestive heart failure or liver failure. Nausea, vomiting, and cardiac dysrhythmias can occur more frequently when levels exceed 20 μg/ml. Seizures may occur when serum levels exceed 30 μg/ml.

2. Aminophylline (85% theophylline)	**Short action** (q6h doses): Tabs: 100,200 mg Liquid: 105 mg/5 ml **Sustained release:** Phyllocontin: Tab: 225 mg **Parenteral:** Available for dilution in common IV solutions.	<u>IV:</u> Loading dose of 3-6 mg of aminophylline over 20 mg, then maintenance infusion of 0.1 to 0.5 mg/kg/h. <u>PO:</u> Maintenance dose of 500-1100 mg/day in divided doses.	Maintenance dose is adjusted to maintain serum theophylline levels between 10-20 μg/ml. Lower maintenance dose should be used in patients with congestive heart failure or liver failure. Nausea, vomiting, and cardiac dysrhythmias can occur more frequently when levels exceed 20 μg/ml. Seizures may occur when serum levels exceed 30 μg/ml.

SEDATIVES

DRUG	SUPPLIED	DOSE/ROUTE	REMARKS
Diphenhydramine hydrochloride (Benadryl)	Caps: 25,50 mg Oral elixir: 12.5 mg/5 ml Oral solution: 12.5,13.3 mg/5 ml Tabs: 25,50 mg Vials: 10,50 mg/ml Topical cream: 1,2% Topical lotion: 1%	ADULTS: Oral and Parenteral: 25-50 mg po/im/iv q 6 h. Topical: 1-2% applied to area tid or qid. CHILDREN: Oral and Parenteral: 5 mg/kg daily in 3 or 4 divided doses.	Adverse reactions include CNS depression and other CNS disturbances, CNS tract disturbances. Use with caution in patients with angle-closure glaucoma, prostatic hypertrophy, stenosing peptic ulcer, pyloroduodenal obstruction or bladder neck obstruction, asthma, COPD, increased intraocular pressure, hyperthyroidism, cardiovascular disease and hypertension. Contraindications include patients with acute asthma attacks and hypersensitivity to drug. May cause CNS stimulant effect, especially in children.
Hydroxyzine hydrochloride and pamoate (Vistaril, Atarax)	Caps: 25,50,100 mg Tabs: 10,25,50,100 mg Tabs (film-coated): 10,25,50,100 mg Oral solution: 10 mg/5 ml Oral susp: 25 mg/5 ml Vials: 25,50 mg/ml	ADULTS: Oral: Pruritis: 25-50 mg po qid. Sedation: 50-100 mg po qid. Parenteral (IM only): 25-100 mg qid. CHILDREN: Oral: Pruritis and sedation: < 6 years old: 50 mg daily; > 6 years old: 50-100 mg daily in divided doses. Parenteral (IM only): Pre-op: 0.6 mg/kg.	Use 2-track technique for IM administration. Do not give IV. Adverse reactions include CNS depression and other CNS disturbances, local discomfort and sterile abscesses with IM injections.
Chloral hydrate	Caps: 250,500 mg Oral solution: 250,500 mg/5 ml Supp: 325,500,650 mg	ADULTS: Oral and Rectal: Sedation: 250 mg po/pr tid. Hypnotic: 500-1000 mg po/pr at bedtime; increase dose gradually up to 2 g per dose. CHILDREN: Oral and Rectal: Sedation: 8.3 mg/kg po/pr tid (up to 500 mg tid). Hypnotic: 50 mg/kg po/pr (up to 1 g dose).	Adverse reactions include GI tract disturbances, CNS disturbances. Contraindications include patients with marked hepatic or renal disease, and patients with hypersensitivity or idiosyncratic reactions to chloral hydrate. Use with caution in patients on warfarin therapy. May interfere with some urine glucose tests.

SEDATIVES (continued)

DRUG	SUPPLIED	DOSE/ROUTE	REMARKS
Pentobarbital (Nembutal)	Caps: 50,100 mg Oral elixir: 18.2 mg/5 ml Vials: 50 mg/ml Supp: 30,60,120, 200 mg	ADULTS (Oral, Parenteral, Rectal): Sedation: 20-40 mg po/iv/im/pr bid or qid. Hypnotic: 100-200 mg po/iv/im/pr at bedtime. CHILDREN (Oral, Parenteral, Rectal): Sedation: 2-6 mg/kg daily in 3 divided doses (up to 100 mg daily).	Rate of IV administration should not exceed 50 mg/min. Gradual withdrawal of pentobarbital is recommended after prolonged use. Do *not* administer more than 250 mg or 5 ml at any given site. See phenobarbital for additional comments.
Scopolamine (Transderm-Scop)	Transcutaneous: 0.5 mg/2.5 cm²/3 day	ADULTS: Topical: apply to post-auricular skin at least 4 h before anti-emetic effect is required and leave on for up to 72 h.	*Contraindicated* in glaucoma and hypersensitivity to scopolamine.

SERUMS

DRUG	SUPPLIED	DOSE/ROUTE	REMARKS
Hepatitis B immune globulin (H-BIG, Hep-B-Gammagee)	Vial: 5 ml	0.06 ml/kg IM within 24-48 h of exposure, and also 1 month later.	Post-exposure prophylaxis is recommended following either needle stick or direct mucous membrane inoculation or oral ingestion involving HB$_s$-Ag-positive materials such as blood, plasma, serum. Confirmation of HB$_s$-Ag in the donor is *essential* and anti-HB$_s$ screening of the potential recipient is desirable prior to receipt of HBIG. 5 ml vial costs $135-$150.
Immune globulin (IG) for Hepatitis A	Vial: 5 ml	Pre-exposure: Travelers to endemic areas: Residence for < 3 months: 0.02 ml/kg IM one-time dose. Residence for > 3 months: 0.06 ml/kg IM q 5 months. Post-exposure — *close* contact: 0.02 ml/kg IM one-time dose. In cases of common source exposure, IG is *not* recommended once cases have begun to occur.	

SKELETAL MUSCLE RELAXANTS

DRUG	SUPPLIED	DOSE/ROUTE	REMARKS
Pancuronium bromide (Pavulon)	Amps: 2 mg/ml Vials: 1 mg/ml	**ADULTS AND CHILDREN** (> 1 month old): Parenteral: 0.04-0.1 mg/kg iv; additional doses of 0.01 mg/kg may be administered at 25 and 60 min intervals. **NEONATES** (< 1 month old): Parenteral: test dose 0.02 mg/kg iv, then as above.	Non-depolarizing neuromuscular blocking agent. Adverse reactions include tachycardia, increase in blood pressure. Use with *caution* in renal disease. *Contraindications* include hypersensitivity to pancuronium and/or bromides. Doses may be reduced depending on anesthetic agent used.
Tubocurarine chloride (d-tubocurarine chloride)	Vials: 3 mg/ml (3 mg = 20 units)	**ADULTS:** Parenteral: 6-9 mg iv, followed by 3-4.5 mg in 3-5 min if necessary. For prolonged procedures, additional doses of 3 mg may be given (0.165 mg/kg). **Diagnosis of myasthenia gravis:** 0.004-0.033 mg/kg iv.	Non-depolarizing neuromuscular blocking agent. Doses may be reduced depending on anesthetic agent used. Rapid IV administration or high doses may cause hypotension. Use with *caution* in myasthenia gravis, renal disease, impaired cardiovascular, hepatic, pulmonary or endocrine function. *Contraindications* include hypersensitivity to tubocurarine. Adverse reactions include histamine release effects.
Atracurium besylate (Tracrium)	Amps: 10 mg/ml	**ADULTS AND CHILDREN** (> 2 years old): Parenteral (IV push): Initial dose: 0.4-0.5 mg/kg iv for intubation. Maintenance dose: 0.08-0.1 mg/kg iv as necessary.	Non-depolarizing neuromuscular blocking agent. Adverse reactions include histamine release effects and cardiovascular changes. Use with *extreme caution* in myasthenia gravis. *Contraindications* include hypersensitivity to atracurium. Doses may be reduced depending on anesthetic agent used.
Gallamine triethiodide (Flaxedil)	Vials: 20,100 mg/ml	**ADULTS AND CHILDREN** (> 1 month old): Parenteral: 1 mg/kg iv (up to 100 mg); additional doses of 0.5-1 mg/kg may be needed at 40 min intervals. **NEONATES** (< 2 month old): Parenteral: 0.25-0.75 mg/kg iv initially; additional doses of 0.1-0.5 mg/kg.	Non-depolarizing neuromuscular blocking agent. Contraindications include patients with renal dysfunction, shock, severe tachycardia, hypersensitivity to gallamine or iodides, and myasthenia gravis. Doses may be reduced depending on anesthetic agent used.

SKELETAL MUSCLE RELAXANTS (continued)

DRUG	SUPPLIED	DOSE/ROUTE	REMARKS
Vecuronium bromide (Norcuron)	Vials: 10 mg for reconstitution + 5 ml sterile water (2 mg/ml)	ADULTS AND CHILDREN (> 10 years old): Parenteral: Inhalation: 0.08-0.1 mg/kg iv. Maintenance: Balanced anesthesia: 0.01-0.015 mg/kg iv; Inhalation anesthesia: 0.008- 0.012 mg/kg iv. CHILDREN (< 10 years old): 1-9 years old: may require higher initial doses; < 1 year old: more susceptible to the drug.	Non-depolarizing neuromuscular blocking agent. Adverse reactions include cardiovascular changes. Use with *caution* in liver dysfunction and in patients with myasthenia gravis. *Contraindications* include hypersensitivity to vecuronium. Doses may be reduced depending on anesthetic agent used.
Succinylcholine chloride	Amps: 50 mg/ml Vials: 20,100/mg/ml Powder for injection: 100,500,1000 mg per vial.	ADULTS: Parenteral: Test dose: 0.1 mg/kg iv. Short procedures: 0.6 mg/kg iv over 10-30 sec (0.3-1.1 mg/kg). Prolonged procedures: 2.5 mg/min iv infusion (0.5-10 mg/min) or 2.5-4 mg/kg im (up to 150 mg). CHILDREN: Parenteral: 1-2 mg/kg iv or 2.5-4 mg/kg im.	Depolarizing neuromuscular blocking agent. Doses may be reduced depending on anesthetic agent used. Adverse reactions include brady-cardia, hypotension and cardiac arrhythmias. Use with *extreme caution* in patients recovering from severe trauma, patients with electrolyte imbalances, patients on quinidine or digitalis, patients with pre-existing hyperkalemia, para-plegia, extensive or severe burns, extensive denervation of skeletal muscle, head trauma, degenerative or dystrophic neuromuscular disease, during ocular surgery, and glaucoma. *Contraindications* include hypersensitivity to succinylcholine, genetically determined disorders of plasma pseudocholinesterase, myopathies associated with elevated serum creatine kinase values, angle-closure glaucoma, or penetrating eye injuries.

STEROIDS — CLINICAL USES (see also "Preoperative Preparation" page 77)

1. Physiological replacement.
   a. Glucocorticoid.
      1) Hydrocortisone: 12.5 mg/M²/day IM or IV, qd; 25.0 mg/M²/day po in 3 divided doses.
      2) Cortisone acetate:15-16 mg/M²/day IM or IV, qd; 30-32 mg/M²/day po in 3 divided doses.
   b. Mineralocorticoid.
      1) Deoxycorticosterone acetate (DOCA): 1.0-2.0 mg/day IM (in oil), single dose.
      2) 9-alpha-fluoro-cortisol (Florinef): 0.05-0.15 mg/day po.
2. Acute adrenal insufficiency.
   a. Hydrocortisone: 100 mg IV push loading dose, then 100 mg IVPB q 8 h.
3. Chronic adrenal insufficiency.
   a. Hydrocortisone: 30 mg qd po in divided doses (20 mg po a.m., 10 mg po p.m.).
4. Hypercalcemia.
   a. Hydrocortisone: 250-500 mg/day po or IV q 8 h initially, then prednisone 10-30 mg/day for long-term maintenance.
5. Sclerosing cholangitis.
   a. Prednisone: 40-50 mg po qd.
6. Myasthenia gravis.
   a. Prednisone: 10-100 mg po qd (tapering dose regimen).
7. Acute myasthenic crisis.
   a. ACTH (corticotropin): 40 I.U. IV q 12 h.
8. Breast carcinoma.
   a. Prednisolone: 30 mg po qd.
9. Rheumatic carditis.
   a. Prednisolone: 40 mg po qd.
10. Ulcerative colitis.
    a. ACTH (corticotropin): 40 I.U. IV q 12 h.
    b. Prednisone: 60-120 mg po qd (tapering dose).
    c. Prednisolone: 100 mg/day, continuous IV infusion.
    d. Methylprednisolone: 40 mg retention enema HS.
    e. Hydrocortisone: 100 mg retention enema HS for 3 weeks or until clinical remission occurs.
11. Cerebral edema.
    a. Dexamethasone: 10 mg IV loading dose, then 4 mg IV q 4-6 h for 36-72 h.
12. Sarcoidosis.
    a. Prednisone: 40 mg po qd.
13. Acute polymeuritis.
    a. Prednisone: 40 mg po qd.
14. Polymyositis and dermatomyositis.
    a. Prednisone: 40-60 mg po qd.

STEROIDS – CLINICAL USES (continued)

15. Anti-inflammatory.
   a. Prednisone: less than 100 mg/day.
   b. Dexamethasone: 3-6 mg/kg IV bolus, then 3-6 mg/kg IVPB q 2 h until positive response, or up to 3 doses.
16. Shock (debatable).
   a. Methylprednisolone: 15-30 mg/kg IV bolus, then 15-30 mg/kg IVPB q 2-4 h up to 3 doses or until positive response.
17. ARDS (debatable).
   a. Methylprednisolone: 30 mg/kg IVPB q 6 h for 48 h.
18. Aspiration (debatable).
   a. Prednisone: 50-100 mg po qd for 3 days.
19. Organ transplant (variable protocols).
   a. Prednisone: 50-100 mg po qd (tapering doses).
20. Idiopathic thrombocytopenia.
   a. Prednisone: 1.0-2.0 mg/kg/day po.
21. Chronic obstructive pulmonary disease (variable protocols).
   a. Prednisone: 5-10 or more mg/day (response dependent).
22. Nephrotic syndrome.
   a. Prednisone: 2 mg/kg/day po (based on edema-free "ideal" weight).
23. Periarteritis nodosa.
   a. Prednisone: 40-60 mg po qd.
24. Wegener's granulomatosis.
   a. Prednisone: 60 mg po qd.
25. Systemic lupus erythematosis.
   a. Prednisone: 40-60 mg po qd.
26. Pemphigus vulgaris.
   a. Prednisone: 80-300 mg po qd.
27. Keloids, intraarticular administration.
   a. Dexamethasone suspension (8 mg/ml vial).
      1) Large joints: 2-4 mg.
      2) Small joints: 0.8-1.0 mg.
      3) Soft tissue infiltration: 2-6 mg.
      4) Ganglia: 1-2 mg.
      5) Tendon sheaths: 0.4-1.0 mg.
   b. Triamcinolone hexacetonide (Aristospan): 5 mg or 20 mg/ml, or triamcinolone acetonide (Kenalog).
      1) Soft tissue infiltration up to 0.5 mg/m².
      2) Intraarticular 2-20 mg (depending on joint size and degree of inflammation) q 3-4 weeks.
      3) Up to 1 ml of 1% lidocaine may be administered simultaneously to promote immediate relief.

TOPICALS, ANTISEPTICS, DISINFECTANTS

DRUG	SUPPLIED	DOSE/ROUTE	REMARKS
Gamma benzene (Kwell)	Cream: 1% Lotion: 1% Shampoo: 1%	Topical: 1 oz lotion or 30 g cream.	Wash off after 8 h. For scabies, lice, crabs, gnats. *Contraindicated* in pregnancy and in infants due to LNS toxicity from cutaneous absorption. Apply neck to toes; *avoid* urethral meatus and mucous membranes.
Hexachlorophene (Phisohex)	Solution	Topical	Bacteristatic. Systemic toxicity under conditions permitting absorption (e.g., skin of premature infants).
Chlorhexidine gluconate (Hibiclens, Hibitane, Hibistat)	Hibiclens: 4% in base Hibitane: 0.5% weight/ volume tincture in 70% isopropanol Hibistat: 0.5% weight/ weight chlorhexidine in 70% isopropanol with emollients	Topical	For wound antisepsis, general skin cleansing and surgical scrubs. pH range 5–8. Effective against gram-positives (10 μg/ml), gram-negatives (50 μg/ml) and fungi (200 μg/ml). Rapid acting, considerable residual adherence, low potential for contact- and photosensitivity; poorly absorbed.
Hydrogen peroxide H_2O_2	3% H_2O_2 solution	Topical	When H_2O_2 comes in contact with catalase, it rapidly decomposes into H_2O and O_2 in wounds and on mucous membranes, loosening and debriding infectious detritus. Solutions diluted with mouthwash are used for stomatitis and gingivitis. *Never* use H_2O_2 in closed body cavities or abscesses.
Gentian violet (Genapax)	Topical solution: 1%, 2% Vaginal tampons: 5 mg	Topical application bid to tid for 3 days	Stains; may tattoo if applied to granulation tissue. Do *not* use on face. Usually used against cutaneous or mucocutaneous *Candida albicans* infection. Can cause esophagitis, tracheitis, laryngitis if swallowed or aspirated. Effective against gram-positives (*Staph.*) and fungi (*Candida*). Not effective against gram-negatives, AFB, or spores.

TOPICALS, ANTISEPTICS, DISINFECTANTS (continued)

DRUG	SUPPLIED	DOSE/ROUTE	REMARKS
Povidone-iodine (Betadine, Pharmadine)	Ointment, solution	Topical	Bactericidal, antifungal. May be painful and can facilitate debridement of contaminated wounds. Metabolic acidosis; some absorption. *Avoid in* iodine allergics.
Alexis–Carrel Henry Dakin Solution	0.5% sodium hypochlorite adjusted to neutral pH with $NaHCO_3$	Topical	Use 1/4 to 1/2 strength solution in treatment of suppurative wounds; solvent action in debridement of wounds.
Tincture of iodine	2-7% solution of I_2 in aqueous alcohol	Topical	Bactericidal (see Povidone-iodine).
Nitrofurazone (Furacin)	Cream: 0.2% Ointment: 0.2% Solution: 0.2%	Topical	Used as topical agent for skin infections and burn wounds. Bactericidal for many gram-positive and gram-negative organisms, but most *Pseudomonae* and *Proteus* are resistant. *Avoid* in renal failure. Can cause GI disturbances, rash, pruritus; occasionally causes drug fever and neuropathy.
Podophyllin resin [*Keratolytic agent*] (Podoben)	Solution: 11.5%, 2.5%	Topical: applied and washed off within 1-4 h (not longer than 4-6 h); repeat weekly for up to 4 applications.	For condylomata acuminata; if no regression after 4 weekly applications, use alternative treatment such as cryo, electro or laser therapy, 5FU intravenously.
Silver nitrate	Ophthalmic solution: 1%	2 drops in each eye.	Prophylaxis of gonococcal ophthalmia neonatorum.
Mafenide acetate (Sulfamylon)	Cream: 8.5% Solution: 5%	Topical	Broad spectrum. Hypertonic; painful; readily absorbed; metabolic acidosis; carbonic anhydrase inhibitor; pulmonary toxicity. Inhibits epithelialization and, although it can delay eschar separation in burn wounds, it penetrates eschar well. Discontinue use for 24-48 hours if acid-base disturbances occur.

TOPICALS, ANTISEPTICS, DISINFECTANTS (continued)

DRUG	SUPPLIED	DOSE/ROUTE	REMARKS
Silver sulfadiazine (Silvadene)	Cream: 1%	Topical to burn wounds, with dressing changes qd or bid.	Isomolar. Poorly absorbed, but blood levels sufficient to inhibit phagocyte chemotaxis may occur.
Isopropyl alcohol	Liquid: 70% solution	Topical	Disinfectant.
Neomycin	Cream or ointment: 0.5% Solution	Apply qd to tid topically. Apply to soak gauze dressings bid to tid.	Aminoglycoside; bactericidal. Active against aerobic gram-negatives and some aerobic gram-positives. Inactive against viruses, fungi and most anaerobes, *E. coli, H. influenza, Proteus* sp., *Staph* sp., and *Serratis*. Minimally active against *Strep* sp.; no activity against *Pseudomonas*. Not absorbed from intact skin, but readily absorbed from denuded areas. Can be a contact sensitizer in 5-15% of patients treated. Hypersensitivity reactions dermatitis and urticaria. Cross allergenicity has been observed with other aminoglycosides. Ototoxicity, nephrotoxicity, and neuromuscular blockade have been seen following topical application to large areas of altered skin integrity (e.g., burns).
Bacitracin preparations	Powder, ointment: 500 units/g	Topical application qd to tid	For the treatment of superficial skin infections. May lead to fungal overgrowth, especially *Candida*. Bacitracin is active against many gram-positives. Bacteriostatic or bacteriostatic. Not absorbed in any appreciable amount from skin, denuded skin, wounds or mucous membranes. Low toxicity topically, but anaphylactoid reactions have occurred Local irritation, itching or burning should lead to discontinuation of the preparation.

1. Bacitracin 400 or 500 units/g plus Polymyxin B sulfate 5000 units/g (Clinicydin, Neo-thrycex)
2. Bacitracin zinc 400 units/g plus Neomycin sulfate 0.5% plus Polymyxin B sulfate 5000 units/g (Neosporin, Neomixin)
3. Hydrocortisone 1.0% plus all the medications in #2 above (Cortisporin).
4. Bacitracin zinc 500 units/g plus Polymyxin B sulfate 10,000 units/g (Polysporin ointment [PSO]).

URINARY ANTI-INFECTIVES

DRUG	SUPPLIED	DOSE/ROUTE	REMARKS
Methenamine mandelate (Mandelamine)	Granules: 500 mg, 1 g Susp: 250,500 mg/5 ml Tabs: 500 mg, 1 g	PO: 1 g q 6 h (480 mg methenamine) after meals and at bedtime.	Effective against most organisms *in vitro*. Active principle is formaldehyde. Should *not* be used in tissue infection (pyelonephritis). Urine pH must be kept below 5.5 for effect; co-administer ascorbic acid to acidify the urine. Can cause nausea, vomiting, skin rash, dysuria in 3%. Not effective in systemic bacterial infections or tissue outside the urinary tract.
Methenamine hippurate (Hiprex, Urex)	Tabs: 1 g	PO: 1 g q 12 h	
Nalidixic acid (NegGram)	Susp: 250 mg/5 ml Tabs: 250,500,1000 mg	PO: 1 g q 6 h for 1-2 weeks.	For gram-negative urinary tract pathogens (*Enterobacteriaceae*) except *Pseudomonas*. High degree of resistance may develop during therapy. Avoid in children, pregnancy, lactation. Can cause GI hypersensitivity, fever, eosinophilia, photosensitivity, neurological disturbances, hemolytic anemia, thrombocytopenia, false elevation of urinary 17-ketosteroids. Administer 1 h before meals. Not effective in systemic bacterial infection.
Nitrofurantoin (Furadantin, Macrodantin)	Caps (macrocrystals): 25,50,100 mg Caps (microcrystals): 50,100 mg Susp: 25 mg/5 ml Tabs (microcrystals): 50,100 mg	PO: 50-100 mg q 6 h	May be administered with food. Macrocrystals may cause less GI upset. Covers many gram-positive and gram-negative organisms. In the urinary tract, it is not effective against *Pseudomonas* and some *Klebsiella*-enterobacter and *Proteus* species. Neuropathy with high dose or renal failure. Absorption increased with meals. Causes hemolytic anemia in G6PD deficiency. Do *not* use in infants < 1 month old. Increased activity in acid urine. *Contraindicated* in renal failure. Treatment of urinary tract infections only. May turn urine a dark yellow or brown color.

URINARY ANTI-INFECTIVES (continued)

DRUG	SUPPLIED	DOSE/ROUTE	REMARKS
Trimethoprim (Proloprim)	Tabs: 100,200 mg	PO: 100 mg q 12 h or 200 mg qd.	Active against most common gram-negative bacteria associated with urinary tract infections, except *Pseudomonas aeruginosa*. Questionable efficacy in urinary tract infections when used alone vs. in combination with sulfamethoxazole.
Neomycin-polymycin (Neosporin GU irrigant).	200,000 units of polymixin B per ml with Neomycin sulfate 57 mg/ml	1 liter/day irrigating at a continuous rate with triple lumen foley catheter.	Some bacterial stains are resistant and may be selected out. Use for treatment of uncomplicated bladder infections due to susceptible organisms or prophylaxis of infection when frequent catheter opening is necessary (e.g., after transurethral surgery).
Acetic acid 0.25% in normal saline	0.25% solution	1 liter/day continuous irrigation. (Bladder irrigation)	Mainly for *Pseudomonas*. Less effective against other gram-negatives.

VACCINES

DRUG	SUPPLIED	DOSE/ROUTE	REMARKS
Hemophilus b polysaccharide virus (b-Capsa 1)	Vial: Powder for injection	0.5 ml (25 μg) sc	Immunization of children 24 months to 6 years of age against diseases caused by Hemophilus influenza b.
Hepatitis B virus vaccine inactivated (Heptavax-B)	Vial: 20 μg/ml	20 μg IM in 3 doses; first 2 doses are spaced 1 month apart, and 3rd dose at 6 months.	High-risk populations: 1. Medical and lab personnel who have frequent contact with hepatitis B-positive blood or blood products. 2. Hemodialysis patients. 3. Male homosexuals. 4. Neonates of chronic HB$_s$Ag carriers. Anti-HB$_s$ or anti-HB$_c$ screening tests should be done on all potential recipients of the vaccine who are at high risk prior to administration. Cost of vaccine approximately $100 for 3 doses.

VACCINES (continued)

DRUG	SUPPLIED	DOSE/ROUTE	REMARKS
Influenza virus vaccine 1985-86 (subvirion) (Fluogen, Fluzone)	Vial: 5 ml	0.5 ml IM in 2 doses 4 weeks apart	Formulated annually based on specifications of the U.S. Public Health Service.
Influenza virus vaccine 1985-86 (whole virion) (Fluzone)	Vial: 5, 25 ml	0.5 ml IM as a single dose	High-risk populations: 1. Geriatric patients. 2. Adults and children with chronic disorders of the cardiovascular, pulmonary, and/or renal systems, metabolic diseases, severe anemia, and/or compromised immune function. 3. Medical personnel who have extensive contact with high-risk patients. 4. Residents of chronic-care facilities. Subvirion vaccine should be used in children 12 years or younger; whole virion vaccine should be used in adults.
Pneumococcal vaccine, polyvalent (Pneumovax 23)	Vial: 0.5 ml Syringe: 0.5 ml	0.5 ml IM/SC as a single dose	Current vaccine contains 23 capsular poly-saccharide types of Streptococcus pneumonia. Recommended in: (1) Adults with chronic disease (cardiovascular & pulmonary) who present with increased morbidity with respiratory infections; (2) Adults with increased risk for pneumococcal disease (i.e., splenic dysfunction or anatomic asplenia). Booster doses not recommended.

VASOCONSTRICTORS

DRUG	SUPPLIED	DOSE/ROUTE	REMARKS
Metaraminol (Aramine)	Vial: 10 mg/ml	IV: titrate to desired hemodynamic effects. IM: 2-10 mg, followed by additional doses q 10 min.	Primary effect is on α-adrenergic receptors with β_1-adrenergic receptor activity as well. Can decrease renal blood flow, especially in hypovolemic patients.
Methoxamine (Vasoxyl)	Vial: 20 mg/ml	IVP: 3-5 mg and, if necessary, titrate with continuous infusion. IM: 5-20 mg, followed q 15 min by additional doses if necessary.	Predominantly direct effect on α-adrenergic receptors only. Can decrease renal blood flow, especially in hypovolemic patients.

VASOCONSTRICTORS (continued)

DRUG	SUPPLIED	DOSE/ROUTE	REMARKS
Norepinephrine (Levophed)	Amp: 4 mg/4 ml	Initial IV dose: 1-4 $\mu g/min$ up to 8-12 $\mu g/min$ or more as needed to maintain a low-normal blood pressure (80-100 mm Hg systolic)	Predominant α-agonist; some β-adrenergic (β_1) activity. Powerful peripheral vasoconstrictor. Also causes visceral, renal and mesenteric vasoconstriction. Contraindicated in hypovolemia and with cyclopropane and halothane. Extravasation can lead to tissue sloughing.
Phenylephrine HCl (Neo-synephrine)	Amp: 10 mg/ml	Initial dose: 0.01 mg/min; dose is highly variable – titrate to effect.	Stimulates primarily α-receptors; powerful peripheral vasoconstriction. Deleterious if vasoconstriction already present. Contraindicated in severe hypertension, hypovolemia, ventricular tachycardia and hypersensitivity to phusions in patients with GI hemorrhage. If bleeding is well-controlled by peripheral infusion, the infusion rate should be left at the controlling dose for 12 hrs, then tapered every 8-12 hrs. Also used in the treatment of diabetes insipidus.
Vasopressin (Pitressin)	Vials: 20 units/ml (Vasopressin) Susp: 5 units/ml (Vasopressin tannate)	GI hemorrhage (Vasopressin): Initial IV dose (same as intra-arterial dose): 0.2 units/min, then up to maximum safe dose of 0.6 units/ml. Diabetes insipidus (Vasopressin): 5-10 units IM/SQ 2-4 times daily as needed.	Portal pressure can be reduced by giving either systemically or with selective SMA infusions in patients with GI hemorrhage. If bleeding is well-controlled by peripheral infusion, the infusion rate should be left at the controlling dose for 12 hrs, then tapered every 8-12 hrs. Also used in the treatment of diabetes insipidus.

VASODILATORS

DRUG	SUPPLIED	DOSE/ROUTE	REMARKS
Alpha methyldopa (Aldomet)	Vial: 250 mg/5 ml Tabs: 125,250,500 mg Susp: 250 mg/5 ml	250-500 mg IV or po q 6 h. Initial adult PO: 250 mg bid/tid 2x/day, then increase or decrease until adequate response achieved. Maintenance adult PO: 500-2000 mg/day given in 2-4 divided doses.	Stimulates central α-adrenergic receptors. Often requires 24-48 h to achieve its effect. Contraindicated in active hepatic disease and hypersensitivity to methyldopa. Drowsiness is fairly common.

VASODILATORS (continued)

DRUG	SUPPLIED	DOSE/ROUTE	REMARKS
Diazoxide (Hyperstat)	Amp: 300 mg/20 ml	1-3 mg/kg (max 150 mg) q 5-15 min until adequate response is achieved; then at 4-24 h intervals as needed.	Smooth muscle relaxation in peripheral arterioles. Rapid reduction in blood pressure with 4-6 h effect. Most effective when combined with a "loop" diuretic secondary to sodium and water retaining effects. Increases blood glucose by inhibiting pancreatic insulin secretion.
Diltiazem HCl (Cardizem)	Tabs: 30,60 mg	PO: 30 mg 4 times/day and increased at 1-2 day intervals as needed.	Slows sinoatrial and atrioventricular nodal conduction. Used in management of Prinzmetal's variant angina and chronic stable angina pectoris. May increase digoxin plasma concentrations.
Hydralazine (Apresoline)	Amp: 20 mg/ml Tabs: 10,25,50,100 mg	Initially: PO: 10 mg 4 times/day for 2-4 days, then prn increase to 25-50 mg 4 times/day IV: 10-20 mg and repeated prn in severe hypertension or hypertensive emergencies.	Vascular smooth muscle relaxant, primarily arterioles. Potent antihypertensive; reduces systemic vascular resistance in CHF. Contraindicated in hypovolemia. Can lead to tachycardia. Has been associated with rheumatoid states and S.L.E. in high doses. Can cause increased pulmonary artery pressure in mitral valve disease. 75-100 mg PO hydralazine is equivalent to 20-25 mg IV hydralazine.
Labetalol HCl (Trandate, Normodyne)	Tabs: 100,200,300 mg Vial: 5 mg/ml	Oral: initially 100 mg po bid, adjusted in 100 mg 2/day q 2-3 days until optimal blood pressure achieved. Usual dose is 200-400 mg po bid. Parenteral: initially 20 mg IV push, then 20-80 mg IV push q 10 min until desired effect is achieved (up to 300 mg (total), or continuous infusion at initial rate of 2 mg/min; adjust rate according to blood pressure response.	Non-selective β-adrenergic blocker and selective α1-adrenergic blocker. β-blocker activity is 3:1 (oral) and 7:1 (IV). Decrease in heart rate is minimal secondary to α-blockade. IV administration requires patients to be kept supine to avoid a substantial fall in blood pressure. Useful in treatment of coexisting systemic and intracranial hypertension.

VASODILATORS (continued)

DRUG	SUPPLIED	DOSE/ROUTE	REMARKS
Sodium nitroprusside (Nipride)	Vial: 50 mg	Initial dose: 0.5–10 μg/kg/min. Solution must be protected from light.	Direct venous and arterial vascular smooth muscle relaxant resulting in peripheral vasodilation. Useful in cardiogenic shock, post open-heart surgery, control of peripheral vascular resistance in low-flow states, hypertensive crisis, mitral regurgitation, reduction of pulmonary vascular resistance, induced hypotension. *Contraindicated* in hypovolemia and acute myocardial ischemia. Must monitor cyanide levels, especially when used in high doses for prolonged periods of time. Signs of cyanide toxicity include progressive acidosis, tachyphylaxis, resistance to nitroprusside, and hypotension.
Nitroglycerin	Cutaneous paste 2% Sublingual tabs: 0.15, 0.3, 0.4, 0.6 mg Vial: 0.5 mg/ml (5 mg) Transdermal system: 2.5 μg; 5, 7.5, 10, 15 mg	Initial IV dose: 10 μg/min; titrate to response. Sublingual tabs: variable dosing. Topical: variable dosing.	Vascular smooth muscle relaxant with predominant venous capacitance activity. Can antagonize coronary artery spasm and increase coronary blood flow. Reduce LVEDP by reducing preload. Alleviates myocardial ischemia induced by coronary spasm or subendocardial ischemia seen with an elevation of LVEDP. Can reduce blood pressure. *Contraindicated* in hypovolemia.
Phentolamine (Regitine)	Vial: 5 mg	**Diagnosis of pheochromocytoma:** IVP or IM: 5 mg **Hypertension in pheochromocytoma:** 5 mg IM/IV q 1–2 h. **Extravasation:** 5–10 mg in 10 ml 0.9% NaCl infiltrated into the affected area.	Competitively blocks α-adrenergic receptors. However, activity is relatively transient. Minimal β-adrenergic receptor activity. Used primarily in diagnosis of pheochromocytoma and immediately prior to or during pheochromocytomectomy to improve or control paroxysmal hypertension. Also used to prevent dermal necrosis following IV extravasation of norepinephrine and dopamine.

VASODILATORS (continued)

DRUG	SUPPLIED	DOSE/ROUTE	REMARKS
Nifedipine (Procardia)	Caps: 10, 20 mg	PO: 10 mg 3 times/day; usual maintenance dose is 30-60 mg given in 3 divided doses.	Used in the management of Prinzmetal's variant angina and chronic stable angina pectoris. No effect on sinoatrial and atrioventricular nodal conduction. Principal effect is vasodilation of main coronary and systemic arteries. Monitor blood pressure initially.
Trimethaphan camsylate (Arfonad)	Amps: 500 mg/5 ml	Initial dose: 0.5-2 mg/min, with adjustment as needed.	Predominant sympathetic and parasympathetic ganglionic blocker which aids in blood pressure reduction and is especially used when augmentation of cardiac contractility is not needed. Useful in treatment of coexisting systemic and intracranial hyperextension in aorta dissection. *Contraindicated* in hypovolemia and in cases where tachycardia is potentially harmful. Can cause early tachyphylaxis. Excessive dosage can cause potential neuromuscular paralysis.

PART V

REFERENCE DATA

NORMAL LAB VALUES AT THE
UNIVERSITY OF CINCINNATI MEDICAL CENTER

Test	Units	Specimen Type	Norms
5-Nucleotidase	MIU/ML	Blood	3.0 - 11.0
Acid Phos., Total	MIU/ML	Blood	0.0 - 6.0
Acetylcholine Recept Ab	NMOL/L	Blood	< 0.5
Albumin	GM/DL	Blood	3.5 - 5.0
Aldolase	MIU/ML	Blood	1.0 - 6.0
Aldosterone, Urine	MCG/24 HR	Urine	2.0 - 14.0
Alkaline Phosphatase	MIU/ML	Blood	8.0 - 240.0
Alpha-1-Antitrypsin	MG/DL	Blood	0.0 - 470.0
Alpha-Feto Protein	NG/ML	Blood	< 10
Ammonia	MCMOL/L	Blood	8.0 - 72.0
Amylase, Serum	MIU/ML	Blood	0.0 - 200.0
Amylase, Urine, Fluid	U/TVOL	Urine	0.0 - 1250.0
APTT	SEC	Blood	4.0 - 34.0
Arsenic, Blood	MCG/L	Blood	0.0 - 20.0
Arylsulfatase, Urine	UNITS/L	Urine	> 1.0 U/L
B-2-Microglobulin	MG/L	Blood	0.0 - 3.0
Beta-2-Microglobulin	MCG/L	Urine	0.0 - 270.0
Bile Acid	MCMOL/ML	Blood	0.0 - 1.3
Bilirubin, Direct	MG/DL	Blood	0.0 - 0.4
Bilirubin, Total	MG/DL	Blood	0.1 - 1.1
Bleeding Time	MIN		≤ 9.5
Bromide	MCG/ML	Blood	0.0 - 1500.0
BUN	MG/DL	Blood	5.0 - 20.0
C-Reactive Protein	MG/DL	Blood	< 0.8
C3 Binding		Blood	Negative
Calcitonin	PG/ML	Blood	0.0 - 107.0
Calcium, Serum	MG/DL	Blood	8.5 - 10.5
Calcium, Urine, Fluid	MG/TVOL	Urine	0.0 - 250.0
Candida Titer	DILUTION TITER	Blood	Negative
Cannabinoid Screen	PRESENCE or ABSENCE	Urine	Negative
Carbamazepine	MCG/ML	Blood	4.0 - 12.0
Carboxyhemoglobin	%	Blood	< 5% (Non-Smoker) < 10% (Smoker)
Carotene	MCG/DL	Blood	0.0 - 650.0
Catecholamines, Pl.	FRPG/ML	Blood	0.0 - 625.0

NORMAL LAB VALUES (continued)

Test	Units	Specimen Type	Norms
Ceruloplasmin	MG/DL	Blood	0.0 - 60.0
Chlordiazepoxide	MCG/ML	Blood	1.0 - 3.0
Chloride	MEQ/ML	Blood	5.0 - 110.0
Chloride, Urine, Fluid	MEQ/TVOL	Urine	0.0 - 250.0
Cholinesterase	MIU/ML	Blood	0.0 - 4800.0
Chromium, Serum	MCG/L	Blood	0.0 - 28.0
Cir. Immune Complexes	% BIND	Blood	0.0 - 3.9
Clot. Retraction	%	Blood	8.0 - 93.0
CO_2, Total	MEQ/L	Blood	1.0 - 33.0
Cold Agglutinin	DILUTION	Blood	Neg. - 1:16
Complement, Total Serch50	U	Blood	4.0 - 192.0
Copper, Urine	MCG/TVOL	Urine	< 40 - 60
CPK-MB%	%	Blood	0.0 - 6.0
Creatinine	MG/DL	Blood	0.7 - 1.4
Creatinine, Urine, Fluid	GM/VOL	Urine	1.0 - 1.8
CSF Glucose	MG/DL	CSF	0.0 - 70.0
CSF Protein	MG/DL	CSF	5.0 - 45.0
Cyanide	MCG/ML	Blood	1.0 - 10.0
D-Xylose, Serum	MMOL/L	Blood	Adult > 1.66
D-Xylose, Urine	GM/5 HR	Urine	> 4
Delta Aminolevulinic	MG/24 HR	Urine	7 mg/24 hr
Digitoxin	NG/ML	Blood	0.0 - 26.0
Digoxin	NG/ML	Blood	0.5 - 2.0
DNA Single Strand Bld.	% BIND	Blood	1.0 - 15.0
Eosinophil Count, Blood	CUMM	Blood	0.0 - 450.0
Factor VIII Multimers		Blood	0.0 - 150.0
Factor II Assay	%	Blood	0.0 - 150.0
Factor IX	% of NORMAL	Blood	0.0 - 150.0
Factor V	% of NORMAL	Blood	0.0 - 150.0
Factor VII	% of NORMAL	Blood	0.0 - 150.0
Factor VIII Antigen	%	Blood	0.0 - 150.0
Factor VIII C	% of NORMAL	Blood	0.0 - 150.0
Factor VIII VWF	% of NORMAL	Blood	0.0 - 150.0
Factor X	% of NORMAL	Blood	0.0 - 150.0
Factor XI	% of NORMAL	Blood	0.0 - 150.0
Factor XII	% of NORMAL	Blood	0.0 - 150.0
Factor XIII	% of NORMAL	Blood	0.0 - 150.0
Fecal Fat	GM/72 HR	Stool	< 15.0
Ferritin, Serum	NG/ML	Blood	0.0 - 200.0
Fibrin Degradation	PMCG/ML	Blood	< 16
Fibrinogen	MG/DL	Blood	0.0 - 400.0

NORMAL LAB VALUES (continued)

Test	Units	Specimen Type	Norms
Folate Level, Serum	NG/ML	Blood	0.0 - 500.0
Fr. Eryth. Protoporph.	MCG/GM h	Blood	0.0 - 1.56
FTA-ABS		Blood	ON-REACT
Furosemide	MCG/ML	Blood	1.0 - 2.0
G-6-PD Quant.	U/GM HGB	Blood	4.5 - 10.1
Gamma GT	MIU/ML	Blood	8.0 - 40.0
Gastrin Level, Serum	PG/ML	Blood	6.0 - 97.0
Globulin Synth. Ratio		Blood	.85 - 1.15
Glucose	MG/DL	Blood	0.0 - 100.0
Glutethimide	MCG/ML	Blood	1.0 - 10.0
Glycohemoglobin	%	Blood	5.5 - 8.5
Haptoglobin	MG/DL	Blood	7.0 - 139.0
Hematocrit	%	Blood	Adult: Male 47±7 Female 42±5
Hemoglobin	GM/DL	Blood	Adult: Male 16.0±2.0 Female 14.0±2.0
Hemoglobin, Plasma	MG/DL	Blood	0.0 - 10.0
IgA	MG/DL	Blood	0.0 - 290.0
IgD	MG/DL	Blood	0.0 - 14.0
IgE, Total	IU/ML	Blood	< 250
IgG	MG/DL	Blood	0.0 - 1420.0
IgM	MG/DL	Blood	0.0 - 375.0
IgM Neonatal		Blood	< 23
Ionized Calcium	MG/DL	Blood	4.5 - 5.3
Iron, Urine	MG/24 HR	Urine	0.2 MG/TV
Ketone		Blood	Negative
LE Preparation		Blood	One Seen
Lactic Acid	MEQ/L	Blood	0.0 - 2.0
Lactate Dehydrogenase (LDH)	U/L	Blood	110 - 200
Lead, Blood	MG/DL	Blood	0.0 - 40.0
Leukocyte Alk. Phos.		Blood	5.0 - 85.0
Lipase, Serum	CC/U	Blood	0.0 - 1.0
Lithium	MEQ/L	Blood	0.0 - 1.4
Magnesium, Serum	MG/DL	Blood	1.5 - 2.5
Magnesium, Urine, Fluid	MG/TVOL	Urine	0.0 - 800.0
Mercury, Blood	MCG/L	Blood	0.0 - 20.0
Methemoglobin	%	Blood	0.0 - 2.0
Methylmalonic Acid	UMCG/MG C	Urine	0.0 - 5.0
Monotest		Blood	Negative

NORMAL LAB VALUES (continued)

Test	Units	Specimen Type	Norms
Muramidase, Serum	MCG/ML	Blood	5.0 - 20.0
Muramidase, Urine	MCG/ML	Urine	0.0 - 5.0
Myoglobin, Urine	MCG/ML	Urine	Negative
Neutrophil Adherence	% ADHERE	Blood	3.0 - 71.0
O2 Saturation	%	Blood	2.0 - 99.0
Osmolality, Serum	MOSM/L	Blood	0.0 - 305.0
Osmolality, Urine	MOSM/L	Urine	0.0 - 1200.0
Oxalate	MG/24 HR	Urine	40 MG/24 hr
P50 & 2,3 DPG	MM HG	Blood	4.8 - 26.4
Panc. Glucagon 1	PG/ML	Blood	1.0 - 220.0
Panc. Glucagon 10-20	PG/ML	Blood	1.0 - 220.0
Panc. Glucagon 2-4	PG/ML	Blood	1.0 - 220.0
Panc. Glucagon 5-9	PG/ML	Blood	1.0 - 220.0
Panc. Polypeptide 10-20	PG/ML	Blood	30 UG/TV
Panc. Polypeptide 1	PG/ML	Blood	2.0 - 220.0
Panc. Polypeptide 2-4	PG/ML	Blood	2.0 - 220.0
Panc. Polypeptide 5-9	PG/ML	Blood	2.0 - 220.0
Phenobarbital	MCG/ML	Blood	5.0 - 40.0
Phenytoin	MCG/ML	Blood	0.0 - 20.0
Phosphate, Urine, Fluid	MG/TVOL	Urine	0.0 - 1600.0
Phosphorus, Serum	MG/DL	Blood	2.5 - 4.5
Plasminogen	%	Blood	9.0 - 131.0
Platelet Count	THOUS/CU	Blood	0.0 - 375.0
Porphobilinogen Quant.	MG/24 HR	Urine	0.0 - 2.0
Potassium	MEQ/L	Blood	3.5 - 5.0
Potassium, Urine, Fluid	MEQ/TVOL	Urine	0.0 - 65.0
Protein C Antigen	% of NORMAL	Blood	0.0 - 130.0
Protein, Total	GM/DL	Blood	6.0 - 8.0
Protein, Urine, Fluid	MG/TVOL	Urine	0.0 - 100.0
Prothrombin Time	SEC	Blood	1.4 - 13.0
Protoporphyrin RBC	MCG/DL	Blood	60 MCG/DL
PTH Mid-Molecule	NG/ML	Blood	0.3 - 1.08
PTH, Intact	MCLEQ/ML	Blood	0.0 - 117.0
Ratnoff Fibrinogen	MG/DL	Blood	0.0 - 1000.0
Reticulocyte Count	%	Blood	0.2 - 2.0
Retinol Binding Protein	MG/DL	Blood	3.0 - 6.0
Salicylate	MCG/ML	Blood	0.0 - 200.0
Scleroderma Antibody	TITER	Blood	Negative
Serum Protime	SEC	Blood	0.0 - 20.0
SGOT	MIU/ML	Blood	0.0 - 30.0
SGPT	MIU/ML	Blood	7.0 - 35.0

NORMAL LAB VALUES (continued)

Test	Units	Specimen Type	Norms
Sickle Screen		Blood	Negative
Sjogren's Antibodies	TITER	Blood	Negative
Sodium	MEQ/L	Blood	3.0 - 145.0
Sodium, Urine, Fluid	MEQ/TVOL	Urine	0.0 - 200.0
T3 Resin Uptake	%	Blood	4.0 - 117.0
T3, Reverse	NG/DL	Blood	9.0 - 157.0
T4 RIA			6.5 - 13.5
TOT Assay	NG/10E8	Bone Marrow	0.0 - 50.0
Teichoic Acid AB		Blood	EG - 1:2
Theophylline	MCG/ML	Blood	0.0 - 20.0
Thiocyanate	MCG/ML	Blood	0.0 - 100.0
Thyroglobulin	NG/ML	Blood	Up to 50
Thyroxine Binding Glob.	MCG T4/D	Blood	1.0 - 27.0
Tocainide	MCG/ML	Blood	4.0 - 10.0
Total Glucagon 1	PG/ML	Blood	9.0 - 240.0
Total Glucagon 10-20	PG/ML	Blood	9.0 - 240.0
Total Glucagon 2-4	PG/ML	Blood	9.0 - 240.0
Total Glucagon 5-9	PG/ML	Blood	9.0 - 240.0
Transferrin	MG/DL	Blood	5.0 - 355.0
Trypsin	MCEQ/ML	Duodenal	0.0 - 4.0
TSH	uU/ML	Blood	0 - 7
Urea, Urine or Fluid	GM/VOL	Urine	7.0 - 16.0
Urine Free Cortisol	MCG/24 HR	Urine	9.0 - 140.0
Uroporphyr-I-Synth.	NMOL/ML	Blood	8.0 - 50.0
Valproic Acid	MCG/ML	Blood	0.0 - 120.0
Vaso. Int. Polypep. 10-20	PG/ML	Blood	0.0 - 132.0
Vaso. Int. Polypep. 1	PG/ML	Blood	0.0 - 132.0
Vaso. Int. Polypep. 2-4	PG/ML	Blood	0.0 - 132.0
Vaso. Int. Polypep. 5-9	PG/ML	Blood	0.0 - 132.0
Vitamin A	MCG/DL	Blood	0.0 - 90.0
Vitamin B-12 Level	PG/ML	Blood	0.0 - 900.0
Vitamin B1	MCG/DL	Blood	1.6 - 4.0
Vitamin B6	NG/ML	Blood	3.6 - 18.0
Vitamin D (25-OH)	NG/DL	Blood	1.7 - 68.0
Vitamin E	MG/DL	Blood	0.5 - 2.5
Warfarin	MCG/ML	Blood	1.0 - 10.0
Zinc, Serum	MCG/DL	Blood	0.0 - 95.5

POUNDS TO KILOGRAMS
(1 kg = 2.2 lb; 1 lb = 0.45 kg)

lb	kg	lb	kg	lb	kg	lb	kg	lb	kg
5	2.3	50	22.7	95	43.1	140	63.5	185	83.9
10	4.5	55	25.0	100	45.4	145	65.8	190	86.2
15	6.8	60	27.2	105	47.6	150	68.0	195	88.5
20	9.1	65	29.5	110	49.9	155	70.3	200	90.7
25	11.3	70	31.7	115	52.2	160	72.6	205	93.0
30	13.6	75	34.0	120	54.4	165	74.8	210	95.3
35	15.9	80	36.3	125	56.7	170	77.1	215	97.5
40	18.1	85	38.6	130	58.9	175	79.4	220	99.8
45	20.4	90	40.8	135	61.2	180	81.6		

FEET AND INCHES TO CENTIMETERS
(1 cm = 0.39 in; 1 in = 2.54 cm)

ft	in	cm	ft	in	cm	ft	in	cm
0	6	15.2	3	0	91.4	4	8	142.2
1	0	30.5	3	1	93.9	4	9	144.7
1	6	45.7	3	2	96.4	4	10	147.3
1	7	48.3	3	3	99.0	4	11	149.8
1	8	50.8	3	4	101.6	5	0	152.4
1	9	53.3	3	5	104.1	5	1	154.9
1	10	55.9	3	6	106.6	5	2	157.5
1	11	58.4	3	7	109.2	5	3	160.0
2	0	61.0	3	8	111.7	5	4	162.6
2	1	63.5	3	9	114.2	5	5	165.1
2	2	66.0	3	10	116.8	5	6	167.6
2	3	68.6	3	11	119.3	5	7	170.2
2	4	71.1	4	0	121.9	5	8	172.7
2	5	73.6	4	1	124.4	5	9	175.3
2	6	76.1	4	2	127.0	5	10	177.8
2	7	78.7	4	3	129.5	5	11	180.3
2	8	81.2	4	4	132.0	6	0	182.9
2	9	83.8	4	5	134.6	6	1	185.4
2	10	86.3	4	6	137.1	6	2	188.0
2	11	88.8	4	7	139.6	6	3	190.5

FAHRENHEIT/CELSIUS TEMPERATURE CONVERSION
[F = 9/5 C + 32; C = 5/9 (F – 32)]

F		C	F		C
90	=	32.2	100	=	37.8
91	=	32.8	101	=	38.3
92	=	33.3	102	=	38.9
93	=	33.9	103	=	39.4
94	=	34.4	104	=	40.0
95	=	35.0	105	=	40.6
96	=	35.6	106	=	41.1
97	=	36.1	107	=	41.7
98	=	36.7	108	=	42.2
99	=	37.2	109	=	42.8

METRIC SYSTEM PREFIXES
(Small Measurement)

k	kilo–	10^3
c	centi–	10^{-2}
m	milli–	10^{-3}
μ	micro–	10^{-6}
n	nano– (formerly millicro, $m\mu$)	10^{-9}
p	pico– (formerly micromicro, $\mu\mu$)	10^{-12}
f	fento–	10^{-15}
a	atto–	10^{-18}

APOTHECARY EQUIVALENTS

30	g	....	1	oz		20	mg	....	1/3	gr
6	g	....	90	gr		15	mg	....	1/4	gr
5	g	....	75	gr		12	mg	....	1/5	gr
4	g	....	60	gr		10	mg	....	1/6	gr
3	g	....	45	gr		8	mg	....	1/8	gr
2	g	....	30	gr		6	mg	....	1/10	gr
1.5	g	....	22	gr		5	mg	....	1/12	gr
1	g	....	15	gr		4	mg	....	1/15	gr
0.75	g	....	12	gr		3	mg	....	1/20	gr
0.6	g	....	10	gr		1.5	mg	....	1/40	gr
0.4	g	....	6	gr		1.2	mg	....	1/50	gr
0.3	g	....	5	gr		1	mg	....	1/60	gr
0.25	g	....	4	gr		0.8	mg	....	1/80	gr
0.2	g	....	3	gr		0.6	mg	....	1/100	gr
0.15	g	....	21/2	gr		0.5	mg	....	1/120	gr
0.12	g	....	2	gr		0.4	mg	....	1/150	gr
0.1	g	....	11/2	gr		0.3	mg	....	1/200	gr
75	mg	....	11/4	gr		0.25	mg	....	1/250	gr
60	mg	....	1	gr		0.2	mg	....	1/300	gr
50	mg	....	3/4	gr		0.15	mg	....	1/400	gr
40	mg	....	2/3	gr		0.12	mg	....	1/500	gr
30	mg	....	1/2	gr		0.1	mg	....	1/600	gr
25	mg	....	3/8	gr						

NOMOGRAM FOR THE DETERMINATION OF
BODY SURFACE AREA OF CHILDREN AND ADULTS

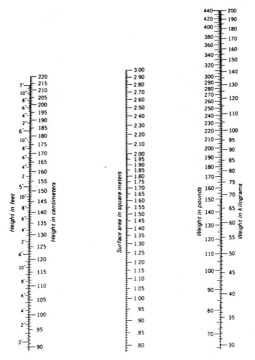

Ref: Way LW (ed): *Current Surgical Diagnosis and Treatment*, 7th ed. Lange Medical Publications, Los Altos, CA, 1985, p. 1188, with permission.

NOMOGRAM FOR THE DETERMINATION OF BODY SURFACE AREA OF CHILDREN

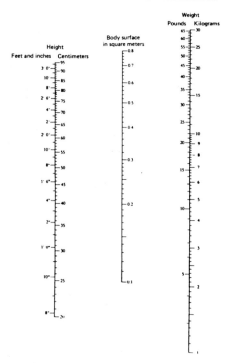

Ref: Way LW (ed): *Current Surgical Diagnosis and Treatment*, 7th ed. Lange Medical Publications, Los Altos, CA, 1985, p. 1188, with permission.

OXYHEMOGLOBIN DISSOCIATION CURVES
FOR WHOLE BLOOD

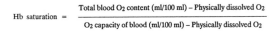

$$\text{Hb saturation} = \frac{\text{Total blood } O_2 \text{ content (ml/100 ml)} - \text{Physically dissolved } O_2}{O_2 \text{ capacity of blood (ml/100 ml)} - \text{Physically dissolved } O_2}$$

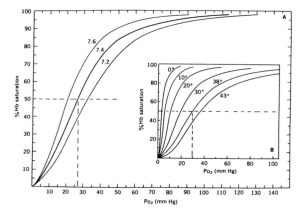

Large diagram indicates influence of change in acidity of blood on affinity of blood for O_2. Curves are based on studies by Dill and by Bock *et al.* on blood of one man (A.V. Bock). At a particular P_{O_2} (e.g., 40 mm Hg), acidification of blood results in release of O_2. Action of changes in P_{CO_2} appear due in part to their effect on pH and in part to formation of carbamino compounds, displacing 2,3–DPG from Hb. Inset shows, for blood of sheep, influence of temperature change on P_{O_2}–% HbO_2 relationships; an increase in temperature (as in working muscle) aids in "unloading" O_2 from HbO_2; during hypothermia, hemoglobin has increased affinity for O_2.

Reproduced by permission from C.J. Lambertsen, "Transport of oxygen, carbon dioxide, and inert gases by the blood," in *Medical Physiology*, 14th ed., V.B. Mountcastle, editor. St. Louis, 1980, The C.V. Mosby Co., p. 1725.

HENDERSON – HASSELBACH NOMOGRAM

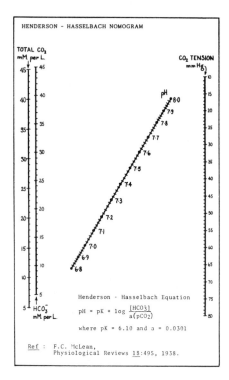

Ref: *The Harriet Lane Handbook*, 12th ed. (M.G. Greene, ed.). St. Louis: Mosby–Year Book, 1990. Reproduced by permission.

Index